Handbook of Hepato-Pancreato-Biliary Surgery

Handbook of Hepato-Pancreato-Biliary Surgery

Edited by Isaac Stanton

hayle
medical

New York

Hayle Medical,
750 Third Avenue, 9th Floor,
New York, NY 10017, USA

Visit us on the World Wide Web at:
www.haylemedical.com

ISBN: 978-1-63241-770-1

Cataloging-in-Publication Data

Handbook of hepato-pancreato-biliary surgery / edited by Isaac Stanton.
    p. cm.
Includes bibliographical references and index.
ISBN 978-1-63241-770-1
1. Liver--Surgery. 2. Pancreas--Surgery. 3. Biliary tract--Surgery. I. Stanton, Isaac.
RD546 .H35 2019
617.556 205 92--dc23

Contents

Preface

Hepato-pancreato-biliary surgery is the medical and surgical care for the treatment of diseases and disorders of the liver, pancreas, biliary tract and duodenum. It provides treatment to patients with primary and metastatic cancers of the liver, pancreas, bile duct and gallbladder, as well as benign conditions such as cysts, bile duct injuries and biliary strictures. The investigation, diagnosis and recommendation of effective treatment strategies, as well as operative procedures and provision of preoperative, perioperative and late postoperative care are within the scope of this field. HPB surgery can include laparoscopic procedures, resections, transplantation surgeries and reconstruction surgeries. A number of specialists may be involved in HPB surgery such as hepatobiliary and transplant surgeons, hepatologists, interventional radiologists and diagnostic radiologists. This book is a compilation of chapters that discuss the most vital concepts and emerging trends in the field of hepato-pancreato-biliary surgery. It consists of contributions made by international experts. Through this book, we attempt to further enlighten the readers about the new concepts in this field.

This book is a result of research of several months to collate the most relevant data in the field.

When I was approached with the idea of this book and the proposal to edit it, I was overwhelmed. It gave me an opportunity to reach out to all those who share a common interest with me in this field. I had 3 main parameters for editing this text:

1. Accuracy – The data and information provided in this book should be up-to-date and valuable to the readers.

2. Structure – The data must be presented in a structured format for easy understanding and better grasping of the readers.

3. Universal Approach – This book not only targets students but also experts and innovators in the field, thus my aim was to present topics which are of use to all.

Thus, it took me a couple of months to finish the editing of this book.

I would like to make a special mention of my publisher who considered me worthy of this opportunity and also supported me throughout the editing process. I would also like to thank the editing team at the back-end who extended their help whenever required.

Editor

Venous Outflow Reconstruction in Adult Living Donor Liver Transplant: Outcome of a Policy for Right Lobe Grafts without the Middle Hepatic Vein

Mohamed Ghazaly,[1,2] Mohamad T. Badawy,[1] Hosam El-Din Soliman,[1] Magdy El-Gendy,[1] Tarek Ibrahim,[1] and Brian R. Davidson[2]

[1] *Liver Transplant Department, National Liver Institute, Menoufiya University, Shebeen El-Koum, Egypt*
[2] *University Department of Surgery and Liver Transplant Unit, Royal Free Hospital Trust and Royal Free and University College School of Medicine, Hampstead Campus, Pond Street, London NW3 2QG, UK*

Correspondence should be addressed to Mohamed Ghazaly; mohamed.ghazaly79@yahoo.com

Academic Editor: Shu-Sen Zheng

Introduction. The difficulty and challenge of recovering a right lobe graft without MHV drainage is reconstructing the outflow tract of the hepatic veins. With the inclusion or the reconstruction of the MHV, early graft function is satisfactory. The inclusion of the MHV or not in the donor's right lobectomy should be based on sound criteria to provide adequate functional liver mass for recipient, while keeping risk to donor to the minimum. *Objective.* Reviewing the results of a policy for right lobe grafts transplant without MHV and analyzing methods of venous reconstruction related to outcome. *Materials and Methods.* We have two groups Group A (with more than one HV anast.) ($n = 16$) and Group B (single HV anast.) ($n = 24$). Both groups were compared regarding indications for reconstruction, complications, and operative details and outcomes, besides describing different modalities used for venous reconstruction. *Results.* Significant increase in operative details time in Group A. When comparison came to complications and outcomes in terms of laboratory findings and overall hospital stay, there were no significant differences. Three-month and one-year survival were better in Group A. *Conclusion.* Adult LDLT is safely achieved with better outcome to recipients and donors by recovering the right lobe without MHV, provided that significant MHV tributaries (segments V, VIII more than 5 mm) are reconstructed, and any accessory considerable inferior right hepatic veins (IRHVs) or superficial RHVs are anastomosed.

1. Introduction

Chronic liver disease and cirrhosis are important causes of morbidity and mortality in the world. Moreover, the burden of chronic liver disease is projected to increase due in part to the increasing prevalence of end-stage liver disease and HCC secondary to NAFLD and HCV. Liver transplantation is the best treatment option for end-stage liver disease, including early HCC associated with advanced cirrhosis. However, the application of liver transplantation is severely limited by the shortage of deceased donor grafts; hence many patients die from progression of the disease while waiting for a graft [1].

The shortage of cadaveric livers has sparked an interest in living donor liver transplantation (LDLT). LDLT may increase the liver graft pool and reduce waiting list mortality [2, 3]. In adults, right hemiliver graft can satisfy the demands of the recipient's metabolism and prevent small-for-size syndrome. The difficulty and challenge of LDLT without MHV drainage is providing adequate venous drainage of the graft [4, 5]. Obstruction of venous outflow leads to graft congestion and failure [6].

The major controversy with right lobe LDLT lies in the necessity for including the MHV in the graft and in concerns for the safety of the donor. The MHV carries out important venous drainage for the right anterior segment and is essential for perfect graft function in nearly 85% of right lobe LDLTs [7]. In the absence of the MHV, the right anterior segment of the liver graft may suffer from congestion and damage with subsequent diffuse mechanical injury to the right posterior segment, and the liver graft becomes effectively of small size. With the inclusion or the reconstruction of the MHV, early graft function is satisfactory. The inclusion of the MHV or not in the donor's right lobectomy should be based on sound criteria to provide adequate functional liver mass for the recipient, while keeping the risk to the donor to the minimum [8].

De Villa et al. [9] described the Kaohsiung principle based on the donor-to-recipient body weight ratio, the volume of the donor's right lobe to the recipient's standard liver volume and the size of MHV tributaries from the anterior segment. Later, the Kyoto group, using the three-dimensional reconstructed images of the hepatic vascular anatomy, divided the right lobe graft morphologically into two types: one is a right hepatic vein dominant graft and the other is a MHV dominant graft [7, 10].

Regarding taking the right lobe graft with or without the MHV, we adopted a policy where we used to leave RHV within the donor guided by right lobe (mainly segments 5 and 8 have adequate venous drainage radiologically) and GRWR is 0.8 or more. If GRWR < 0.8 or MHV is the main drainage for the right lobe (provided that remaining liver volume is adequate for the donor, which is >35% of total liver volume) and there are no other donors available, we have to harvest the graft with MHV.

Our aim is to review the results of a policy for right lobe grafts without MHV and to analyze the methods of venous reconstruction related to outcome.

2. Patients and Methods

Over the period from January 2009 to January 2011, 40 patients underwent live donor liver transplant using a right lobe liver graft without the middle hepatic vein in the National Liver Institute, Menoufiya University, Egypt. This study has analyzed the results of these 40 cases.

Detailed data of all 40 donors and recipients were collected, tabulated, and analyzed with special concerns on clinical and demographic data of the donors including sex, age, body mass index (BMI) and relationship to recipient; history of medical diseases (especially hepatic diseases including Child-Pugh score and MELD score); examination: body build (weight and height) and abdominal examination for any scar of previous operation and any abnormalities by inspection and palpation.

The donor and recipient characteristics are given in Tables 1, 2. The selected donors were generally young (mean 24 years) with a low BMI (24.7). All donors were within the third degree relation of consanguinity as we generally do not accept unrelated donations for medicolegal issues, with sons presenting the highest percentage of 17 donors (42.5%) and cousins the lowest with 3 donors (7.5%).

All donors underwent liver biopsy. Four donors (10%) had steatosis and 2 donors (5%) had mild periportal fibrosis. These percentages are still within the accepted criteria for transplantation according to our policy and in most of the literature, besides these were the only available donors.

TABLE 1: 40 Donors data.

Donors data (40 donors)	
Age	Mean 24.55 + SD 5.35389
BMI	Mean 24.7275 + SD 3.73699
Sex	
Male	30 donors (75%)
Female	10 donors (25%)
Liver biopsy	
Normal	34 (85%)
Steatosis (maximum 10%)	4 (10%)
Very mild PPF	2 (5%)

TABLE 2: 40 Recipients data.

Recipients data (40 patients)	
Age	Mean 47.325 + SD 8.6362
Weight	Mean 78.2 + SD 12.20593
MELD score	Mean 16.3 + SD 4.40396
GRWR	Mean 1.09525 + SD 0.21211

TABLE 3: Indication for liver transplant.

Indication for liver transplant	Number (%)
HCV	19 (47.5%)
HCC	13 (32.5%)
Cryptogenic cirrhosis	5 (12.5%)
Alcoholic	1 (2.5%)
Budd chiari syndrome	1 (2.5%)
HBV	1 (2.5%)

The recipients were aged from 24 to 60 years with a mean MELD of (16.3 + 4.4). Commonest etiology of the liver disease was HCV+/−HCC presenting up to (80%) Table 3. The graft-to-recipient weight ratios (GRWR) were above 0.8, ranged from a minimum of 0.84 to 1.9 (mean 1.09525 + 0.21).

Laboratory: complete blood picture, liver function tests, renal function tests, coagulation profile, blood sugar, electrolytes, HLA typing, crossmatching, tumor markers (AFP, CEA, CA19-9, and CA50), arterial blood gases, urine and stool analysis, and proteins S and C; serology: HBV DNA, antibody for HCV (PCR), HIV, CMV, EBV, varicella and rubella viruses, and liver biopsy.

Preoperative assessment of the donor anatomy: ultrasound and Doppler US: with special emphasis on liver parenchyma (steatosis and any lesion) and hepatic veins including distribution, number, caliber, and the presence of accessory veins. Triphasic computed tomography (CT): a serial coronal section view is especially useful to evaluate the hepatic veins variants and the volumetry of the graft and remnant liver.

3. CT Volumetry

A contrast material-enhanced CT examination of the abdomen was included in the evaluation and was required for

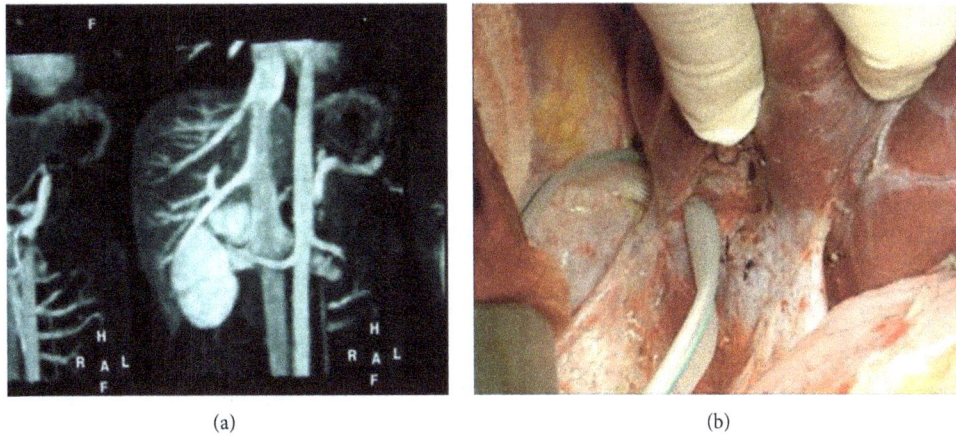

(a)   (b)

FIGURE 1: Big inferior right hepatic vein (IRHV) on MRV enography (a) and operative picture (b).

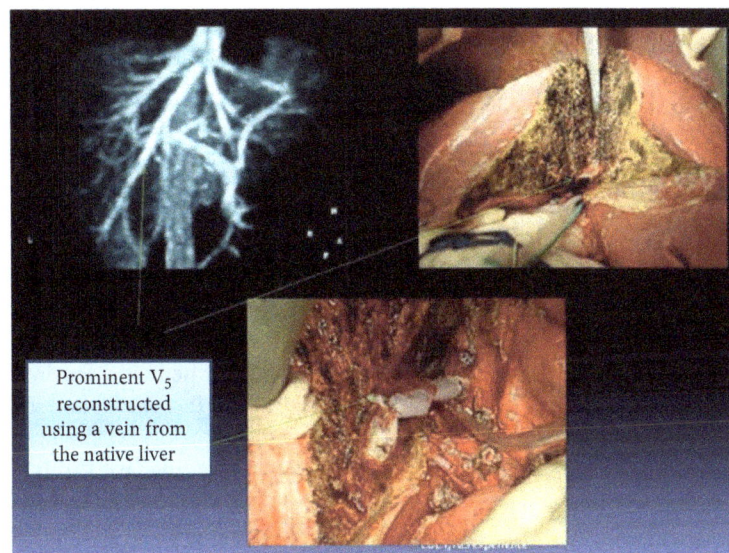

Prominent V$_5$ reconstructed using a vein from the native liver

FIGURE 2: Big V5 vein in MRV: V5 in the graft during donor hepatotomy and after reconstruction in the recipient.

the analysis of morphologic characteristics, the vascular status of the liver, and the evaluation of the hepatic parenchyma.

Magnetic resonance angiography and venography were done to evaluate the vascular variants of HA, HV, and PV.

3.1. MR Venography. MRV was done using Philips Achieva 1.5 T machine. The following findings were recorded: (1) tributaries of the middle hepatic veins (MHV) including segments V and VIII veins; (2) the presence of accessory inferior right hepatic vein (IRHV) or superficial right hepatic vein (SRHV); (3) the variable entering patterns of the RHV, MHV, and IRHV into IVC, and (4) the diameter of the veins at their point of connection to the major veins. A comparison of the findings from the preoperative MR venography and the operative findings was made in an attempt to establish an accurate picture of the donor hepatic venous anatomy and plan the method of venoplasty, if at all required see Figures 1 and 2.

The intraoperative anatomical evaluation of biliary system is done by intraoperative cholangiography.

4. Surgical Procedures of LDLT

4.1. Donor Hepatectomy. LDLT was done through a bilateral subcostal incision with an upward midline extension. Intraoperative cholangiography via cystic duct was required to study the anatomy of the bile duct. Right hilar dissection was then performed to isolate the right hepatic artery, right portal vein, and right hepatic duct. Then the right lobe of the liver was rotated toward the left side for division of the ligaments on the right side of the liver and the minute hepatic venous branches. The liver was transected at a plane just to the right of the middle hepatic vein using an ultrasonic dissector. The transection plane was determined by intraoperative US and temporary occlusion of the right portal vein and right hepatic artery. When the transection approached the liver hilum, the right hepatic duct together with the surrounding Glission sheath was encircled. Then, the right hepatic duct was divided near the confluence of the hepatic ducts by scissors.

The transection was carried down to the junction of the right hepatic vein with the inferior vena cava. The right hepatic artery was then divided. The right hepatic vein was clamped at the junction with the inferior vena cava and divided. The stumps of the right portal vein and right hepatic vein were closed with continuous nonabsorbable sutures. The falciform ligament was sutured to the anterior abdominal wall. A drain was inserted into the right subphrenic cavity before wound closure.

4.2. Graft and Back Table. We perfused the grafts via the right PV with 2 liters of 4-degree histidine-tryptophan-ketoglutarate (HTK) solution which was also used to flush the biliary tract. The right hepatic vein orifice was inspected and all additional hepatic vein branches were identified and reconstructed, whenever indicated, using the criteria mentioned in the results section (Table 5). The size of all veins was measured using specific rulers. The grafts were weighed and graft to recipients weight ratio was calculated.

4.3. Operative Techniques in Recipients. The operative procedures were performed via chevron incision with upper midline extension.

When resecting recipients' liver, we attentively reserved posteriorhepatic inferior vena cava's (IVC) integrality, dissociated right hepatic vein cling to IVC, and reserved the orifices of right hepatic vein (RHV), along with the end axis enlarged IVC downward, making it suitable for donor's RHV and anastomosis. It was necessary to make ellipsed incision on suitable parts of IVC when the orifices of crassitude tributaries of right hepatic inferior vein or MHV were jointed with IVC by interpositioning the recipient portal vein, great saphenous vein, or cryopreserved cadaveric blood vessels. We adopted end-to-end anastomosis of grafts' right tributaries of PV to recipient's PV trunk, then opened blood flow in hepatic vein and PV, and ended nonhepatic phase period. Bypass was not used in all of our cases, as we only did partial IVC clamping. With loupe, we finished hepatic artery anastomosis and adopted end-to-end anastomosis of right hepatic duct to common hepatic duct, or Roux-en-Y choledochojejunostomy. If right hepatic duct had many tributaries and their caliber ≤2 mm, biliary tracts should be reconstructed under microscope. Splenectomy was performed at the same time if recipients suffered from splenomegaly and hypersplenism (blood platelet $\leq 30 \times 10^9/\text{L}$). If PV pressure was >25 cm H_2O, splenic artery ligation was performed for recipients in order to alleviate PV pressure.

Intraoperative Doppler US: a routine surveillance intraoperative US study entails grayscale assessment of the liver parenchyma and biliary tree and Doppler evaluation of the vasculature.

4.4. Postoperative Monitoring of Donor and Recipient

4.4.1. Donor. Recovery: In ICU for two days. Medications: Receiving IV antibiotics, IV fluid for 3–5 days and then converting to oral feeding; pain killer and low molecular weight anticoagulant for 10 days s.c with daily followup by Doppler US, Lab (LFTs, RFTs, coagulation profile and CBS). Outcome: complications: acute rejection episodes, renal impairment, portal vein thrombosis, hepatic artery thrombosis, and biliary complications. Mortality: causes, rate, and analysis of survival. Discharge: 10–15 days after operation.

4.4.2. Recipient. Recipient was in ICU for 1 week and then transferred for the transplant unit. Postoperative anticoagulant therapy: in most of the cases, heparin was used in more than 50 u/kg/day infusion. The dose was increased according to need to keep the INR between 2 and 3 for at least 10 days. Then the antiplatelets, persantin is given for one month. Postoperative Doppler US followup: Doppler US was used routinely for followup and was done twice for the first 10 days then once daily for detection of any early vascular and biliary problem and graft dysfunction.

We use broad spectrum antibiotics, mainly a combination of Meropenem and Metronidazole and then we do serial culture and sensitivity tests (from our infection control unit), then we might need to change regimen according to it. We also use Diclofenac (Fluconazole) as an antifungal prophylaxis for 7 days. In our antiviral regimen, we use Zovirax (Acyclovir) 200 mg tds starting from the 7th day postoperative till 6 months, and if there is CMV infection we use Ganciclovir (Cymevene vial) for 2 weeks. We used no prophylaxis for hepatitis. For immunotherapy, we use either Ciclosporin or Tacrolimus and steroids for 3 months. Regarding coagulopathy in recipients, especially in patients who had severe bleeding, we use blood, FFP, cryopreservation, and platelets transfusion and in some cases we use Factor 7 (Novo seven vial). We use prophylactic heparinization for 10 days, and then we shift for low molecular weight heparin (LMWH).

4.4.3. Outcome. We compare both groups regarding laboratory findings (total bilirubin), overall hospital stay, three-month survival, and one-year survival. Long term outcome and survival analysis: calculation of outcome was done using Kaplan-Meier method.

4.4.4. Statistical Analysis. Descriptive statistics were based on percentage for categorical data and on means, median, standard deviation, and range summarizing data distribution for continuous measures. Numerical data were presented as mean and standard deviation (SD). All data were analyzed using the SPSS package for windows. The following tests were used: Student's t-test, to test for significance when comparing the means of two sets of quantitative data, and the P (probability) value was considered to be of statistical significance if it was less than 0.05. Survival analysis was performed according to the Kaplan-Meier method from the date of surgery to that of death or event or to the most recent clinic visit.

5. Results

60% of grafts had a single right hepatic vein Table 4 and were directly anastomosed to the IVC. For all of our cases, we used to make longitudinal enlargement of the orifice of the right hepatic vein stump by the incising an anterior slit, down to its junction with the inferior vena cava (IVC) in order to guarantee wide and patent anastomosis.

At the time of transplant 16 of the 40 grafts (40%) were found to have more than 1 hepatic vein. The additional vessels and the methods of reconstruction are shown in Table 5. See Figures 3, 4, and 5.

Of the 16 patients with additional hepatic veins in the right lobe graft, 4 had interposition grafts and two venous patches to the anterior wall of RHV.

Special consideration had to be paid to accessory hepatic veins draining separately into the IVC, especially if the vein caliber is larger than 5 mm and there is a gap between the opening of this accessory vein and the main right hepatic vein. In that situation, it was necessary to make another IVC opening for extra separate anastomosis. That was the case in 14 cases out of the 16 cases with more than one single hepatic vein.

According to the source of the graft, there were 5 cases where we used portal vein of the recipient, and in the other one, we used recipient umbilical vein.

Two out of these six patients had acute rejection episodes in the early postoperative period; both of them had tolerated it and gradually improved with the proper postoperative care and adjusting the dose of immunotherapy.

The patency of the graft was followed up postoperatively with Doppler US for all of them, and they were all patent.

5.1. Postoperative Outcome. The cold ischemia time was significantly longer in those undergoing hepatic vein reconstruction Table 6 (mean = 68.75 (35–130) versus 51.25 (20–90)), P = 0.04688 as was the warm ischaemia time (mean 57.875 (30–80) versus 43.33 (25–75)), P = 0.00145. Finally, the HV anastomosis time in minutes had a mean = 34.6875 (15–65) for Group A and 17.70833 (15–30) for Group B with a P value of P = 0.0001.

The major complications in both groups Table 7 were mainly in the form of acute rejection episodes in 8 cases (20%); out of these eight patients, only one died early postoperative due to graft rejection, but the other seven patients tolerated it and gradually improved with the proper postoperative care and adjusting the dose of immunotherapy.

Renal impairment was 7 cases (17.5%); four out of them died early postoperative (almost all of them died within 2 months) due to the presence of other comorbidities in the form of HAT, biliary leak and sepsis, and heart failure, and one case with early graft dysfunction as well, while the other three passed it.

Portal vein thrombosis was in one case only (2.5%); portal vein thrombosis was diagnosed by color Doppler US; medical treatment in the form of increasing the dose of anticoagulants and changing from oral anticoagulant into injectable form was tried. Hepatic artery thrombosis was in 3 cases (7.5%); two of them had surgical reconstruction and did well and the

third one died early postoperative as he had hepatic artery and portal vein thrombosis as well.

Biliary complications were in 16 cases (40%) with no significant difference between both groups; out of these sixteen cases, eight cases (20%) developed anastomotic leaks and the other eight cases developed biliary strictures. Out of these eight cases, six cases were managed conservatively, and two cases required surgical intervention.

5.2. Overall Morbidity and Survival Table 8. Again, when the comparison came to the outcomes in terms of laboratory findings (total Bilirubin on three-day levels and one-month levels), overall hospital stay, three-month survival, and one-year survival there were no significant differences between both groups, where the total bilirubin level after one month had a median of 0.8 +range (0.2–5.5) for Group A and a median of 1 + range (0.5–27) for Group B. The hospital stay in days had a median of 27 + range (13–51) for Group A and a median of 25 + range (5–84) for Group B.

The three-month survival was slightly better for Group A where it was 15 (93.75%) for Group A and 19 (79.16%) for Group B. The one-year survival as well was better for Group A with 14 patients out of 16 alive (87.5%) versus 17 patients out of 24 (70.83%) for Group B. The overall 1-year survival for our series was 31 cases out of 40 (77.5%).

6. Discussion

In our study, all the forty grafts were right lobe grafts without the middle hepatic vein with exception only in two cases. The number of cases with more than one graft hepatic vein present intraoperative was sixteen cases (40%). Out of these sixteen cases, there were fourteen cases which actually required more than one hepatic vein anastomosis. All cases had only two vessel anastomoses (some of them after adjustment and refashioning of graft hepatic veins on the back table and this was to decrease warm ischemia time as much as possible).

Our results came in agreement with Marcos et al. 1999 who performed 25 right lobe living donor liver transplants without the MHV, with an excellent patient survival rate of 88% [11].

The Kyoto group, using the three-dimensional reconstructed images, divided the right lobe graft morphologically into two types: one is a right hepatic vein dominant graft in which the territory draining into the MHV is less than 40% of the right lobe graft, and the other is a MHV dominant graft [10]. Their indication for a right lobe graft with or without the MHV is based on dominancy of the hepatic vein, graft-to-recipient weight ratio, and remnant liver volume [7]. The group performed 217 right lobe LDLTs successfully according to this algorithm [12].

Right liver grafts with the MHV trunk (extended right lobe grafts) were first performed by the Hong Kong Group in 1996, as left lobe grafts from relatively small volunteer donors will not meet the metabolic demand of larger recipients [13]. Seven LDLTs, using this technique, were initially performed under high urgency situations. Although a high postoperative

TABLE 4: Results of preoperative MR venography and operative findings of venous anatomy.

No.	MRI venography	No. of HV in MRV	No. of graft HVs (intraoperative)	Use venous graft	Actual diameter of HV in mm (intraop.)	No. of HV anastomosis
1	*RHV & V8*	*2*	*2*	*Yes*	*22 & 9*	*1*
2	*RHV & V5*	*2*	*2*	*Yes*	*30 & 15*	*2*
3	*RHV & IRHV*	*2*	*2*	*No*	*20 & 21*	*2*
4	**RHV**	**1**	**2**	**No**	**24 & 8**	**2**
5	**RHV & IRHV**	**2**	**3**	**Yes**	**29 & 16 & 11**	**2**
6	*RHV & IRHV*	*2*	*2*	*No*	*33 & 18*	*2*
7	**RHV & V8 & IRHV**	**3**	**4**	**Yes**	**24 & 18 & 11 & 10**	**2**
8	*RHV & V8 & V5*	*3*	*3*	*No*	*31, 2 less than 5 mm*	*1*
9	*RHV & IRHV*	*2*	*2*	*No*	*26 & 13*	*2*
10	*RHV & IRHV*	*2*	*2*	*No*	*26 & 13*	*2*
11	*RHV & IRHV*	*2*	*2*	*No*	*36 & 15*	*2*
12	**RHV + MHV**	**2**	**3**	**Yes**	**23—20—14**	**2**
13	**RHV**	**1**	**2**	**No**	**28—14**	**2**
14	*RHV & IRHV*	*2*	*2*	*No*	*35—18*	*2*
15	*RHV & IRHV + MHV*	*3*	*3*	*Yes*	*20—27—21*	*2*
16	*RHV & IRHV*	*2*	*2*	*No*	*32—15*	*2*
1	RHV	1	1	No	33	1
2	RHV	1	1	No	27	1
3	RHV	1	1	No	31	1
4	RHV	1	1	No	32	1
5	RHV	1	1	No	29	1
6	RHV	1	1	No	26	1
7	**RHV & V8**	**2**	**1**	**No**	**29**	**1**
8	**RHV & PRHV**	**2**	**1**	**No**	**33**	**1**
9	RHV	1	1	No	36	1
10	RHV	1	1	No	33	1
11	RHV	1	1	No	24	1
12	RHV	1	1	No	30	1
13	RHV	1	1	No	28	1
14	RHV	1	1	No	30	1
15	RHV	1	1	No	29	1
16	RHV	1	1	No	30	1
17	RHV	1	1	No	32	1
18	RHV	1	1	No	32	1
19	RHV	1	1	No	28	1
20	RHV	1	1	No	29	1
21	RHV	1	1	No	33	1
22	RHV	1	1	No	27	1
23	**RHV & V8**	**2**	**1**	**No**	**32**	**1**
24	RHV	1	1	No	33	1

[*] Highlighted (in bold) eight cases where the intra-operative findings were different from the pre-operative MRI venography recordings.
[*] Upper 16 italic cases: cases that had more than one graft hepatic vein intraoperatively.

complication rate was reported (donors 29%, recipients 86%), the results are comparable to the best possible outcome in cadaveric transplantation for patients with similar status [14]. Meanwhile, another kind of right lobe liver grafts without the MHV (modified right lobe graft) emerged [11, 15] because the surgeons feared donor risk and important ethical issues. The extended right lobe grafts were too extensive as an operation for the donor [16, 17], and sufficient size of the remnant liver

Venous Outflow Reconstruction in Adult Living Donor Liver Transplant: Outcome of a Policy...

7

TABLE 5: Hepatic venous variations in donor (actual intraoperative findings) and their reconstruction.

Hepatic venous variations in donor	Number of cases	Reconstruction	Method of reconstruction
Single IRHV	11	All	All IRHVs were anastomosed to IVC through an opening separate of that of RHV
2 IRHV	1	Yes	Interposition graft between 2 IRHVs into one opening into IVC
V5	1	Yes	Interposition graft between V5 and RHV into one opening into IVC
V8	1	Yes	Interposition graft between V8 and RHV into one opening into IVC
V5 + V8	1	Neither of them	—
2 IRHV + V8	1	Both	Interposition graft between 2 IRHVs into one opening into IVC, V8 to RHV

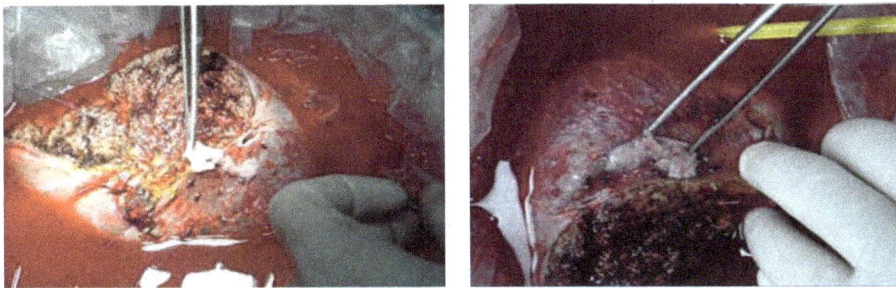

FIGURE 3: Multiple inferior hepatic veins (IHV) reconstructed into one opening using recipient PV graft.

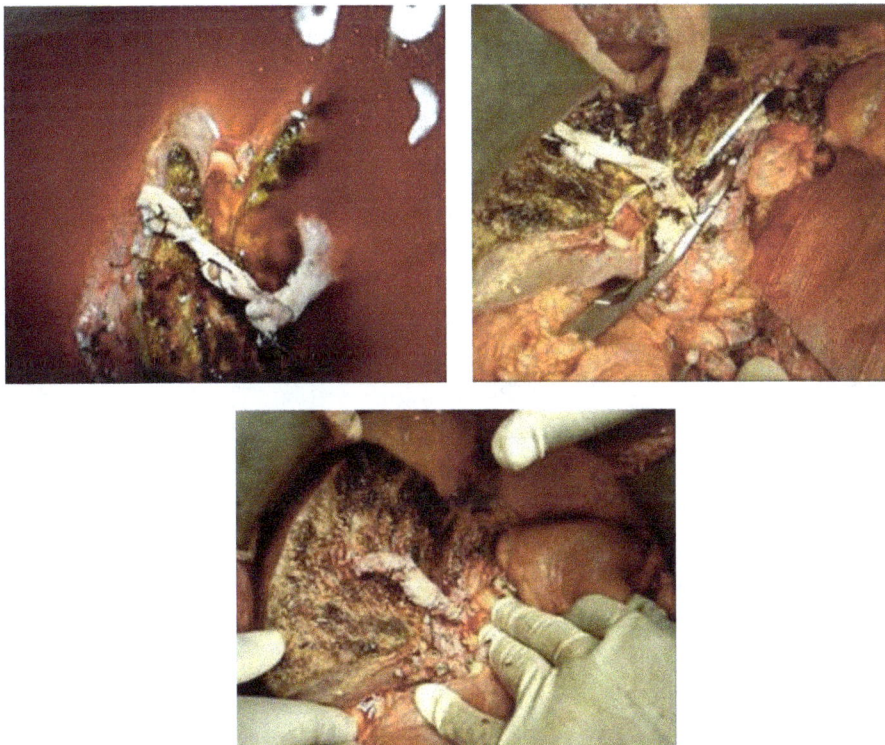

FIGURE 4: Multiple veins in graft: V5 reconstructed with PV graft with inferior right hepatic vein (IRHV) and RHV.

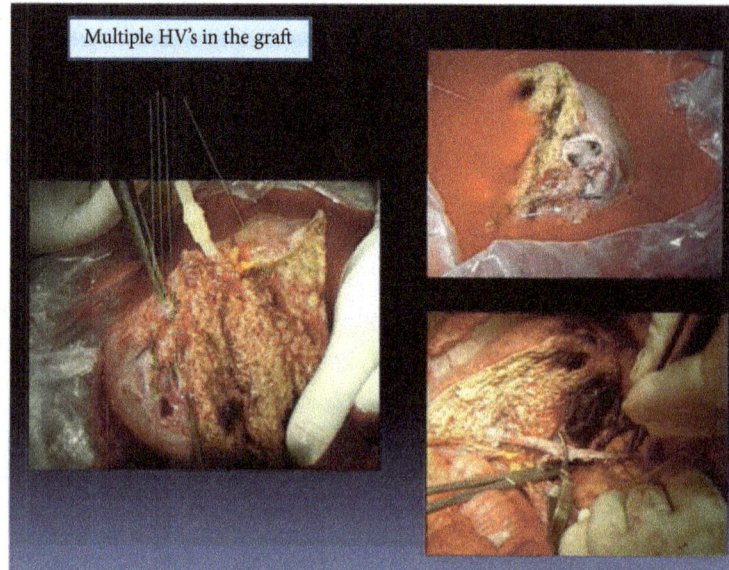

FIGURE 5: Multiple hepatic veins (HV) openings; V5, right hepatic vein (RHV), big posterior HV and inferior right hepatic vein (IRHV), and V5 reconstructed using PV graft to IVC.

TABLE 6: Operative details.

Parameters	Group A (reconstruction patients with more than one HV anast.) ($n = 16$)	Group B (patients with single HV anast.) ($n = 24$)	P value
Cold ischemia time	Mean = 68.75 (35–130)	Mean = 51.25 (20–90)	0.04688
Warm ischemia time	Mean = 57.875 (30–80)	Mean = 43.33 (25–75)	0.00145
HV anastomosis time/min.	Mean = 34.6875 (15–65)	Mean = 17.70833 (15–30)	0.0001

The cold ischemia time was significantly longer in those undergoing hepatic vein reconstruction (mean = 68.75 (35–130) versus 51.25 (20–90)), $P = 0.04688$ as was the warm ischaemia time (mean 57.875 (30–80) versus 43.33 (25–75)), $P = 0.00145$. Finally, the HV anastomosis time in minutes had a mean = 34.6875 (15–65) for Group A and 17.70833 (15–30) for Group B with a P value of $P = 0.0001$.

TABLE 7: Major complications in both groups.

Complications	Group A (reconstruction patients with more than one HV anast.) ($n = 16$)	Group B (patients with single HV anast.) ($n = 24$)
Acute rejection episodes	4 (25%)	4 (16.6%)
Renal impairment	2 (12.5%)	5 (20.8%)
Portal vein thrombosis	1 (6.25%)	0 (0 %)
Hepatic artery thrombosis	1 (6.25%)	2 (8.3%)
Biliary complications	5 (31.25%)	11 (45.8%)

TABLE 8: Outcome in terms of laboratory findings (total bilirubin), overall hospital stay, three-month survival, and one-year survival.

Parameters	Group A (reconstruction patients with more than one HV anast.) ($n = 16$)	Group B (patients with single HV anast.) ($n = 24$)
Total bilirubin		
3-day level (mg/dL)	Median 3.25 + range (1.6–6)	Median 2.25 + range (0.3–10)
1-month level (mg/dL)	Median 0.8 + range (0.2–5.5)	Median 1 + range (0.5–27)
Hospital stay (days)	Median 27 + range (13–51)	Median 25 range (5–84)
Three-month survival	15 (93.75%)	19 (79.16%)
One-year survival	14 (87.5%)	17 (70.83%)

[18] as well as drainage of the segment 4 in the donor could not be guaranteed [5].

Some centers have introduced their experience in determining the extent of donor hepatectomy either with or without the MHV. de Villa et al. [9] described the Kaohsiung principle based on the donor-to-recipient body weight ratio, the volume of the donor's right lobe to the recipient's standard liver volume and the size of MHV tributaries from the anterior segment. This principle was applied in 25 living donor liver transplant operations and procured successful outcomes in both donors and recipients [12].

Adham et al. had 33 patients who received 34 cadaveric right split liver grafts. According to the type of recipient pairs (adult/adult or adult/child), the right liver graft was deprived of the MHV or not. They concluded that adult right SLT without the MHV is safe and associated with similar long-term results as compared with those of the right graft including the MHV, despite that early liver function recovered more slowly [19].

In our series, 40% of cases had atypical hepatic venous anatomy and showed more than one single right hepatic vein only within the right lobe graft. Fan Cheng et al.'s study showed that comparing MR venography with intraoperative surgical findings yielded clear visualization of the right, middle, and left hepatic veins in all cases, 100%. For those essential minor branches, which were equal to or larger than 5 mm in diameter, they obtained 88.2% accuracy [20]. The results of our study also illustrate that the MR venography has an accuracy of at least 87.5% of detecting accessory and minor hepatic veins and are in agreement with the literature supporting the use of MR venography for the definition of hepatic veins anatomy.

Since January 2006, Tashiro et al. have applied vascular closure staple technique successfully during liver transplantation in seven patients. They used this technique in reconstruction of the V8 and V5 tributaries in six and three patients, respectively, using the recipient's own middle hepatic vein. None of the patients experienced vascular complications and all had good venous flow postoperatively with excellent results [21].

To prevent RHV anastomotic stenosis, various methods of enlarging the RHV orifice have been introduced. Rather than constructing a standard end-to-end anastomosis between the orifices of the RHVs, Lee carried out simple enlargement of the orifice of the recipient vein by the creation of an anterior slit, down to its junction with the inferior vena cava (IVC), because the caliber of the recipient's RHV or caval orifice should be larger than the caliber of the liver graft's RHV for a wide and long-patent anastomosis [8]. That was the same strategy we adapted in our cases.

Marcos et al. introduced complete cavoplasty at the orifice of the RHV by creating an elliptical defect approximately 1.5 to 2.0 times the diameter of the donor RHV in the IVC [22].

Sugawara et al. introduced a new reconstruction method by which the anastomosis is lengthened by adding a venous patch. Long preservation of the recipient's RHV allowed the formation of a reservoir between the liver graft and the recipient's IVC. A transverse slit incision to the anterior wall of the RHV across the IVC orifice, and patch plasty

with a U-shaped recipient portal vein, hepatic vein, or thick saphenous vein will enlarge the RHV orifice and allow reservoir formation [23]. We have also applied the same technique in two cases which had short right hepatic vein stump using a recipient portal vein.

The diamond shaped patch method carried out by the Tokyo group also allows for the widening of the RHV anastomotic orifice and for reservoir formation [23].

New strategies for HV reconstruction that would be tolerable to the compression of venous anastomotic sites by the regenerating liver graft were therefore suggested, one by the Tokyo group, using a cryopreserved large vein [24] and one by the Asan group, using an autogenous vein [25]. The Tokyo group introduced the double VC technique, using the cryopreserved VC to create a "common large opening" reconstruction when multiple major SHVs (caliber, ≥5 mm) were present. The Asan group has formulated a technique using the recipient's own autogenous vein instead of a cryopreserved VC. If the recipient portal vein showed no associated portal vein thrombosis and stenosis, the major SHVs were anastomosed to the interpositioned portal vein reservoir, which would prevent the compression occlusion of the anastomotic site by the enlarging liver graft [8].

Lee et al. [26] reported a good result of reconstruction of MHV tributaries of the anterior segment using the great saphenous vein. Cattral et al. [27] also described their successful use of the recipient's left portal vein as an interposition graft.

Regarding the type of the venous graft, we mainly used portal vein of the recipient in 5 cases, and in the other one, we used recipient's umbilical vein. Up to now, many types of vein grafts have been used for the reconstruction of the MHV, including the saphenous vein [6], umbilical vein, left portal vein, mainly from the recipient, and the inferior mesenteric vein and iliac vein, mainly from the donor [12]. Recently, some cryopreserved veins have been introduced for hepatic vein reconstruction [28]. This type of vein grafts might be the best way to keep outflow and make the reconstruction technically simple, but such vein grafts may have the problem of obstruction in the long-term observation period [29]. In WU Hong's study, they used the great saphenous vein as an interposition graft and formulated a strategy for reconstructing outflow in right liver grafts without the MHV [6].

Yu et al. (Hangzhou, China) in their institution, also mainly used the recipient's portal vein (main portal vein and its branch) as the interpositional MHV graft [12]. This kind of vein graft has several advantages over other vessels. Firstly, it is always available and easy to expose after the resection of the liver and eliminates the extensive dissection in the recipient or donor. Secondly, the suitable caliber, thick wall, and natural curvature of the portal vein can reduce the risk of thrombosis [27] after transplantation.

The European experience of adult LDLT summarized by Broelsch et al. [30] reported on 11 centers in 8 countries that performed 105 pediatric and 123 adult living donations, 111 of which were right lobe allografts. Recipient and allograft survival were 86% and 83%, respectively. Two large single center reports from France and Germany reported 1-year graft survival ranging from 75% to 85% [31, 32]. Marcos [33] reported that the survival rate of the first 20 recipients was 80% and improved to 95% in the next 20 recipients. We had very similar results with an overall 1-year survival for our series of 31 cases out of 40 (77.5%).

Bak et al. [34] of the University of Colorado reported 85% recipient survival in an initial series of 20 right lobe allografts. The primary causes of graft failure were primary nonfunction and vascular thrombosis. Their LDLT results in this series showed graft survival of 90.9%.

Adham et al. had 33 patients who received 34 cadaveric right split liver grafts. The first group (GI, $n = 15$) included grafts with only the right hepatic vein (RHV) outflow; the second (GII, $n = 18$) included grafts with both right and MHV outflows. The 2 groups were similar in patient demographics, initial liver disease, and donor characteristics. At one year, patient survival was 94% for both groups [19]. In our series, the one-year survival rates were better for Group A (reconstruction patients with more than one HV anastomosis, $n = 16$) 87.5%) with 87.5% versus 70.83% for Group B (patients with single HV anastomosis). All of the six patients with venous grafts are alive till now and doing well.

In Wu et al. series, recipients' survival rate was 89.1% (49/55) at median followup of 10 months (range, 1 to 26 months). Six patients (10.9%) died of small-for-size syndrome (1), renal failure (1), multiple organ failure (3) within 3 months after transplantation, and recurrent HCC (1) within 13 months after transplantation. The overall graft survival rate was 90.9% (50/55). Causes of graft failure were hepatic vein stricture (1), small-for-size syndrome (2), vascular thrombosis (1), and sepsis (1). One late death caused by tumor recurrence was not considered graft failure in this analysis [6]. In a study by Bin Liu's et al. consisting of 47 cases using right lobe graft without middle hepatic vein (MHV) and 3 cases using dual grafts (one case using two left lobe, 2 using one right lobe and one left lobe), among 50 adult recipients, 4 cases (8%) died postoperatively within 3 months. Their 1-year actual survival rate was 92% [6].

In summary, hepatic venous reconstruction in right lobe LDLT is technically challenging. A custom-made strategy in individuals may be necessary depending on whether significant MHV tributaries and major SHVs are present, although there is no consensus regarding the optional strategy for outflow reconstruction in LDLT without the use of the MHV. The most serious problem of adult LDLT without MHV is the obstruction of V5 or V8 outflow. The appropriate length of the reconstructed RHV is still controversial; a technique to secure an RHV anastomosis of adequate length and width may be a better option than a stretched, short anastomosis to prevent outflow obstruction. In our institute, we believe that adult LDLT is safely achieved with better outcome to both recipients and donors by harvesting the right lobe graft without MHV, provided that significant MHV tributaries (segments V and VIII more than 5 mm) are reconstructed, and any accessory considerable inferior right hepatic veins (IRHVs) or superficial RHVs are anastomosed.

Acknowledgments

Study results were tabulated, analyzed, and reviewed under Professor Brian Davidson's supervision, Liver Transplant Department, Royal Free Hospital, University College London, London, UK (under a UK/Egyptian joint Ph.D. supervision Scheme). The main study was performed in National Liver Institute, Menoufiya University, Egypt (Grant no. 30-2009/2010 Tanta University/Ministry of Higher Education).

References

[1] Y.-S. Lim and W. R. Kim, "The global impact of hepatic fibrosis and end-stage liver disease," *Clinics in Liver Disease*, vol. 12, no. 4, pp. 733–746, 2008.

[2] X.-H. Wang, L.-N. Yan, F. Zhang et al., "Early experiences on living donor liver transplantation in China: multicenter report," *Chinese Medical Journal*, vol. 119, no. 12, pp. 1003–1009, 2006.

[3] L.-N. Yan, B. Li, Y. Zeng et al., "Modified techniques for adult-to-adult living donor liver transplantation," *Hepatobiliary and Pancreatic Diseases International*, vol. 5, no. 2, pp. 173–179, 2006.

[4] H. Oya, Y. Sato, S. Yamamoto et al., "Surgical procedures for decompression of excessive shear stress in small-for-size living donor liver transplantation: new hepatic vein reconstruction," *Transplantation Proceedings*, vol. 37, no. 2, pp. 1108–1111, 2005.

[5] S.-G. Lee, "Asian contribution to living donor liver transplantation," *Journal of Gastroenterology and Hepatology*, vol. 21, no. 3, pp. 572–574, 2006.

[6] H. Wu, J.-Y. Yang, L.-N. Yan et al., "Hepatic venous outflow reconstruction in adult right lobe living donor liver transplantation without middle hepatic vein," *Chinese Medical Journal*, vol. 120, no. 11, pp. 947–951, 2007.

[7] T. Kaneko, K. Kaneko, H. Sugimoto et al., "Intrahepatic anastomosis formation between the hepatic veins in the graft liver of the living related liver transplantation: Observation by Doppler ultrasonography," *Transplantation*, vol. 70, no. 6, pp. 982–985, 2000.

[8] S.-G. Lee, "Techniques of reconstruction of hepatic veins in living-donor liver transplantation, especially for right hepatic vein and major short hepatic veins of right-lobe graft," *Journal of Hepato-Biliary-Pancreatic Surgery*, vol. 13, no. 2, pp. 131–138, 2006.

[9] V. H. de Villa, C.-L. Chen, Y.-S. Chen et al., "Right lobe living donor liver transplantation: addressing the middle hepatic vein controversy," *Annals of Surgery*, vol. 238, no. 2, pp. 275–282, 2003.

[10] K. Tanaka and T. Yamada, "Living donor liver transplantation in Japan and Kyoto University: what can we learn?" *Journal of Hepatology*, vol. 42, no. 1, pp. 25–28, 2005.

[11] A. Marcos, R. A. Fisher, J. M. Ham et al., "Right lobe living donor liver transplantation," *Transplantation*, vol. 68, no. 6, pp. 798–803, 1999.

[12] P.-F. Yu, J. Wu, and S.-S. Zheng, "Management of the middle hepatic vein and its tributaries in right lobe living donor

liver transplantation," *Hepatobiliary and Pancreatic Diseases International*, vol. 6, no. 4, pp. 358–363, 2007.

[13] C.-M. Lo, S.-T. Fan, C.-L. Liu et al., "Extending the limit on the size of adult recipient in living donor liver transplantation using extended right lobe graft," *Transplantation*, vol. 63, no. 10, pp. 1524–1528, 1997.

[14] N. L. Ascher, J. R. Lake, J. C. Emond, and J. P. Roberts, "Liver transplantation for fulminant hepatic failure," *Archives of Surgery*, vol. 128, no. 6, pp. 677–682, 1993.

[15] M. E. Wachs, T. E. Bak, F. M. Karrer et al., "Adult living donor liver transplantation using a right hepatic lobe," *Transplantation*, vol. 66, no. 10, pp. 1313–1316, 1998.

[16] S.-T. Fan, V. H. De Villa, T. Kiuchi, S.-G. Lee, and M. Makuuchi, "Right anterior sector drainage in right-lobe live-donor liver transplantation," *Transplantation*, vol. 75, no. 3, supplement, pp. S25–S27, 2003.

[17] S.-T. Fan, C.-M. Lo, C.-L. Liu, W.-X. Wang, and J. Wong, "Safety and necessity of including the middle hepatic vein in the right lobe graft in adult-to-adult live donor liver transplantation," *Annals of Surgery*, vol. 238, no. 1, pp. 137–148, 2003.

[18] H. Yamamoto, Y. Maetani, T. Kiuchi et al., "Background and clinical impact of tissue congestion in right-lobe living-donor liver grafts: a magnetic resonance imaging study," *Transplantation*, vol. 76, no. 1, pp. 164–169, 2003.

[19] M. Adham, J. Dumortier, A. Abdelaal, P. Sagnard, C. Boucaud, and O. Boillot, "Does middle hepatic vein omission in a right split graft affect the outcome of liver transplantation? A comparative study of right split livers with and without the middle hepatic vein," *Liver Transplantation*, vol. 13, no. 6, pp. 829–837, 2007.

[20] Y. F. Cheng, C. L. Chen, T. L. Huang et al., "Single imaging modality evaluation of living donors in liver transplantation: magnetic resonance imaging," *Transplantation*, vol. 72, no. 9, pp. 1527–1533, 2001.

[21] H. Tashiro, T. Itamoto, H. Ohdan et al., "Reconstruction of the middle hepatic vein tributaries draining segments V and VIII of a right liver graft by using the recipient's own middle hepatic vein and vascular closure staples," *Surgery Today*, vol. 38, no. 3, pp. 289–291, 2008.

[22] A. Marcos, M. Orloff, L. Mieles, A. T. Olzinski, J. F. Renz, and J. V. Sitzmann, "Functional venous anatomy for right-lobe grafting and techniques to optimized outflow," *Liver Transplantation*, vol. 7, no. 10, pp. 845–852, 2001.

[23] Y. Sugawara, M. Makuuchi, H. Imamura, J. Kaneko, T. Ohkubo, and N. Kokudo, "Outflow reconstruction in recipients of right liver graft from living donors," *Liver Transplantation*, vol. 8, no. 2, pp. 167–168, 2002.

[24] Y. Sugawara, M. Makuuchi, H. Imamura, J. Kaneko, and N. Kokudo, "Outflow reconstruction in extended right liver grafts from living donors," *Liver Transplantation*, vol. 9, no. 3, pp. 306–309, 2003.

[25] S. Hwang, S.-G. Lee, K.-M. Park et al., "Quilt venoplasty using recipient saphenous vein graft for reconstruction of multiple short hepatic veins in right liver grafts," *Liver Transplantation*, vol. 11, no. 1, pp. 104–107, 2005.

[26] S. G. Lee, K. M. Park, S. Hwang et al., "Modified right liver graft from a living donor to prevent congestion," *Transplantation*, vol. 74, no. 1, pp. 54–59, 2002.

[27] M. S. Cattral, P. D. Greig, D. Muradali, and D. Grant, "Reconstruction of middle hepatic vein of a living-donor right lobe liver graft with recipient left portal vein," *Transplantation*, vol. 71, no. 12, pp. 1864–1866, 2001.

[28] T. Hashimoto, Y. Sugawara, Y. Kishi et al., "Superior vena cava graft for right liver and right lateral sector transplantation," *Transplantation*, vol. 79, no. 8, pp. 920–925, 2005.

[29] Y. Sugawara, M. Makuuchi, N. Akamatsu et al., "Refinement of venous reconstruction using cryopreserved veins in right liver grafts," *Liver Transplantation*, vol. 10, no. 4, pp. 541–547, 2004.

[30] C. E. Broelsch, M. Malago, G. Testa, and C. Valentin-Gamazo, "Living donor liver transplantation in adults: outcome in Europe," *Liver Transplantation*, vol. 6, supplement 2, no. 6, pp. S64–S65, 2000.

[31] O. Boillot, J. Belghiti, D. Azoulay, J. Gugenheim, O. Soubrane, and D. Cherqui, "Initial French experience in adult-to-adult living donor liver transplantation," *Transplantation Proceedings*, vol. 35, no. 3, pp. 962–963, 2003.

[32] M. Malago, G. Testa, A. Frilling et al., "Right living donor liver transplantation: an option for adult patients: single institution experience with 74 patients," *Annals of Surgery*, vol. 238, no. 6, pp. 853–862, 2003.

[33] A. Marcos, "Right lobe living donor liver transplantation: a review," *Liver Transplantation*, vol. 6, pp. 3–20, 2000.

[34] T. Bak, M. Wachs, J. Trotter et al., "Adult-to-adult living donor liver transplantation using right-lobe grafts: results and lessons learned from a single-center experience," *Liver Transplantation*, vol. 7, pp. 680–686, 2001.

The Preoperative Assessment of Hepatic Tumours: Evaluation of UK Regional Multidisciplinary Team Performance

M. G. Wiggans,[1,2] S. A. Jackson,[1] B. M. T. Fox,[1] J. D. Mitchell,[1] S. Aroori,[1] M. J. Bowles,[1] E. M. Armstrong,[1] J. F. Shirley,[1] and D. A. Stell[1,2]

[1] Plymouth Hospitals NHS Trust, Derriford Hospital, Derriford Road, Plymouth, Devon PL6 8DH, UK
[2] Plymouth University, Peninsula College of Medicine and Dentistry, John Bull Building, Plymouth, Devon PL6 8BU, UK

Correspondence should be addressed to D. A. Stell; david.stell@nhs.net

Academic Editor: Shu-Sen Zheng

Introduction. In the UK, patients where liver resection is contemplated are discussed at hepatobiliary multidisciplinary team (MDT) meetings. The aim was to assess MDT performance by identification of patients where radiological and pathological diagnoses differed. *Materials and Methods.* A retrospective review of a prospectively maintained database of all cases undergoing liver resection from March 2006 to January 2012 was performed. The presumed diagnosis as a result of radiological investigation and MDT discussion is recorded at the time of surgery. Imaging was reviewed by specialist gastrointestinal radiologists, and results were agreed on by consensus. *Results.* Four hundred and thirty-eight patients were studied. There was a significant increase in the use of preoperative imaging modalities ($P \leq 0.01$) but no change in the rate of discrepant diagnosis over time. Forty-two individuals were identified whose final histological diagnosis was different to that following MDT discussion (9.6%). These included 30% of patients diagnosed preoperatively with hepatocellular carcinoma and 25% with cholangiocarcinoma of a major duct. *Discussion.* MDT assessment of patients preoperatively is accurate in terms of diagnosis. The highest rate of discrepancies occurred in patients with focal lesions without chronic liver disease or primary cancer, where hepatocellular carcinoma was overdiagnosed and peripheral cholangiocarcinoma underdiagnosed, where particular care should be taken. Additional care should be taken in these groups and preoperative multimodality imaging considered.

1. Introduction

Cancer care in the UK has undergone a major change in recent years with the centralisation of care in a network of cancer centres [1]. This has led to the establishment of regional hepatopancreaticobiliary (HPB) units where patients in whom liver resection is contemplated are discussed at a multidisciplinary team (MDT) meeting in the presence of radiologists, oncologists, surgeons, and physicians. This is intended to provide greater clinical input into the diagnosis of the wide spectrum of disease processes for which liver resection is appropriate [2]. During the same period increasing awareness of the complimentary role of different imaging modalities in diagnosing liver disease [3–5] has led to many patients having multiple investigations prior

to surgery. Although the accuracy of single imaging modalities including ultrasound [3, 6, 7], computerised tomography (CT) [3, 7, 8], magnetic resonance imaging (MRI) [3, 7, 9], and positron emission tomography (PET) [3, 8] scans in assessing hepatic malignancies has been well described, the performance of MDT review of multiple preoperative imaging techniques with input from clinicians in the diagnosis of malignancy and planning of treatment has not been described.

The Peninsula HPB unit was founded in July 2005 to serve the Devon and Cornwall region of England (population 1.7 million). Imaging from referring hospitals is imported and discussed in a weekly MDT meeting, and treatment recommendations are made and recorded. After resection histology of the excised sample is also discussed at the MDT meeting. Despite MDT assessment, we have experienced cases either where the histological diagnosis has differed from the presumed preoperative diagnosis or where the available imaging does not allow a certain diagnosis to be made. In this situation a list of differential diagnoses is made from which treatment is recommended. Furthermore, despite advanced imaging techniques, some patients undergo surgery without proceeding to resection due to unexpected operative findings. The primary aim of this study was to identify patients where the diagnosis determined by the MDT differed from the final histological diagnosis. A secondary aim was to identify recurring areas of confusion to guide future MDT assessment and to determine if the rate of inaccurate diagnosis of liver tumours and assessments of resectability of liver lesions has changed over time.

2. Materials and Methods

The Peninsula HPB unit has maintained a prospective database since the inception of the unit where the outcome of MDT discussion is recorded prior to surgery. A review of all patients undergoing surgery from March 2006 to January 2012 was performed. Details of preoperative diagnosis, imaging modalities performed, operative findings, and final histology were retrieved. Patients were identified where the MDT was unable to make a definitive diagnosis leading to differential options. All imaging was re-reviewed by a specialist gastrointestinal radiologist and results agreed by consensus. For comparison of utilisation of imaging modalities, the group was split into two halves consisting of 219 patients each. The dataset was also divided to compare the earlier with later experience. Statistical analysis was performed using a chisquare test or Mann-Whitney U test, and a P value of <0.05 was considered statistically significant. Analyses were performed using SPSS version 20 (IBM, New York, USA).

3. Results

3.1. *Patient Population.* Four hundred and thirty-eight patients were identified including 248 males and 190 females with median age 65 years (range 21–90). The indications for surgery are shown in Table 1. Four hundred and seventeen patients underwent liver resection (95%), and 21 patients (5%) underwent surgery without resection. Details of the group not proceeding to resection are shown in Table 2.

3.2. *Imaging Performed.* In total 969 imaging investigations (excluding repeat images of the same modality) were performed for the 438 patients including CT, MRI, PET, US, and ERCP. Only five patients did not have a CT scan. The number of MRI scans undertaken increased from 96 in the first half of the study (219 patients) to 131 in the second the second ($P = 0.001$). Similarly the number of PET scans undertaken increased from 85 to 115 ($P = 0.005$). In a minority of patients ERCP or Octreotide scans were performed where indicated.

The total number of investigations performed increased significantly during the study period from 442 in the first half to 525 in the second. Similarly, the median number of scans performed per patient increased from two (1–4) to three (1–4) ($P < 0.001$).

3.3. *Correlation of MDT Assessment with Operative Findings.* A decision not to resect was made in 21 patients (4.8%) either because of peritoneal disease, tumour progression or because no malignant lesion could be identified (Table 2).

There was no change in the rate of nonresection over time (10/219 versus 11/219). MDT assessment of operability was most accurate for CRM where only 7/270 patients (2.6%) were not resected and least accurate for patients with hilar cholangiocarcinomas where 4/23 patients were not resected ($P < 0.001$).

3.4. *Correlation of MDT Diagnosis with Final Pathology.* Of the 438 patients operated on in this period 42 individuals were identified whose final histological diagnosis was different to the outcome of the MDT discussion (9.6%) (Table 1). There was no change in the rate of discrepant diagnosis over time (23/219 versus 19/219) (Table 3). The median number of lesions per patient was one in both the first (range 0–9) and second (range 0–20) halves of the series ($P = 0.057$). Similarly there was no difference in maximum tumour size with a median of 35 mm (range 6–210) in the first half and 35 mm (range 3–230) in the second ($P = 0.936$). The median number of imaging modalities used was three in patients with discrepant diagnoses compared to two in those with correct diagnoses ($P = 0.003$). The only difference occurred in the use of MRI where 31/42 (73.8%) patients with discrepant diagnoses had additional MRI compared to 196/396 (49.5%) patients where the diagnosis was correct ($P = 0.003$). In total twenty-two patients (5%) underwent hepatic resection for what proved to be benign disease having been diagnosed with malignancy preoperatively. The difficult areas of MDT assessment fell into the following categories.

3.5. *Hepatocellular Cancer.* Thirteen of 44 patients diagnosed as having hepatoma at MDT and proceeding to resection had different histological diagnoses after surgery, of which three were benign. There was no significant difference in the rate of discrepant diagnosis in those with and without a history of chronic liver disease (CLD) (6/19 versus 7/25) (Table 4). In six patients with CLD the final histology revealed a mixed type of tumour with features of both hepatoma and cholangiocarcinoma. For the purposes of this study these have been classed as correct diagnoses.

3.6. *Cholangiocarcinoma of Major Hepatic Duct.* All patients with suspected cholangiocarcinoma of a major hepatic duct underwent cholangiography (percutaneous, endoscopic, or MR) in addition to cross-sectional imaging. Seven of 28 patients diagnosed with cholangiocarcinoma at MDT had a different histological diagnosis after resection (Table 3). There was no significant difference in the rate of incorrect diagnosis in those who presented with obstructive jaundice (3/19) and those without (4/9). Of those patients diagnosed with cholangiocarcinoma without obstructive jaundice, the diagnosis was confirmed in five patients on final histology.

TABLE 1: MDT indications for resection and number with discrepant histological diagnoses.

Primary MDT diagnosis	Number (%)		Median age (range)		Male/female	Discrepant diagnosis (%)	
Colorectal liver metastases (CRM)	279	(64)	67	(33–90)	176/103	10	(3.6)
Hepatoma	44	(10)	63	(33–84)	31/13	13	(30)
Hilar cholangiocarcinoma	28	(7)	67	(32–77)	14/14	7	(25)
Other metastases	24	(5)	62	(32–76)	8/16	1	(4)
Gall bladder carcinoma	20	(5)	61	(41–82)	5/15	1	(5)
Neuroendocrine tumour (NET)	11	(3)	51	(41–77)	8/3	0	—
Metastasis of unknown origin	6	(1)	63	(43–73)	4/2	5	(83)
Biliary cystadenoma	6	(1)	34	(21–43)	0/6	0	—
Focal nodular hyperplasia (FNH)	5	(1)	34	(30–38)	0/5	0	—
Hepatocellular adenoma	4	(<1)	31	(30–39)	0/4	0	—
Benign cyst	3	(<1)	52	(47–65)	0/3	1	(33)
Breast metastases	3	(<1)	67	(45–78)	0/3	3	(100)
Peripheral cholangiocarcinoma	3	(<1)	70	—	2/1	1	(33)
Primary sarcoma	1	(<1)	71	—	0/1	0	—
Haemangioma	1	(<1)	33	—	0/1	0	—
Total	438		65	(21–90)	248/190	42	(9.8)

TABLE 2: Reasons for nonresection.

Final diagnosis	Number (%)		Peritoneal disease	Disease progression	No/benign disease
Colorectal metastases (CRM)	7/270	(2.6)	4	3	0
Hepatoma	2/33	(6)	0	2	0
Hilar cholangiocarcinoma	4/23	(17)	0	4	0
Gall bladder carcinoma (GBC)	2/19	(11)	2	0	0
Other metastases	3/30	(10)	1	2	0
Neuroendocrine tumour (NET)	1/13	(8)	0	1	0
Haemangioma	1/9	(11)	0	0	1
Normal liver	1	—	0	0	1
Total	21	(4.8)	7	12	2

3.7. Colorectal Metastases. All patients diagnosed with CRM had a history of colorectal cancer, but 10 (3.6%) had different histological diagnoses after resection (Table 3), of which six were benign. Six of these were metachronous lesions and four were synchronous with their colorectal cancer diagnosis ($P = 0.539$).

3.8. Solid Liver Lesions with No History of Chronic Liver Disease or Primary Malignancy. Thirty-four patients underwent resection of peripheral liver lesions (including hepatomas) with no history of CLD or primary malignancy of whom 13 had discrepant diagnoses (Table 4).

Peripheral cholangiocarcinoma was rarely diagnosed correctly preoperatively. Of eleven patients with a diagnosis of peripheral cholangiocarcinoma at histology, only two had been diagnosed correctly preoperatively, both by percutaneous biopsy. The remainder were inaccurately diagnosed as hepatomas or metastases (Table 3).

3.9. Adenoma/FNH/Hepatocellular Carcinoma. A group of 10, predominantly young, female patients (median age 33,

range 33–63) was identified in whom the MDT differential list included FNH, adenoma, or hepatocellular carcinoma. After resection all patients had a histological diagnosis that was included in the alternatives made at MDT. In five patients histology revealed hepatic adenoma, four revealed FNH, and one a hepatoma.

4. Discussion

This study reveals a number of important features of the MDT assessment of patients with focal liver lesions during the six-year development of a regional HPB unit. Firstly there has been a 50% increase in the number of imaging modalities used in the assessment of these patients over a short time interval. This has been caused by an increased utilisation of PET scans and MRI due to an increased awareness of their role and improved access. Although PET scans have poor sensitivity for detecting multiple liver lesions, they are valuable in the preoperative assessment of patients with hepatic CRM to exclude extrahepatic disease [10, 11]. MRI scans with diffusion-weighted imaging have been shown to

TABLE 3: Discrepant diagnoses in 42 patients.

MDT diagnosis	Total discrepant	Histological diagnosis																
		Angiomyolipoma* (1)	Benign cyst* (4)	Benign fibrosis* (3)	Bile duct papilloma* (1)	Breast metastasis (3)	Peripheral cholangiocarcinoma (11)	CRM (270)	FNH* (6)	Focal fat* (2)	Haemangioma* (9)	Hepatoma (34)	NET (13)	No lesion* (2)	Sarcoma (4)	Chronic inflammation* (1)	Ovarian metastasis (5)	Xanthogranulomatous cholecystitis* (1)
Hepatoma (44)	13	1	—	—	—	—	5	1	—	1	2	—	2	—	—	1	—	—
Colorectal metastases (CRM) (279)	10	—	—	—	—	2	1	—	—	—	4	1	—	2	—	—	—	—
Hilar cholangiocarcinoma (31)	7	—	2	3	1	1	—	—	—	—	—	—	—	—	—	—	—	—
Metastases of unknown origin (6)	5	—	—	—	—	—	3	—	—	—	1	—	—	—	1	—	—	—
Breast metastases (3)	3	—	—	—	—	—	—	—	—	1	1	1	—	—	—	—	—	—
Peripheral cholangiocarcinoma (3)	1	—	—	—	—	—	—	—	1	—	—	—	—	—	—	—	—	—
Anal metastases (7)	1	—	—	—	—	—	—	—	—	—	—	1	—	—	—	—	—	—
Benign cyst (3)	1	—	—	—	—	—	—	—	—	—	—	—	—	—	—	—	1	—
Gall bladder carcinoma (20)	1	—	—	—	—	—	—	—	—	—	—	—	—	—	—	—	—	1
Total	42	1	2	3	1	3	9	1	1	2	8	3	2	2	1	1	1	1

Total number of each diagnosis in the series (438) shown in brackets.

All MDT diagnoses of neuroendocrine tumours (NET) (11), focal nodular hyperplasia (FNH) (5), biliary cystadenoma (6), primary sarcoma (1), and haemangioma (1) were confirmed on histology.

* Benign pathology.

TABLE 4: MDT and histological diagnoses of 34 patients with peripheral liver lesions and no history of CLD or malignancy.

MDT diagnosis	Histology								
	Hepatoma	Peripheral cholangio-carcinoma	Haem-angioma	Neuroendocrine tumour	Metastasis of unknown origin (MUO)	Hepatic sarcoma	Focal nodular hyperplasia	Fat	Total
Hepatoma	18	4	1	1	—	—	—	1	25
Metastases of unknown origin	—	3	1	—	1	1	—	—	6
Peripheral cholangiocarcinoma	—	2	—	—	—	—	1	—	3
Total	18	9	2	1	1	1	1	1	34

have greater sensitivity than CT in the detection of CRM [8, 12], hepatoma [13], and metastatic NET [14], although these scans have only been available to this department since 2011. The policy of this unit is not to biopsy potentially resectable liver lesions due to the potential risk of tumour seeding [15, 16].

In this series 21 patients (5%) did not undergo surgical resection, and the rate of non-resection did not change significantly over time. The rate of non-resection of liver lesions following assessment has been described previously with reported rates of 3–12% [17, 18]. The commonest cause of non-resection in our series was disease progression. The time interval between imaging and surgery may have a major impact on this outcome, limiting the value of modern imaging. Peritoneal disease was noted in seven of the unresected patients, which is not readily identified by any imaging modality [19].

The highest rate of discrepancies in our series occurred in the group of patients with focal liver lesions without a history of chronic liver disease or primary cancer. This finding emphasises the importance of assessing imaging in the context of the clinical history (13/34). Two observations arise from this group of significance in clinical practice. Firstly the majority of patients (5/6) diagnosed with metastases of unknown origin (MUO) have defined histology after resection, of which the most common is peripheral cholangiocarcinoma. These lesions typically have hypovascular appearances on imaging with ring-like enhancement [20] and can easily be misdiagnosed as colorectal or breast metastases [21]. Recently published guidelines for the management of MUO recommend a range of chemotherapy regimens [22], none of which have been shown to be of benefit in the treatment of cholangiocarcinoma, whereas surgical resection of peripheral cholangiocarcinoma is of proven benefit [23] but is rarely appropriate in the treatment of MUO. Similarly 4/25 patients diagnosed as having hepatoma in this setting are ultimately shown to have peripheral cholangiocarcinoma. Peripheral cholangiocarcinoma is less common than hepatocellular carcinoma [24] which may lead to a low index of suspicion in MDT diagnosis.

In patients with a history of CLD and focal liver lesions, there remains a high rate of patients found not to have hepatoma after excision (7/19). These include neuroendocrine metastases which are hypervascular lesions having similar radiological appearances to hepatoma. This has implications for this patient group where treatment is often recommended without a histological diagnosis.

The commonest indication for liver resection in our series has been CRM, and the rate of discrepant diagnoses for this group is low (3.6%). The most common alternative diagnosis after resection in this group was haemangioma. The radiological characteristics of this group have been described elsewhere [25] and can be difficult to distinguish from metastases. Interestingly two patients in this group were found to have breast cancer metastases after primary breast surgery two and ten years previously. Breast metastases can have similar radiological features to CRM and can occur many years after the primary diagnosis. A further breast metastasis occurred as an obstructing lesion of the left hepatic duct sixteen years after primary surgery and was diagnosed as a hilar cholangiocarcinoma.

The high rate of discrepant diagnoses in patients with major duct cholangiocarcinoma has been shown previously [26–28]. These lesions are usually sclerosing adenocarcinomas causing biliary obstruction and are often not visible as a mass lesion [20]. In this situation the presence of the lesion is inferred by the radiological finding of ductal dilation along with clinical features of obstruction. The most common alternative diagnosis in this series was ductal fibrosis. This condition may be a manifestation of an autoimmune process and can have similar radiological features to cholangiocarcinoma [29]. Peribiliary cysts can often be diagnosed preoperatively by the presence of multiple cysts but can also mimic cholangiocarcinoma [20] as in the two cases experienced in this series. The most difficult lesions to assess and make treatment recommendations for are peripheral ductal lesions which do not cause jaundice but are found coincidentally or cause cholestasis. In these patients often the only finding is a short segment of dilated intrahepatic duct. In this series 5/9 of these patients were found to have a cholangiocarcinoma on final histology, and surgery for these lesions is therefore justified, particularly as these lesions can usually be resected safely without the need for resection of the extrahepatic biliary tree.

A particularly difficult group of patients to assess and make treatment recommendations for is the group of predominantly young women with primary liver lesions where the differential diagnosis includes hepatoma, adenoma, and focal nodular hyperplasia. These lesions are usually single but may be multifocal and often occur on a background of obesity or oral contraceptive use [30]. In this series 6/10 lesions were shown to be neoplastic on final histology (adenoma or hepatoma) and surgery appears justified in this patient group.

Overall 5% of patients underwent surgery for misdiagnosed benign lesions, which is similar to earlier experience [31]. The most common benign lesions were haemangiomas which can be hypo-, iso-, or hyperattenuating on imaging and can sometimes increase in size [25], making distinction from malignant tumours difficult.

In conclusion approximately 10% of patients proceeding to surgery following discussion at the HPB MDT are subsequently shown to have an inaccurate diagnosis and 5% are understaged. Despite an increase in the number of imaging modalities used, there has been no change in this rate over time. These discrepancies must be considered in the context of the risk of overstaging resectable disease or misdiagnosing malignant lesions as benign.

References

[1] R. M. Charnley and S. Paterson-Brown, "Surgeon volumes in oesophagogastric and hepatopancreatobiliary resectional surgery," *British Journal of Surgery*, vol. 98, no. 7, pp. 891–893, 2011.

[2] "Improving outcomes in colorectal cancers improving outcomes in colorectal cancers," National Institute for Health and Clinical Excellence, 2004, http://www.nice.org.uk/nicemedia/live/10895/28833/28833.pdf.

[3] D. V. Sahani and S. P. Kalva, "Imaging the liver," *Oncologist*, vol. 9, no. 4, pp. 385–397, 2004.

[4] S. Bipat, M. S. van Leeuwen, J. N. M. Ijzermans, P. M. M. Bossuyt, J.-W. Greve, and J. Stoker, "Imaging and treatment of patients with colorectal liver metastases in the Netherlands: a survey," *Netherlands Journal of Medicine*, vol. 64, no. 5, pp. 147–151, 2006.

[5] K. O. Ong and E. Leen, "Radiological staging of colorectal liver metastases," *Surgical Oncology*, vol. 16, no. 1, pp. 7–14, 2007.

[6] J. Choi, "Imaging of hepatic metastases," *Cancer Control*, vol. 13, no. 1, pp. 6–12, 2006.

[7] W. Schima, C. Kulinna, H. Langenberger, and A. Ba-Ssalamah, "Liver metastases of colorectal cancer: US, CT or MR?" *Cancer Imaging*, vol. 5, pp. S149–156, 2005.

[8] S. Bipat, M. S. van Leeuwen, E. F. I. Comans et al., "Colorectal liver metastases: CT, MR imaging, and PET for diagnosis—meta-analysis," *Radiology*, vol. 237, no. 1, pp. 123–131, 2005.

[9] S. Blyth, A. Blakeborough, M. Peterson, I. C. Cameron, and A. W. Majeed, "Sensitivity of magnetic resonance imaging in the detection of colorectal liver metastases," *Annals of the Royal College of Surgeons of England*, vol. 90, no. 1, pp. 25–28, 2008.

[10] F. G. Fernandez, J. A. Drebin, D. C. Linehan et al., "Five-year survival after resection of hepatic metastases from colorectal cancer in patients screened by positron emission tomography with F-18 fluorodeoxyglucose (FDG-PET)," *Annals of Surgery*, vol. 240, no. 3, pp. 438–450, 2004.

[11] R. H. Huebner, K. C. Park, J. E. Shepherd et al., "A meta-analysis of the literature for whole-body FDG PET detection of recurrent colorectal cancer," *Journal of Nuclear Medicine*, vol. 41, no. 7, pp. 1177–1189, 2000.

[12] R. C. Semelka, W. G. Cance, H. B. Marcos, and M. A. Mauro, "Liver metastases: comparison of current MR techniques and spiral CT during arterial portography for detection in 20 surgically staged cases," *Radiology*, vol. 213, no. 1, pp. 86–91, 1999.

[13] M. Kudo, "Diagnostic imaging of hepatocellular carcinoma: recent progress," *Oncology*, vol. 81, no. 1, pp. 73–85, 2011.

[14] A. G. Rockall, K. Planche, N. Power et al., "Detection of neuroendocrine liver metastases with MnDPDP-enhanced MRI," *Neuroendocrinology*, vol. 89, no. 3, pp. 288–295, 2009.

[15] O. M. Jones, M. Rees, T. G. John, S. Bygrave, and G. Plant, "Biopsy of resectable colorectal liver metastases causes tumour dissemination and adversely affects survival after liver resection," *British Journal of Surgery*, vol. 92, no. 9, pp. 1165–1168, 2005.

[16] A. B. Cresswell, F. K. S. Welsh, and M. Rees, "A diagnostic paradigm for resectable liver lesions: to biopsy or not to biopsy?" *HPB*, vol. 11, no. 7, pp. 533–540, 2009.

[17] W. R. Jarnagin, Y. Fong, A. Ky et al., "Liver resection for metastatic colorectal cancer: assessing the risk of occult irresectable disease," *Journal of the American College of Surgeons*, vol. 188, no. 1, pp. 33–42, 1999.

[18] A. Schepers, S. Mieog, B. B. van de Burg, J. van Schaik, G.-J. Liefers, and P. J. Marang-van de Mheen, "Impact of complications after surgery for colorectal liver metastasis on patient survival," *Journal of Surgical Research*, vol. 164, no. 1, pp. e91–e97, 2010.

[19] C. M. Patel, A. Sahdev, and R. H. Reznek, "CT, MRI and PET imaging in peritoneal malignancy," *Cancer Imaging*, vol. 11, no. 1, pp. 123–139, 2011.

[20] Y. E. Cheung, M. J. Kim, Y. N. Park et al., "Varying appearances of cholangiocarcinoma: radiologic- pathologic correlation," *RadioGraphics*, vol. 29, no. 3, pp. 683–700, 2009.

[21] B. I. Choi, J. M. Lee, and J. K. Han, "Imaging of intrahepatic and hilar cholangiocarcinoma," *Abdominal Imaging*, vol. 29, no. 5, pp. 548–557, 2004.

[22] NICE, "Metastatic malignant disease of unknown primary origin: diagnosis and management of metastatic malignant disease of unknown primary origin," 2010, http://www.nice.org.uk/nicemedia/live/13044/49848/49848.pdf.

[23] J. Bridgewater and C. Imber, "New advances in the management of biliary tract cancer," *HPB*, vol. 9, no. 2, pp. 104–111, 2007.

[24] M.-F. Chen, "Peripheral cholangiocarcinoma (cholangiocellular carcinoma): clinical features, diagnosis and treatment," *Journal of Gastroenterology and Hepatology*, vol. 14, no. 12, pp. 1144–1149, 1999.

[25] J. P. Heiken, "Distinguishing benign from malignant liver tumours," *Cancer Imaging*, vol. 7, pp. S1–S14, 2007.

[26] T. Patel, "Cholangiocarcinoma-controversies and challenges," *Nature Reviews Gastroenterology and Hepatology*, vol. 8, no. 4, pp. 189–200, 2011.

[27] E. Buc, M. Lesurtel, and J. Belghiti, "Is preoperative histological diagnosis necessary before referral to major surgery for cholangiocarcinoma?" *HPB*, vol. 10, no. 2, pp. 98–105, 2008.

[28] B. Boland, A. Kim, N. Nissen, and S. Colquhoun, "Cholangiocarcinoma: aggressive surgical intervention remains justified," *American Surgeon*, vol. 78, no. 2, pp. 157–160, 2012.

[29] H.-C. Oh, M.-H. Kim, K. T. Lee et al., "Clinical clues to suspicion of IgG4-associated sclerosing cholangitis disguised as primary sclerosing cholangitis or hilar cholangiocarcinoma," *Journal of Gastroenterology and Hepatology*, vol. 25, no. 12, pp. 1831–1837, 2010.

3

Iatrogenic Biliary Injuries: Multidisciplinary Management in a Major Tertiary Referral Center

Ibrahim Abdelkader Salama,[1] Hany Abdelmeged Shoreem,[1]
Sherif Mohamed Saleh,[1] Osama Hegazy,[1] Mohamed Housseni,[2] Mohamed Abbasy,[3]
Gamal Badra,[3] and Tarek Ibrahim[1]

[1] Department of Hepatobiliary Surgery, National Liver Institute, Menophyia University, Shiben Elkom, Egypt
[2] Department of Radiology, National Liver Institute, Menophyia University, Shiben Elkom, Egypt
[3] Department of Hepatology, National Liver Institute, Menophyia University, Shiben Elkom, Egypt

Correspondence should be addressed to Ibrahim Abdelkader Salama; ibrahim_salama@hotmail.com

Academic Editor: Christos G. Dervenis

Background. Iatrogenic biliary injuries are considered as the most serious complications during cholecystectomy. Better outcomes of such injuries have been shown in cases managed in a specialized center. *Objective.* To evaluate biliary injuries management in major referral hepatobiliary center. *Patients & Methods.* Four hundred seventy-two consecutive patients with postcholecystectomy biliary injuries were managed with multidisciplinary team (hepatobiliary surgeon, gastroenterologist, and radiologist) at major Hepatobiliary Center in Egypt over 10-year period using endoscopy in 232 patients, percutaneous techniques in 42 patients, and surgery in 198 patients. *Results.* Endoscopy was very successful initial treatment of 232 patients (49%) with mild/moderate biliary leakage (68%) and biliary stricture (47%) with increased success by addition of percutaneous (Rendezvous technique) in 18 patients (3.8%). However, surgery was needed in 198 patients (42%) for major duct transection, ligation, major leakage, and massive stricture. Surgery was urgent in 62 patients and elective in 136 patients. Hepaticojejunostomy was done in most of cases with transanastomotic stents. There was one mortality after surgery due to biliary sepsis and postoperative stricture in 3 cases (1.5%) treated with percutaneous dilation and stenting. *Conclusion.* Management of biliary injuries was much better with multidisciplinary care team with initial minimal invasive technique to major surgery in major complex injury encouraging early referral to highly specialized hepatobiliary center.

1. Introduction

Iatrogenic biliary injuries during cholecystectomy are a serious surgical complication that can have devastating consequences, including a significant risk of early death [1, 2].

Iatrogenic biliary injuries are feared complications reported to occur in approximately 0.2-0.3% in open cholecystectomy Era, but with incidence figures increasing following the introduction of laparoscopic cholecystectomy, with a mean figure of bile duct injuries when including both minor and major injuries up to 0.9% [3, 4]; this is initially attributed to a "learning curve phenomenon" which frequently occurs after introduction of any new procedure or technology [5].

Approximately 17–20% of biliary injuries were recognized intraoperatively [6].

The long-term implications for the patient, surgeon, and healthcare system along with the rising cost of litigation continue to mitigate this otherwise excellent procedure [7].

Traditionally, surgery has been the gold standard for the management of biliary injuries. Recently, various endoscopic and radiological intervention methods have been used as the preferred modalities of these patients [8], as they permitted a less invasive approach with similar or reduced morbidity rates at surgical treatment [9].

The management outcome of iatrogenic biliary injuries when it occurs has been shown to be better when such injuries are managed at specialized hepatobiliary center equipped with multidisciplinary service [10, 11].

The availability of surgical expertise to repair small caliber bile ducts high within the porta-hepatis and the availability of specialized radiological and endoscopic support are the main factors that contribute to the better outcome [12].

The choice of surgical reconstruction and timing of surgical repair are decisive for long-term course. Numerous surgical and interventional treatment modalities that are available require close interdisciplinary cooperation of gastroenterologists, radiologists, and surgeons [13, 14].

In this setting, we analysed the multidisciplinary management approach of iatrogenic bile duct injuries following cholecystectomy with emphasis on the improvement of long-term outcome in a major hepatobiliary referral center.

2. Patients and Methods

This retrospective study included 472 patients with iatrogenic bile duct injuries following cholecystectomy (open and Laparoscopic) referred to the Department of Hepatobiliary Surgery at National Liver Institute, Menophyia University, Egypt (a major tertiary referral center in delta region) from January 2002 to January 2012 and treated by multidisciplinary approach team including hepatobiliary surgeons, gastroenterologists, and interventional radiologists. The multidisciplinary team was established after ethical and scientific approval from Hepatobiliary Department and National Liver Institute committees. All cases of iatrogenic bile duct injuries should undergo this multidisciplinary team approach to set up a road map management of such cases.

All patients complained of postcholecystectomy biliary tract injuries encountered with variable presentation and timing from the surgical insult until they were referred to our center for further evaluation and management.

Cases were subjected to the following:

thorough detailed history taking;

meticulous clinical examination.

Operative details of the previous cholecystectomy should be revised with surgical team of referring hospital.

Investigation needed to diagnose the problems such as liver function tests and abdominal ultrasound were done for all cases as routine preliminary workup.

Computed tomography or magnetic resonance imaging was done in some cases.

Cholangiogram was done for all cases (the gold standard evaluation of biliary injuries) as a trans-tube cholangiogram (with a T-tube in place), an endoscopic cholangiography endoscopic retrograde cholangiopancreatography (ERCP) in most cases, or percutaneous transhepatic cholangiogram in some selected cases in which endoscopic approaches failed.

After receiving patients data by multidisciplinary team, patient condition was categorized through discussion of detailed results of treatment for each category to reach consensus on which type of modality to start with, either endoscopy or intervention radiology as minimal techniques for definitive treatment or bridging technique for definitive

surgery (as complementary tool) prior to surgery or whether surgery still is needed for definitive treatment or surgery is mandatory from the start as definitive treatment.

Also the multidisciplinary team approach gave an outreach service for on-table repair of iatrogenic bile duct injuries to nearby hospitals around the tertiary center in 19 cases after receiving emergency call from the surgical team in those hospitals.

Patients were categorized according to the presentation into the biliary leakage group and the biliary stricture group as diagnosed by previous tools. Each group was managed according to the road map made by multidisciplinary team, starting with the minimally invasive tools (endoscopic treatment alone or in addition to percutaneous interventional radiological manipulation in difficult cases) to more invasive surgical treatment.

Biliary leakage group classified according to the classification of Strasberg et al. [15] was managed by endoscopic sphincterotomy in mild cases and/or stenting in moderate to major leakage, with concomitant stone extraction if present with the common bile duct (CBD) by ERCP.

Biliary stricture group categorized according to the classification of Strasberg et al. [15] was treated initially by endoscopic dilatation and stenting in repeated endoscopic sessions, with upgrading of the stent, until cure was obtained (after full dilatation of the stricture segment as evident by loss of the waist in the cholangiogram).

Percutaneous manipulation was attempted in cases of proximal biliary injuries as in major CBD injuries, transaction, or ligation through percutaneous transhepatic cholangiogram as diagnostic tool prior to surgery, percutaneous manipulations, and guide wire deployment through the CBD prior to combined procedures (Rendezvous) techniques or percutaneous dilatation and stenting for stricture or injuries.

Surgical approaches: surgical intervention was attempted for the cases not fixed by endoscopy or interventional radiology or cases which deserved surgical intervention from the start (transection, ligation, fibrotic stricture of CBD, and postoperative stenotic stricture in bilioenteric anastomosis (redo operation)), with the following surgical maneuvers:

(i) emergency surgery for peritoneal lavage and drainage of biliary peritonitis;

(ii) on-table repair of iatrogenic bile duct injuries in cases diagnosed intraoperatively in our center or as an outreach service in nearby hospitals;

(iii) primary repair on T-tube splint in a minor laceration injury of the CBD;

(iv) choldocholithotomy procedure in associated CBD stones;

(v) undoing CBD ligation;

(vi) bilioenteric anastomosis operations were done as a Roux-En-Y loop depending upon the site of injury, in proximal injuries in porta hepatis (Hepp-Couinaud technique), was capitalized on the extrahepatic course of the left main hepatic duct. Hepaticojejunostomy was done (for the injuries above the biliary confluence) in which the repair was done in the common hepatic duct or at the bile duct confluence with widening the stoma by opening the right and left bile ducts together at site of confluence (stomaplasty), or cholodochojejunostomy was done (in the injuries below the cystic duct insertion and the proximal bile and hepatic duct was not cicatrized or infected). The bilioenteric anastomosis may be side to side or end to side maneuvers depending upon the site and extent of the biliary injuries, and the anastomosis was tension free, mucosa to mucosa, and good wide stoma, with T-tube or biliary splint (specially small ducts) in majority of the cases to decompress the biliary tree in the immediate post-operative period and to obtain postoperative, contrast studies.

3. Results

This study was conducted on 472 cases of postcholecystectomy biliary injuries. The mean age was (46.8 years), with a range of 19–71 years. Out of 472 cases there were 302 cases (64%) females and 170 cases (36%) were males. Biliary injuries cases were 265 (56%) after laparoscope and 207 (44%) after open approach, with most of the cases of the open approach occurring at the late 5 years of study as the learning curve for laparoscopic approach reaches its saturation state and many surgeons, especially the young ones, become master of the laparoscopic technique without gaining good training in the open approach. only 24 cases (5%) were originally operated on in our center and 19 cases (4%) were operated on in the nearby hospitals as part of outreach service program for biliary injuries after urgent consultation from surgical team of those hospitals. Cases presented to our center within a month after operation were considered as early referrals and they were 274 cases (58%) including outstretch service, but the cases presented postoperatively after one month were considered late referrals and they were 208 cases (42%).

Cholangiogram was the main line of the diagnosis in cases of biliary injuries and was done in most of our cases. Also cholangiogram was the method of the diagnosing intraoperatively 5 cases in our center and 19 cases of outreach service program as intraoperative cholangiogram was done for those patients during or after the completion of the repair.

Cholangiography methods were done by endoscopy (endoscopic retrograde cholangiopancreatography (ERCP)) for 346 patients (73.4%), percutaneous transhepatic cholangiogram (PTC) was done for 24 patients (5%), magnetic resonance cholangiopancreatography (MRCP) was done for 61 patients (13%), intraoperative cholangiogram was done in 24 cases (5%), and complementary tests, combination of all these tests, were done for 17 patients (3.6%).

CT scan and MRI of the abdomen were done in most of the cases to detect any abdominal collection.

According to the results of cholangiogram, the injuries can be classified into biliary leakage and stricture group (Table 1).

Biliary leakage group includes 288 (61%).

TABLE 1: Cholangiographic data.

Cholangiogram finding	N	%
Biliary leakage		
Minor leakage	93	19.7%
Major leakage	52	11%
Stricture		
High CBD stricture	26	5.5%
Middle CBD stricture	68	14.4%
Low CBD stricture	24	5%
Complex injuries		
Transection of CBD	17	3.7%
Ligated CBD	31	6.5%
Leakage and stone	69	14.6%
Leakage and stricture	20	4.2%
Stricture and stone	18	3.8%
Postoperative anastomotic stricture (stenosis)	17	3.7%
No abnormalities were detected	37	7.8%
Total	472	100%

CBD: common bile duct.

Cholangiogram demonstrated the following injuries:

minor leakage in 93 patients (19.7%);

major leakage in 52 patients (11%);

possible transaction of CBD in 17 patients (3.6%);

leakage with CBD stone shadow in 69 patients (14.6%);

leakage with CBD stricture in 20 patients (4.2%);

undetected leakage by cholangiography in 37 patients (7.8%) that may be due to minor leakage from bile ductules or gall bladder bed;

biliary stricture group includes 184 patients (39%).

Cholangiogram demonstrated the following injuries:

possible CBD ligation in 31 patients (6.5%);

stricture in CBD

(i) high stricture in 26 patients (5.5%),
(ii) middle stricture in 68 patients (14.4%),
(iii) low stricture in 24 patients (5%),

stricture and stone in 18 cases (3.8%);

postoperative bilioenteric stoma stricture in 17 patients (3.7%).

Treatment was done by either endoscopic approach (ERCP) alone or in conjunction with percutaneous approach or percutaneous approach alone or surgical approach after failing of the endoscopic or percutaneous approach or surgery from the start according to patient condition assessed by multidisciplinary team.

TABLE 2: Endoscopic treatment of biliary injuries.

	N	%
Endoscopic treatment		
Endoscopic sphincterotomy only for minor leakage	31	6.5%
Endoscopic sphincterotomy and stenting for mild leakage	47	10%
Endoscopic sphincterotomy and stenting for marked leakage	22	4.6%
Endoscopic sphincterotomy and stenting for transaction injuries	4	0.8%
Endoscopic sphincterotomy, stone extraction, and stenting for leakage with stones	51	10.8%
Endoscopic sphincterotomy with dilatation and stenting for leakage with stricture	8	1.7%
Endoscopic sphincterotomy and dilatation of ampullary stricture	13	2.8%
Endoscopic repeated dilatation with 8 French stents to 12 French stents		
Single stent (in CBD and CHD)	38	8%
Double stents (right and left hepatic ducts)	11	2.3%
Endoscopic dilatation of CBD stricture, stone extraction, and stenting for CBD stricture with stone	7	1.5%
Total	232	49%

CBD: common bile duct. CHD: common hepatic duct.

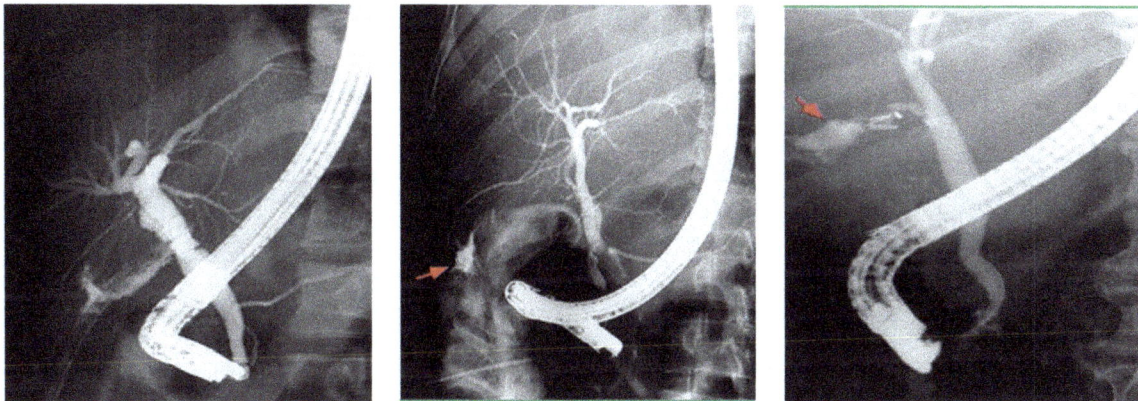

FIGURE 1: Endoscopic retrograde cholangiopancreatography showing minor biliary leakage from cystic duct stump and aberrant RHD radical, treated by sphincterotomy and stenting.

3.1. Endoscopic Treatment of Biliary Injuries (232 Cases (49%)). Endoscopy was attempted in 232 patients (49%) using a side viewing videoscope, with regular instruments that were used in sphincterotomy and balloon dilatation and sphincteroplasty. Endoscopic treatments include sphincterotomy in mild cases and/or stenting in moderate to major biliary leakage, with concomitant stone extraction if present within the CBD (retrieval using basket, balloon extractor, or manual mechanical lithotripsy), and also dilatation and stenting in repeated endoscopic sessions with upgrading of stents until a cure was obtained (after full dilatation of the stricture segment as evident by loss of the waist in the repeated follow-up cholangiogram) (Table 2 and Figures 1, 2, and 3).

3.2. Percutaneous Manipulations Treatment of Biliary Injuries (42 Patients (9%)). This approach was done in 42 patients after endoscopic failure in delineation of the proximal biliary tree as in the major CBD injuries, transection, or ligation through percutaneous transhepatic cholangiogram prior to surgery. Percutaneous manipulations and guide wire deployment through the CBD prior to combined procedures with

conjunction with endoscopy (Rendezvous technique) in 18 patients or with other percutaneous techniques in the rest of the cases were attempted, where therapeutic dilatation and stenting for stricture or injuries were used in 14 cases and diagnostic PTC prior to surgery was used in the other 10 cases (Table 3 and Figures 4, 5, and 6).

3.3. Surgical Treatment of Biliary Injuries (198 Cases (42%)). Surgery was attempted in 198 cases (42%) either as an urgent surgery in 62 patients (including in-table repair in 19 patients in outreach service and 5 patients in our center) or as an elective surgery in 136 patients. In urgent surgery (62 patients) slipped cystic duct was ligated in 12 cases while peritoneal drainage and external biliary stents were inserted in 30 cases prior to further definitive treatment; however, it was a definitive treatment in 20 patients (17 patients in outreach service and 3 patients in our center).

The surgical maneuvers involved the following (Table 4 and Figures 7, 8, 9, and 10):

(i) peritoneal lavage and drainage for biliary peritonitis;

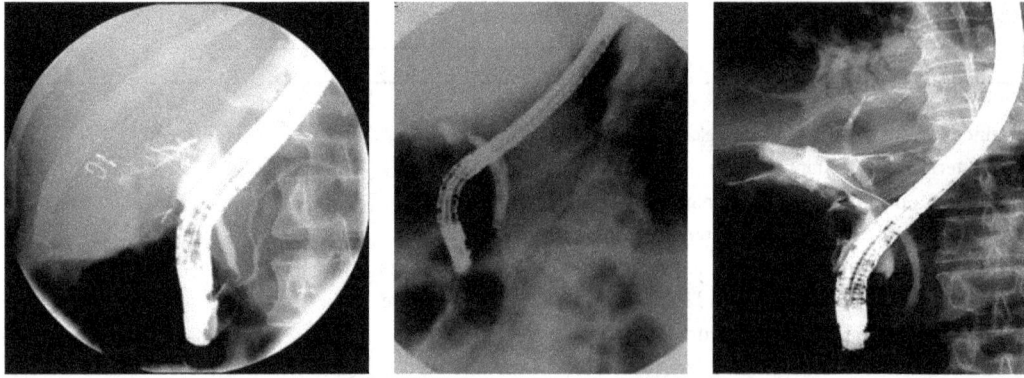

FIGURE 2: Endoscopic retrograde cholangiopancreatography showing a clipped, ligated common bile duct and a transection common bile duct with major biliary leakage.

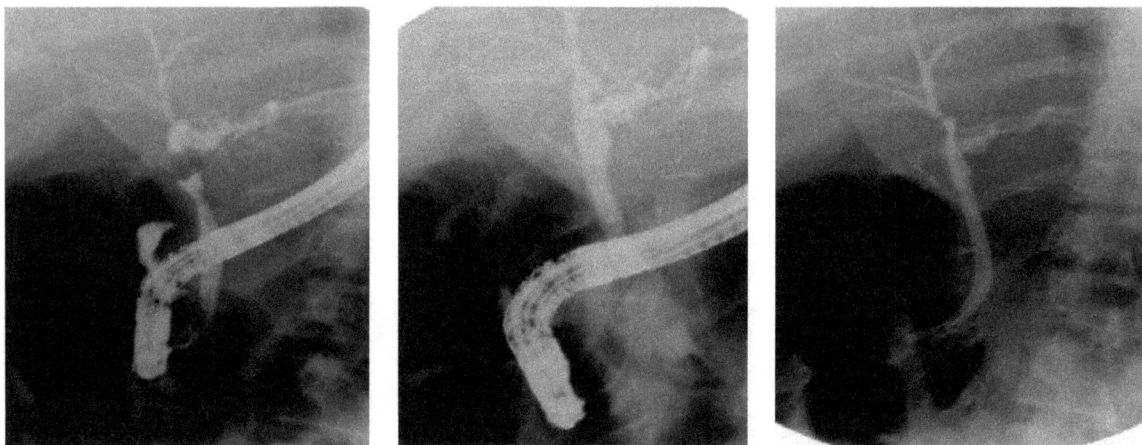

FIGURE 3: Endoscopic retrograde cholangiopancreatography showing common bile duct stricture treated by dilation and stenting.

(ii) drainage and ligation of slipped cystic duct ligature or clip;

(iii) CBD repair on a T-tube splint in a minor lacerations injury in the CBD;

(iv) choledocholithotomy procedure in associated CBD stones;

(v) undoing ligation and strictureplasty with a T-tube splint if CBD ligation is discovered early;

(vi) bilioenteric anastomosis by Roux-en-Y hepaticoje-junostomy.

3.4. Management and Follow-Up after Procedure. Routine postoperative management was carried out as follow. Endoscopically and percutaneously treated cases were regaining oral feeding 6 hours after the procedure and were discharged at the next day after the patient's condition became stable. Surgical cases were followed up in surgical ICU overnight and transferred to the surgical ward for a variable period prior to discharge (7–13 days). All cases were followed up for a period of 1.5–5 years after procedure.

3.5. Morbidity and Mortality. There was one (0.5%) mortality postsurgical maneuver due to biliary sepsis with secondary biliary cirrhosis due to long standing biliary stricture and obstruction. Complications were reported in each group of treatment optionally, postendoscopic maneuver complications were cholangitis, pancreatitis, and stent obstruction, and postpercutaneous manipulation complications were bleeding from PTC/PTD, biliary leakage around PTD, or slipped PTD catheter commonly reported; however, postsurgical complications were mainly wound infection, postoperative bile leakage in early postoperative period and postoperative intrahepatic stones, postoperative biliary stricture, and incisional hernia in the long-term follow-up (Table 5).

4. Discussion

Iatrogenic bile duct injuries pose a complex challenge to the treating physicians [16]. Simon wrote that "too many common bile ducts are still being cut during cholecystectomy" [17]. After decades of advent of laparoscopic cholecystectomy we still have too many common bile ducts injured during this operation. Obviously and luckily, bile duct injuries rate during cholecystectomy has fallen to more encouraging rate of 0.2% [18].

TABLE 3: Percutaneous radiological treatment of biliary injuries.

	N	%
Radiological treatment		
Diagnostic PTC prior to surgery for major CBD injuries	10	2.1%
PTC and stenting for stricture and leakage	3	0.6%
Rendezvous technique plus endoscopy for failed cases or stricture dilation and stenting	18	3.8%
PTD for ligated CBD in bad patient condition prior to surgery	5	1%
PTC and percutaneous dilatation and stenting for postoperative anastomotic stricture or stenosis	6	1.3%
Total	42	9%

PTC: percutaneous transhepatic cholangiogram. CBD: common bile duct. PTD: percutaneous transhepatic drainage.

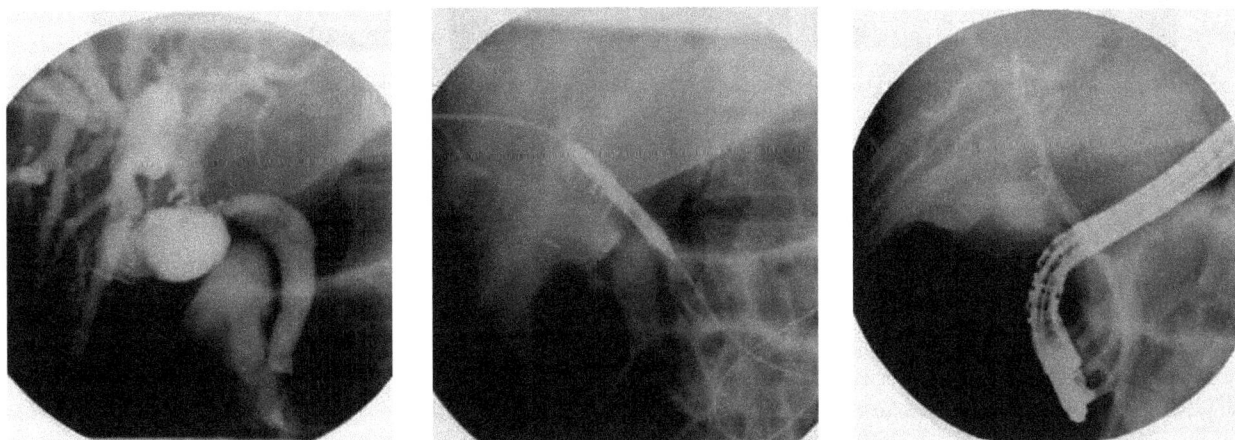

FIGURE 4: Rendezvous technique that followed PTC by dilatation and stenting of the CBD.

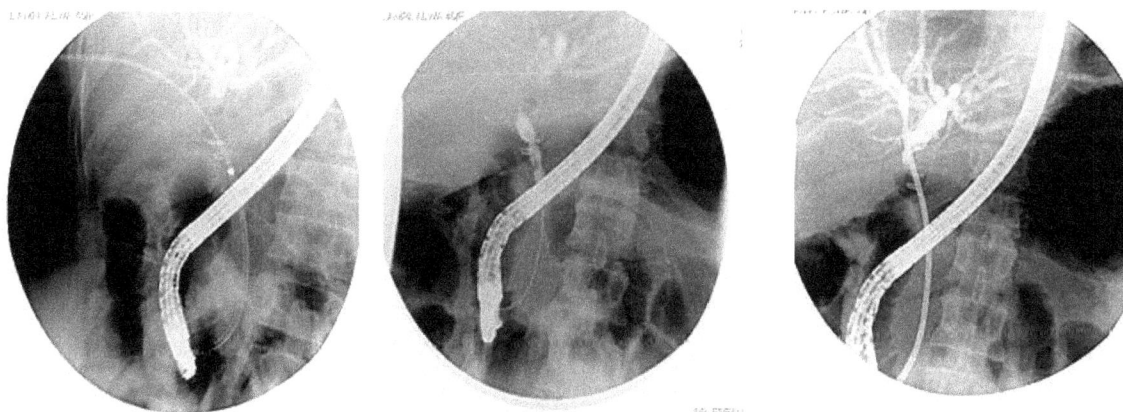

FIGURE 5: Rendezvous techniques with endoscopic stenting for common bile duct stricture.

Inadequate management of bile duct injuries led to severe complications, such as biliary peritonitis leading to sepsis and multiple organ failure in early phase, and biliary cirrhosis during long-term follow-ups, and eventually the need for liver transplantation [19].

Not all forms of diagnostic workup and specialized treatments are available in all hospitals and there should be a low barrier for referral. Unfortunately, lesions will occur, but suboptimal treatment of biliary injuries is not accepted nowadays.

Our institute is a major referral center for hepatobiliary surgery with an increase in the flow of referral cases of postcholecystectomy biliary injuries. We adapted the multidisciplinary management approach program to deal with all cases of postcholecystectomy biliary injuries.

All cases of biliary injuries were reviewed by the multidisciplinary team following the steps of diagnosis and treatment.

In this series, all cases were subjected to a variety of diagnostic workups for diagnosis and delineation of biliary tract before any therapeutic intervention. In 7.8% of the

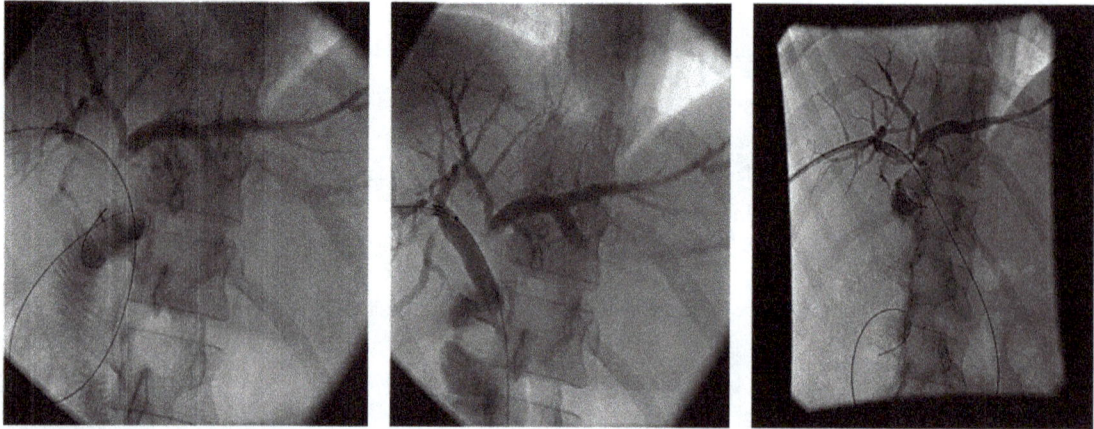

FIGURE 6: Percutaneous transhepatic dilation and stenting of the postoperative anastomotic stricture.

TABLE 4: Surgical management of biliary injuries.

Surgical procedure	N	%
Urgent surgery (62 patients)		
Ligated slipped cystic duct (open or laparoscopic)	12	2.5%
Peritoneal lavage and external biliary stent	30	6.4%
CBD repair over T-tube in cases of injuries detected intraoperatively (on-table repair)	13	2.7%
Bilioenteric anastomosis in cases of injuries detected intraoperatively (on-table repair)	7	1.5%
Elective surgery (136 patients)		
Choledocholithotomy and CBD repair over T-tube splint	8	1.7%
Choledocholithotomy, strictureplasty, and T-tube splint	12	2.5%
CBD strictureplasty and repair over T-tube splint	9	2%
Bilioenteric anastomosis by Roux-en-Y hepaticojejunostomy (96 patients)		
Bismuth I injuries	40	8.5%
Bismuth II injures	31	6.6%
Bismuth III injuries (Hepp-Couinaud hepaticojejunostomy)	18	3.8%
Bismuth IV injuries with		
2-duct anastomosis with transanastomotic stent	4	0.8%
3-duct anastomosis with transanastomotic stent	3	0.6%
Redo surgery		
Repeated bilioenteric anastomosis for postoperative stricture and stenosis	11	2.3%
Total	198	42%

CBD: common bile duct.

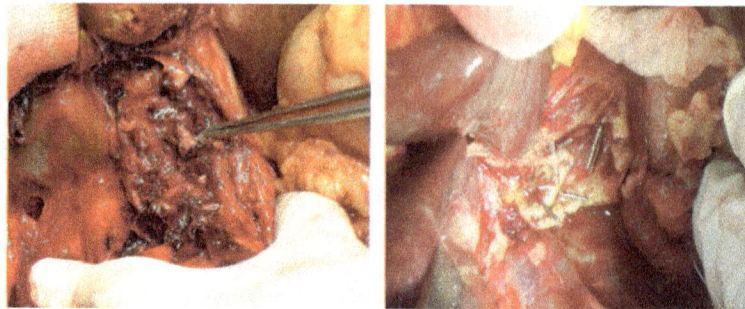

FIGURE 7: Operative photograph of ligated common bile duct with ligature (open) and clip (Laparoscopic).

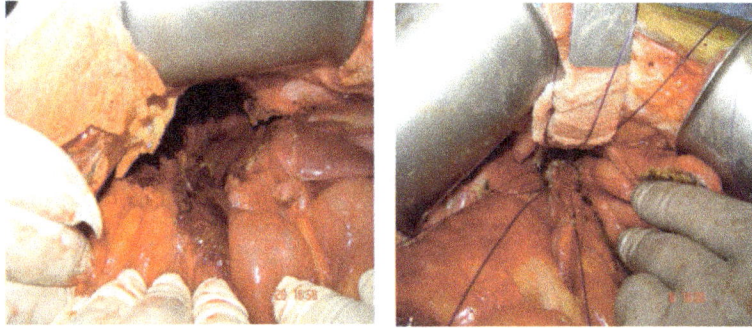

FIGURE 8: Operative photograph of meticulous dissection in porta hepatis to expose biliary injuries.

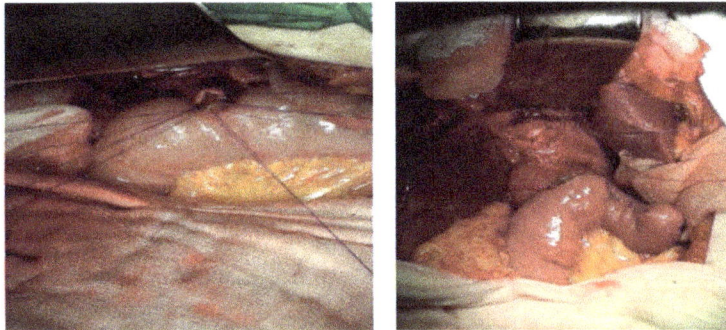

FIGURE 9: Operative dissections of hepatic ducts with Roux-en-Y loop hepaticojejunostomy anastomosis.

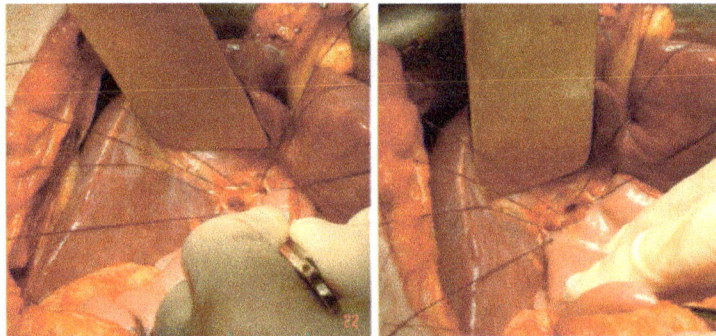

FIGURE 10: Operative hepaticojejunostomy and anastomosis of jejunum with single ostomy of both right and left hepatic ducts after operative stomaplasty.

cases diagnostic workup did not reveal any abnormalities which were considered as minor injuries and were treated conservatively without any intervention.

Management of biliary injuries detected during cholecystectomy is mainly dependent on the local expertise. If a competent hepatobiliary surgeon is not available, biliary drainage should be performed without exploration and patients should be referred to a highly specialized center as further exploration could lead to proximal extension of the lesion, sacrificing the normal healthy duct tissues, with having a negative impact on its reconstruction in the near future.

Multidisciplinary team has outreach service to nearby hospitals around our institute for immediate on-table repair of biliary injuries. In this series, 19 cases (4%) were treated as outreach service. In 17 cases, definitive treatment by repair

of the bile duct over T-tube splint and hepaticojejunostomy anastomosis were performed with good long-term follow-up, while in other 2 cases biliary drainage was done for later further definitive treatment.

The advantages of immediate on-table repair of biliary injuries include single anesthesia, surgical procedure for the patient, and shorter hospital stay. When a hepatobiliary surgeon provides the service of on-table repair as an outreach service, in addition to the added advantage of better surgical outcome, the need to transfer the patient to a tertiary center is also abolished.

As opposed to a delayed repair, an immediate on-table repair nullifies the need for prolonged external biliary drainage and associated increases risk of sepsis. The disadvantages of such an outreach on-table repair of bile duct

TABLE 5: Morbidity and mortality.

Procedure	N	%
Endoscopic maneuvers (232 cases)	29	12.5%
Cholangitis	9	7.7%
Pancreatitis	3	2.6%
Stent occlusion	8	14.6%
Bad patient compliance	9	5.2%
Mortality	0	0
Percutaneous maneuvers (42 cases)	5	12%
Biliary leakage around the PTD	2	4.8%
Bleeding from PTC and PTD	1	2.4%
Slipped PTD catheter	2	4.8%
Mortality	0	0
Surgical procedures (198 cases)	22	11%
Postoperative bile leakage	7	3.5%
Wound infection	8	4.5%
Postoperative intrahepatic stones	2	1.5%
Postoperative biliary stricture and stenosis	3	1.5%
Incisional hernia	2	1%
Mortality	1	0.5%

PTD: percutaneous transhepatic drainage.

injures are that these injuries are often complex, requiring high hepaticojejunostomy reconstruction for nondilated, normal diameter (usually 3–8 mm) ducts with thin wall.

With our experience in living liver transplant at our center since 2003, our surgical team used to operate on normal bile ducts and becoming familiar with access to the site of injury was achieved satisfactorily since our outreach team brought a long suitable abdominal wall retractor and other instruments that are used for hepatobiliary surgery.

The extent of the ischaemic injury suffered by the bile duct is less apparent in the immediate repair setting [20, 21]. To reduce this, the proximal bile duct was divided up into a level where good blood from the cut surface of the duct occurred. This may explain why out of 17 cases of outreach service repair 2 cases developed late stricture of the hepaticojejunostomy requiring radiological dilatation.

The higher rate of injuries with laparoscopic method was initially attributed to the learning curve. This has, however, remained the same, a decade after the wide spread acceptance of the procedure [22, 23].

In this series, biliary injuries after laparoscopic approach were 56% of the total cases and 44% for open approach, with most of the cases of open approach occurring at the late 5 years of study as the learning curve for laparoscopic approach reaches its saturation state and many surgeons, especially the young ones, become masters of the laparoscopic technique without gaining good training in the open approach.

Bile leakage was a common presentation among our patients (61%), usually the leakage that originated from the liver bed or biliary injuries as documented by various studies [24], and can be explained also as the sphincter of Oddi creates a pressure gradient that results in bile spillage to outside rather than in the duodenum [25].

Bile leakage was demonstrated by cholangiogram in most of the cases (251 of 288 patients); however, the spillage was very mild and not evident by contrast injection in 37 cases (12.8%), such minimal bile leakage was resolved spontaneously which is concomitant to the stated facts in other literatures [26].

Endoscopic treatment in this series was applied in 232 (49%) cases of biliary leakage and stricture.

In this series, endoscopic treatment was achieved in mild and moderate cases up to 96–100%, as explained in the literatures that endoscopic treatment accelerates the healing period by decompressing the biliary system; in addition, it closes the defect physically and acts as a bridge at the site of extravasation. Stenting also acts as a mold and prevents stricture formations during recovery period and should be the preferred treatment [27].

In major leakage (type D&E) Strasberg classification endoscopic treatment with sphincterotomy and stenting was successful in 65% (34 out 52 cases) only. This result was compatible with other reports in [28–30].

Out of 34 cases 10 cases developed later stricture which was treated with upgrading the size of the stent; our results are also comparable with other literature reports [27].

Common bile duct stones were found to be exacerbating the bile leakage in 69 cases and were successfully treated by sphincterotomy and stone extraction in conjunction with stenting in 61 cases (88%) out of 69 cases. This result was in agreement with other reports [31, 32]. Also, common bile duct stricture found with leakage was treated by appropriate boogies or balloon dilatation and stenting in 8 cases out of 20 cases, in agreement with findings by other authors [33, 34].

In biliary strictures after biliary injuries the endoscopic treatment was successful in 67 patients with sphincterotomy, boogies or balloon dilatation, and convenient stenting. It was performed in conjunction with common bile duct stone extraction in 7 cases out of 18 cases and in repeated ERCP sessions to replace or subsequently upgrade the stent in 49 cases, in agreement with other previous reports stating that ERCP and stenting have good results with lower rates of morbidity and mortality [30, 33, 34].

Endoscopy is the preferable initial therapy in biliary leakage and stricture [35, 36], but it needs a long period (about 24 months) and repeated endoscopic sessions with progressive increase in the number of the stents to better calibrate the stricture [37].

Stents should be replaced every 3 months before possible clogging could cause cholangitis, and the patient should be informed about the risk of stenting and duration of the treatment [38–40].

Otherwise, surgery is indicated as the treatment of choice, especially in surgically suitable patient [37]. However, Davids and colleagues [35] reported equal relapse of 17% of both treatments.

Unfortunately, the role of endoscopy is weak in common bile duct transection injuries with leakage as only 4 cases out of 17 patients were endoscopically treated, in agreement with other studies demonstrating this low incidence of endoscopic treatment of such problems [30, 37].

Diagnostic percutaneous transhepatic cholangiography (PTC) was done in 10 cases prior to surgery in high proximal injuries not delineated by endoscopy and percutaneous transhepatic drainage (PTD) was inserted for 5 patients in bad condition for preoperative preparation for surgery in high ligation of common bile duct.

Stenting of stricture with leakage in high proximal injuries was done in 3 patients out of 20 patients. However, Rendezvous techniques plus endoscopy were performed in cases which failed endoscopy in 18 cases, in agreement with other reports in [41, 42].

Percutaneous dilatation and stenting for stenosis and stricture in post-bilioenteric repair was successfully performed in 6 cases out 17 cases with good long-term results, in agreement with several reports of the treatment of such postoperative biliary stricture at stoma side in bilioenteric anastomosis [41, 42].

Surgery was done in 198 cases (42%) of this series as an urgent surgery for the 62 cases, ligated slipped cystic duct (open or laparoscopic)was done in 12 cases, and peritoneal lavage with external biliary drainage was carried out in 30 cases; however, the surgery was definitive (on table-repair) in 20 cases and 13 cases were common bile duct repair over T-tube and in 7 cases bilioenteric anastomosis was done on-table repair as practiced by other authors [43, 44].

On other hand, surgery was needed as elective in 136 patients, especially after failure of other minimal invasive techniques (endoscopy and interventional radiology), and surgery was effective in common bile duct repair over a T-tube splint, choledocholithotomy, and common bile duct repair over T-tube splint, choledocholithotomy, stricture-plasty and T-tube splint, and bilioenteric anastomosis, which was done in 96 cases as the operation of choice in most documented studies [45–47].

In this series, we used transanastomotic stents, the rationale that leaks of small bilioenteric anastomosis promote stricture and the rationale that both lowering of the intraductal pressure and adequate flow through the anastomosis were warranted by stents, as practiced by other authors [45, 48, 49].

Redo surgery in the post-bilioenteric anastomotic stricture or stenosis was done in 11 cases out of 17 cases with good long-term outcome.

The operation of choice in this series is Roux-en-Y hepaticojejunostomy as good long-term surgical results are obtained in this type of technique as documented in most literatures [45–47].

No mortality occurred in this series after endoscopic treatment, which is consistent with most reports in the literature [50]. But some minor complications were seen as cholangitis, pancreatitis, stent clogging, and bad patient compliance. Unfortunately, one death occurred following surgery (due to biliary sepsis leading to multiorgans failure) as well as some complications such as wound infection, bile leakage, incisional hernia and postanastomotic stenosis and strictures which were encountered in 3 cases only as our results are less than those of the reported in the literatures which state that stenosis occurs in about 10% of the cases after bilioenteric anastomosis [38, 45, 46, 48, 49].

All complication were treated conservatively except incisional hernia which was treated with hernia repair with mesh and postoperative anastomotic stricture, managed by percutaneous dilatation and stenting as it is very beneficial in such cases documented by other authors [41, 42].

5. Conclusion

The management of patients with biliary injuries should be ideally performed/discussed in a multidisciplinary team approach that consists of a gastroenterologist, radiologist, and surgeon. Better outcomes of such cases are mainly the result of multidisciplinary care and changes in technical aspects which have changed considerably through the time of learning curve with growing experience of the team. Early referral to high volume tertiary care center with experienced hepatobiliary surgeon, skilled gastroenterologist, and interventional radiologist would appear to be necessary to assure optimal results and should be encouraged.

References

[1] D. R. Flum, A. Cheadle, C. Prela, E. P. Dellinger, and L. Chan, "Bile duct injuries during cholecystectomy and survival in medicare beneficiaries," *Journal of the American Medical Association*, vol. 290, no. 16, pp. 2168–2173, 2003.

[2] B. Törnqvist, Z. Zheng, W. Ye, A. Waage, and M. Nilsson, "Long-term effects of iatrogenic bile duct injury during cholecystectomy," *Clinical Gastroenterology and Hepatology*, vol. 7, no. 9, pp. 1013–1018, 2009.

[3] J. K. Sicklick, M. S. Camp, K. D. Lillemoe et al., "Surgical management of bile duct injuries sustained during laparoscopic cholecystectomy: perioperative results in 200 patients," *Annals of Surgery*, vol. 241, no. 5, pp. 786–795, 2005.

[4] A. Waage and M. Nilsson, "Iatrogenic bile duct injury: a population-based study of 152 776 cholecystectomies in the Swedish inpatient registry," *Archives of Surgery*, vol. 141, no. 12, pp. 1207–1213, 2006.

[5] M. H. Khan, T. J. Howard, E. L. Fogel et al., "Frequency of biliary complications after laparoscopic cholecystectomy detected by ERCP: experience at a large tertiary referral center," *Gastrointestinal Endoscopy*, vol. 65, no. 2, pp. 247–252, 2007.

[6] K. Ludwig, J. Bernhardt, H. Steffen, and D. Lorenz, "Contribution of intraoperative cholangiography to incidence and outcome of common bile duct injuries during laparoscopic cholecystectomy," *Surgical Endoscopy and Other Interventional Techniques*, vol. 16, no. 7, pp. 1098–1104, 2002.

[7] B. J. Carroll, M. Birth, and E. H. Phillips, "Common bile duct injuries during laparoscopic cholecystectomy that result in litigation," *Surgical Endoscopy*, vol. 12, no. 4, pp. 310–314, 1998.

[8] V. Singh, K. L. Narasimhan, G. R. Verma, and G. Singh, "Endoscopic management of traumatic hepatobiliary injuries," *Journal of Gastroenterology and Hepatology (Australia)*, vol. 22, no. 8, pp. 1205–1209, 2007.

[9] Z. Volgyi, T. Fischer, M. Szenes, and B. Gasztony, "Endoscopic management of post-operative biliary tract injuries," *Clinical and Experimental Medical Journal (CEMED)*, vol. 4, no. 1, pp. 153–162, 2010.

[10] A. Frilling, J. Li, F. Weber et al., "Major bile duct injuries after laparoscopic cholecystectomy: a tertiary center experience," *Journal of Gastrointestinal Surgery*, vol. 8, no. 6, pp. 679–685, 2004.

[11] A. Savar, I. Carmody, J. R. Hiatt, and R. W. Busuttil, "Laparoscopic bile duct injuries: management at a tertiary liver center," *The American Surgeon*, vol. 70, no. 10, pp. 906–909, 2004.

[12] M. A. Silva, C. Coldham, A. D. Mayer, S. R. Bramhall, J. A. C. Buckels, and D. F. Mirza, "Specialist outreach service for on-table repair of iatrogenic bile duct injuries—a new kind of "travelling surgeon"," *Annals of the Royal College of Surgeons of England*, vol. 90, no. 3, pp. 243–246, 2008.

[13] H. Bismuth and P. E. Majno, "Biliary strictures: classification based on the principles of surgical treatment," *World Journal of Surgery*, vol. 25, no. 10, pp. 1241–1244, 2001.

[14] D. O. Olsen, "Bile duct injuries during laparoscopic cholecystectomy: a decade of experience," *Journal of Hepato-Biliary-Pancreatic Surgery*, vol. 7, no. 1, pp. 35–39, 2000.

[15] S. M. Strasberg, M. Hertl, and N. J. Soper, "An analysis of the problem of biliary injury during laparoscopic cholecystectomy," *Journal of the American College of Surgeons*, vol. 180, no. 1, pp. 101–125, 1995.

[16] C. A. Langenbuch, "Ein fall von exstirpation der gallenblase wegen chronischer cholelithiasis," *Heilung, Berliner Klinische Wohenschrift*, vol. 19, pp. 725–727, 1882.

[17] M. M. Simon, "Pitfalls to be avoided in cholecystectomy," *The American Journal of Surgery*, vol. 66, no. 3, pp. 367–381, 1944.

[18] J. J. Roslyn, G. S. Binns, E. F. X. Hughes, K. Saunders-Kirkwood, M. J. Zinner, and J. A. Cates, "Open cholecystectomy: a contemporary analysis of 42,474 patients," *Annals of Surgery*, vol. 218, no. 2, pp. 129–137, 1993.

[19] C. Loinaz, E. M. González, C. Jiménez et al., "Long-term biliary complications after liver surgery leading to liver transplantation," *World Journal of Surgery*, vol. 25, no. 10, pp. 1260–1263, 2001.

[20] S. B. Archer, D. W. Brown, C. D. Smith, G. D. Branum, and J. G. Hunter, "Bile duct injury during laparoscopic cholecystectomy: results of a national survey," *Annals of Surgery*, vol. 234, no. 4, pp. 549–559, 2001.

[21] M. A. Mercado, C. Chan, H. Orozco, M. Tielve, and C. A. Hinojosa, "Acute bile duct injury: the need for a high repair," *Surgical Endoscopy and Other Interventional Techniques*, vol. 17, no. 9, pp. 1351–1355, 2003.

[22] S. J. Savader, K. D. Lillemoe, C. A. Prescott et al., "Laparoscopic cholecystectomy-related bile duct injuries: a health and financial disaster," *Annals of Surgery*, vol. 225, no. 3, pp. 268–273, 1997.

[23] R. M. Walsh, J. M. Henderson, D. P. Vogt et al., "Trends in bile duct injuries from laparoscopic cholecystectomy," *Journal of Gastrointestinal Surgery*, vol. 2, no. 5, pp. 458–462, 1998.

[24] A. J. McMahon, G. Fullarton, J. N. Baxter, and P. J. O'Dwyer, "Bile duct injury and bile leakage in laparoscopic cholecystectomy," *British Journal of Surgery*, vol. 82, no. 3, pp. 307–313, 1995.

[25] A. N. Barkun, M. Rezieg, S. N. Mehta et al., "Postcholecystectomy biliary leaks in the laparoscopic era: risk factors, presentation, and management," *Gastrointestinal Endoscopy*, vol. 45, no. 3, pp. 277–282, 1997.

[26] S. N. Mehta, E. Pavone, J. S. Barkun, G. A. Cortas, and A. N. Barkun, "A review of the management of post-cholecystectomy biliary leaks during the laparoscopic era," *The American Journal of Gastroenterology*, vol. 92, no. 8, pp. 1262–1267, 1997.

[27] E. Parlak, B. Çiçek, S. Dişibeyaz, S. Ö. Kuran, D. Oğuz, and B. Şahin, "Treatment of biliary leakages after cholecystectomy and importance of stricture development in the main bile duct injury," *Turkish Journal of Gastroenterology*, vol. 16, no. 1, pp. 21–28, 2005.

[28] A. Abdel-Raouf, E. Hamdy, E. El-Hanafy, and G. El-Ebidy, "Endoscopic management of postoperative bile duct injuries: a single center experience," *Saudi Journal of Gastroenterology*, vol. 16, no. 1, pp. 19–24, 2010.

[29] J. M. Sarmiento, M. B. Farnell, D. M. Nagorney et al., "Quality of life assessment of surgical reconstruction after laparoscopic cholecyctectomy-induced bile duct injuries: what happens at 5 years and beyond?" *Archives of Surgery*, vol. 139, no. 5, pp. 483–489, 2004.

[30] A. Csendes, C. Navarrete, P. Burdiles, and J. Yarmuch, "Treatment of common bile duct injuries during laparoscopic cholecystectomy: endoscopic and surgical management," *World Journal of Surgery*, vol. 25, no. 10, pp. 1346–1351, 2001.

[31] A. Cuschieri, E. Croce, A. Faggioni et al., "EAES ductal stone study. Preliminary findings of multi-center prospective randomized trial comparing two-stage vs single-stage management," *Surgical Endoscopy*, vol. 10, no. 12, pp. 1130–1135, 1996.

[32] D. G. Maxton, D. E. F. Tweedle, and D. F. Martin, "Retained common bile duct stones after endoscopic sphinctertomy; temporary and long-term treatment with biliary stenting," *Gastrointestinal Endoscopy*, vol. 44, pp. 105–106, 1996.

[33] M. A. Al-Karawi and F. M. Sanai, "Endoscopic management of bile duct injuries in 107 patients: experience of a Saudi referral center," *Hepato-Gastroenterology*, vol. 49, no. 47, pp. 1201–1207, 2002.

[34] P. Draganov, B. Hoffman, W. Marsh, P. Cotton, and J. Cunningham, "Long-term outcome in patients with benign biliary strictures treated endoscopically with multiple stents," *Gastrointestinal Endoscopy*, vol. 55, no. 6, pp. 680–686, 2002.

[35] P. H. P. Davids, A. K. F. Tanka, E. A. J. Rauws et al., "Benign biliary strictures: surgery or endoscopy?" *Annals of Surgery*, vol. 217, no. 3, pp. 237–243, 1993.

[36] G. Costamagna, M. Pandolfi, M. Mutignani, C. Spada, and V. Perri, "Long-term results of endoscopic management of postoperative bile duct strictures with increasing numbers of stents," *Gastrointestinal Endoscopy*, vol. 54, no. 2, pp. 162–168, 2001.

[37] I. N. Do, J. C. Kim, S. H. Park et al., "The outcome of endoscopic treatment in bile duct injury after cholecystectomy," *The Korean Journal of Gastroenterology*, vol. 46, no. 6, pp. 463–470, 2005 (Korean).

[38] J. J. G. H. M. Bergman, L. Burgemeister, M. J. Bruno et al., "Long-term follow-up after biliary stent placement for postoperative bile duct stenosis," *Gastrointestinal Endoscopy*, vol. 54, no. 2, pp. 154–161, 2001.

[39] G. C. Vitale, T. C. Tran, B. R. Davis, M. Vitale, D. Vitale, and G. Larson, "Endoscopic management of postcholecystectomy bile duct strictures," *Journal of the American College of Surgeons*, vol. 206, no. 5, pp. 918–923, 2008.

[40] F. Palacio-Velez, A. Gastro-Mendoza, and A. R. Oliver-Guerra, "Results of 21 years of surgery for related iatrogenic bile duct injuries," *Revista de Gastroenterología de México*, vol. 67, pp. 76–81, 2002 (Spanish).

[41] A. R.-D. la Medina, S. Misra, A. J. Leroy, and M. G. Sarr, "Management of benign biliary strictures by percutaneous interventional radiologic techniques (PIRT)," *HPB*, vol. 10, no. 6, pp. 428–432, 2008.

[42] H.-U. Laasch, "Obstructive jaundice after bilioenteric anastomosis: transhepatic and direct percutaneous enetral stent insertion for afferent loop occlusion," *Gut and Liver*, vol. 4, supplement 1, pp. S89–S95, 2010.

[43] V. Singh, G. Singh, G. R. Verma, and R. Gupta, "Endoscopic management of postcholecystectomy biliary leakage," *Hepatobiliary and Pancreatic Diseases International*, vol. 9, no. 4, pp. 409–413, 2010.

[44] J. K. Sicklick, M. S. Camp, K. D. Lillemoe et al., "Surgical management of bile duct injuries sustained during laparoscopic cholecystectomy: perioperotive results in 200 patients," *Annals of Surgery*, vol. 241, no. 5, pp. 786–795, 2005.

[45] M. A. Mercado, C. Chan, H. Orozco et al., "To stent or not to stent bilioenteric anastomosis after iatrogenic injury: a dilemma not answered?" *Archives of Surgery*, vol. 137, no. 1, pp. 60–63, 2002.

[46] R. M. Walsh, J. M. Henderson, D. P. Vogt, and N. Brown, "Long-term outcome of biliary reconstruction for bile duct injuries from laparoscopic cholecystectomies," *Surgery*, vol. 142, no. 4, pp. 450–457, 2007.

[47] J. Li, K. Zhou, and D. Wu, "Mucosa improved biliary-enteric anastomosis end to side in a small-caliber choledochojejunostomy application," *Journal of Jiangsu University*, vol. 15, article 4124, 2005.

[48] M. G. House, J. L. Cameron, R. D. Schulick et al., "Incidence and outcome of biliary strictures after pancreaticoduodenectomy," *Annals of Surgery*, vol. 243, no. 5, pp. 571–576, 2006.

[49] M. Abdel Wahab, G. El-Ebiedy, A. Sultan et al., "Postcholecystectomy bile duct injuries: experience with 49 cases managed by different therapeutic modalities," *Hepato-Gastroenterology*, vol. 43, no. 11, pp. 1141–1147, 1996.

[50] G. D. de Palma, G. Persico, R. Sottile et al., "Surgery or endoscopy for treatment of postcholecystectomy bile duct strictures?" *The American Journal of Surgery*, vol. 185, no. 6, pp. 532–535, 2003.

4

Aggressive Treatment of Patients with Metastatic Colorectal Cancer Increases Survival: A Scandinavian Single-Center Experience

Kristoffer Watten Brudvik,[1,2,3] Simer Jit Bains,[1,2]
Lars Thomas Seeberg,[3] Knut Jørgen Labori,[3] Anne Waage,[3] Kjetil Taskén,[1,2,4]
Einar Martin Aandahl,[1,2,5] and Bjørn Atle Bjørnbeth[3]

[1] Centre for Molecular Medicine Norway, University of Oslo, 0318 Oslo, Norway
[2] Biotechnology Centre, University of Oslo, 0317 Oslo, Norway
[3] Department of Hepato-Pancreato-Biliary Surgery, Oslo University Hospital, 0424 Oslo, Norway
[4] Department of Infectious Diseases, Oslo University Hospital, 0424 Oslo, Norway
[5] Department of Transplantation Surgery, Oslo University Hospital, 0424 Oslo, Norway

Correspondence should be addressed to Bjørn Atle Bjørnbeth; bbjoer@ous-hf.no

Academic Editor: Olivier Farges

Background. We examined overall and disease-free survivals in a cohort of patients subjected to resection of liver metastasis from colorectal cancer (CRLM) in a 10-year period when new treatment strategies were implemented. *Methods.* Data from 239 consecutive patients selected for liver resection of CRLM during the period from 2002 to 2011 at a single center were used to estimate overall and disease-free survival. The results were assessed against new treatment strategies and established risk factors. *Results.* The 5-year cumulative overall and disease-free survivals were 46 and 24%. The overall survival was the same after reresection, independently of the number of prior resections and irrespectively of the location of the recurrent disease. The time intervals between each recurrence were similar (11 ± 1 months). Patients with high tumor load given neoadjuvant chemotherapy had comparable survival to those with less extensive disease without neoadjuvant chemotherapy. Positive resection margin or resectable extrahepatic disease did not affect overall survival. *Conclusion.* Our data support that one still, and perhaps to an even greater extent, should seek an aggressive therapeutic strategy to achieve resectable status for recurrent hepatic and extrahepatic metastases. The data should be viewed in the context of recent advances in the understanding of cancer biology and the metastatic process.

1. Introduction

The incidence of colorectal cancer (CRC) is increasing and is now the fourth leading cause of cancer deaths worldwide [1]. Twenty percent of the patients present with synchronous liver metastases and another 30–40% develop liver metastases during followup [2]. Hepatic resection remains the only potentially curable treatment and is now offered to 20–25% of the patients whereas only 10% were selected for this treatment ten years ago [3]. The main exclusion criteria for liver resection of colorectal liver metastases (CRLMs)

are nonresectable liver metastasis (tumor growth into both portal branches and/or into both left and right liver vein), inadequately functioning residual liver parenchyma, or nonresectable extrahepatic disease. These exclusion criteria have all been challenged in recent years. Close followup after primary CRC (early detection of metastasis), implementation of new surgical techniques including two-stage hepatectomy with portal vein embolization [4, 5] and transplantation methods, and the introduction of new chemotherapy and biological agents capable of converting inoperable cases to a resectable status by tumor downsizing have increased the number of patients eligible for resection of liver metastases [6, 7]. As a consequence, reresection of patients with recurrent disease is now offered to an increasing number of selected patients [8, 9].

A cohort of 239 patients with CRC and synchronous or metachronous CRLMs eligible for liver resection with curative intent was followed from 2002 to 2011. The aim of the study was to examine overall and disease-free survivals related to number of resections, therapeutic downsizing, surgical technique, and other factors considered to have prognostic value.

2. Patients and Methods

2.1. Patients Selection and Management. All patients were considered preoperatively by a multidisciplinary team. The assessment included computed tomography (CT) of the abdomen and chest with the addition of magnetic resonance (MR) or ultrasonography with contrast when resectability could not be determined after CT. Positron emission tomography (PET) became available in 2009 and was used to assess extrahepatic disease in selected cases. Intraoperative contrast-enhanced ultrasonography (CEU) was used in every procedure after 2007 to assess resectability and tumor expansion as previously described [10]. Preoperative carcinoembryonic antigen (CEA) levels were determined in all patients in the most recent 5-year period.

The Brisbane terminology was applied to classify the liver resections [11]. Laparoscopic resection was introduced during the last 4-year period for selected patients with small, subcapsular lesions or lesions in the lateral or lower segments (segments II, III, IVb, V, and VI). The term two-stage hepatectomy was used where the first surgical step included nonanatomical resection on one side combined with postoperative portal vein embolization of the most affected side, followed by a second step with formal resection of the side with remaining disease.

2.2. Data Collection and Statistics. Information was retrieved from medical records, including operation, radiology, and pathology reports. Followup was performed in our outpatient clinic at 4, 8, and 12 months and from the second postoperative year at 6-month intervals for a total of 5 years. Size of the largest tumor and number of metastases were used to compare tumor load between subgroups and the tumor load was calculated by points based on the worst score for each parameter in the Basingstoke Predictive Index (8 points if diameter of the largest tumor >10 cm; adapted to 8 points/cm and 4 points if >3 metastases; adapted to 1 point/number of metastases and multiplied by 10 to produce a score where size and load are equally representative). We assessed our results against established risk factors reported by others [12–14] (see supplemental Figure S1 in Supplementary Material available online at http://dx.doi.org/10.1155/2013/727095).

Filemaker Pro 9.0 (Santa Clara, CA, USA) was used to register data that were analyzed in SPPS 16.0 (Chicago, IL, USA). Graphs were made in SigmaPlot 11.0 (San Jose, CA, USA). Kaplan-Meier plots and log-rank (Mantel-Cox) comparisons were used to compute cumulative survival data. Pearson's chi-square test was used to compare ratios. Group means were compared using Student's *t*-test if the variables passed a normality test; otherwise medians where compared with rank-sum test. The study and database were approved by the Oslo University Hospital Data Protection Officer for Research.

3. Results

Patients undergoing surgery for CRLMs (adenocarcinoma) were registered partly prospectively and partly retrospectively in a database from October 2002 to August 2011. In the study period, a total of 268 patients were initially included. Of these, 27 patients were deemed inoperable intraoperatively due to extensive hepatic or extrahepatic metastatic disease and excluded from the study. Five of these patients were scheduled for two-stage hepatectomy [15] but were inoperable at the 2nd surgical step. In addition, two patients in the original database received liver transplants [16] and were excluded resulting in a total of 239 patients analyzed in the present study.

The cohort of 239 patients with metastatic colorectal cancer patients resected for liver metastasis was examined for overall and disease-free survivals. Characteristics of the patient cohort and primary tumor are presented in supplemental Table S1.

3.1. Liver Resection. Liver resection of the CRLMs was successfully accomplished in 90.7% ($n = 214$) of the planned single-stage procedures and in 83.3% ($n = 25$) of the planned two-stage procedures (mean age 64.3 years, range 26–89 years; 118 females; Table 1). A total of 353 surgical procedures were registered in the cohort, representing primary resections ($n = 239$), secondary resections ($n = 65$), and tertiary resections ($n = 21$); 2nd step of two-stage hepatectomy ($n = 25$) and 2nd step of single-stage surgery converted to two-stage without embolization ($n = 3$; see supplemental Table S2 for details of the surgical procedures). In 16 patients with rectum cancer (after 2008), a liver-first approach was chosen [17]. The type of resection and details are presented in supplemental Table S2.

3.2. Overall and Oncologic Outcome. Intraoperative mortality was zero; however three (1.3%) died within 30 days after the surgical procedure (day 17, 29, and 29, resp.). At a median observation time of 24 months (range 1–108 months by October 2011) 99 of the 239 patients (41.1%) were alive and disease-free, and 64 (26.8%) of the patients were alive with recurrent disease and were currently receiving palliative treatment or were undergoing evaluation for re-resection. Furthermore, 66 of the patients (27.6%) had died of the disease and 10 (4.2%) had died of unrelated reasons or of unknown cause. The cumulative overall 5- and 9-year survivals were 46.0 and 34.9%, respectively, and comparable to that of other centers (36 to 58% and 23 to 36% for 5- and 10-year survivals, respectively [12, 13, 18–23]). The disease-free survivals were 24.0 and 20.0% for 5- and 7-year follow-up periods, respectively (Figure 1(a)). The locations of recurrent

TABLE 1: Characteristics of liver metastases.

	Value
Age (range)	64.3 (26–89)
Female/male	118/121
BPI score (range) ($n = 94$)	5.98 (0–27)
Metachronous/synchronous metastases	133/106
Number of tumors in the liver	
1/2/3/4/5/6 or more	87/52/31/14/12/18
Missing	25
Size diameter mm (mean/median/min/max)	29/22/2/155
Missing	15
Number of segments involved	
1/2/3/4/5/6 or more	63/70/40/29/13/6
Missing	18
CEA ($n = 140$)	55.5 (0.7–1400.0)
Extra hepatic disease	19
Neoadjuvant chemotherapy	
Yes/no/na	112/127/0
Adjuvant chemotherapy	
Yes/no/na	128/89/22

disease are presented in supplemental Table S3 and show a shift in target organ as the disease continues to recur.

3.3. Resection of Recurring Metastases. In the observation period 146 patients presented with a second recurrent disease and surgery with curative intent was performed in 65 (44.8%) of them. A third recurrent disease presented in 69 patients and surgery with curative intent was performed in 21 (30.4%). Overall survival appeared to be the same after the first, second, and third resections and the disease-free survival was similar in the groups resected once and twice (Figure 1(a)). Furthermore, survival after the second resection was comparable independently of whether the location of the recurrent disease was to the liver, lung, or elsewhere (Figure 1(b) and supplement Table S3). The average time from surgery of the primary tumor to resection of the first CRLM was 11.7 months; the average time from surgery for the CRLM to the presentation of a second recurrent disease (irrespective of localization) was 10.1 whereas the mean time from the second to the third recurrence was 11.0 months.

3.4. Downsizing and Neoadjuvant Chemotherapy. Preoperative (neoadjuvant) chemotherapy was given to 46.9% of the patients ($n = 112$, Table 1). The indications for neoadjuvant chemotherapy changed during the study period. In the first 5-year period (2002–2006, $n = 24$; 32.9%), neoadjuvant therapy was primarily given to nonresectable patients. In the last 5-year period (2007–2011, $n = 88$; 53.0%), the indications were broader and included patients with high tumor load (3 or more metastases *or* large metastasis above 30 mm (diameter) *or* synchronous metastases) and from January 2010 young patients *with* elevated CEA *and* ECOG performance status 0-1 [24]. The cumulative overall 5-year survival of patients receiving neoadjuvant chemotherapy was 36.1% versus 52.6%

in the nonneoadjuvant group ($P = 0.008$) whereas survival between the two groups appeared similar during past 80 months (Figure 2(a)). The 5-year disease-free survival was 21.0% in the neoadjuvant group versus 26.5% in the non-neoadjuvant group ($P = 0.025$). Tumor load was significantly higher in the neoadjuvant group (Figure 2(a), insert).

Stratification of neoadjuvant chemotherapy combined with tumor load revealed that the survival in patients with high tumor load receiving preoperative chemotherapy was increased compared to that of patients not receiving chemotherapy. In contrast, patients with low tumor load who did not receive neoadjuvant chemotherapy had increased survival compared to the survival of those who received chemotherapy.

3.5. Two-Stage Hepatectomy. Thirty patients received two-stage hepatectomy from 2008 due to bilateral disease. Five of them (16.7%) were inoperable at the second surgical step and excluded from the study and results. Patients selected for two-stage hepatectomy had a higher risk of developing recurrence as all patients in this group presented with recurrent disease within 2 years compared to a 60.7% recurrence in patients subject to a single-stage procedure in the same time interval (Figure 2(b)). Nonetheless, the overall survival in the group that received two-stage hepatectomy appeared comparable to that of the single-stage procedure group with the limited data available. Of the 25 patients who underwent the two-stage procedure, six (24.0%) were alive with a mean observation time of 17 months (range 6–45) and were reported to be disease-free at the time of examination of the cohort.

3.6. Laparoscopic Surgery. Since the introduction of laparoscopic resection in 2008, 60 patients have been selected for this procedure of which 48 were successfully completed (20.0% conversion rate). In addition, the first step of planned two-stage surgery was performed laparoscopically in two patients. Patients selected for a laparoscopic approach had a better outcome than patients selected for open surgery (Figure 2(c)) and lower tumor load (insert).

3.7. Prognostication of Colorectal Liver Metastasis. Primary tumor lymph node status, histological differentiation grade, synchronous or metachronous disease, tumor size (metastasis), numbers of metastases, affected liver segments, and CEA levels turned out to be prognostic markers affecting survival (supplemental Figure S1). Furthermore, we found ascending age to be a positive prognostic marker for disease-free survival (Figure 3(a)). In contrast, examining the overall survival, we observed an apparent higher mortality in the older patient group. Extrahepatic disease ($n = 19$, Figure 3(c)) and positive hepatic resection margin (R1/R2, $n = 31$, Figure 3(b)) impaired disease-free survival. However, overall survival was not affected by resectable extrahepatic disease or positive resection margins.

In the present material, men had better overall outcome and rectum cancer correlated positively with overall and disease-free survivals (supplemental Figure S1a and b).

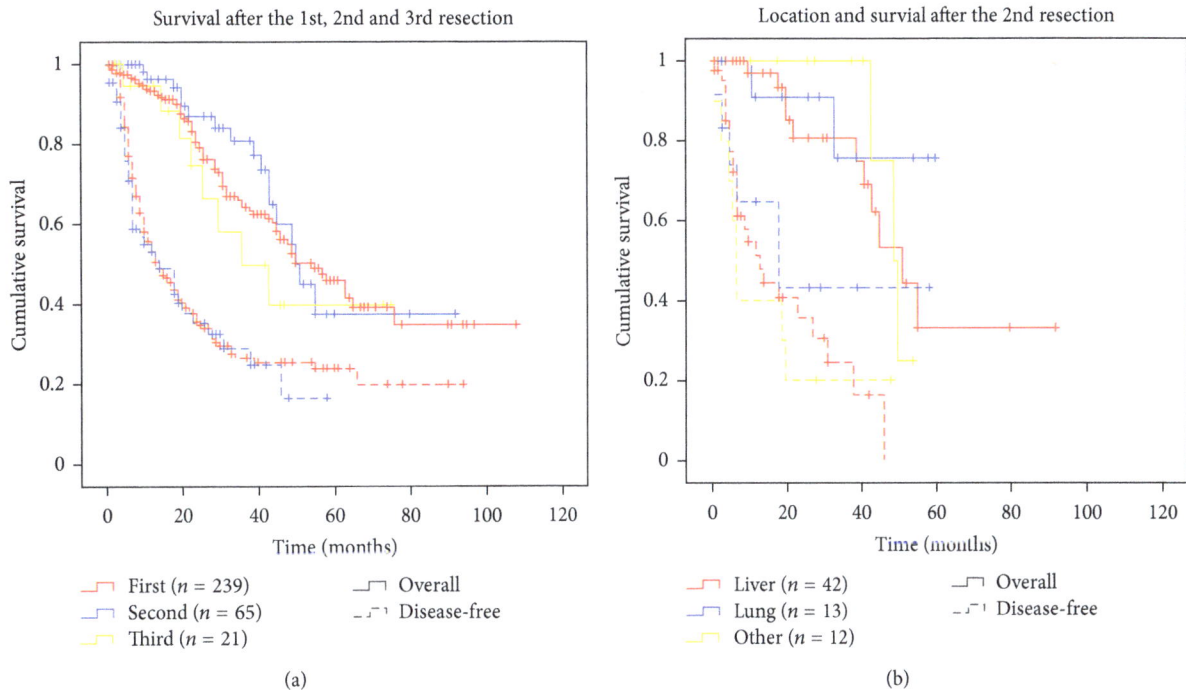

FIGURE 1: Overall and disease-free survivals of colorectal cancer patients following liver resection of primary or recurring metastasis. (a) The Kaplan-Meier plots showing overall (full line) and disease-free (dashed line) survivals in the total population and after the first, second, and third resections. +: censored cases. (b) Survival after a second resection of colorectal metastases at different locations (67 procedures in 65 patients; one patient resected for liver and lung; one patient resected for liver and lymph recurrent disease), data presented as in (a).

4. Discussion

Surgical treatment of CRLMs is offered to an increasing number of patients with metastatic CRC [3]. This has opened several new avenues in the treatment of this patient group, and as a consequence fundamental questions in tumor biology and clinical strategies are now being challenged. Recent reports on survival following re-resection of CRLMs and resection of extrahepatic metastases support a more aggressive treatment practice [8, 25–27]. Neoadjuvant chemotherapy to downsize CRLMs increases the number of resectable cases and provides the opportunity to target a larger patient population. In the present study patients who received neoadjuvant chemotherapy to downsize CRLMs reached a long-term overall survival comparable to that of primary resectable patients, despite widespread disease. It is, in this connection, important to note that tumor load calculations were performed based on information in the pathology reports and are therefore postneoadjuvant chemotherapy which means that they underreport the initial tumor load.

Here we report that second and third resections of recurring CRLMs should be considered when possible and that resection also should be assessed in patients with extrahepatic recurrences as their prognosis does not appear to be worse, but for strict recommendations randomized clinical trials would be needed. Patients selected for laparoscopic approach had a better outcome than patients selected for open surgery (Figure 2(c)), which may be related to the selection criteria and tumor load. A recent report indicates laparoscopic results

comparable to those of open surgery when the selection criteria are identical for the two procedures [28]. Females are reported to have a better prognosis after liver resection for CRLMs than males and colon cancer to have better prognosis than rectum cancer [14]. However, in the present material, men had better overall outcome and a primary rectum cancer correlated positively with overall and disease-free survivals (supplemental Figure S1a and b). The latter may reflect observations that neoadjuvant radiochemotherapy and a more radical surgical technique, total mesorectal excision (TME), have improved survival after treatment for rectum cancer. Ascending age has been reported to be both negatively and positively correlated with survival [12, 14, 29]. We found ascending age to be a positive prognostic marker for disease-free survival (Figure 3(a)), which may be related to more aggressive tumor biology in younger patients. A higher proportion of the young patients presented with recurrent disease and the recurrence occurred more rapidly than in older patients. Interestingly, the overall survival curves were inverted compared to disease-free survival with respect to the different age groups (Figure 3(a)). This could be explained by increased surgical and adjuvant efforts towards young and otherwise healthy patients. If this is the case, this in itself could be proof that an aggressive approach could produce long-term survivors.

Recent genetic and molecular studies of metastatic malignant disease indicate that metastases often develop in parallel to the primary tumor from an early stage, and that the tumor biology of the metastases is not necessarily more aggressive

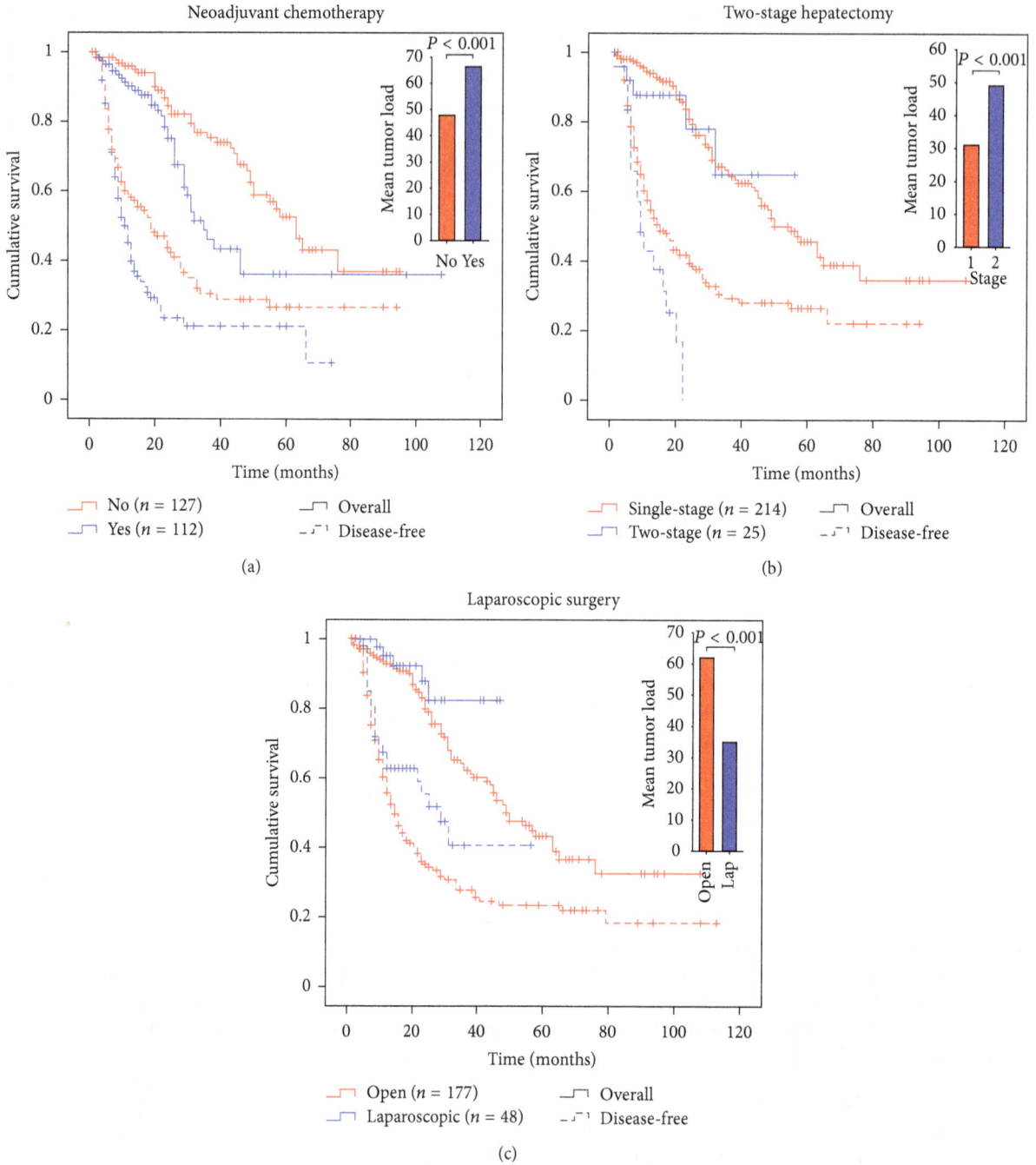

FIGURE 2: Overall and disease-free survivals after neoadjuvant chemotherapy and the first resection for colorectal metastases (a), after two-stage hepatectomy with portal vein embolization (b), or after laparoscopic surgery (c). Data presented as in Figure 1(a). Bar charts (top left corners) show mean *tumor load score* calculated as indicated in the Patients and Methods section. Independent *t*-test was used to compare mean tumor load in subgroups.

than that of the primary tumor [30, 31]. Previous studies addressing the growth rate of various malignant tumors including CRC indicate that the tumor volume doubling time (TVDT) of the metastases is comparable to that of the primary tumor [32]. This may suggest that metastases identified late and removed in re-resection procedures could represent tumors that were not recognized at the time of surgery of the primary tumor or the first metastasis due to their small

size, rather than progressively developing and increasingly aggressive metastases. In our cohort, this may be reflected in the observation that overall survival and oncologic outcome were comparable in patients with successful outcome of the first resection and those who required a second or third resection. In line with this thinking, "recurrent disease" may be a misnomer as the disease may not be recurring but continues to deliver earlier established metastases growing in

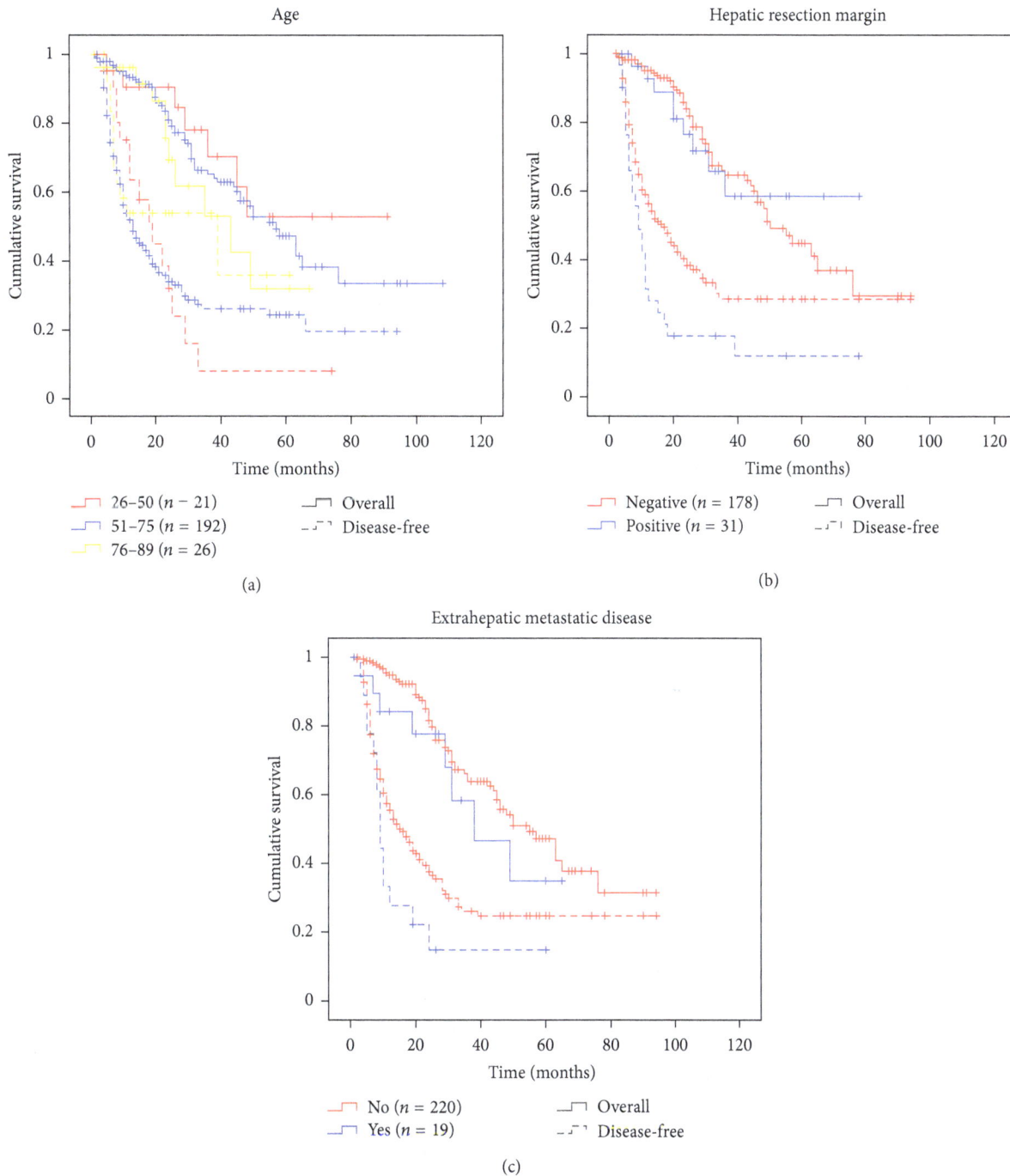

FIGURE 3: Overall and disease-free survivals stratified on risk factors. Data presented by the Kaplan-Meier plots with overall (solid line) and disease-free (dashed line). Age group (a), hepatic resection margin (b), and extrahepatic disease at the time point of surgery, as indicated.

parallel and reaching a size that allows diagnosis at different time points following the primary surgery. Thus, resection of metastases may in many cases represent incremental tumor-reductive surgery rather than treatment of recurrent disease. This may also help to explain why the discrimination between R0 and R1/R2 resections of CRC metastases is not crucial with respect to overall survival (our data and [33]). These findings are in contrast to expected results from current scoring systems [12, 14]. In conclusion, metastatic disease is systemic or multifocal in its nature and may encompass unrecognized foci at the time of surgery in most if not all patients irrespectively of the presentation at diagnosis. Eradication of all tumor tissue may therefore not be conceivable in the majority of the patients. However, this recognition should not preclude an aggressive treatment approach with repeated resections that continue to reduce tumor load.

Extrahepatic metastatic spread has previously been considered an end-stage disease. In recent years, however, combined liver and lung resections have produced long-time survivors. Consequently, pulmonary metastasis alone is no longer considered an exclusion criterion for surgery [34]. Six patients in our cohort presented with concomitant pulmonary lesions with uncertain malignant potential; resection of CRLMs was performed with a "wait and watch" approach taken with respect to the development of pulmonary metastases. In four patients the pulmonary metastases progressed but were accessible by lung resection and three of these were alive and had remained disease-free until the time of examination of the cohort. It is also interesting to observe that patients resected for recurrent disease to the lung after first having performed hepatic resection had comparable and maybe even better survival compared to those repeatedly resected for recurrent disease in the liver, and as such, pulmonary metastases may not be a sign of an explosive metastatic spread [35].

5. Conclusion

The presented results indicate that surgical treatment, when possible with or without neoadjuvant treatment, significantly prolongs life and may in some cases cure the disease, even when extensive. Hence, efforts to identify or induce technically resectable cases are crucial and include early detection of metastatic spread, improved surgical techniques, and neoadjuvant chemotherapy to downsize the metastases. Patients that become resectable after neoadjuvant therapy appear to reach the same survival rate as that of as patients that are primary resectable. Furthermore, neoadjuvant therapy may also be used for selection of patients with the best prognosis after surgical resection, as patients that progress during ongoing treatment will probably not benefit from surgical treatment. The present report adds to the current knowledge base of the outcome of an aggressive treatment approach to metastatic CRC. Although metastatic CRC has a poor prognosis, surgical treatment has clear patient benefit and strategies to make patients resectable and available for surgery should be pursued.

Acknowledgments

The work was funded by the Norwegian Cancer Society and Oslo University Hospital. Kristoffer Watten Brudvik is a fellow of the Norwegian Cancer Society.

References

[1] L. V. Karsa, T. A. Lignini, J. Patnick, R. Lambert, and C. Sauvaget, "The dimensions of the CRC problem," *Best Practice and Research: Clinical Gastroenterology*, vol. 24, no. 4, pp. 381–396, 2010.

[2] M. P. Legolvan and M. Resnick, "Pathobiology of colorectal cancer hepatic metastases with an emphasis on prognostic factors," *Journal of Surgical Oncology*, vol. 102, no. 8, pp. 898–908, 2010.

[3] C. Penna and B. Nordlinger, "Surgery of liver metastases from colorectal cancer: new promises," *British Medical Bulletin*, vol. 64, pp. 127–140, 2002.

[4] R. Adam, A. Laurent, D. Azoulay, D. Castaing, and H. Bismuth, "Two-stage hepatectomy: a planned strategy to treat irresectable liver tumors," *Annals of Surgery*, vol. 232, no. 6, pp. 777–785, 2000.

[5] D. Jaeck, E. Oussoultzoglou, E. Rosso et al., "A two-stage hepatectomy procedure combined with portal vein embolization to achieve curative resection for initially unresectable multiple and bilobar colorectal liver metastases," *Annals of Surgery*, vol. 240, no. 6, pp. 1037–1051, 2004.

[6] R. Adam, V. Delvart, G. Pascal et al., "Rescue surgery for unresectable colorectal liver metastases downstaged by chemotherapy: a model to predict long-term survival," *Annals of Surgery*, vol. 240, no. 4, pp. 644–658, 2004.

[7] K. Lehmann, A. Rickenbacher, A. Weber, B. C. Pestalozzi, and P.-A. Clavien, "Chemotherapy before liver resection of colorectal metastases: friend or foe?" *Annals of Surgery*, vol. 255, no. 2, pp. 237–247, 2012.

[8] R. Adam, G. Pascal, D. Azoulay, K. Tanaka, D. Castaing, and H. Bismuth, "Liver resection for colorectal metastases: the third hepatectomy," *Annals of Surgery*, vol. 238, no. 6, pp. 871–884, 2003.

[9] H. Petrowsky, M. Gonen, W. Jarnagin et al., "Second liver resections are safe and effective treatment for recurrent hepatic metastases from colorectal cancer: a bi-institutional analysis," *Annals of Surgery*, vol. 235, no. 6, pp. 863–871, 2002.

[10] A. Schulz, J. B. Dormagen, A. Drolsum, B. A. Bjornbeth, K. J. Labori, and N. E. Klow, "Impact of contrast-enhanced intraoperative ultrasound on operation strategy in case of colorectal liver metastasis," *Acta Radiologica*, vol. 53, pp. 1081–1087, 2012.

[11] S. M. Strasberg, "Nomenclature of hepatic anatomy and resections: a review of the Brisbane 2000 system," *Journal of Hepato-Biliary-Pancreatic Surgery*, vol. 12, no. 5, pp. 351–355, 2005.

[12] M. Rees, P. P. Tekkis, F. K. S. Welsh, T. O'Rourke, and T. G. John, "Evaluation of long-term survival after hepatic resection for metastatic colorectal cancer: a multifactorial model of 929 patients," *Annals of Surgery*, vol. 247, no. 1, pp. 125–135, 2008.

[13] Y. Fong, J. Fortner, R. L. Sun, M. F. Brennan, and L. H. Blumgart, "Clinical score for predicting recurrence after hepatic resection for metastatic colorectal cancer: analysis of 1001 consecutive cases," *Annals of Surgery*, vol. 230, no. 3, pp. 309–321, 1999.

[14] M. W. Kattan, M. Gönen, W. R. Jarnagin et al., "A nomogram for predicting disease-specific survival after hepatic resection for metastatic colorectal cancer," *Annals of Surgery*, vol. 247, no. 2, pp. 282–287, 2008.

[15] M. Narita, E. Oussoultzoglou, D. Jaeck et al., "Two-stage hepatectomy for multiple bilobar colorectal liver metastases," *British Journal of Surgery*, vol. 98, no. 10, pp. 1463–1475, 2011.

[16] M. Hagness, A. Foss, P. D. Line et al., "Liver transplantation for nonresectable liver metastases from colorectal cancer," *Annals of Surgery*, vol. 257, pp. 800–806, 2013.

[17] A. E. van der Pool, J. H. de Wilt, Z. S. Lalmahomed, A. M. Eggermont, J. N. Ijzermans, and C. Verhoef, "Optimizing the outcome of surgery in patients with rectal cancer and

synchronous liver metastases," *British Journal of Surgery*, vol. 97, no. 3, pp. 383–390, 2010.

[18] E. K. Abdalla, J.-N. Vauthey, L. M. Ellis et al., "Recurrence and outcomes following hepatic resection, radiofrequency ablation, and combined resection/ablation for colorectal liver metastases," *Annals of Surgery*, vol. 239, no. 6, pp. 818–827, 2004.

[19] M. A. Choti, J. V. Sitzmann, M. F. Tiburi et al., "Trends in long-term survival following liver resection for hepatic colorectal metastases," *Annals of Surgery*, vol. 235, no. 6, pp. 759–766, 2002.

[20] L. C. Cummings, J. D. Payes, and G. S. Cooper, "Survival after hepatic resection in metastatic colorectal cancer: a population-based study," *Cancer*, vol. 109, no. 4, pp. 718–726, 2007.

[21] F. G. Fernandez, J. A. Drebin, D. C. Linehan, F. Dehdashti, B. A. Siegel, and S. M. Strasberg, "Five-year survival after resection of hepatic metastases from colorectal cancer in patients screened by positron emission tomography with F-18 fluorodeoxyglucose (FDG-PET)," *Annals of Surgery*, vol. 240, no. 3, pp. 438–450, 2004.

[22] J. Figueras, J. Torras, C. Valls et al., "Surgical resection of colorectal liver metastases in patients with expanded indications: a single-center experience with 501 patients," *Diseases of the Colon and Rectum*, vol. 50, no. 4, pp. 478–488, 2007.

[23] T. M. Pawlik, C. R. Scoggins, D. Zorzi et al., "Effect of surgical margin status on survival and site of recurrence after hepatic resection for colorectal metastases," *Annals of Surgery*, vol. 241, no. 5, pp. 715–724, 2005.

[24] B. Nordlinger, H. Sorbye, B. Glimelius et al., "Perioperative chemotherapy with FOLFOX4 and surgery versus surgery alone for resectable liver metastases from colorectal cancer (EORTC Intergroup trial 40983): a randomised controlled trial," *The Lancet*, vol. 371, no. 9617, pp. 1007–1016, 2008.

[25] S. Nakamura, S. Sakaguchi, R. Nishiyama et al., "Aggressive repeat liver resection for hepatic metastases of colorectal carcinoma," *Surgery Today*, vol. 22, no. 3, pp. 260–264, 1992.

[26] R. Adam, H. Bismuth, D. Castaing et al., "Repeat hepatectomy for colorectal liver metastases," *Annals of Surgery*, vol. 225, no. 1, pp. 51–62, 1997.

[27] C. W. Pinson, J. K. Wright, W. C. Chapman, C. L. Garrard, T. K. Blair, and J. L. Sawyers, "Repeat hepatic surgery for colorectal cancer metastasis to the liver," *Annals of Surgery*, vol. 223, no. 6, pp. 765–776, 1996.

[28] A. M. Kazaryan, I. P. Marangos, B. I. Røsok et al., "Laparoscopic resection of colorectal liver metastases: surgical and long-term oncologic outcome," *Annals of Surgery*, vol. 252, no. 6, pp. 1005–1012, 2010.

[29] R. J. de Haas, D. A. Wicherts, C. Salloum et al., "Long-term outcomes after hepatic resection for colorectal metastases in young patients," *Cancer*, vol. 116, no. 3, pp. 647–658, 2010.

[30] C. A. Klein, "Parallel progression of primary tumours and metastases," *Nature Reviews Cancer*, vol. 9, no. 4, pp. 302–312, 2009.

[31] N. H. Stoecklein and C. A. Klein, "Genetic disparity between primary tumours, disseminated tumour cells, and manifest metastasis," *International Journal of Cancer*, vol. 126, no. 3, pp. 589–598, 2010.

[32] S. Friberg and S. Mattson, "On the growth rates of human malignant tumors: implications for medical decision making," *Journal of Surgical Oncology*, vol. 65, pp. 284–297, 1997.

[33] N. Ayez, Z. S. Lalmahomed, A. M. M. Eggermont et al., "Outcome of microscopic incomplete resection (R1) of colorectal liver metastases in the era of neoadjuvant chemotherapy," *Annals of Surgical Oncology*, vol. 19, no. 5, pp. 1618–1627, 2012.

[34] D. R. Carpizo and M. D'Angelica, "Liver resection for metastatic colorectal cancer in the presence of extrahepatic disease," *The Lancet Oncology*, vol. 10, no. 8, pp. 801–809, 2009.

[35] J. S. Spratt Jr. and T. L. Spratt, "Rates of growth of pulmonary metastases and host survival," *Annals of Surgery*, vol. 159, pp. 161–171, 1964.

5

Effects of a Preconditioning Oral Nutritional Supplement on Pig Livers after Warm Ischemia

Arash Nickkholgh,[1] Zhanqing Li,[1] Xue Yi,[1] Elvira Mohr,[1] Rui Liang,[1] Saulius Mikalauskas,[1] Marie-Luise Gross,[2] Markus Zorn,[3] Steffen Benzing,[4] Heinz Schneider,[5] Markus W. Büchler,[1] and Peter Schemmer[1]

[1] *Department of General and Transplant Surgery, Ruprecht-Karls University, 69120 Heidelberg, Germany*
[2] *Institute of Pathology, Ruprecht-Karls University, 69120 Heidelberg, Germany*
[3] *Central Laboratory, Ruprecht-Karls University, 69120 Heidelberg, Germany*
[4] *Fresenius Kabi Deutschland GmbH, 61440 Oberursel, Germany*
[5] *HealthEcon AG, 4051 Basel, Switzerland*

Correspondence should be addressed to Peter Schemmer, peter.schemmer@med.uni-heidelberg.de

Academic Editor: John J. Lemasters

Background. Several approaches have been proposed to pharmacologically ameliorate hepatic ischemia/reperfusion injury (IRI). This study was designed to evaluate the effects of a preconditioning oral nutritional supplement (pONS) containing glutamine, antioxidants, and green tea extract on hepatic warm IRI in pigs. *Methods.* pONS (70 g per serving, Fresenius Kabi, Germany) was dissolved in 250 mL tap water and given to pigs 24, 12, and 2 hrs before warm ischemia of the liver. A fourth dose was given 3 hrs after reperfusion. Controls were given the same amount of cellulose with the same volume of water. Two hours after the third dose of pONS, both the portal vein and the hepatic artery were clamped for 40 min. 0.5, 3, 6, and 8 hrs after reperfusion, heart rate (HR), mean arterial pressure (MAP), central venous pressure (CVP), portal venous flow (PVF), hepatic arterial flow (HAF), bile flow, and transaminases were measured. Liver tissue was taken 8 hrs after reperfusion for histology and immunohistochemistry. *Results.* HR, MAP, CVP, HAF, and PVF were comparable between the two groups. pONS significantly increased bile flow 8 hrs after reperfusion. ALT and AST were significantly lower after pONS. Histology showed significantly more severe necrosis and neutrophil infiltration in controls. pONS significantly decreased the index of immunohistochemical expression for TNF-α, MPO, and cleaved caspase-3 ($P < 0.001$). *Conclusion.* Administration of pONS before and after tissue damage protects the liver from warm IRI via mechanisms including decreasing oxidative stress, lipid peroxidation, apoptosis, and necrosis.

1. Introduction

During liver surgery, the inflow occlusion maneuver to prevent blood loss as well as the liver manipulation itself have been shown to induce a cascade of molecular events, referred to as ischemia-reperfusion injury (IRI). IRI leads to the activation of Kupffer cells (KCs), the release of reactive oxygen species (ROS) and proinflammatory cytokines, microcirculatory disturbances, and eventually liver dysfunction and failure [1–10]. Different strategies have been proposed to prevent or ameliorate IRI. Among others, pharmacological preconditioning has been shown to be effective via mechanisms including, but not limited to, the direct neutralization of ROS, upregulation of anti-inflammatory, and downregulation of proinflammatory signaling pathways [11–27].

During IRI, intestinal endotoxins (LPS) leak through the altered gut membrane into the portal circulation and enhance the phagocytosis in hepatic KCs [28–35]. This interrelation between intestinal LPS and hepatic KCs makes the gastrointestinal tract an attractive target for the pharmacological preconditioning strategies against hepatic IRI. We hypothesized that an oral pharmacological preconditioning supplement, tailored not only to exert direct ROS-scavenging activity but also to stabilize the gut epithelium during IRI, would tackle the warm hepatic IRI in a porcine model. To the best of our knowledge, this work is the first report of an oral pharmacological preconditioning against hepatic IRI in a larger animal model.

2. Materials and Methods

2.1. Animal Care. German landrace pigs (32.3 ± 0.9 kg) were given access to standard laboratory chow (ssniff R/M-H, ssniff Spezialdiäten, Soest, Germany) and tap water *ad libitum* before experiments. All experimental procedures were reviewed and approved by the responsible authority (Regierungspräsidium Karlsruhe, Baden-Württemberg, Germany) according to the animal welfare legislation (§ 8 Abs. 1 Tierschutzgesetz (TierSchG) dated 18 May, 2006 (BGBI. I S. 1206)) and were performed according to institutional guidelines at the Ruprecht-Karls University of Heidelberg.

2.2. Experimental Procedure. Pigs underwent general anesthesia. After premedication with Azaperone (Stresnil, Janssen-Cilag Pharma, Wien, Austria, 1-2 mg/kg, i.m.) and midazolamhydrochloride (Dormicum 15 mg/3 mL, Roche, Grenzach-Wyhlen, Germany, 0.5–0.7 mg/kg, i.m.), anesthesia was induced with Esketaminhydrochloride (KETANEST S 25 mg/mL, Parke-Davis, Berlin, Germany, 10 mg/kg i.v.) and midazolam hydrochloride (1–1.4 mg/kg i.v.). After endotracheal intubation, animals were ventilated with a mixture of 1.5–2.0 L/min oxygen, 0.5–1.0 L/min air, and 0.75%–1.5% isoflurane (Isofluran-Baxter, Baxter, Unterschleißheim, Germany, semiopen ventilation). For analgesia, Piritramide (Dipidolor, Janssen-Cilag, Neuss, Germany, 3.75 mg/h intravenously) was administered. Body temperature was maintained using warming blankets (WarmTouch, Maleinckrodt Medical GmbH, Hennet/Sieg, Germany) and monitored by continuous rectal temperature probes. Systemic hemodynamic parameters, including mean arterial pressure (MAP) and central venous pressure (CVP), were measured continuously (Stetham Transducer, Hellige Monitoring, Freiburg, Germany) by indwelling polypropylene catheters (Braun, Melsungen, Germany) in the common carotid artery and internal jugular vein, respectively. Heart rate (HR) was monitored by body surface electrocardiogram recordings. Experimental groups were given a preconditioning oral nutritional supplement (pONS, 70 g per serving, Fresenius Kabi, Germany) containing glutamine, green tea extract (the resource, method of extraction, and composition of green tea extract has been published elsewhere [36]), vitamin C, vitamin E, beta carotene, selenium, zinc, and carbohydrates (1 sachet = 70 g) (Table 1) dissolved in 250 mL tap water 24 hrs (p.o.) and 12 hrs (p.o.) before the operation. The animals were then fasted overnight. On the day of operation and after performing a midline laparotomy, a third dose of pONS was applied via a jejunostomy tube. The portal vein and common hepatic artery were then mobilized and encircled by elastic bands. Two hrs after the administration of the third dose of pONS, the portal vein and the common hepatic artery were closed with Yasargil clamps (Aesculap, Tübingen, Germany) for 40 min to induce warm ischemia. Common bile duct was cannulated to collect

TABLE 1: Composition of the pONS.

Component	Dry weight per sachet (g)
Glutamine	15
Antioxidants	
Green tea extract	1
Vitamin C	0.75
Vitamin E	0.25
ß-carotene	0.005
Selenium	0.00015
Zinc	0.01
Carbohydrates	50

1 sachet of pONS was dissolved in 250 mL tap water before use. Conditions as mentioned in Materials and Methods. pONS: preconditioning oral nutritional supplement.

bile continuously. After 40 min, the liver was reperfused by removing the clamps. A fourth dose of pONS was given 3 hrs after reperfusion. Controls were given the same amount of cellulose with the same volume of water. Serial blood samples were drawn and spun at 0.5, 3, 6, and 8 hrs after reperfusion and serum samples were kept at −20°C for the analysis of transaminases (aspartate aminotransferase (AST) and alanine aminotransferase (ALT)) serum concentrations with standard enzymatic methods [37]. The changes in bile production during each time interval were documented and the amount of the newly produced bile was plotted at the end of each time interval to assess the bile flow rate over time. Liver tissue was taken 8 hrs after reperfusion for histology (hematoxylin and eosin (H&E) staining) and immunohistochemistry (TNF-α, myeloperoxidase, cleaved caspase-3). Hemodynamic parameters (HR, MAP, CVP, PVF, HAF) were continuously monitored throughout the experiments; ultrasonic probes (Transsonic System Inc, New York, NY, USA) were used for the measurement of portal venous flow (PVF) and hepatic arterial flow (HAF). The experimental design is outlined in Figure 1. After the completion of experimental procedures 8 hrs after reperfusion, animals were sacrificed in deep anesthesia through the intravenous application of a high dose of potassium chloride.

2.3. Histology. Liver samples were fixed by perfusion with 5% paraformaldehyde in Krebs-Henseleit bicarbonate buffer (118 mmol/L NaCl, 25 mmol/L NaHCO3, 1.2 mmol/L KH2PO4, 1.2 mmol/L MgSO4, 4.7 mmol/L KCl, and 1.3 mmol/L CaCl2) at pH 7.6, embedded in paraffin, and processed for light microscopy (H&E) 8 hrs after warm ischemia. In order to assess the histomorphological changes, 40 areas of 0.15 mm^2 were evaluated per slide using a point-counting method as described previously [38]: grade 0, minimal or no evidence of injury; grade 1, mild injury, including cytoplasmic vacuolation and focal nuclear pyknosis; grade 2, moderate to severe injury with extensive nuclear pyknosis, cytoplasmic hypereosinophilia, and loss of intercellular borders; grade 3, severe necrosis with disintegration of hepatic cords, hemorrhage, and neutrophil infiltration. To describe leukocyte infiltration

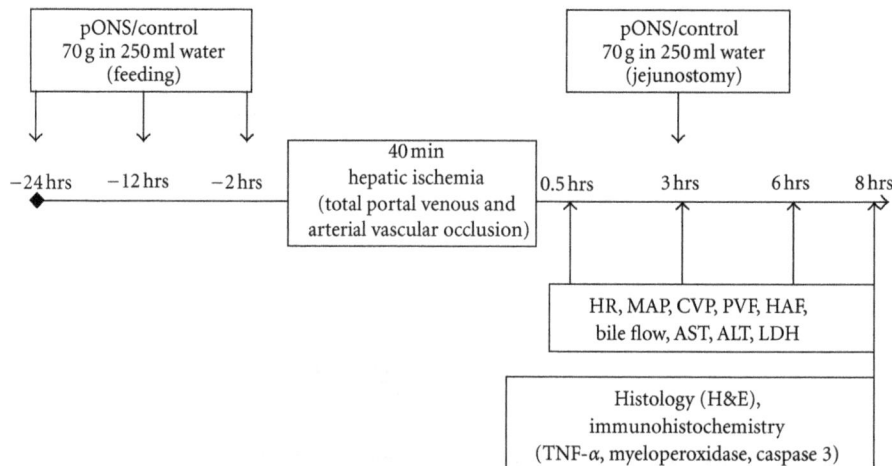

FIGURE 1: Experimental design. pONS (70 g in 250 mL tap water) was given to overnight-fasted German Landrace pigs 24, 12, and 2 hrs before warm ischemia of the liver. A fourth dose was given 3 hrs after reperfusion. Controls were given the same amount of cellulose. Two hrs after administration of the third dose, both the portal vein and the hepatic artery were clamped for 40 min. After reperfusion, hemodynamic parameters, bile production, and transaminases were measured serially. Liver tissue was taken 8 hrs after reperfusion for histology (H&E) and immunohistochemistry (TNF-a, myeloperoxidasby the Mann-Whitney rank sume, cleaved caspase-3) as described in Materials and Methods. pONS: preconditioning oral nutritional supplement; hrs: hours; min: minutes; PR: pulse rate; MAP: mean arterial pressure; CVP: central venous pressure; PVF: portal venous flow; HAF: hepatic artery flow; AST: aspartate aminotransferase; ALT: alanine aminotransferase.

into the hepatic tissue, a scale from 1 to 4 was used: grade 1, <10 leukocytes/field (focal infiltration); grade 2, 10–20 (mild infiltration); grade 3, 21–50; grade 4, >50 leukocytes/field.

2.4. Immunohistochemistry. Paraffin sections from liver tissue obtained 8 hrs after reperfusion were deparaffinized in xylene and rehydrated with graded ethanol. Antigen retrieval was performed via microwave pretreatment in EDTA buffer (pH 9.0) three times for 5 min. The specimens were then cooled and treated with 30% hydrogen peroxidase (H_2O_2) in phosphate-buffered saline (PBS)—final H_2O_2 concentration: 1%—to block endogenous peroxidases. Nonspecific antibody binding was blocked by normal rabbit serum. Sections were incubated with rabbit polyclonal anti-mouse tumor necrosis factor-alpha (TNF-α) antibody (Biosource Europe, Nivelles, Belgium) at the dilution of 1 : 500, and rabbit polyclonal anti-cleaved caspase-3 antibody (DCS, Hamburg, Germany) at a 1 : 200 dilution. After incubation, secondary biotinylated polyclonal rabbit anti-mouse immunoglobulin (Dako, Hamburg, Germany) was applied at a dilution of 1 : 200 for 1 hr followed by streptavidin-biotin complex. For myeloperoxidase (MPO) immunohistochemistry analysis, the sections were pretreated with proteinase K (1 : 40 dilution) and then blocked with bovine serum albumin. They were then incubated with the primary antibody, a polyclonal rabbit anti-MPO antibody (Dako, Carpinteria, CA, USA) at a dilution of 1 : 200, for 60 min at room temperature. A biotinylated swine anti-rabbit antibody (diluted 1 : 300) was used as the secondary antibody.

Positive cells for immunohistochemistry were counted in 10 microscopic fields per slide and slides were evaluated with a semiquantitative technique, relating the score of 0 to 4 points to the fraction of stained cells: scale 0, 0% cells; 1, <5%

cells; 2, 5%–20% cells; 3, >20%–40% cells; 4, >40% positive cells as described elsewhere [12].

2.5. Statistics. Mean values ± SEM were compared using one-way ANOVA with the Students-Newman-Keuls post hoc test for the analysis of differences in hemodynamic values, vascular flow measurements, bile production, and transaminases. Differences in histological grading of injury as well as in immunohistochemical staining were tested by the Mann-Whitney rank sum test. $P < 0.05$ was selected prior to the investigation as the criterion for significance of differences between groups.

3. Results

3.1. General and Hemodynamic Data. Hematocrit, body weight, and temperature were not different between control and pONS groups ($n = 6$ in each group) (Table 2). Continuous postperfusion monitoring of the hemodynamic parameters (HR, MAP, CVP, PVF, HAF) also showed no significant differences between the two groups (Table 2).

3.2. Liver Injury and Bile Production. While serum ALT increased in controls after warm ischemia/reperfusion to the liver, pONS prevented this effect; the difference between the two groups started to be significant 6 hours after reperfusion (49 ± 3 U/L in controls versus 35 ± 3 U/L in pONS; $P = 0.01$). This difference continued to exist until the end of experiments, 8 hrs after perfusion (50 ± 3 U/L in controls versus 33 ± 4 U/L in pONS; $P = 0.02$). pONS had the same effect on serum AST levels after reperfusion. The difference between the groups was significant 8 hrs after reperfusion (140 ± 52 U/L in controls versus 46 ± 7 U/L in pONS;

(a)

(b)

(c)

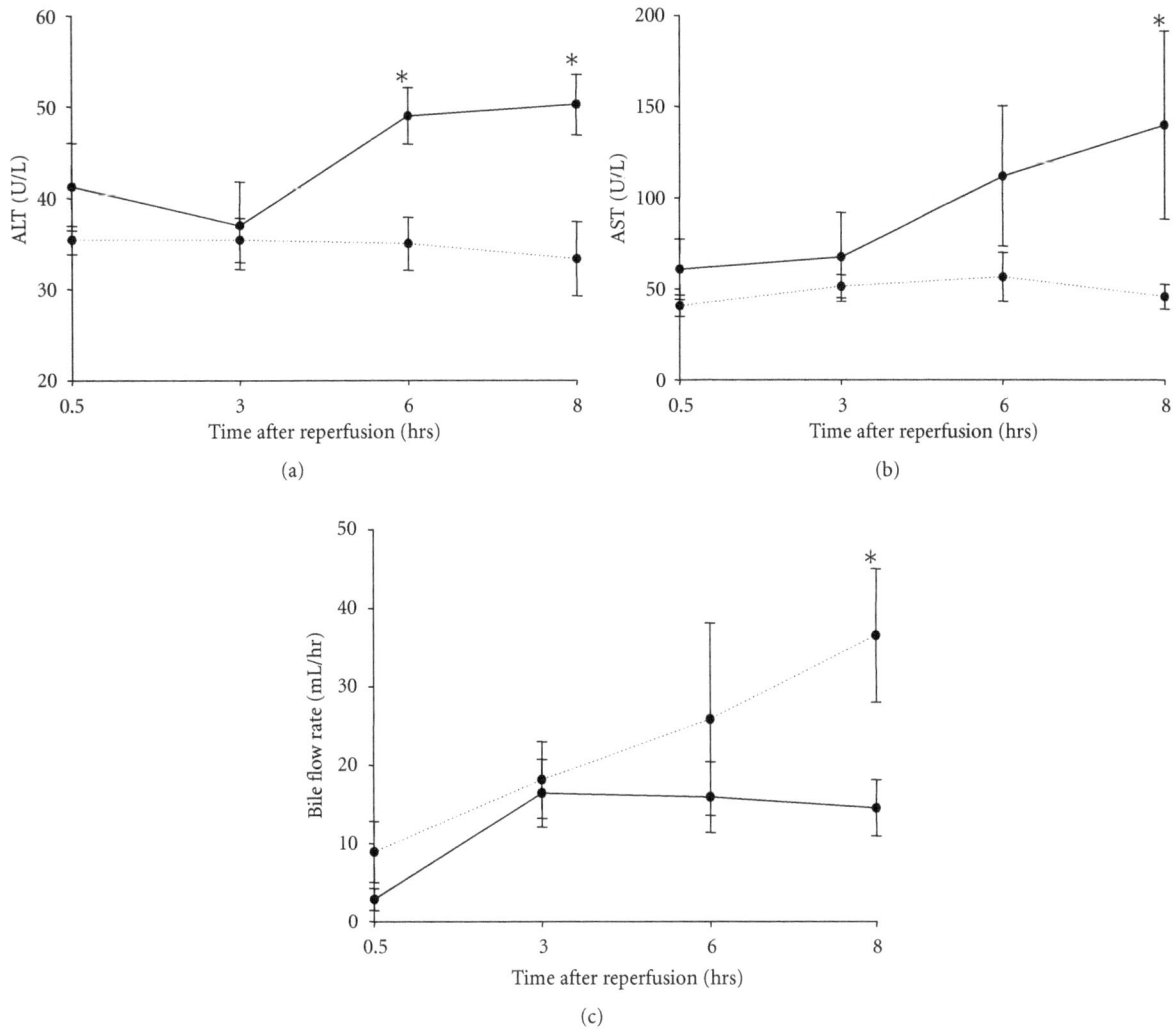

FIGURE 2: Effects of pONS on serum transaminases and bile production after reperfusion. ((a), (b)) Serial measurement of transaminases was performed after reperfusion as described in Materials and Methods. (c) Bile flow rate (mL/hr) has been depicted over time after reperfusion. Values are mean ± SEM ($P < 0.05$ by one-way ANOVA with Students-Newman-Keuls post hoc test, $n = 6$ per group); *$P < 0.05$ for comparison to controls; AST: aspartate aminotransferase; ALT: alanine aminotransferase; pONS: preconditioning oral nutritional supplement.

TABLE 2: Basic parameters.

	Control ($n = 6$)	pONS ($n = 6$)	P
Body weight (kg)	33.1 ± 1.7	31.4 ± 0.8	0.4
Temperature (°C)	36.9 ± 0.2	36.8 ± 0.2	0.7
Respiratory rate (/min)	12 ± 1	12 ± 1	0.9
Hct (%)	30 ± 0.9	33 ± 1.7	0.1
HR (/min)	177 ± 10	185 ± 9	0.6
MAP (mmHg)	90 ± 4.1	91 ± 3.7	0.9
CVP (mmHg)	15 ± 1.7	14.8 ± 0.5	0.9
PVF (L/min)	1.4 ± 0.6	1.9 ± 0.2	0.3
HAF (dL/min)	114 ± 22	117 ± 12	0.9

Table shows basic parameters (body weight, temperature, and respiratory rate) as well as postperfusion data for hematocrit (Hct), heart rate (HR), mean arterial pressure (MAP), central venous pressure (CVP), portal venous flow (PVF), and hepatic arterial flow (HAF). Values are mean ± SEM.

$P = 0.01$) (Figure 2). There was significantly more severe necrosis with disintegration of hepatic cords, hemorrhage, and neutrophil infiltration (the median grade for necrosis and leukocyte infiltration were 3 and 4, resp.) in control tissue taken 8 hrs after reperfusion. pONS decreased the severity of the above-mentioned histomorphological changes in the liver (the median grade of necrosis and leukocyte infiltration of 1; $P < 0.001$) (Figure 3). Bile flow rate (mL/hr) was significantly higher in the pONS group 8 hrs after reperfusion (Figure 2).

3.3. Immunohistochemistry. The immunohistochemical analysis of sections obtained 8 hrs after reperfusion indicated positive staining for TNF-α, MPO, and cleaved Caspase-3. pONS reduced the number of positively stained hepatocytes against all of three above enzymes (Figure 4).

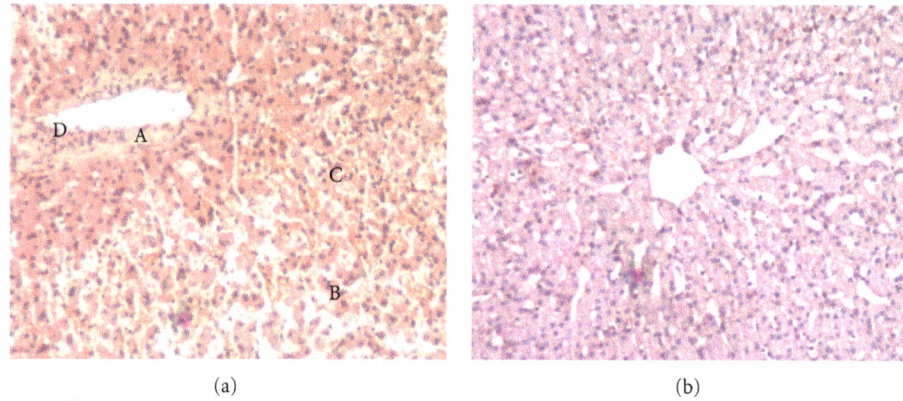

(a)   (b)

FIGURE 3: Liver injury eight hours after reperfusion. Liver tissue was taken 8 hrs after reperfusion and processed for light microscopy by H&E staining. (a), control; (b), pONS; controls displayed severe focal necrosis (A) with disintegration of hepatic cords (B), hemorrhage (C), and neutrophil infiltration (D) 8 hrs after reperfusion; this effect was significantly blunted by pONS. Pictures depict typical pattern of pathology; pONS: preconditioning oral nutritional supplement.

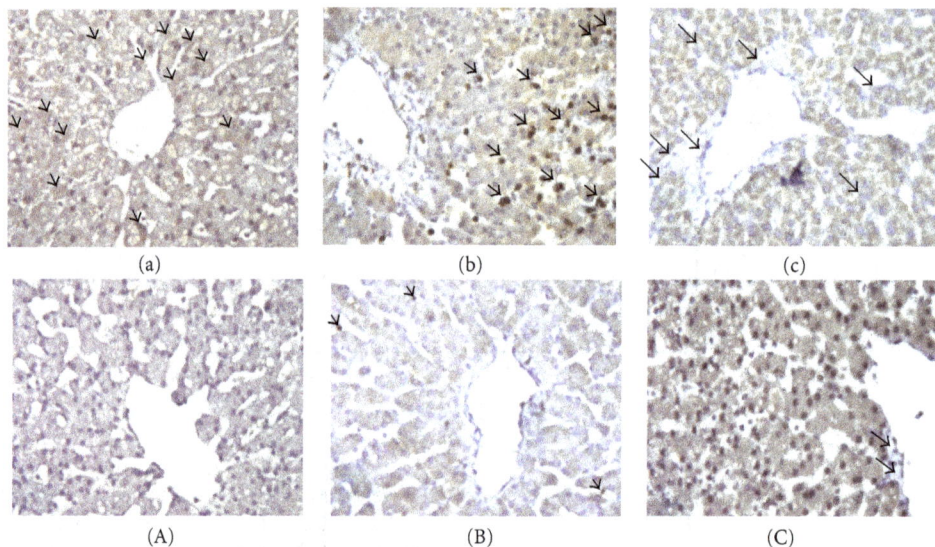

(a)   (b)   (c)

(A)   (B)   (C)

FIGURE 4: Immunohistochemistry for TNF-α ((a), (A)), MPO ((b), (B)), and cleaved Caspase-3 ((c), (C)). Conditions as described in Materials and Methods. Eight hrs after reperfusion, tissue was collected and processed for immunohistochemical analysis with light microscopy. The intensity of TNF-α expression (brown staining, black arrows), MPO expression (brown staining, black arrows), and cleaved Caspase-3 (blue halo, black arrows) was significantly higher in controls ((a), (b), (c), resp.) compared to their pONS counterparts ((A), (B), (C), resp.). Pictures depict typical pattern of staining (original magnification: $\times 200$). TNF-α: tumor necrosis factor-alpha; MPO: myeloperoxidase; pONS: preconditioning oral nutritional supplement.

The quantitative assessment of immunohistochemical findings is presented in Table 3.

4. Discussion

The manipulation of the liver during hepatic surgery activates Kupffer cells, which leads to the release of proinflammatory cytokines, including tumor necrosis factor-alpha (TNF-α) and interlukin-1 (IL-1) as well as free radicals, thus initiating an inflammatory cascade [2–7]. This phenomenon is usually further complicated through the application of the Pringle maneuver (hepatic inflow occlusion) in an attempt to prevent blood loss during the hepatic transection [39]. The

cumulative effect induces warm IRI to the liver, which results, depending on the duration of ischemia, in microcirculatory disturbances, liver cell damage, and—in severe cases—liver failure [40]. Several approaches have been proposed to pharmacologically tackle hepatic IRI; none, however, has found its way into clinical routine yet.

To prevent IRI, it is important to neutralize reactive oxygen and nitrogen species, either by administering radical scavengers or by enhancing the capacity of endogenous redox defense systems [41]. A vast variety of dietary constituents can exert radical scavenging effects in vivo. Among all, hydrophilic ascorbic acid (vitamin C) and lipophilic α-tocopherol (vitamin E) are the important components of

TABLE 3: Quantitative assessment of immunohistochemical findings.

Expression	Control ($n = 6$)				pONS ($n = 6$)				P
	n	median	25%	75%	n	median	25%	75%	
TNF-α	84	2	2	3	102	1	1	1	<0.001
MPO	79	4	3	4	99	2	2	3	<0.001
Caspase-3	81	4	3	4	100	2	1	2	<0.001

Conditions as described in Materials and Methods; $n = 6$ in each group; median values of indices for immunohistochemical expression of TNF-α, MPO, and cleaved caspase-3 with interquartile range 8 hrs after warm ischemia/reperfusion have been compared with Mann-Whitney rank sum. TNF-α: tumor necrosis factor-alpha; MPO: myeloperoxidase; pONS: preconditioning oral nutritional supplement.

the human antioxidant system [42]. Carotenoids, the principal dietary source of vitamin A in humans [43], polyphenolic compounds in green tea extract [36, 44], selenium [45], and zinc [46] all exert antioxidant action; a synergism among the different antioxidants as part of an antioxidant network has been shown [47–49].

Large amounts of Gram-negative bacteria and endotoxins (LPS) are normally present in the intestines. A reduction in splanchnic blood flow and ischemia damages the intestinal wall and changes the permeability of the gut membrane, leading to excessive leakage of LPS and bacterial translocation into the portal circulation. It has been shown that LPS can activate KCs directly [50]. Scavenger receptors, including the scavenger receptor cystein-rich (SRCR) superfamily members that are expressed on KCs, are involved in the bactericidal action by binding and endocytosis of endotoxin [51, 52]. The CD11/CD18 receptor of KCs, the pattern recognition receptors (PRRs) CD14, and the Toll-like receptor 4 (TLR4) in combination with the adaptor protein MD2 are reported to be essentially involved in the LPS-associated KC activation [50, 53]. This may reflect an evolutionary adaptation by KCs to their local hepatic environment and strategic anatomic position in the portal circuit, which is optimal for the removal of endotoxin and, thus, for the protection of the host [54]. Glutamine has been shown to have a positive impact on the intestinal barrier by reducing permeability and bacterial translocation and preserving mucosal integrity [55, 56]. It can, therefore, prevent Kupffer cell activation and results in a more favorable outcome [57].

However, we did not measure blood LPS levels or histology of intestine, which might have further documented the protective effects of pONS on intestine.

In many models of liver injury, TNF-α levels are elevated and correlate with injury; the inhibition of TNF-α activity can attenuate liver injury, protect hepatic morphology, and decrease mortality [54]. MPO has been shown to be largely responsible for the neutrophil-induced parenchymal cell killing [58]. Released from the neutrophil's azurophilic granules, MPO can generate hypochlorous acid, a diffusible oxidant and chlorinating agent that gives rise to other toxic species, such as chloramines [59]. Apoptotic cell death can trigger neutrophil transmigration, severely aggravating apoptotic cell injury; caspase inhibitors can have a significant overall protective effect on hepatic IRI [60]. In the present study, we have shown that the oral administration of consecutive doses of a preconditioning supplement in experimental pigs significantly reduced the transaminases

compared to controls after hepatic warm IRI. Furthermore, pONS resulted in significantly milder histological changes as well as a significant increase in bile production. The milder histological changes as well as improved sinusoidal bile production after pONS represents reduced postreperfusion injury. This has been further proved by the immunohistochemical analysis of the tissues obtained 8 hrs postreperfusion; pONS reduced the expression of TNF-α, MPO, and cleaved Caspase-3. pONS most likely exerts these protective effects via different mechanisms including direct antioxidative effects of its various antioxidant constituents including vitamin C, vitamin E, β-carotene, polyphenolic compounds in green tea extract, selenium and zinc. Furthermore, pONS most likely exerts an inhibitory effect on LPS-associated KC activation through glutamine.

To the best of our knowledge, this work is the first report of an oral pharmacological preconditioning against hepatic IRI in a larger animal model. The application of an oral nutritional substance in pigs is safe, reproducible, and well-deals with the current obstacles faced within the context of hepatic surgery and warm IRI. Tailoring such clinically-oriented experiments may finally help improve bench-to-bedside preconditioning protocols.

Acknowledgments

A. Nickkholgh together with Z. Li, R. Liang, and S. Mikalauskas carried out the experiments; A. Nickkholgh wrote the paper. E. Mohr performed the histological and immunohistochemical preparations. X. Yi and M.-L. Gross reviewed the histological and immunohistochemical part of the study. H. Schneider and S. Benzing supported the study regarding the experimental product and the design. M. Zorn was consulted regarding the biochemical measurements. M. Büchler and P. Schemmer supported the design of the study with their knowledge and experience. Further, P. Schemmer conceived and designed the study based on his experimental experience. The paper has been seen and approved by all authors listed above. The authors thank Katherine Hughes for editing the paper as a native speaker. The authors have declared no conflict of interest.

References

[1] C. Bremer, B. U. Bradford, K. J. Hunt et al., "Role of Kupffer cells in the pathogenesis of hepatic reperfusion injury," *American Journal of Physiology*, vol. 267, no. 4, pp. 630–636, 1994.

[2] P. Schemmer, R. Schoonhoven, J. A. Swenberg, H. Bunzendahl, and R. G. Thurman, "Gentle in situ liver manipulation during organ harvest decreases survival after rat liver transplantation: role of Kupffer cells," *Transplantation*, vol. 65, no. 8, pp. 1015–1020, 1998.

[3] P. Schemmer, H. D. Connor, G. E. Arteel et al., "Reperfusion injury in livers due to gentle in situ organ manipulation during harvest involves hypoxia and free radicals," *Journal of Pharmacology and Experimental Therapeutics*, vol. 290, no. 1, pp. 235–240, 1999.

[4] P. Schemmer, B. U. Bradford, M. L. Rose et al., "Intravenous glycine improves survival in rat liver transplantation," *American Journal of Physiology*, vol. 276, no. 4, pp. 924–932, 1999.

[5] P. Schemmer, R. Schoonhoven, J. A. Swenberg et al., "Gentle organ manipulation during harvest as a key determinant of survival of fatty livers after transplantation in the rat," *Transplant International*, vol. 12, no. 5, pp. 351–359, 1999.

[6] P. Schemmer, H. Bunzendahl, J. A. Raleigh, and R. G. Thurman, "Graft survival is improved by hepatic denervation before organ harvesting," *Transplantation*, vol. 67, no. 10, pp. 1301–1307, 1999.

[7] P. Schemmer, N. Enomoto, B. U. Bradford et al., "Activated Kupffer cells cause a hypermetabolic state after gentle in situ manipulation of liver in rats," *American Journal of Physiology*, vol. 280, no. 6, pp. 1076–1082, 2001.

[8] B. K. Hanboon, W. Ekataksin, G. Alsfasser et al., "Microvascular dysfunction in hepatic ischemia-reperfusion injury in pigs," *Microvascular Research*, vol. 80, no. 1, pp. 123–132, 2010.

[9] P. Schemmer, M. Golling, T. Kraus et al., "Extended experience with glycine for prevention of reperfusion injury after human liver transplantation," *Transplantation Proceedings*, vol. 34, no. 6, pp. 2307–2309, 2002.

[10] P. Schemmer, A. Mehrabi, T. Kraus et al., "New aspect on reperfusion injury to liver—impact of organ harvest," *Nephrology Dialysis Transplantation*, vol. 19, no. 4, pp. 26–35, 2004.

[11] S. P. Luntz, K. Unnebrink, M. Seibert-Grafe et al., "HEGPOL: randomized, placebo controlled, multicenter, double-blind clinical trial to investigate hepatoprotective effects of glycine in the postoperative phase of liver transplantation [ISRCTN69350312]," *BMC Surgery*, vol. 5, article 18, 2005.

[12] P. Schemmer, R. Liang, M. Kincius et al., "Taurine improves graft survival after experimental liver transplantation," *Liver Transplantation*, vol. 11, no. 8, pp. 950–959, 2005.

[13] M. Kincius, R. Liang, A. Nickkholgh et al., "Taurine protects from liver injury after warm ischemia in rats: the role of Kupffer cells," *European Surgical Research*, vol. 39, no. 5, pp. 275–283, 2007.

[14] C. Jahnke, A. Mehrabi, M. Golling et al., "Evaluation of microperfusion disturbances in the transplanted liver after Kupffer cell destruction using GdCl3: an experimental porcine study," *Transplantation Proceedings*, vol. 38, no. 5, pp. 1588–1595, 2006.

[15] A. Nickkholgh, H. Schneider, J. Encke, M. W. Büchler, J. Schmidt, and P. Schemmer, "PROUD: effects of preoperative long-term immunonutrition in patients listed for liver transplantation," *Trials*, vol. 8, article 20, 2007.

[16] A. Nickkholgh, M. Barro-Bejarano, R. Liang et al., "Signs of reperfusion injury following CO_2 pneumoperitoneum: an *in vivo* microscopy study," *Surgical Endoscopy and Other Interventional Techniques*, vol. 22, no. 1, pp. 122–128, 2008.

[17] P. Schemmer, A. Nickkholgh, H. Schneider et al., "PORTAL: pilot study on the safety and tolerance of preoperative melatonin application in patients undergoing major liver resection:

[18] X. Guan, G. Dei-Anane, R. Liang et al., "Donor preconditioning with taurine protects kidney grafts from injury after experimental transplantation," *Journal of Surgical Research*, vol. 146, no. 1, pp. 127–134, 2008.

[19] R. Liang, A. Nickkholgh, K. Hoffmann et al., "Melatonin protects from hepatic reperfusion injury through inhibition of IKK and JNK pathways and modification of cell proliferation," *Journal of Pineal Research*, vol. 46, no. 1, pp. 8–14, 2009.

[20] Z. Li, A. Nickkholgh, X. Yi et al., "Melatonin protects kidney grafts from ischemia/reperfusion injury through inhibition of NF-kB and apoptosis after experimental kidney transplantation," *Journal of Pineal Research*, vol. 46, no. 4, pp. 365–372, 2009.

[21] R. Liang, H. Bruns, M. Kincius et al., "Danshen protects liver grafts from ischemia/reperfusion injury in experimental liver transplantation in rats," *Transplant International*, vol. 22, no. 11, pp. 1100–1109, 2009.

[22] X. Guan, G. Dei-Anane, H. Bruns et al., "Danshen protects kidney grafts from ischemia/reperfusion injury after experimental transplantation," *Transplant International*, vol. 22, no. 2, pp. 232–241, 2009.

[23] K. Hoffmann, M. W. Büchler, and P. Schemmer, "Supplementation of amino acids to prevent reperfusion injury after liver surgery and transplantation—where do we stand today?" *Clinical Nutrition*, vol. 30, no. 2, pp. 143–147, 2011.

[24] H. Bruns, I. Watanpour, M. M. Gebhard et al., "Glycine and taurine equally prevent fatty livers from Kupffer cell-dependent injury: an *in vivo* microscopy study," *Microcirculation*, vol. 18, no. 3, pp. 205–213, 2011.

[25] G. O. Ceyhan, A. K. Timm, F. Bergmann et al., "Prophylactic glycine administration attenuates pancreatic damage and inflammation in experimental acute pancreatitis," *Pancreatology*, vol. 11, no. 1, pp. 57–67, 2011.

[26] S. Mikalauskas, L. Mikalauskiene, H. Bruns et al., "Dietary glycine protects from chemotherapy-induced hepatotoxicity," *Amino Acids*, vol. 40, no. 4, pp. 1139–1150, 2011.

[27] A. Nickkholgh, H. Schneider, M. Sobirey et al., "The use of high-dose melatonin in liver resection is safe: first clinical experience," *Journal of Pineal Research*, vol. 50, no. 4, pp. 381–388, 2011.

[28] J. P. Nolan, "Endotoxin, reticuloendothelial function, and liver injury," *Hepatology*, vol. 1, no. 5, pp. 458–465, 1981.

[29] K. B. Cowper, R. T. Currin, T. L. Dawson, K. A. Lindert, J. J. Lemasters, and R. G. Thurman, "A new method to monitor Kupffer-cell function continuously in the perfused rat liver: dissociation of glycogenolysis from particle phagocytosis," *Biochemical Journal*, vol. 266, no. 1, pp. 141–147, 1990.

[30] P. Schemmer, N. Enomoto, B. U. Bradford, H. Bunzendahl, J. A. Raleigh, and R. G. Thurman, "Autonomic nervous system and gut-derived endotoxin: involvement in activation of Kupffer cells after in situ organ manipulation," *World Journal of Surgery*, vol. 25, no. 4, pp. 399–406, 2001.

[31] K. Monden, S. Arii, S. Itai et al., "Enhancement of hepatic macrophages in septic rats and their inhibitory effect on hepatocyte function," *Journal of Surgical Research*, vol. 50, no. 1, pp. 72–76, 1991.

[32] R. L. Schultze, A. Gangopadhyay, O. Cay, D. Lazure, and P. Thomas, "Tyrosine kinase activation in LPS stimulated rat Kupffer cells," *Cell Biochemistry and Biophysics*, vol. 30, no. 2, pp. 287–301, 1999.

[33] R. Tokyay, S. T. Zeigler, D. L. Traber et al., "Postburn gastrointestinal vasoconstriction increases bacterial and endotoxin

translocation," *Journal of Applied Physiology*, vol. 74, no. 4, pp. 1521–1527, 1993.

[34] S. E. Morris, N. Navaratnam, C. M. Townsend, and D. N. Herndon, "Decreased mesenteric blood flow independently promotes bacterial translocation in chronically instrumented sheep," *Surgical Forum*, vol. 40, pp. 88–91, 1989.

[35] M. Golling, C. Jahnke, H. Fonouni et al., "Distinct effects of surgical denervation on hepatic perfusion, bowel ischemia, and oxidative stress in brain dead and living donor porcine models," *Liver Transplantation*, vol. 13, no. 4, pp. 607–617, 2007.

[36] R. Liang, A. Nickkholgh, M. Kern et al., "Green tea extract ameliorates reperfusion injury to rat livers after warm ischemia in a dose-dependent manner," *Molecular Nutrition and Food Research*, vol. 55, no. 6, pp. 855–863, 2011.

[37] H. U. Bergmeyer, *Methods of Enzymatic Analysis*, Academic Press, New York, NY, USA, 1988.

[38] R. G. Thurman, I. Marzi, G. Seitz, J. Thies, J. J. Lemasters, and F. Zimmerman, "Hepatic reperfusion injury following orthotopic liver transplantation in the rat," *Transplantation*, vol. 46, no. 4, pp. 502–506, 1988.

[39] N. N. Rahbari, M. N. Wente, P. Schemmer et al., "Systematic review and meta-analysis of the effect of portal triad clamping on outcome after hepatic resection," *British Journal of Surgery*, vol. 95, no. 4, pp. 424–432, 2008.

[40] H. Jaeschke and A. Farhood, "Kupffer cell activation after no-flow ischemia versus hemorrhagic shock," *Free Radical Biology and Medicine*, vol. 33, no. 2, pp. 210–219, 2002.

[41] G. K. Glantzounis, H. J. Salacinski, W. Yang, B. R. Davidson, and A. M. Seifalian, "The contemporary role of antioxidant therapy in attenuating liver ischemia-reperfusion injury: a review," *Liver Transplantation*, vol. 11, no. 9, pp. 1031–1047, 2005.

[42] M. K. Sharma and G. R. Buettner, "Interaction of vitamin C and vitamin E during free radical stress in plasma: an ESR study," *Free Radical Biology and Medicine*, vol. 14, no. 6, pp. 649–653, 1993.

[43] E. Nagel, A. Meyer zu Vilsendorf, M. Bartels, and R. Pichlmayr, "Antioxidative vitamins in prevention of ischemia/reperfusion injury," *International Journal for Vitamin and Nutrition Research*, vol. 67, no. 5, pp. 298–306, 1997.

[44] Z. Zhong, M. Froh, H. D. Connor et al., "Prevention of hepatic ischemia-reperfusion injury by green tea extract," *American Journal of Physiology*, vol. 283, no. 4, pp. 957–964, 2002.

[45] C. Zapletal, S. Heyne, R. Breitkreutz, M. M. Gebhard, and M. Golling, "The influence of selenium substitution on microcirculation and glutathione metabolism after warm liver ischemia/reperfusion in a rat model," *Microvascular Research*, vol. 76, no. 2, pp. 104–109, 2008.

[46] Y. Horie, R. Wolf, S. C. Flores, J. M. McCord, C. J. Epstein, and D. N. Granger, "Transgenic mice with increased copper/zinc-superoxide dismutase activity are resistant to hepatic leukostasis and capillary no-reflow after gut ischemia/reperfusion," *Circulation Research*, vol. 83, no. 7, pp. 691–696, 1998.

[47] S. Vertuani, A. Angusti, and S. Manfredini, "The antioxidants and pro-antioxidants network: an overview," *Current Pharmaceutical Design*, vol. 10, no. 14, pp. 1677–1694, 2004.

[48] M. H. Wijnen, R. M. H. Roumen, H. L. Vader, and R. J. A. Goris, "A multiantioxidant supplementation reduces damage from ischaemia reperfusion in patients after lower torso ischaemia. A randomised trial," *European Journal of Vascular and Endovascular Surgery*, vol. 23, no. 6, pp. 486–490, 2002.

[49] G. Schindler, M. Kincius, R. Liang et al., "Fundamental efforts toward the development of a therapeutic cocktail with a manifold ameliorative effect on hepatic ischemia/reperfusion injury," *Microcirculation*, vol. 16, no. 7, pp. 593–602, 2009.

[50] G. L. Su, S. M. Goyert, M. H. Fan et al., "Activation of human and mouse Kupffer cells by lipopolysaccharide is mediated by CD14," *American Journal of Physiology*, vol. 283, no. 3, pp. 640–645, 2002.

[51] E. S. van Amersfoort, T. J. C. van Berkel, and J. Kuiper, "Receptors, mediators, and mechanisms involved in bacterial sepsis and septic shock," *Clinical Microbiology Reviews*, vol. 16, no. 3, pp. 379–414, 2003.

[52] M. van Oosten, E. van de Bilt, T. J. C. van Berkel, and J. Kuiper, "New scavenger receptor-like receptors for the binding of lipopolysaccharide to liver endothelial and Kupffer cells," *Infection and Immunity*, vol. 66, no. 11, pp. 5107–5112, 1998.

[53] A. Tsung, R. A. Hoffman, K. Izuishi et al., "Hepatic ischemia/reperfusion injury involves functional TLR4 signaling in nonparenchymal cells," *Journal of Immunology*, vol. 175, no. 11, pp. 7661–7668, 2005.

[54] B. Vollmar and M. D. Menger, "The hepatic microcirculation: mechanistic contributions and therapeutic targets in liver injury and repair," *Physiological Reviews*, vol. 89, no. 4, pp. 1269–1339, 2009.

[55] R. G. dos Santos, M. L. Viana, S. V. Generoso, R. E. Arantes, M. I. Davisson Correia, and V. N. Cardoso, "Glutamine supplementation decreases intestinal permeability and preserves gut mucosa integrity in an experimental mouse model," *Journal of Parenteral and Enteral Nutrition*, vol. 34, no. 4, pp. 408–413, 2010.

[56] J. Schroeder, B. Alteheld, P. Stehle, M. C. Cayeux, R. L. Chioléro, and M. M. Berger, "Safety and intestinal tolerance of high-dose enteral antioxidants and glutamine peptides after upper gastrointestinal surgery," *European Journal of Clinical Nutrition*, vol. 59, no. 2, pp. 307–310, 2005.

[57] M. Kul, S. Vurucu, E. Demirkaya et al., "Enteral glutamine and/or arginine supplementation have favorable effects on oxidative stress parameters in neonatal rat intestine," *Journal of Pediatric Gastroenterology and Nutrition*, vol. 49, no. 1, pp. 85–89, 2009.

[58] H. Jaeschke, "Mechanisms of liver injury. II. Mechanisms of neutrophil-induced liver cell injury during hepatic ischemia-reperfusion and other acute inflammatory conditions," *American Journal of Physiology*, vol. 290, no. 6, pp. 1083–1088, 2006.

[59] J. El-Benna, P. M. C. Dang, M. A. Gougerot-Pocidalo, and C. Elbim, "Phagocyte NADPH oxidase: a multicomponent enzyme essential for host defenses," *Archivum Immunologiae et Therapiae Experimentalis*, vol. 53, no. 3, pp. 199–206, 2005.

[60] H. Jaeschke, "Molecular mechanisms of hepatic ischemia-reperfusion injury and preconditioning," *American Journal of Physiology*, vol. 284, no. 1, pp. 15–26, 2003.

6

Glycemic Control after Total Pancreatectomy for Intraductal Papillary Mucinous Neoplasm: An Exploratory Study

Laith H. Jamil,[1] Ana M. Chindris,[2] Kanwar R. S. Gill,[1] Daniela Scimeca,[1] John A. Stauffer,[3] Michael G. Heckman,[4] Shon E. Meek,[2] Justin H. Nguyen,[5] Horacio J. Asbun,[3] Massimo Raimondo,[1] Timothy A. Woodward,[1] and Michael B. Wallace[1]

[1] Division of Gastroenterology and Hepatology, Mayo Clinic, Jacksonville, FL 32224, USA
[2] Division of Endocrinology, Mayo Clinic, Jacksonville, FL 32224, USA
[3] Department of Surgery, Mayo Clinic, Jacksonville, FL 32224, USA
[4] Biostatistics Unit, Mayo Clinic, Jacksonville, FL 32224, USA
[5] Department of Transplantation, Mayo Clinic, Jacksonville, FL 32224, USA

Correspondence should be addressed to Michael B. Wallace, wallace.michael@mayo.edu

Academic Editor: Christos G. Dervenis

Background. Glycemic control following total pancreatectomy (TP) has been thought to be difficult to manage. Diffuse intraductal papillary mucinous neoplasm (IPMN) is a potentially curable precursor to pancreatic adenocarcinoma, best treated by TP. *Objective.* Compare glycemic control in patients undergoing TP for IPMN to patients with type 1 diabetes mellitus (DM). *Design/Setting.* Retrospective cohort. *Outcome Measure.* Hemoglobin A1C(HbA1C) at 6, 12, 18, and 24 months after TP. In the control group, baseline was defined as 6 months prior to the first HbA1c measure. *Results.* Mean HgbA1C at each point of interest was similar between TP and type I DM patients (6 months (7.5% versus 7.7%, $P = 0.52$), 12 months (7.3% versus 8.0%, $P = 0.081$), 18 months (7.7% and 7.6%, $P = 0.64$), and at 24 months (7.3% versus 7.8%, $P = 0.10$)). Seven TP patients (50%) experienced a hypoglycemic event compared to 65 type 1 DM patients (65%, $P = 0.38$). *Limitations.* Small number of TP patients, retrospective design, lack of long-termfollowup. *Conclusion.* This suggests that glycemic control following TP for IPMNcan be well managed, similar to type 1 DM patients. Fear of DM following TP for IPMN should not preclude surgery when TP is indicated.

1. Introduction

Diabetes mellitus (DM) induced by total pancreatectomy (TP), often termed "Pancreatogenic Diabetes," is often thought to be difficult to manage [1–4]. The notion that TP could cause brittle diabetes in up to 25% of patients may adversely influence the decision to perform the surgery. In addition, the overall quality of life will likely be affected by such intervention [5]. More recent data suggests that glycemic control following TP may not be as challenging as initially thought [6]. Intraductal papillary mucinous neoplasm (IPMN) is a distinct pathological entity comprised of a papillary proliferation of mucin-producing epithelial cells that may produce excessive mucus and may cause cystic dilation of the pancreatic duct [7]. IPMN has a broad histological spectrum, ranging from minimal mucinous hyperplasia or adenoma to invasive carcinoma [8]. Criteria for pancreatic resections in IPMN, including TP, have been proposed [9]. IPMN involvement of the main pancreatic duct has been shown to be a risk factor for prevalent and incident cancers and therefore is a leading cause for recommending surgical resection [8]. Recent evidence reports that TP for IPMN is gaining popularity [10–14].

Many published studies evaluating glycemic control post-TP have included all patients undergoing TP regardless of etiology [5, 6]. Blanchet et al. reported a series of 10 patients in which glycemic control was achieved successfully after TP for mucinous pancreatic tumors; seven of those patients had IPMN [15].

It is unknown whether the underlying pancreatic disease has any impact on insulin production prior to TP, which may affect glycemic control after surgery.

Most studies evaluating glycemic control in these patients were performed prior to the availability of more advanced treatment modalities of DM such as insulin pumps [1–5].

The aim of this exploratory study was to evaluate glycemic control in patients undergoing TP for IPMN and compare them to a control group of patients with type 1 DM, who were being followed during the same period. This included both long-term control, through measuring HbA1c, as well as occurrence of reported glycemic control-related complications such as hypoglycemia and hyperglycemia. We also evaluated the outcome of these reported episodes. This data stemmed and was expanded from a previously published study where we examined the outcome of TP for various indications [16].

2. Methods

We performed a retrospective chart review of all patients who underwent TP for IPMN between July 2004 and July 2008 at Mayo Clinic, in Jacksonville, Florida. We identified 29 patients. Follow-up data was available in 19 patients. Patients were included if they had at least one HbA1c measurement at any of the 4 time points of interest (6 [±3], 12 [±3], 18 [±3], or 24 [±3] months after TP). Such data was available for 14 of the 29 patients (48%). Sample sizes at each of the four time points were $N = 10$, $N = 9$, $N = 7$, and $N = 6$, respectively. The date of TP was considered as the baseline time point in TP patients. Of the 14 patients included in this study, 2 had type 2 DM prior to surgery. When comparing the 14 included TP patients with the 15 patients who were excluded due to insufficient data, no significant difference regarding age at surgery, gender, weight, BMI, pancreatic enzyme supplement use, or insulin regimen was noted (all $P \geq 0.11$).

Type I DM patients were included if at baseline, which was defined as 6 months prior to the first HbA1c measure, their duration of disease was at least 2 years. HbA1c measures in controls were considered at the same four time points as the TP patients (6 [±3], 12 [±3], 18 [±3], or 24 [±3] months after baseline). We identified 366 patients with an ICD code corresponding to type 1 diabetes mellitus (medical record numbers in arithmetical order) from our outpatient clinic. We selected every 5th patient on the list; after that, we continued with every 5th patient from the remaining list and so on until we identified 100 patients that we used as controls. Patients who were found to have type 2 DM during chart review were excluded. These patients were treated in our clinic within the same timeframe as the IPMN patients, between July 2003 and July 2006 and therefore had access to the same therapeutic means as our patient population. All patients had HbA1C measured within the interval studied.

2.1. Total Pancreatectomy Insulin Regimens and Doses. All patients were started on an insulin infusion following surgery and were discharged on meal time insulin Aspart (Novo Nordisk, Bagsvaerd, DN) with a correction scale. In addition, patients were given either Recombinant Insulin Glargine (Sanofi-Aventis, Bridgewater, N.J.) (13 patients) or Insulin Detemir (Novo Nordisk, Bagsvaerd, DN) (one patient),

based on the preference of their endocrinologist. Their most current insulin regimens were Recombinant Insulin Glargine2-24 units once a day along with Insulin Aspart per sliding scale for meal coverage in 10 patients, Insulin pump in 3 patients, and Insulin Detemir12 units in the morning and four units in the evening along with Insulin Aspart per sliding scale for meal coverage in 1 patient.

2.2. Statistical Analysis. Patient characteristics at baseline were compared between TP patients and type I DM patients using a Wilcoxon rank-sum test or Fisher's exact test. In the primary analysis, we compared mean HbA1c values between TP patients and type I DM patients using a two-sample t-test separately at each time point. We also estimated the difference in mean HbA1c between groups along with a 95% confidence interval (CI). Additionally, we examined the sensitivity of the results to the adjustment for potentially confounding variables in multivariable linear regression analysis, adjusting for any variable that differed significantly ($P \leq 0.05$) between TP patients and type I DM patients. In secondary analysis, again separately at each time point, we estimated the proportion of patients with a HbA1c level of less than 7% for TP patients and type I diabetes patients using exact binomial 95% CI and compared these proportions using Fisher's exact test. We estimated the difference in this proportion between groups along with a 95% small sample CI using Newcombe's score method [17]. No adjustment for potentially confounding variables was made in this secondary analysis, owing to the limitations on the number of variables that can be reasonably adjusted for in a regression model involving a dichotomous outcome as opposed to a continuous outcome [18]. We also evaluated trends in HbA1c values over time, separately in TP and type I DM patients, using mixed effects linear regression models including a random effect for patient. P-values less than or equal to 0.05 were considered statistically significant. All statistical analyses were performed using SPLUS (version 8.0.1; Insightful Corporation, Seattle, Washington).

3. Results

3.1. Patient Characteristics. Patient characteristics at baseline for TP and type I DM patients are shown in Table 1. TP patients were older (median: 72 years versus 52 years, $P < 0.001$), while the control group had more men (52% versus 14%, $P = 0.01$), more years of education (median: 16 years versus 12 years, $P = 0.034$), and were heavier at baseline (median: 78 kg versus 60 kg, $P = 0.028$) when compared to type I DM patients. BMI was not significantly different between the two groups (median: 26 versus 24, $P = 0.47$). The median duration of disease in type I DM patients was 26 years (range: 2 years–55 years). The indication for TP was diffuse involvement of the pancreas in 11 patients and positive margins during surgery in the remaining three patients. On pathology, mucinous adenocarcinoma was noted in one patient, noninvasive carcinoma in eight patients, adenoma in four patients, and one patient had borderline findings for malignancy. None had lymphovascular invasion. There was

TABLE 1: Patient characteristics at baseline.

Variable	TP ($N = 14$)	Type I DM ($N = 100$)	P value
Age at baseline (years)	72 (57–78)	52 (21–84)	<0.001
Gender			0.010
Male	2 (14%)	52 (52%)	
Female	12 (86%)	48 (48%)	
Weight at baseline (kg)	60 (50–105)	78 (49–130)	0.028
BMI at baseline	24 (20–36)	26 (20–40)	0.47
Years of education	12 (12–17)	16 (8–18)	0.034
Pancreatic enzyme supplement	13 (93%)	N/A	N/A
Duration of disease (years)	N/A	26 (2–55)	N/A

The sample median (minimum-maximum) is given for numerical variables. Information was unavailable for years of education ($N = 9$). P-values result from a Wilcoxon rank sum test or Fisher's exact test. (TP: total pancreatectomy; DM: diabetes mellitus).

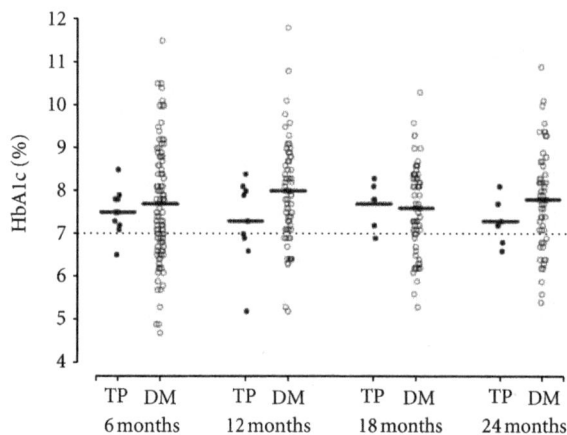

FIGURE 1: HbA1c values after baseline in TP and type I diabetes mellitus patients. The sample mean is shown with a solid horizontal line.

no recurrence of disease noted in these patients during their followup.

3.2. Glycemic Control. Mean HbA1c was similar between TP and type I DM patients at six months (7.5% versus 7.7%, $P = 0.74$), 12 months (7.3% versus 8.0%, $P = 0.11$), 18 months (7.7% and 7.6%, $P = 0.79$), and at 24 months (7.3% versus 7.8%, $P = 0.31$) (Table 2). These findings remained consistent when adjusted for age at baseline, gender, weight at baseline, and years of education (Table 2), all of which differed significantly between groups. There was no evidence of a difference in HbA1c values between the 6-month, 12-month, 18-month, and 24-month time points in TP patients ($P = 0.37$) or type I DM patients ($P = 0.46$).

Differences in the proportion of patients with an HbA1c less than 7% at each time point of interest after baseline were also not significant (all $P \geq 0.42$) between TP and control patients (10% versus 33% at 6 months, 33% versus 21% at 12 months, 14% versus 25% at 18 months, and 33% versus 28% at 24 months) (Table 3). The individual HbA1c values for TP patients and controls for the different time periods are shown in Figure 1.

3.3. Glycemic Control-Related Complications. When considering the presence of a symptomatic hypoglycemic event at any point during the study period after baseline, seven TP patients (50%) experienced a hypoglycemic episode compared to 65 type I DM patients (65%) ($P = 0.38$). Six out of seven TP patients (86%) who experienced a hypoglycemic episode treated the episode themselves at home, compared to 59 type I DM patients (91%). The remaining 6 type I DM patients (9%) received treatment at a hospital compared to 1 TP patient who required admission to the emergency room, where she was treated with intravenous Dextrose 50% and discharged home. No patient reported a hyperglycemic episode that required hospitalization or evaluation in the emergency department.

3.4. Pancreatic Insufficiency. Following hospital discharge, 13 of 14 TP patients continued on pancreatic enzyme supplements to avoid malabsorption, with its potential negative effects on glycemic control. Only two patients continued to complain of steatorrhea because of intolerance of medications (one patient) and inadequate dosing (one patient).

4. Discussion

The findings of our exploratory study suggest that glycemic control following TP may be manageable, with control and complication rates similar to that of typical type 1 DM patients who have not undergone pancreatectomy. Our focus on IPMN patients offered a more homogenous patient population with a relatively reduced list of comorbidities that could influence the results.

The endocrine abnormalities accompanying TP include both glucagon and pancreatic polypeptide (PP) deficiency in addition to insulin and thus are considered to be different than conventional type 1 and type 2 DM. TP patients have been thought to be more vulnerable to severe hypoglycemic episodes, tend to be resistant to ketosis, and have a higher plasma level of gluconeogenic precursors, which include lactate and alanine because of glucagon absence [19, 20]. As for pancreatic polypeptide, it has been suggested that it plays a key role in the induction of hepatic sensitivity to insulin and insulin receptor regulation [21, 22]. Following TP, insulin

TABLE 2: Comparison of HbA1c values after baseline between total pancreatectomy and type I diabetes mellitus patients.

Time after baseline	TP-HbA1c (%)			Type I DM-HbA1c (%)			TP-Type I DM			
							Single variable analysis*		Multivariable analysis[†]	
	Median (min–max)	Mean ± SD	N	Median (min–max)	Mean ± SD	N	Difference in means (95% CI)	P value	Difference in means (95% CI)	P value
6 months	7.5 (6.5–8.5)	7.5 ± 0.5	10	7.4 (4.7–11.5)	7.7 ± 1.4	100	−0.14 (−1.00, 0.72)	0.74	−0.05 (−1.05, 0.95)	0.93
12 months	7.3 (5.2–8.4)	7.3 ± 1.0	9	8.0 (5.2–11.8)	8.0 ± 1.2	68	−0.69 (−1.54, 0.15)	0.11	−0.67 (−1.57, 0.23)	0.14
18 months	7.8 (6.9–8.3)	7.7 ± 0.5	7	7.6 (5.3–10.3)	7.6 ± 1.0	65	0.11 (−0.69, 0.90)	0.79	−0.05 (−0.94, 0.84)	0.91
24 months	7.3 (6.6–8.1)	7.3 ± 0.6	6	7.8 (5.4–10.9)	7.8 ± 1.2	58	−0.50 (−1.47, 0.48)	0.31	−0.78 (−1.87, 0.31)	0.16

*Estimates of differences in means and P values result from a two-sample t-test. [†]Estimates of differences in means and P-values result from linear regression models adjusted for age at baseline, gender, weight, and years of education, all of which differed between TP patients and type I diabetes mellitus patients with a P-value of 0.05 or less. (TP: total pancreatectomy; DM: diabetes mellitus).

TABLE 3: Comparison of presence of HbA1c <7% after baseline between total pancreatectomy and type I diabetes mellitus patients.

Time after baseline	TP		Type I DM		TP-Type I DM	
	Fraction (%) with HbA1c <7%	95% CI	Fraction (%) with HbA1c <7%	95% CI	Difference in proportions (95% CI)	P value
6 months	1/10 (10%)	0%–45%	33/100 (33%)	24%–43%	−23% (−36%, 9%)	0.17
12 months	3/9 (33%)	7%–70%	14/68 (21%)	12%–32%	13% (−11%, 45%)	0.42
18 months	1/7 (14%)	0%–58%	16/65 (25%)	15%–37%	−10% (−27%, 28%)	1.00
24 months	2/6 (33%)	4%–78%	16/58 (28%)	17%–41%	6% (−21%, 44%)	1.00

P-values result from Fisher's exact test. (TP: total pancreatectomy; DM: diabetes mellitus).

receptors are unregulated peripherally, rendering patients uniquely sensitive to insulin replacement [23], resulting in problematic glycemic control and increased susceptibility to both hyper- and hypoglycemia.

The underlying pancreatic disease may play a role in glycemic control subsequent to TP. Previous studies have shown that patients with chronic pancreatitis tended to have a poorer diabetic outcome [24]. There has been a recent increase in performing TP for malignant diseases of the pancreas [25], benign pancreatic disease [26], patients with genetic abnormalities [27] and premalignant pancreatic disease, mainly IPMN [10–14, 28]. More recent studies looking at outcome after TP show more favorable outcome with both quality of life [5, 29] and in glycemic control [6, 15]. None of these studies focused on IPMN patients.

The improved overall results seen in the past decade may also be multifactorial. Improvements in glucose monitoring systems, insulin delivery systems, and insulin formulations may contribute to superior glycemic control for these patients [30].

Since the first description of IPMN in 1982 by Ohashi et al. [31], IPMN is being increasingly recognized in all parts of the world [32–37]. IPMN has a broad histological spectrum, ranging from minimal mucinous hyperplasia or adenoma to invasive carcinoma [12]. IPMNs are believed to have typical adenoma-carcinoma sequence. The estimated time for this progression is thought to be approximately 5 years [12]. However, it remains a difficult task to determine which IPMN may have malignancy based only on imaging characteristics. This has led to an international consensus on guidelines for management of IPMN including when surgery should be considered [9].

The frequency of malignancy (in situ and invasive) also varies, depending on the type of IPMN. In main duct IPMN, the frequency of malignancy ranges between 60 and 92%, with a mean of 70%. Approximately two-thirds of these malignant neoplasms are invasive [12, 37–44], while in branch duct IPMN, the frequency of malignancy is significantly less, ranging from 6 to 46% [12, 38–44].

One of the main reasons to consider TP in IPMN patients is the increase in survival for those with pancreatic cancer arising in the background of IPMN versus sporadic pancreatic cancer after surgical resection [8]. Another reason is the increased survival in patients with noninvasive IPMN compared to those with invasive IPMN [11, 12, 14, 28, 45, 46], where it can be as low as 24% at 2.5 years [46].

Recurrence of tumor after resection is not uncommon. In a study by Chari et al, 8% of noninvasive IPMNs recurred after partial pancreatectomy compared to none after TP [11]. Interestingly, recurrence was found to be noninvasive in three patients and invasive in two patients [11]. This is in sharp contrast to patients who had invasive IPMN, where recurrence rates after partial pancreatectomy were 67% and after TP were 62% [11]. This emphasizes the need for early detection and aggressive therapy prior to the development of invasive cancer.

Islet cell autotransplants in patients undergoing TP for chronic pancreatitis have shown to have durable function and extended insulin-independence rates, despite a lower beta-cell mass [47]. The fear of infusion of occult carcinoma cells in the islet preparation has limited the use of this procedure for patients with pancreatic adenocarcinoma, although there have been a few published case reports [48, 49]. In one study, islet cell autotransplant was performed in two patients with IPMN, one who underwent TP, and another underwent partial pancreatectomy, in which IPMN was confined to the pancreatic body on imaging, with no evidence of recurrence at one-year followup [50]. IPMN may occur within or away from the intraductal component [51] thus the multicentric nature of IPMN raises a question concerning the suitability of islet cell autotransplantation as an option in the management of these tumors.

The HbA1c levels seen in our post-TP and control patients are comparable to published studies, including those seen in patients after TP [5, 6, 29], in patients with type 1 DM [52, 53], and to type 2 DM patients in the United Kingdom Prospective Diabetes Study (UKPDS) [54].

Hypoglycemia is a feared complication of pancreatogenic diabetes, due to the loss of the counterregulatory mechanism offered by glucagon. The percentage of hypoglycemic episodes in TP patients in our study was similar to that of type 1 DM patients, and none required hospital admission.

Similar to the study by Jethwa et al. [6], we were unable to find specific reasons for why keeping diabetes under control in this group did not seem to be any more difficult than in patients with autoimmune type 1 diabetes. Better patient understanding of consequences of TP, early education on diabetes (all patients were seen by an endocrinologist immediately following their operation), advances in medical therapy, and blood glucose monitoring could all be contributory factors.

Although use of various types of insulin among patients within both groups made it impossible to make direct comparison, all regimens used were within current guidelines and had the potential to offer excellent glucose control.

Diabetes control is mainly patient driven. Excellent control has been achieved with various insulin regimens, including those used by the patients included in this study.

In addition to improved endocrine control, exocrine insufficiency may be improved by modern pancreatic enzyme formulations. This is important to avoid malabsorption, with its potential negative effects on glycemic control.

This study is not without its limitations. This is a retrospective study conducted at a single center. The length of followup was short; however, this study did not intend to assess long-term glycemic control and complications. Also, hypo- and hyperglycemia were self-reported and therefore, subject to recall bias.

The chief limitation of this study is the small sample size, particularly the small number of TP patients, which resulted in very low power to detect differences between the TP group and the type I DM patients. TP patients were included if they had HbA1c values available at any one of the four time points we considered, and thus our sample size of 14 TP patients was further reduced at each given post-TP time point. Thus, the possibility of a type II error is important to acknowledge.

5. Conclusion

These findings suggest that glycemic control following TP for IPMN can be well managed and controlled with a variety of insulin therapy regimens. If these findings are validated in a prospective study that involves a larger number of TP patients, implications are that fear of DM following TP for IPMN should not preclude surgery.

6. Study Highlights

(1) What is the current knowledge.

Glycemic control following total pancreatectomy has been thought to be difficult to manage with potential life-threatening complications.

(2) What is new here.

(a) Glycemic control following total pancreatectomy for intraductal papillary mucinous neoplasm can be well managed and controlled with a variety of insulin therapy regimens.

(b) The mean HbA1c was similar between patient undergoing total pancreatectomy for intraductal papillary mucinous neoplasm and type I DM patients.

References

[1] T. Kiviluoto, T. Schroder, and S. L. Karonen, "Glycemic control and serum lipoproteins after total pancreatectomy," *Annals of Clinical Research*, vol. 17, no. 3, pp. 110–115, 1985.

[2] C. M. Dresler, J. G. Fortner, K. McDermott, and D. R. Bajorunas, "Metabolic consequences of (regional) total pancreatectomy," *Annals of Surgery*, vol. 214, no. 2, pp. 131–140, 1991.

[3] F. Duron and J. J. Duron, "Pancreatectomy and diabetes," *Annales de Chirurgie*, vol. 53, no. 5, pp. 406–411, 1999.

[4] A. Sauvanet, "Functional results of pancreatic surgery," *Revue du Praticien*, vol. 52, no. 14, pp. 1572–1575, 2002.

[5] B. J. Billings, J. D. Christein, W. S. Harmsen et al., "Quality-of-life after total pancreatectomy: is it really that bad on long-term follow-up?" *Journal of Gastrointestinal Surgery*, vol. 9, no. 8, pp. 1059–1067, 2005.

[6] P. Jethwa, M. Sodergren, A. Lala et al., "Diabetic control after total pancreatectomy," *Digestive and Liver Disease*, vol. 38, no. 6, pp. 415–419, 2006.

[7] G. Kloppel, D. Longnecker, C. Capella, and L. Sobin, *Histological Typing of Tumors of the Exocrine Pancreas*, World Health Organization International, 2nd edition, 1996.

[8] T. A. Sohn, C. J. Yeo, J. L. Cameron, C. A. Iacobuzio-Donahue, R. H. Hruban, and K. D. Lillemoe, "Intraductal papillary mucinous neoplasms of the pancreas: an increasingly recognized clinicopathologic entity," *Annals of Surgery*, vol. 234, no. 3, pp. 313–322, 2001.

[9] M. Tanaka, S. Chari, V. Adsay et al., "International consensus guidelines for management of intraductal papillary mucinous neoplasms and mucinous cystic neoplasms of the pancreas," *Pancreatology*, vol. 6, no. 1-2, pp. 17–32, 2006.

[10] J. Bendix Holme, N. O. Jacobsen, M. Rokkjaer, and A. Kruse, "Total pancreatectomy in six patients with intraductal papillary mucinous tumour of the pancreas: the treatment of choice," *Journal of the International Hepato Pancreato Biliary*, vol. 3, no. 4, pp. 257–262, 2001.

[11] S. T. Chari, D. Yadav, T. C. Smyrk et al., "Study of recurrence after surgical resection of intraductal papillary mucinous neoplasm of the pancreas," *Gastroenterology*, vol. 123, no. 5, pp. 1500–1507, 2002.

[12] T. A. Sohn, C. J. Yeo, J. L. Cameron et al., "Intraductal papillary mucinous neoplasms of the pancreas: an updated experience," *Annals of Surgery*, vol. 239, no. 6, pp. 788–799, 2004.

[13] K. Yamaguchi, H. Konomi, K. Kobayashi et al., "Total pancreatectomy for intraductal papillary-mucinous tumor of the pancreas: reappraisal of total pancreatectomy," *Hepato-Gastroenterology*, vol. 52, no. 65, pp. 1585–1590, 2005.

[14] A. D. Yang, L. G. Melstrom, D. J. Bentrem et al., "Outcomes after pancreatectomy for intraductal papillary mucinous neoplasms of the pancreas: an institutional experience," *Surgery*, vol. 142, no. 4, pp. 529–537, 2007.

[15] M. C. Blanchet, F. Andreelli, J. Y. Scoazec et al., "Total pancreatectomy for mucin-producing tumor of the pancreas," *Annales de Chirurgie*, vol. 127, no. 6, pp. 439–448, 2002.

[16] J. A. Shtauffer, J. H. Nguyen, M. G. Heckman et al., "Patient outcomes after total pancreatectomy: a single centre contemporary experience," *Journal of the International Hepato Pancreato Biliary*, vol. 11, no. 6, pp. 483–492, 2009.

[17] R. G. Newcombe, "Interval estimation for the difference between independent proportions: comparison of eleven methods," *Statistics in Medicine*, vol. 17, no. 8, pp. 873–890, 1998.

[18] F. E. Harrell Jr., *Regression Modeling Strategies: With Application to Linear Models, Logistic Regression, and Survival Analysis*, 2001.

[19] R. H. Unger, "Glucagon physiology and pathophysiology," *The New England Journal of Medicine*, vol. 285, no. 8, pp. 443–449, 1971.

[20] H. Karmann, F. Laurent, and P. Mialhe, "Pancreatic hormones disappearance after total pancreatectomy in the duck: correlation between plasma glucagon and glucose," *Hormone and Metabolic Research*, vol. 19, no. 11, pp. 538–541, 1987.

[21] N. E. Seymour, C. Brunicardi, R. L. Chaiken et al., "Reversal of abnormal glucose production after pancreatic resection by pancreatic polypeptide administration in man," *Surgery*, vol. 104, no. 2, pp. 119–129, 1988.

[22] L. A. Slezak and D. K. Andersen, "Pancreatic resection: effects on glucose metabolism," *World Journal of Surgery*, vol. 25, no. 4, pp. 452–460, 2001.

[23] R. Nosadini, S. Del Prato, A. Tiengo et al., "Insulin sensitivity, binding, and kinetics in pancreatogenic and type I diabetes," *Diabetes*, vol. 31, no. 4, part 1, pp. 346–355, 1982.

[24] F. P. Gall, C. Gebhardt, and H. Zirngibl, "Chronic pancreatitis, results in 116 consecutive partial duodenopancreatectomies combined with occlusion of the pancreatic duct," *Fortschritte der Medizin*, vol. 99, no. 47-48, pp. 1967–1972, 1981.

[25] H. Nathan, C. L. Wolfgang, B. H. Edil et al., "Peri-operative mortality and long-term survival after total pancreatectomy for pancreatic adenocarcinoma: a population-based perspective," *Journal of Surgical Oncology*, vol. 99, no. 2, pp. 87–92, 2009.

[26] G. Garcea, J. Weaver, J. Phillips et al., "Total pancreatectomy with and without islet cell transplantation for chronic pancreatitis: a series of 85 consecutive patients," *Pancreas*, vol. 38, no. 1, pp. 1–7, 2009.

[27] D. K. Bartsch, "Familial pancreatic cancer," *British Journal of Surgery*, vol. 90, no. 4, pp. 386–387, 2003.

[28] S. C. Kim, K. T. Park, Y. J. Lee et al., "Intraductal papillary mucinous neoplasm of the pancreas: clinical characteristics and treatment outcomes of 118 consecutive patients from a single center," *Journal of Hepato-Biliary-Pancreatic Surgery*, vol. 15, no. 2, pp. 183–188, 2008.

[29] M. W. Müller, H. Friess, J. Kleeff et al., "Is there still a role for total pancreatectomy?" *Annals of Surgery*, vol. 246, no. 6, pp. 966–974, 2007.

[30] D. G. Heidt, C. Burant, and D. M. Simeone, "Total pancreatectomy: indications, operative technique, and postoperative sequelae," *Journal of Gastrointestinal Surgery*, vol. 11, no. 2, pp. 209–216, 2007.

[31] K. Ohashi, Y. Murakami, and M. Maruyama, "Four cases of mucin producing cancer of the pancreas on specific findings of the papilla of Vater," *Digestive Endoscopy*, vol. 20, pp. 348–351, 1982.

[32] Y. Itai, K. Ohhashi, and H. Nagai, "'Ductectatic' mucinous cystadenoma and cystadenocarcinoma of the pancreas," *Radiology*, vol. 161, no. 3, pp. 697–700, 1986.

[33] M. Yamada, S. Kozuka, K. Yamao, S. Nakazawa, Y. Naitoh, and Y. Tsukamoto, "Mucin-producing tumor of the pancreas," *Cancer*, vol. 68, no. 1, pp. 159–168, 1991.

[34] K. Yamaguchi, Y. Ogawa, K. Chljiiwa, and M. Tanaka, "Mucin-hypersecreting tumors of the pancreas: assessing the grade of malignancy preoperatively," *American Journal of Surgery*, vol. 171, no. 4, pp. 427–431, 1996.

[35] E. V. Loftus Jr., B. A. Olivares-Pakzad, K. P. Batts et al., "Intraductal papillary-mucinous tumors of the pancreas: clinicopathologic features, outcome, and nomenclature," *Gastroenterology*, vol. 110, no. 6, pp. 1909–1918, 1996.

[36] M. Sugiyama, Y. Atomi, and J. Hachiya, "Intraductal papillary tumors of the pancreas: evaluation with magnetic resonance cholangiopancreatography," *American Journal of Gastroenterology*, vol. 93, no. 2, pp. 156–159, 1998.

[37] R. Salvia, C. Fernández-Del Castillo, C. Bassi et al., "Main-duct intraductal papillary mucinous neoplasms of the pancreas: clinical predictors of malignancy and long-term survival following resection," *Annals of Surgery*, vol. 239, no. 5, pp. 678–687, 2004.

[38] M. Kobari, S. I. Egawa, K. Shibuya et al., "Intraductal papillary mucinous tumors of the pancreas comprise 2 clinical subtypes. Differences in clinical characteristics and surgical management," *Archives of Surgery*, vol. 134, no. 10, pp. 1131–1136, 1999.

[39] B. Terris, P. Ponsot, F. Paye et al., "Intraductal papillary mucinous tumors of the pancreas confined to secondary ducts show less aggressive pathologic features as compared with those involving the main pancreatic duct," *American Journal of Surgical Pathology*, vol. 24, no. 10, pp. 1372–1377, 2000.

[40] R. Doi, K. Fujimoto, M. Wada, and M. Imamura, "Surgical management of intraductal papillary mucinous tumor of the pancreas," *Surgery*, vol. 132, no. 1, pp. 80–85, 2002.

[41] T. Matsumoto, M. Aramaki, K. Yada et al., "Optimal management of the branch duct type intraductal papillary mucinous neoplasms of the pancreas," *Journal of Clinical Gastroenterology*, vol. 36, no. 3, pp. 261–265, 2003.

[42] B. S. Choi, T. K. Kim, A. Y. Kim et al., "Differential diagnosis of benign and malignant intraductal papillary mucinous tumors of the pancreas: MR cholangiopancreatography and MR angiography," *Korean Journal of Radiology*, vol. 4, no. 3, pp. 157–162, 2003.

[43] Y. Kitagawa, T. A. Unger, S. Taylor et al., "Mucus is a predictor of better prognosis and survival in patients with intraductal papillary mucinous tumor of the pancreas," *Journal of Gastrointestinal Surgery*, vol. 7, no. 1, pp. 12–18, 2003.

[44] M. Sugiyama, Y. Izumisato, N. Abe, T. Masaki, T. Mori, and Y. Atomi, "Predictive factors for malignancy in intraductal papillary-mucinous tumours of the pancreas," *British Journal of Surgery*, vol. 90, no. 10, pp. 1244–1249, 2003.

[45] C. P. Raut, K. R. Cleary, G. A. Staerkel et al., "Intraductal papillary mucinous neoplasms of the pancreas: effect of invasion and pancreatic margin status on recurrence and survival," *Annals of Surgical Oncology*, vol. 13, no. 4, pp. 582–594, 2006.

[46] M. Raimondo, I. Tachibana, R. Urrutia, L. J. Burgart, and E. P. DiMagno, "Invasive cancer and survival of intraductal papillary mucinous tumors of the pancreas," *American Journal of Gastroenterology*, vol. 97, no. 10, pp. 2553–2558, 2002.

[47] D. E. R. Sutherland, A. C. Gruessner, A. M. Carlson et al., "Islet autotransplant outcomes after total pancreatectomy: a contrast to islet allograft outcomes," *Transplantation*, vol. 86, no. 12, pp. 1799–1802, 2008.

[48] S. Förster, X. Liu, U. Adam, W. D. Schareck, and U. T. Hopt, "Islet autotransplantation combined with pancreatectomy for treatment of pancreatic adenocarcinoma: a case report," *Transplantation Proceedings*, vol. 36, no. 4, pp. 1125–1126, 2004.

[49] F. Alsaif, M. Molinari, A. Al-Masloom, J. R. T. Lakey, T. Kin, and A. M. J. Shapiro, "Pancreatic islet autotransplantation with completion pancreatectomy in the management of uncontrolled pancreatic fistula after whipple resection for ampullary adenocarcinoma," *Pancreas*, vol. 32, no. 4, pp. 430–431, 2006.

[50] B. W. Lee, J. H. Jee, J. S. Heo et al., "The favorable outcome of human islet transplantation in Korea: experiences of 10 autologous transplantations," *Transplantation*, vol. 79, no. 11, pp. 1568–1574, 2005.

[51] S. Miyakawa, A. Horiguchi, M. Hayakawa et al., "Intraductal papillary adenocarcinoma with mucin hypersecretion and coexistent invasive ductal carcinoma of the pancreas with apparent topographic separation," *Journal of Gastroenterology*, vol. 31, no. 6, pp. 889–893, 1996.

[52] R. P. L. M. Hoogma, P. J. Hammond, R. Gomis et al., "Comparison of the effects of continuous subcutaneous insulin infusion (CSII) and NPH-based multiple daily insulin injections (MDI) on glycaemic control and quality of life: results of the 5-nations trial," *Diabetic Medicine*, vol. 23, no. 2, pp. 141–147, 2006.

[53] D. Bruttomesso, D. Crazzolara, A. Maran et al., "In Type 1 diabetic patients with good glycaemic control, blood glucose variability is lower during continuous subcutaneous insulin infusion than during multiple daily injections with insulin glargine," *Diabetic Medicine*, vol. 25, no. 3, pp. 326–332, 2008.

[54] "Intensive blood-glucose control with sulphonylureas or insulin compared with conventional treatment and risk of complications in patients with type 2 diabetes (UKPDS 33). UK Prospective Diabetes Study (UKPDS) Group," *The Lancet*, vol. 352, no. 9131, pp. 837–853, 1998.

7

Renal Dysfunction Is an Independent Risk Factor for Mortality after Liver Resection and the Main Determinant of Outcome in Posthepatectomy Liver Failure

M. G. Wiggans,[1,2] **G. Shahtahmassebi,**[3] **M. J. Bowles,**[1] **S. Aroori,**[1] **and D. A. Stell**[1,2]

[1] Hepatobiliary Surgery, Plymouth Hospitals NHS Trust, Derriford Hospital, Derriford Road, Plymouth, Devon PL6 8DH, UK
[2] Peninsula College of Medicine and Dentistry, University of Exeter and Plymouth University, John Bull Building, Plymouth, Devon PL6 8BU, UK
[3] School of Science and Technology, Nottingham Trent University, Nottingham NG1 4BU, UK

Correspondence should be addressed to D. A. Stell; david.stell@nhs.net

Academic Editor: Vito R. Cicinnati

Introduction. The aim of this study was to assess the interaction of liver and renal dysfunction as risk factors for mortality after liver resection. *Materials and Methods.* A retrospective analysis of 501 patients undergoing liver resection in a single unit was undertaken. Posthepatectomy liver failure (PHLF) was defined according to the International Study Group of Liver Surgery (ISGLS) definition (assessed on day 5) and renal dysfunction according to RIFLE criteria. 90-day mortality was recorded. *Results.* Twenty-three patients died within 90 days of surgery (4.6%). The lowest mortality occurred in patients without evidence of PHLF or renal dysfunction (2.7%). The mortality rate in patients with isolated PHLF or renal dysfunction was 20% compared to 45% in patients with both. Diabetes ($P = 0.028$), renal dysfunction ($P = 0.030$), and PHLF on day 5 ($P = 0.011$) were independent predictors of 90-day mortality. *Discussion.* PHLF and postoperative renal dysfunction are independent predictors of 90-day mortality following liver resection but the predictive value for mortality is significantly higher when failure of both organ systems occurs simultaneously.

1. Introduction

Despite advances in both operative technique and perioperative care liver resection is associated with mortality rates of 0 to 22% (median 3.7%) and morbidity rates of 12.5% to 66% (median 36%) [1] including liver [2, 3] and renal dysfunction [4]. Liver dysfunction is a major contributor to both morbidity and mortality with an incidence between 1.2% and 32% in published series [5–12]. Renal dysfunction has also been shown to be associated with mortality following liver resection [13], with a reported incidence between 5 and 15% [4, 14]. Posthepatectomy renal failure may occur in conjunction with liver failure when maldistributive circulatory changes occur causing intravascular hypovolaemia [4, 15] but is also related to operative stress and blood loss [16, 17].

Postoperative liver dysfunction has been defined by the "50-50 criteria" as a prothrombin index of less than 50% (mean normal prothrombin time (PT) divided by patient's observed PT) and a serum bilirubin of >50 μmol/L on the fifth postoperative day, which has been shown to predict liver failure and death after hepatectomy [2]. More recently posthepatectomy liver failure (PHLF) has been defined by the International Study Group of Liver Surgery (ISGLS) as a postoperatively acquired deterioration in the ability of the liver to maintain its synthetic, excretory, and detoxifying functions, characterized by an increased INR (or need of clotting factors to maintain normal INR) and hyperbilirubinaemia on or after postoperative day five [18]. The ability of this newer definition of PHLF, using lower measures of dysfunction, to predict mortality has not been thoroughly assessed.

The aim of this study was to assess the utility of the ISGLS definition of PHLF on postoperative day 5 as a predictor of mortality and to determine the interaction of liver and renal dysfunction in predicting 90-day mortality after liver resection.

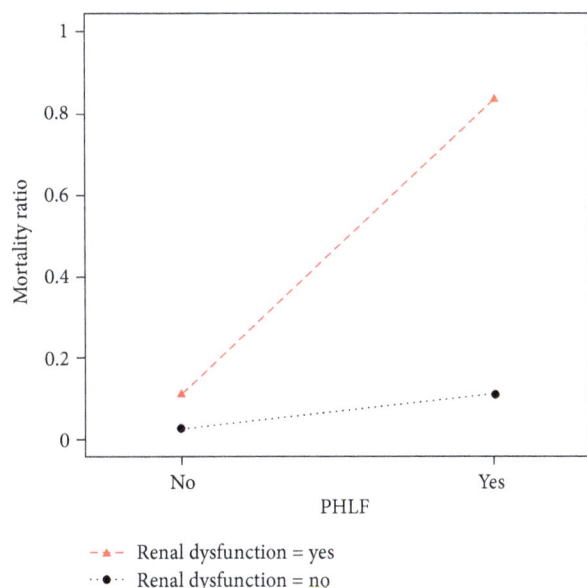

FIGURE 1: Mortality ratio of combined liver and renal dysfunction in 495 patients undergoing liver resection.

2. Materials and Methods

A retrospective analysis of a prospectively maintained database of all patients undergoing liver resection in this unit between July 2005 and September 2012 was undertaken. Five hundred and one patients were studied. Patient characteristics, laboratory data, and intraoperative details were retrieved. Liver resections were defined according to the Brisbane classification [19] and undertaken using standard techniques. Prior to resection the operating surgeon makes a visual assessment of the condition of the liver parenchyma and records this as normal or abnormal. Hepatic inflow occlusion was used in a minority of cases where there was excessive blood loss. The POSSUM scoring system was used to calculate the preoperative physiological risk score [20].

All patients were followed up for a minimum of 90 days and mortality was recorded along with details of the cause of death. The cause of death was determined from case-sheet review, radiological and laboratory data, and death certificates. Patients who died with jaundice and/or radiological evidence of ascites and/or encephalopathy in the absence of any other clear diagnosis were determined to have died of liver failure. Patients who died within 24 hours of surgery were excluded from further analysis as these deaths were most likely due to perioperative complications. Patients were also excluded if no postoperative blood tests were available.

Serum biochemistry tests and coagulation assays were performed on patients in the first 24 postoperative hours and the tests repeated according to clinical course. The peak measurement of bilirubin, prothrombin time (PT), and creatinine were recorded and used for analysis and patients with PHLF were identified as having an increased PT and serum bilirubin on postoperative day five according to the ISGLS definition [18]. In patients with preoperatively increased PT or serum bilirubin concentration PHLF was defined as an

TABLE 1: Preoperative and intraoperative characteristics of 501 patients undergoing hepatic resection.

$n = 501$	Median (range)	Count (%)
Age	65 (21–90)	
Gender		
Female		223 (45)
Male		278 (55)
Indication for surgery		
Benign		46 (9)
Primary		
Hepatocellular carcinoma		39 (8)
Cholangiocarcinoma		31 (6)
Others		28 (6)
Secondary		
Colorectal metastases		308 (61)
Other metastases		49 (10)
Liver directed chemotherapy		
Yes		176 (35)
No		325 (65)
Diabetes		
Yes		55 (11)
No		446 (89)
BMI	26 (16–54)	
ASA Grade		
1		51 (10)
2		323 (64)
3		124 (25)
4		2 (0.4)
Not recorded		1 (0.2)
Physiologic risk score	16 (12–32)	
Operative risk score	24 (14–35)	
Estimated P-POSSUM mortality (%)	7.7 (0.9–69.3)	
Confirmed fibrosis/cirrhosis		
Yes		22 (4)
No		479 (96)
Preoperative bilirubin (μmol/L)	9 (2–162)	
Preoperative haemoglobin (g/dL)	13.2 (8.6–17.0)	
Preoperative white cell count (/L)	6.9 (2.7–25.0)	
Preoperative albumin (g/L)	44 (24–53)	
Preoperative alkaline phosphatase (U/L)	95 (34–1190)	
Preoperative creatinine (μmol/L)	78 (40–430)	
Preoperative glomerular filtration rate (GFR)		
>90 mL/min		163 (33)

TABLE 1: Continued.

$n = 501$	Median (range)	Count (%)
<90 mL/min		326 (65)
Not measured		12 (2)
Preoperative neutrophil lymphocyte ratio (NLR)	2.5 (0.3–17.3)	
NLR > 5		
Yes		59 (12)
No		442 (88)
Open or laparoscopic approach		
Open		453 (90)
Laparoscopic		48 (10)
Radio frequency ablation (RFA) included		
Yes		23 (5)
No		478 (95)
Wedge resection included		
Yes		189 (38)
No		312 (62)
Operation		
Right hemihepatectomy		173 (35)
Extended right hemihepatectomy		34 (7)
Left hemihepatectomy		64 (13)
Extended left hemihepatectomy		17 (3)
Left lateral sectorectomy		48 (10)
Wedge resection only		133 (27)
Other		32 (6)
Bile duct reconstruction included		
Yes		46 (9)
No		455 (91)
Synchronous bowel procedure		
Yes		23 (5)
No		478 (95)
Operation number		
1st resection		465 (93)
2nd resection		31 (6)
3rd resection		5 (1)
Number of segments resected	4 (1–6)	
Number of procedures	1 (1–10)	
Surgeon's assessment of liver parenchyma		
Normal		323 (64)
Abnormal		171 (34)
Not recorded		7 (1)
Blood loss		

TABLE 1: Continued.

$n = 501$	Median (range)	Count (%)
<500 mL		246 (49)
500–999 mL		175 (35)
≥1000 mL		76 (15)
Not recorded		4 (0.8)
Units transfused	0 (0–26)	

increasing serum bilirubin concentration and increasing PT on postoperative day 5 compared with the values of the previous day. It was not necessary to administer clotting factors to any surviving patients between postoperative days (POD) 1–5. Renal dysfunction was defined as an increase in serum creatinine of ≥1.5-fold from the preoperative baseline within the first five postoperative days, according to RIFLE criteria [21].

To determine potential associations between patient characteristics, operative factors, and organ dysfunction with 90-day mortality univariate logistic regression or chi-square test at the level of $P < 0.25$ [22] was performed, as appropriate. Significant variables in the univariate analysis were included in the multivariate logistic regression model and were considered to be significant if $P < 0.05$. Mortality ratios for organ failure were calculated as the proportion of deaths to proportion of survivors. All analyses were carried out using the statistical package R 2.1.14 [23].

3. Results

Five hundred one patients were studied. The indications for surgery and preoperative and operative details are shown in Table 1. Two patients who died within 24 hours of surgery were excluded from further analysis. One patient died of heart failure after a partially extended right hepatectomy and one died of biliary sepsis and multiorgan failure following an extended right hepatectomy for hilar cholangiocarcinoma. Details of twenty-one patients (4.6%) who died within 90 days of surgery are shown in Table 2. There was no significant difference in the median age of patients who died (71 years) and those who survived (65 years). The median interval to death after surgery was 31 days (7–89 days).

Of the 499 patients studied, blood tests were available in 495 patients (99.2%). Four patients did not have postoperative blood tests, all of whom had minor resections (fewer than three segments) and none of whom died within the study period and were excluded from analysis. A summary of liver and renal function tests in the whole cohort is shown in Table 3 along with the associated mortality.

PHLF occurred in 31 patients of whom two had preexisting liver failure and 12 had extended resections. Seven patients in this group died within 90 days of surgery. Renal dysfunction also occurred in 31 patients, of whom 11 had extended resections. Seven patients in this group died within 90 days of surgery. In 55 patients with diabetes mellitus renal dysfunction occurred in seven patients (12.7%) compared to

TABLE 2: Details of 21 patients who died within 90 days of surgery. (Two patients who died within 24 hours of surgery were excluded.)

Cause of death	Count	Gender		Age	Right hepatectomy	Extended right	Extended left	Minor resection	Interval to death (days)
		Male	Female						
Liver failure	11	9	2	67 (58–76)	3	7	1	0	31 (11–83)
Malignancy	4	2	2	58 (43–76)	2	1	0	1	68.5 (14–86)
Sepsis	1	1	0	71	0	1	0	0	15
PE	1	1	0	71	1	0	0	0	7
Anastomotic leak	1	1	0	80	0	0	0	1	8
Peptic ulcer	1	0	1	81	1	0	0	0	22
Strangulated hernia	1	1	0	76	0	0	0	1	89
Peritonitis	1	1	0	76	0	0	0	1	70

TABLE 3: Postoperative liver and renal dysfunction in 495 patients undergoing hepatic resection (blood tests not performed in four patients).

Laboratory parameters at day 5 ($n = 495$)	Count (%)	90-day mortality (%)	Death due to liver failure
No PHLF or renal dysfunction	444 (89.7)	12 (2.7)	4
PHLF alone	20 (4.0)	2 (10)	2
Renal dysfunction alone	20 (4.0)	2 (10)	2
Renal dysfunction plus PHLF	11 (2.2)	5 (45.5)	3

24 of 440 patients without diabetes (5.5%) ($P = 0.067$). No patient with diabetes and normal preoperative renal function ($n = 12$) developed postoperative renal dysfunction compared to seven of 43 diabetic patients with impaired preoperative renal function ($P = 0.326$).

The lowest mortality (2.7%) occurred in the 444 patients without laboratory evidence of PHLF or renal dysfunction at day five, of whom 12 died, compared to 9 of 51 (17.6%) patients with either or both of these diagnoses. In the first group four of the twelve deaths were due to liver failure compared to seven of the nine deaths in the group with evidence of organ dysfunction at POD 5.

The mortality rate in patients who fulfilled the criteria for PHLF on POD 5 but did not have renal dysfunction was identical (2 of 10 patients) to that of patients with renal dysfunction without PHLF (2 of 10 patients). All four of these patients died of liver failure. Mortality was greatest in the group of eleven patients with both PHLF and renal dysfunction of whom five died. Three of these five patients died of liver failure, one from anastomotic leak, and one from a bleeding peptic ulcer.

Multivariate analysis of potential risk factors for mortality including postoperative organ dysfunction (Table 4) revealed that the only preoperative factor independently associated with 90-day mortality was the presence of diabetes ($P = 0.028$), which more than trebled the risk of 90-day mortality.

Both PHLF on POD 5 and postoperative renal dysfunction were independently associated with 90-day mortality. PHLF at POD 5 increased the risk of 90-day mortality by a factor of 4.5 ($P = 0.011$) and renal dysfunction increased the risk by a factor of 3.6 ($P = 0.030$).

The positive predictive value (PPV) for mortality in patients who fulfilled the criteria for PHLF (including those with and without renal dysfunction) was 22.6%. However within this group the PPV was much lower (10%) if the criteria for PLF were fulfilled with normal renal function (Table 5). The PPV for mortality of fulfilling the criteria for PHLF with concurrent renal dysfunction was 45%.

The effect of developing renal dysfunction in the context of PHLF is demonstrated by the greater than fourfold increase in mortality ratio (Figure 1).

4. Discussion

The principle findings of this study are that PHLF on POD 5 as defined by the ISGLS and postoperative renal dysfunction are independent predictors of 90-day mortality following liver resection. The predictive value for mortality is significantly higher when failure of both organs occurs, with a PPV of 45% and NPV of 97%. Preoperative diabetes mellitus is also an independent predictor of 90-day mortality.

The 90-day mortality (4.6%) in this series is similar to results of other units [1]. An important observation is that half the postoperative deaths in the series occurred between 31 and 90 days after surgery, stressing the importance of reporting 90-day rather than 30-day mortality. Of the 21 postoperative deaths 11 were found to be due to liver failure.

The study confirms the ability of PHLF to predict 90-day mortality. Interestingly however the majority of patients who developed PHLF at POD 5 (24 of 31) recovered whilst six of the eleven patients who died of liver failure did not fulfil the ISGLS definition of PHLF at POD 5. Only one patient in this series fulfilled the "50-50 criteria" of postoperative liver dysfunction, who subsequently recovered. Therefore the "50-50" criteria had no value as a predictor of liver failure or mortality in this series with a PPV of zero. In comparison the ISGLS definition of PHLF has lower thresholds for abnormal bilirubin and PT and is a more clinically useful tool for

TABLE 4: Univariate and multivariate analysis of preoperative and operative factors as well as postoperative blood tests associated with 90-day mortality following liver resection in 495 patients.

n = 495 Factor (preoperative and operative factors and postoperative blood tests)	Univariate		Multivariate	
	Coef (95% CI)	P value	Coef (95% CI)	P value
Age	1.05 (1.01–1.10)	0.029*		0.194
Gender	2.36 (0.91–6.08)	0.077*		0.196
Pathology		0.274		
Liver directed chemotherapy		0.356		
Diabetic	3.09 (1.16–8.20)	0.024*	3.41 (1.14–10.23)	0.028**
BMI		0.444		
ASA grade				
1 versus 2	3.02 (0.70–13.11)	0.139*		0.678
2 versus 3		0.724		
Physiologic score	1.12 (1.03–1.22)	0.010*		0.544
Operative score		0.303		
P-POSSUM mortality	1.04 (1.01–1.07)	0.010*		0.479
Fibrosis/cirrhosis		0.986		
Preoperative bilirubin	1.01 (1.00–1.03)	0.081*		0.652
Preoperative haemoglobin	0.71 (0.55–0.93)	0.012*		0.195
Preoperative white cell count		0.388		
Preoperative albumin	0.90 (0.84–0.96)	0.002*		0.168
Preoperative alkaline phosphatase		0.884		
Preoperative creatinine	1.01 (1.00–1.02)	0.098*		0.764
Preoperative neutrophil lymphocyte ratio	1.13 (0.98–1.31)	0.086*		0.366
Preoperative neutrophil lymphocyte ratio >5	2.18 (0.78–6.11)	0.138*		0.345
Open or laparoscopic resection		0.987		
Radiofrequency ablation (RFA) included		0.991		
Wedge resection included		0.588		
Bile duct reconstruction included	2.96 (1.05–8.39)	0.041*		0.383
Synchronous bowel procedure		0.346		
Operation number		0.549		
Number of segments resected	1.59 (1.18–2.14)	0.003*		0.075
Number of procedures		0.786		
Surgeons assessment of liver parenchyma	2.14 (0.92–4.96)	0.076*		0.494
Blood loss (mL)				
<500 versus >500	2.67 (1.27–5.61)	0.009*		0.716
>500 versus >1000		0.652		
Units of red cells transfused	1.13 (1.02–1.26)	0.023*		0.224
PHLF at POD 5	1.02 (1.01–1.03)	<0.001*	4.51 (1.42–14.40)	0.011**
Renal dysfunction (creatinine rise >1.5x)	1.02 (1.01–1.03)	<0.001*	3.63 (1.13–11.66)	0.030**

*Significant at the level of 0.25 for univariate analysis and included in multivariate analysis.
**Significant at the level of 0.05 for multivariate analysis.

the prediction of 90-day mortality with a PPV of 23% and NPV 97%. This is similar to the findings of the only other study to address this issue, which revealed that the PPV and NPV of PHLF were 32% and 98%, respectively [24]. Simple blood tests therefore have a low positive predictive value for mortality due to liver failure.

Renal dysfunction occurred in 6.3% of patients which is similar to other published series [4, 14]. Renal dysfunction

TABLE 5: Predictive values of PHLF and renal dysfunction within the first five postoperative days in 495 patients undergoing liver resection.

	Positive predictive value (PPV)	Negative predictive value (NPV)
No PHLF or renal dysfunction	0.027	0.824
PHLF alone	0.1	0.970
Renal dysfunction alone	0.1	0.970
PHLF and renal dysfunction	0.455	0.967

following liver resection may occur as a consequence of liver failure and hepatorenal syndrome but may also result from hypovolaemia or damage from inflammatory mediators during surgery [4]. This occurs more commonly in elderly patients with atherosclerosis or hypertension [15]. These mechanisms of renal dysfunction may occur simultaneously. The use of low central venous pressure (CVP) during resection may also increase the risk of postoperative renal dysfunction [25, 26]. The results of this study demonstrate that isolated renal dysfunction is a significant risk factor for mortality independent of the development of PHLF. Interestingly the two patients with isolated renal dysfunction in the first five postoperative days subsequently died of liver failure. This may be attributed to renal dysfunction delaying the onset of hepatic regeneration [27]. The most marked mortality effect of renal dysfunction was seen in conjunction with PHLF, where the mortality rate increased by a factor of four. Therefore, although the ISGLS definition of PHLF is able to predict mortality due to liver failure the development of renal dysfunction in this context is the single most important predictive factor.

The finding of the significance of diabetes as a risk factor for postoperative mortality confirms earlier findings [28]. Insulin is important for hepatic function and regeneration [29] and diabetes is also a risk factor for the development of nonalcoholic fatty liver disease and cirrhosis [30] which may lead to higher rates of PHLF [31]. Diabetic nephropathy is also a major cause of renal dysfunction [32].

In conclusion we have demonstrated that PHLF as defined by the ISGLS on postoperative day five and postoperative renal dysfunction are able to predict 90-day mortality following liver resection, although most patients fulfilling these criteria of organ dysfunction will recover. In addition many patients will succumb to liver failure without fulfilling the PHLF criteria in the early postoperative period. The combination of these two markers of organ dysfunction is the best early predictor of mortality following liver resection and we suggest that PHLF and postoperative renal dysfunction should be used in conjunction when predicting mortality after liver resection.

References

[1] C. D. Mann, T. Palser, C. D. Briggs et al., "A review of factors predicting perioperative death and early outcome in hepatopancreaticobiliary cancer surgery," *HPB*, vol. 12, no. 6, pp. 380–388, 2010.

[2] S. Balzan, J. Belghiti, O. Farges et al., "The "50-50 criteria" on postoperative day 5: an accurate predictor of liver failure and death after hepatectomy," *Annals of Surgery*, vol. 242, no. 6, pp. 824–829, 2005.

[3] T. Schreckenbach, J. Liese, W. O. Bechstein, and C. Moench, "Posthepatectomy liver failure," *Digestive Surgery*, vol. 29, no. 1, pp. 79–85, 2012.

[4] F. Saner, "Kidney failure following liver resection," *Transplantation Proceedings*, vol. 40, no. 4, pp. 1221–1224, 2008.

[5] M. A. J. van den Broek, S. W. M. O. Damink, C. H. C. Dejong et al., "Liver failure after partial hepatic resection: definition, pathophysiology, risk factors and treatment," *Liver International*, vol. 28, no. 6, pp. 767–780, 2008.

[6] O. Farges, B. Malassagne, J. F. Flejou, S. Balzan, A. Sauvanet, and J. Belghiti, "Risk of major liver resection in patients with underlying chronic liver disease: a reappraisal," *Annals of Surgery*, vol. 229, no. 2, pp. 210–215, 1999.

[7] J. Belghiti, K. Hiramatsu, S. Benoist, P. P. Massault, A. Sauvanet, and O. Farges, "Seven hundred forty-seven hepatectomies in the 1990s: an update to evaluate the actual risk of liver resection," *Journal of the American College of Surgeons*, vol. 191, no. 1, pp. 38–46, 2000.

[8] A. Cucchetti, G. Ercolani, M. Vivarelli et al., "Impact of model for end-stage liver disease (MELD) score on prognosis after hepatectomy for hepatocellular carcinoma on cirrhosis," *Liver Transplantation*, vol. 12, no. 6, pp. 966–971, 2006.

[9] S. Dinant, W. de Graaf, B. J. Verwer et al., "Risk assessment of posthepatectomy liver failure using hepatobiliary scintigraphy and CT volumetry," *Journal of Nuclear Medicine*, vol. 48, no. 5, pp. 685–692, 2007.

[10] M. Karoui, C. Penna, M. Amin-Hashem et al., "Influence of preoperative chemotherapy on the risk of major hepatectomy for colorectal liver metastases," *Annals of Surgery*, vol. 243, no. 1, pp. 1–7, 2006.

[11] L. McCormack, H. Petrowsky, W. Jochum, K. Furrer, and P. A. Clavien, "Hepatic steatosis is a risk factor for postoperative complications after major hepatectomy: a matched case-control study," *Annals of Surgery*, vol. 245, no. 6, pp. 923–930, 2007.

[12] J. T. Mullen, D. Ribero, S. K. Reddy et al., "Hepatic insufficiency and mortality in 1,059 noncirrhotic patients undergoing major hepatectomy," *Journal of the American College of Surgeons*, vol. 204, no. 5, pp. 854–862, 2007.

[13] K. Slankamenac, S. Breitenstein, U. Held, B. Beck-Schimmer, M. A. Puhan, and P. Clavien, "Development and validation of a prediction score for postoperative acute renal failure following liver resection," *Annals of Surgery*, vol. 250, no. 5, pp. 720–727, 2009.

[14] T. Armstrong, F. K. S. Welsh, J. Wells, K. Chandrakumaran, T. G. John, and M. Rees, "The impact of pre-operative serum creatinine on short-term outcomes after liver resection," *HPB*, vol. 11, no. 8, pp. 622–628, 2009.

[15] J. G. Abuelo, "Normotensive ischemic acute renal failure," *The New England Journal of Medicine*, vol. 357, no. 8, pp. 797–805, 2007.

[16] W. R. Jarnagin, M. Gonen, Y. Fong et al., "Improvement in perioperative outcome after hepatic resection: analysis of 1,803 consecutive cases over the past decade," *Annals of Surgery*, vol. 236, no. 4, pp. 397–407, 2002.

[17] H. Imamura, Y. Seyama, N. Kokudo et al., "One thousand fifty-six hepatectomies without mortality in 8 years," *Archives of Surgery*, vol. 138, no. 11, pp. 1198–1206, 2003.

[18] N. N. Rahbari, O. J. Garden, R. Padbury et al., "Posthepatectomy liver failure: a definition and grading by the international study group of liver surgery (ISGLS)," *Surgery*, vol. 149, no. 5, pp. 713–724, 2011.

[19] J. Belghiti, P. A. Clavien, E. Gadzijev et al., "The Brisbane 2000 terminology of liver anatomy and resections," *HPB*, vol. 2, no. 3, pp. 333–339, 2000.

[20] G. P. Copeland, D. Jones, and M. Walters, "POSSUM: a scoring system for surgical audit," *The British Journal of Surgery*, vol. 78, no. 3, pp. 355–360, 1991.

[21] R. Bellomo, C. Ronco, J. A. Kellum, R. L. Mehta, and P. Palevsky, "Acute renal failure—definition, outcome measures, animal models, fluid therapy and information technology needs: the second international consensus conference of the acute dialysis quality initiative (ADQI) group," *Critical Care*, vol. 8, no. 4, pp. R204–R212, 2004.

[22] A. Agresti, *An Introduction to Categorical Data Analysis*, John Wiley & Sons, Hoboken, NJ, USA, 2nd edition, 2002.

[23] "'R'—project for statistical computing," 2011, http://www.r-project.org/.

[24] N. N. Rahbari, C. Reissfelder, M. Koch et al., "The predictive value of postoperative clinical risk scores for outcome after hepatic resection: a validation analysis in 807 patients," *Annals of Surgical Oncology*, vol. 18, no. 13, pp. 3640–3649, 2011.

[25] R. M. Jones, C. E. Moulton, and K. J. Hardy, "Central venous pressure and its effect on blood loss during liver resection," *The British Journal of Surgery*, vol. 85, no. 8, pp. 1058–1060, 1998.

[26] R. A. Schroeder, B. H. Collins, E. Tuttle-Newhall et al., "Intraoperative fluid management during orthotopic liver transplantation," *Journal of Cardiothoracic and Vascular Anesthesia*, vol. 18, no. 4, pp. 438–441, 2004.

[27] T. Kawai, Y. Yokoyama, M. Nagino, T. Kitagawa, and Y. Nimura, "Is there any effect of renal failure on the hepatic regeneration capacity following partial hepatectomy in rats?" *Biochemical and Biophysical Research Communications*, vol. 352, no. 2, pp. 311–316, 2007.

[28] S. A. Little, W. R. Jarnagin, R. P. DeMatteo, L. H. Blumgart, and Y. Fong, "Diabetes is associated with increased perioperative mortality but equivalent long-term outcome after hepatic resection for colorectal cancer," *Journal of Gastrointestinal Surgery*, vol. 6, no. 1, pp. 88–94, 2002.

[29] G. K. Michalopoulos, "Liver regeneration," *Journal of Cellular Physiology*, vol. 213, no. 2, pp. 286–300, 2007.

[30] I. R. Wanless and J. S. Lentz, "Fatty liver hepatitis (steatohepatitis) and obesity: an autopsy study with analysis of risk factors," *Hepatology*, vol. 12, no. 5, pp. 1106–1110, 1990.

[31] K. E. Behrns, G. G. Tsiotos, N. F. DeSouza, M. K. Krishna, J. Ludwig, and D. M. Nagorney, "Hepatic steatosis as a potential risk factor for major hepatic resection," *Journal of Gastrointestinal Surgery*, vol. 2, no. 3, pp. 292–298, 1998.

[32] Y. M. Sun, Y. Su, J. Li, and L. F. Wang, "Recent advances in understanding the biochemical and molecular mechanism of diabetic nephropathy," *Biochemical and Biophysical Research Communications*, vol. 433, no. 4, pp. 359–361, 2013.

8

The Impact of Changed Strategies for Patients with Cholangiocarcinoma in This Millenium

Per Lindnér, Magnus Rizell, and Lo Hafström

Transplant Institute, Institute of Clinical Sciences, Sahlgrenska Academy at University of Gothenburg, Sahlgrenska University Hospital, SE-413 45 Gothenburg, Sweden

Correspondence should be addressed to Per Lindnér; per.lindner@surgery.gu.se

Academic Editor: Shu-Sen Zheng

Background. Cholangiocarcinoma is a cancer with a poor prognosis. In this millennium there are new diagnostic and therapeutic strategies for these patients. *Aim.* The aim of this study was to find if these changes influenced survival of individuals with proximal cholangiocarcinoma. *Material.* 627 individuals with a diagnosis of cholangiocarcinoma (not including distal common duct cancer) during the period from 2000 to 2011 were registered in Sweden's Western Region. The material was divided into three consecutive time periods. *Results.* The overall survival curves for individuals with cholangiocarcinoma improved over the three time periods ($n = 627$) ($P = 0.0013$). Median survival increased from 2.6 months in the first period (2000–2003) to 3.6 months in the final four years (2008–2011). Patients with perihilar cholangiocarcinoma (PHC) had longer median survival than those with intrahepatic cholangiocarcinoma (IHC): 6.8 versus 3.2 months ($P = 0.0003$). An improvement in the survival curves over time was seen for those with IHC ($P = 0.034$) but not for patients with PHC ($P = 0.38$). Nine percent of the patients with IHC had potential curative surgical therapy. The three-year survival rate after liver resection for patients with IHC was 35% and 60% after liver transplantation. Among patients with PHC, 15.3% had potential curative bile duct resection with a concomitant liver resection and 6.1% bile duct resection alone. The three-year survival rate for these two groups was 32% and 20%, respectively. *Conclusion.* Overall survival for individuals with PHC was better than for those with IHC. Over time survival in IHC patients improved but not in those with PHC.

1. Introduction

Analysis of a complete population of individuals with a defined cancer diagnosis over a prolonged time period is needed to assess whether new therapeutic strategies have affected the whole population's survival outcome.

Cancers arising from the epithelial lining of the intrahepatic, perihilar, and extrahepatic bile ducts are a heterogeneous group of malignancies. Two major diagnoses are identified by location: the intrahepatic cholangiocellular cancer (IHC) and the perihilar carcinoma (PHC) or Klatskin tumour at the confluence or bifurcation of the left and right hepatic duct proximal to the cystic duct. There is not a clear-cut border between an advanced PHC and an IHC.

The prognosis for individuals with these conditions is poor. An analysis of Netherlands Cancer Registry record for IHC found a three-year survival rate of 8%, but a steady increase over the past decades [1]. This change could be the result of developments in surgery, transplantation, and the introduction of new ablative and molecular targeted therapies.

Bile duct resection with or without liver resection is the hallmark of potentially curative treatment for patients with PHC and 5-year survival is reported among 20–40% after surgical resection [2].

Most of these reports describe highly selective materials subjected to surgery in referral centres and it is difficult to assess if these results affect the whole population with the disease [3–5].

For patients with IHC liver resection can achieve up to 40% five-year survival [6]. With stringent inclusion criteria liver transplantation according to the Mayo protocol has shown impressing long-term results, in PHC, even in multi-institutional setting [6, 7].

The combination of gemcitabine and cisplatinum [8] has demonstrated a survival advantage over treatment with gemcitabine alone, suggesting that certain chemotherapies add to survival [8].

Survival for a complete population of patients with a malignant disease is improving thanks to advancements in diagnostic procedures, patient managements, surgical procedures, and emergence of effective chemotherapeutic agents and molecular target drugs. All of these factors are relevant for the improvements of patients' outcome.

The hypothesis of this study was that there is a continuous improvement in survival for the total population of patients with cholangiocellular carcinoma in this millennium.

The study's goal was further to analyse whether staging and/or therapy options used during the first decade of this century have had an impact on the outcome. The population studied consisted of all individuals diagnosed as having IHC or PHC served by the Western Regional Cancer Centre (RCC) in Sweden. The hypothesis that there is an improvement in survival for patients with cholangiocarcinoma was formulated before data collection.

2. Material

The region served by the RCC has a population of 1.6 million. In this region there is one referral university hospital having a complete liver cancer service, including liver transplantation. All individuals with an established histopathological cancer diagnosis are reported to the RCC. All patients in whom a diagnosis is clinically established are also reported to the register. Included in report data is the stage of the cancer based on clinical and imaging findings, which are translated into TNM criteria (TNM 6 or higher).

In this study's analysis, clinical and pathological information was retrieved from RCC records. Additional information was obtained by reviewing individual patient's charts. When several therapeutic procedures were described the most important therapy was ranked as the instituted therapy. Data on pre- and postoperative adjuvant therapy was not collected. Active palliative treatment (APT) included chemotherapy, TACE (transarterial chemotherapy), sirolimus, sorafenib, and COX-2 inhibitors. Bile duct drainage and radiation therapy of skeleton metastases were considered as best supportive care (BSC).

All curative and active palliative treatments were handled by the liver surgery service at the university hospital.

Cholangiocarcinomas located distally in the bile duct were not included in the analysis.

Between 2000 and 2011 a total of 627 individuals were reported to the RCC as having cancers originating in the epithelial lining of the bile ducts. The 49 individuals, where a diagnosis was not established until the postmortem examination, were also excluded. Available information about the clinical staging, treatment, and survival on the remaining 578 individuals was reviewed. Morphologic diagnosis of cholangiocarcinoma was established when an image of adenocarcinoma was present in the specimen, in combination with immunochemical markers typical for cholangiocarcinoma, including CD7 and CD17. Differentiation between IHC and PHC was based on the location of the tumour within the liver.

A number of patients were at an advanced stage when diagnosed with the cancer and in these patients only minor diagnostic procedures were motivated. These patients were

TABLE 1: (a) Clinical staging for patients with intrahepatic cholangiocarcinoma (IHC) in the three time periods. (b) The treatment for 233 patients with intrahepatic cholangiocarcinoma (IHC) in the three time periods.

(a)

Staging/year	2000–2003	2004–2007	2008–2011	Total
T0	1	0	0	1
T1	2	9	12	23
T2	2	0	4	6
T3	13	10	15	38
T4	1	1	3	5
N1	5	14	15	34
M+	17	19	34	70
Not staged	24	27	5	56
Total	65	80	88	233

(b)

Treatment/year	2000–2003	2004–2007	2008–2011	Total
Curative aim				
Liver resection	2	6	9	17
Transplantation	1	1	3	5
Active palliative				
TACE	0	0	7	7
Chemotherapy	6	14	25	45
Miscellaneous	10	6	1	17
BSC	46	53	43	141
Total	65	80	88	233

registered under the diagnosis of unspecified primary liver cancer ($n = 65$) or unspecified bile duct cancer ($n = 117$) (Table 1). The diagnosis of unspecified primary liver cancer supposedly cholangiocellular (mainly ICD-10: C22.9) used by the register was based on the following: (1) no evidence of a previous or concomitant cancer of no hepatic origin, (2) no underlying liver disease, and (3) no signs of hepatocellular cancer were found. The diagnosis of unspecified bile duct cancer (mainly ICD-10: C24.9) was based on the dominant symptom of stricture(s) in the extra hepatic bile tree above the gallbladder duct that was causing jaundice. These two diagnoses inevitably included mainly cases of IHC and PHC where only best supported care (BSC) was administered and median survival was less than two months. These groups are not further analysed.

In order to explore if there was a continuous progress in the outcome, the material was divided into three equal time cohorts: Period A 2000–2003, Period B 2004–2007, and Period C 2008–2011. No planned changes in the organization of hepatobiliary surgery occurred in the region during 2000–2012, but there was an increased awareness of the disease, which led to more referrals (Table 1).

2.1. Statistics. Survival time was calculated from the date of the report to the RCC, that is, the date a diagnosis was established histopathologically or clinically. Observation time was more than 32 months or till death in all cases. Survival estimates were made using the Kaplan-Meier method

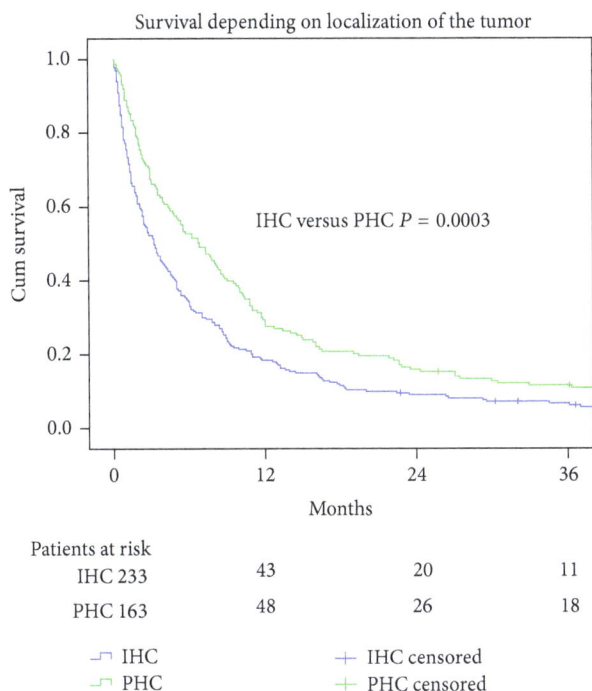

FIGURE 1: Survival curves (Kaplan-Meier log-rank test $P = 0.0003$) for 396 patients with cholangiocarcinoma. Perihilar cancer (PHC) (C 24.0); intrahepatic cancer (C 22.1). Median survival (95% confidence interval) in months: PHC 6.80 (4.81–8.78) and IHC 3.20 (2.30–3.10).

and compared using the log-rank test. All statistics were calculated using SPSS 22 Statistical Software (SPSS, Chicago, IL) and at a significance level of 5%.

2.2. Ethics. The analyses were done at Transplant Institute, Section for Liver Surgery, Sahlgrenska University Hospital, Gothenburg, Sweden, and Regional Cancer Centre of West Sweden, Gothenburg, Sweden. The study was carried out in compliance with the Declaration of Helsinki principles.

3. Results

Overall survival for all individuals with cholangiocarcinoma ($n = 578$) improved over time ($P = 0.0013$). The survival curves for the IHC and PHC are shown in Figure 1.

The median survival for patients with PHC was 6.8 months and for those with IHC 3.0 months ($P = 0.0003$).

The age and sex distribution did not change between the three time periods for neither IHC nor PHC.

3.1. Intrahepatic Cholangiocellular Cancer (IHC). 74% of the individuals with IHC were between 50 and 79 years of age when diagnosed, with an equal number younger (13%) and older (13%) than these age groups. The clinical staging for the 233 individuals with IHC in the three time periods is depicted in Table 1(a). One patient was staged as T0 and was transplanted for primary sclerosing cholangitis and IHC

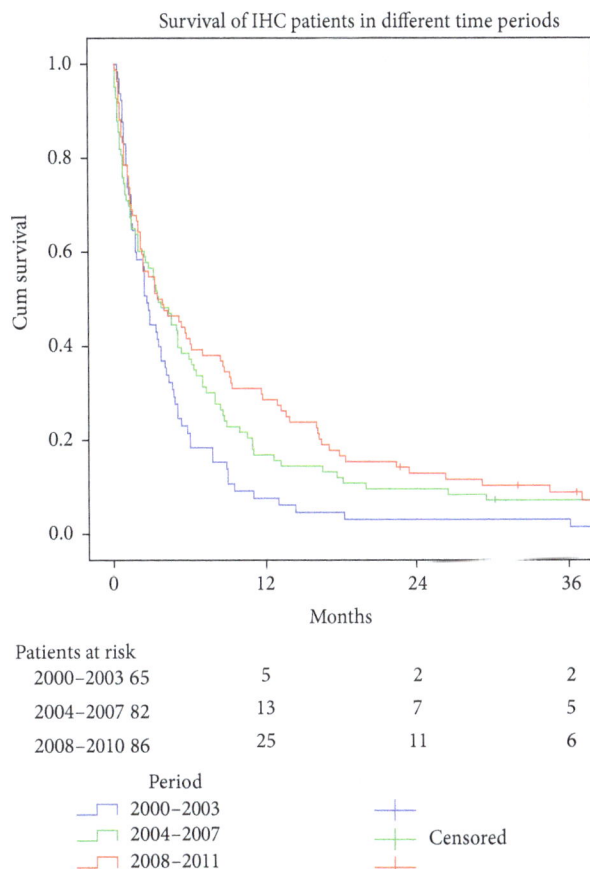

FIGURE 2: Survival curves (Kaplan-Meier log-rank test $P > 0.03$) for 233 patients with intrahepatic cancer (IHC) for three different time periods. Median survival (95% confidence interval) in months: 2000–2003, 2.60 (2.11–3.09); 2004–2007, 3.50 (1.89–5.11); and 2008–2011, 3.40 (0.71–4.07).

was identified in the explanted liver. Over time an increasing number of patients were clinically staged (63% in Period A versus 94% in Period C). Among the staged patients with IHC there was no staging migration over time ($P = 0.27$). In 17% an underlying liver disease was identified. Of those 40 patients ten had primary sclerosing cholangitis (PSC). The diagnosis IHC was established morphologically in 91% of the patients. The diagnosis was in 27% supported by immunochemistry, CD 7 and CD 19.

Overall survival for individuals with IHC was 3.2 months and 6.6% survived more than three years. A significant improvement in overall survival over time was registered for those diagnosed as having IHC ($P = 0.034$) (Figure 2). The one-year survival was significantly higher in the last time period compared to the first period ($P = 0.038$). After two years this difference was no longer significant ($P = 0.34$).

Seventeen of 233 patients (7.3%) had a liver resection and five had a liver transplantation. The three-year overall survival after liver resection was 29% and after liver transplantation 60%. There was a nonsignificant increase in the number of liver resections and transplantations between Periods A and C ($P = 0.064$) (Table 1(b)).

A trend towards a more active palliative therapy was seen with more patients being treated with chemotherapy over time among the three cohorts ($P = 0.06$). When comparing the impact on survival for those treated with chemotherapy, mainly gemcitabine ($n = 45$), the curves for Period A + B ($n = 20$) versus Period C ($n = 25$) were superimposed ($P = 0.96$) and median survival was six months.

A transcatheter arterial chemoembolization, or TACE, was administered during the last period to six patients. A median survival of 18 months for those patients was achieved.

A declining number of individuals got best supportive care (BSC). In Period A it was 69%, in B it was 66%, and in C it was 49% ($P = 0.02$). For these three cohorts, the survival curves were worse for Period C versus Period A + B ($P = 0.04$).

3.2. Perihilar Cholangiocarcinoma (PHC). The diagnosis of PHC was histomorphologically established by brush cytology through an endoscopy or by biopsy in 80% of the patients. In the remaining 20% it was based on radiological findings.

Fifteen percent of patients with PHC were above 79 years of age and 8% were below 50 years.

No significant stage migration was identified over time in the 163 patients with PHC (Table 2(a)). Three patients were staged as T0 as their duct stricture was considered benign. These three patients were from the first period.

The use of Bismuth criteria for staging the cancers in the confluence of the hepatic ducts increased over time from 49% in Period A to 85% in Period C (Table 2(a)). The median survival for the whole PHC-population was 6.8 months and 11% survived more than three years. There was no improvement in survival over time (Figure 3). Twenty patients had underlying liver disease—nine of them had PSC.

Fifteen percent of the patients had curatively aiming bile duct resection with a concomitant liver resection and 5.5% without liver resection. The three-year survival was 32% and 20%, respectively.

Six patients underwent liver transplantation. Three were transplanted according to the Mayo protocol, two of them had survived more than 3 years and three were transplanted outside the protocol and the longest survival was 23 months (Table 2(b)).

There was no increase in number of patients who received active palliative treatment (APT). In the first two periods there were 11 who were given miscellaneous palliative therapy (cox-2 inhibitor $n = 9$, sirolimus $n = 2$).

Median survival from date of diagnosis for the 34 patients that received APT was 8.8 months. The advanced stage of those with PHC is evident as approximately 50% were given best supportive care (BSC) in all periods.

4. Discussion

Biliary malignancies or cholangiocarcinomas are most often asymptomatic until late in the course of the disease and in an advanced stage when the diagnosis is established. In this analysis a great number of patients had their first doctor's consultation when their disease was at such an advanced state that only minor diagnostic procedures were motivated. Even

TABLE 2: (a) Clinical staging and Bismuth staging of 163 patients with perihilar cholangiocarcinoma (PHC) in the three time periods. (b) Therapy for 163 patients with perihilar cholangiocarcinoma (PHC) in the three time periods.

(a)

Staging/year	2000–2003	2004–2007	2008–2011	Total
T0	3	0	0	3
T1	2	5	2	9
T2	3	5	9	17
T3	1	3	5	9
T4	1	1	3	5
N1	9	11	10	30
M+	17	16	20	53
Not staged	13	12	12	37
Total	49	53	61	163
Bismuth staging				
1	13	8	11	32
2	1	0	6	7
3	5	6	14	25
4	5	5	21	31
Not staged	25	34	9	68

(b)

Treatment/year	2000–2003	2004–2007	2008–2011	Total
Curative aim				
Liver resection + bile duct resection	5	11	9	25
Bile duct resection	6	1	3	10
Transplantation	2	0	4	6
Active palliative				
Chemotherapy	2	9	12	23
Miscellaneous	8	3	0	11
BSC	26	29	33	82
Total	49	53	61	163

in patients with advanced disease efforts to get a diagnosis were improved and, consequently, there was a decline over time in the number of individuals for whom diagnosis was established at a postmortem examination. During the study period CT and magnetic resonance imaging (MRI) improved differentiation between hepatocellular carcinoma and IHC [9]. For patients with PHC high-resolution magnetic resonance imaging (MRI) has enabled staging of a cancer in the bile duct confluence according to Bismuth's criteria and is the current preoperative standard to assess PHC with an accuracy around 50% [10].

MRI cholangiography is the golden standard used to delineate the localization and extent of a cancer and the possibility of curative surgery. It has a positive predictive value of 86% [11], but in a recent meta-analysis, Bismuth's criteria had a lower accuracy rate and were of no prognostic value in cases of PHC undergoing resection [9].

The decreasing number of individuals subjected to BSC over time mirrored the increased active therapeutic strategy for patients with IHC. The migration of patients to curative

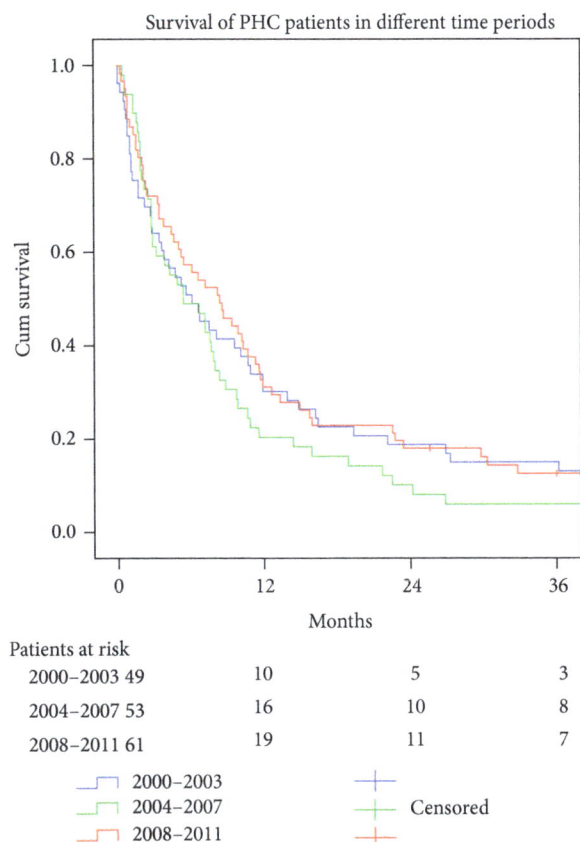

FIGURE 3: Survival curves (Kaplan-Meier log-rank test $P > 0.38$) for 163 patients with perihilar cancer (PHC) for three different time periods. Median survival (95% confidence interval) in months: 2000–2003, 5.50 (2.18–8.82); 2004–2007, 6.20 (2.84–9.56); 2008–2011, 8.50 (4.89–12.11).

and active palliative therapy explains why survival for BSC patients in Period C was worse than in Period A + B.

The improvement in survival over time for patients with ICC could be explained by the fourfold increase in number of patients, from 3 to 12, who had curative surgery (liver resection and liver transplantation) from Period A to Period C contributing in total to 8 patients surviving more than 3 years and 6 to more than five years. If these patients subjected to curative surgery are excluded, there is no significant impact on the survival curves over time ($P = 0.10$). The three-year survival rate after curative surgery was thus 45%, a figure in agreement with what appears in recent reports [12].

The number of patients with ICC that underwent surgery was lower than expected. An explanation could be that in this study we study the whole cohort of patients not only those referred to the surgical clinic. More patients underwent curative surgery over time but the outcome for IHC patients who had curative surgery did not improve between Periods A and B ($n = 10$) versus Period C ($n = 12$). The improvement in survival in the last time period was only observed in those surviving longer than one year.

IHC was considered to be a contraindication for liver transplantation during the whole study period. In the 5 cases where liver transplantation was performed diagnosis

was established first when the liver was explanted in two cases. A multi-institutional analysis in the Nordic countries reported a 5-year survival rate of 58% among those with IHC staged T1N0 and a CA 19-9 of less than 100 who underwent liver transplantation [13]. Based on this figure it has to be asked if there are more patients with IHC who could benefit from liver transplantation. As a recent meta-analysis shows that elevated CA 19-9-levels are associated with a worse prognosis independent of treatment [14], elevated CA 19-9-levels will remain a contraindication to transplantation; even the criteria were expanded.

In this material, preoperatively discovered lymph node metastases beyond the hepatoduodenal ligament were a contraindication for surgery. Even if lymph node metastases are a strong predictor of survival [15], the survival of IHC patients with lymph node involvement can be prolonged with hepatectomy and these cases should not be prematurely deemed noncurative [16].

There was a fourfold increase in number of patients with IHC who were treated with chemotherapy, mainly with gemcitabine. The survival outcome of this therapy did not change over time in this study; this is consistent with others' findings [17, 18].

Among patients selected for TACE in the last period of this study the median survival was 18 months. In comparison, median survival was six months for those receiving systemic chemotherapy. This difference could be explained by a better clinical stage in patients selected for TACE.

For those with PHC there was no improvement in the survival over the three time periods studied (Figure 3). There was no increase in the number treated with curative surgery (27% in Period A to 30% in Period C) and there was no increase in the number of individuals given active palliative treatment between the first and last periods. Despite progress with different treatment options, that is, liver transplantation [6] and chemotherapy [8], the number of patients who benefitted from these treatments was so small that it did not affect the survival rate of the entire population. Based on the present findings it seems reasonable to speculate that progress in treatment of PHC by surgical methods alone is limited. The Mayo protocol with irradiation and chemotherapy and consequent transplantation is reporting a five-year survival of 76% for individuals with PHC [7]. This is an example of how a combination of treatments can improve results. It also raises the question as to whether downsizing PHC and also IHC can increase the number of patients who can benefit from curatively aiming surgery. The role of adjuvant chemotherapy is still debated; a recent meta-analysis did not show any benefit [19], while a registry analysis identified that adjuvant chemotherapy was associated with significant survival benefits among patients with positive nodes or positive margins [20].

A more liberal use of chemotherapy during the last four-year period did not transfer into better outcomes. The presently used drug combinations that are considered effective [8] were not fully adopted even in the last time period; so there may be survival benefit still to be achieved. New protocols with innovative neoadjuvant and adjuvant therapies are needed to further improve long-term outcome following surgery or transplantation for patient with cholangiocarcinoma.

In conclusion, this analysis from a well-defined population in Sweden who had IHC or PHC has found an improvement in survival for patients with IHC. More individuals with IHC were over time treated with curative surgery or chemotherapy. Despite improvements in different treatment options, no changes in outcome were registered for patients with PHC during the first 12 years of this century.

Authors' Contribution

All authors have contributed to the design of the study, analysis of data, and writing of the communication.

Acknowledgments

The study was supported by grants from the Oncological Centre of West Gotaland Region, Sweden. Director Professor Nils Konradi and Assistant Director Susanne Amsler-Nordin of the Oncological Centre have generously supported this analysis. All surgeons in Transplant Institute, Sahlgrenska University Hospital, Gothenburg, Sweden, are acknowledged for their excellent clinical work with study subjects. The English language was reviewed and corrected by Mr. Jonathan Stubbs, professional translator of English medical articles.

References

[1] C. D. M. Witjes, H. E. Karim-Kos, O. Visser et al., "Intrahepatic cholangiocarcinoma in a low endemic area: rising incidence and improved survival," *HPB*, vol. 14, no. 11, pp. 777–781, 2012.

[2] S. A. Khan, H. C. Thomas, B. R. Davidson, and S. D. Taylor-Robinson, "Cholangiocarcinoma," *The Lancet*, vol. 366, no. 9493, pp. 1303–1314, 2005.

[3] W. R. Jarnagin, Y. Fong, R. P. DeMatteo et al., "Staging, resectability, and outcome in 225 patients with hilar cholangiocarcinoma," *Annals of Surgery*, vol. 234, no. 4, pp. 507–519, 2001.

[4] D. J. Rea, M. Munoz-Juarez, M. B. Farnell et al., "Major hepatic resection for hilar cholangiocarcinoma: analysis of 46 patients," *Archives of Surgery*, vol. 139, no. 5, pp. 514–525, 2004.

[5] S. Y. Cho, S.-J. Park, S. H. Kim et al., "Survival analysis of intrahepatic cholangiocarcinoma after resection," *Annals of Surgical Oncology*, vol. 17, no. 7, pp. 1823–1830, 2010.

[6] J. K. Heimbach, G. J. Gores, D. M. Nagorney, and C. B. Rosen, "Liver transplantation for perihilar cholangiocarcinoma after aggressive neoadjuvant therapy: a new paradigm for liver and biliary malignancies?" *Surgery*, vol. 140, no. 3, pp. 331–334, 2006.

[7] S. D. Murad, W. R. Kim, D. M. Harnois et al., "Efficacy of neoadjuvant chemoradiation, followed by liver transplantation, for perihilar cholangiocarcinoma at 12 US centers," *Gastroenterology*, vol. 143, no. 1, pp. 88–98, 2012.

[8] J. Valle, H. Wasan, D. H. Palmer et al., "Cisplatin plus gemcitabine versus gemcitabine for biliary tract cancer," *The New England Journal of Medicine*, vol. 362, no. 14, pp. 1273–1281, 2010.

[9] Y. E. Chung, M.-J. Kim, Y. N. Park et al., "Varying appearances of cholangiocarcinoma: radiologic-pathologic correlation," *Radiographics*, vol. 29, no. 3, pp. 683–700, 2009.

[10] A. Paul, G. M. Kaiser, E. P. Molmenti et al., "Klatskin tumors and the accuracy of the Bismuth-Corlette classification," *American Surgeon*, vol. 77, no. 12, pp. 1695–1699, 2011.

[11] L. Guibaud, P. M. Bret, C. Reinhold, M. Atri, and A. N. Barkun, "Bile duct obstruction and choledocholithiasis: diagnosis with MR cholangiography," *Radiology*, vol. 197, no. 1, pp. 109–115, 1995.

[12] M. Unno, Y. Katayose, T. Rikiyama et al., "Major hepatectomy for perihilar cholangiocarcinoma," *Journal of Hepato-Biliary-Pancreatic Sciences*, vol. 17, no. 4, pp. 463–469, 2010.

[13] S. Friman, A. Foss, H. Isoniemi et al., "Liver transplantation for cholangiocarcinoma: selection is essential for acceptable results," *Scandinavian Journal of Gastroenterology*, vol. 46, no. 3, pp. 370–375, 2011.

[14] S.-L. Liu, Z.-F. Song, Q.-G. Hu et al., "Serum carbohydrate antigen (CA) 19-9 as a prognostic factor in cholangiocarcinoma: a meta-analysis," *Frontiers of Medicine in China*, vol. 4, no. 4, pp. 457–462, 2010.

[15] M. Kiriyama, T. Ebata, T. Aoba et al., "Prognostic impact of lymph node metastasis in distal cholangiocarcinoma," *British Journal of Surgery*, 2015.

[16] T. Adachi, S. Eguchi, T. Beppu et al., "Prognostic impact of preoperative lymph node enlargement in intrahepatic cholangiocarcinoma: a multi-institutional study by the Kyushu study group of liver surgery," *Annals of Surgical Oncology*, 2015.

[17] T. Todoroki, "Chemotherapy for bile duct carcinoma in the light of adjuvant chemotherapy to surgery," *Hepato-Gastroenterology*, vol. 47, no. 33, pp. 644–649, 2000.

[18] T. Takada, H. Amano, H. Yasuda et al., "Is postoperative adjuvant chemotherapy useful for gallbladder carcinoma? A phase III multicenter prospective randomized controlled trial in patients with resected pancreaticobiliary carcinoma," *Cancer*, vol. 95, no. 8, pp. 1685–1695, 2002.

[19] M. N. Mavros, K. P. Economopoulos, V. G. Alexiou, and T. M. Pawlik, "Treatment and prognosis for patients with intrahepatic cholangiocarcinoma: systematic review and meta-analysis," *JAMA Surgery*, vol. 149, no. 6, pp. 565–574, 2014.

[20] M. D. Sur, H. In, S. M. Sharpe et al., "Defining the benefit of adjuvant therapy following resection for intrahepatic cholangiocarcinoma," *Annals of Surgical Oncology*, 2014.

9

The Association between Survival and the Pathologic Features of Periampullary Tumors Varies over Time

Jennifer K. Plichta,[1] Anjali S. Godambe,[2] Zachary Fridirici,[3] Sherri Yong,[2] James M. Sinacore,[4] Gerard J. Abood,[1] and Gerard V. Aranha[1]

[1] Department of Surgery, Loyola University Health Systems, 2160 S. First Avenue, Maywood, IL 60153, USA
[2] Department of Pathology, Loyola University Health Systems, 2160 S. First Avenue, Maywood, IL 60153, USA
[3] Stritch School of Medicine, Loyola University Medical Center, 2160 S. First Avenue, Maywood, IL 60153, USA
[4] Department of Preventive Medicine, Loyola University Medical Center, 2160 S. First Avenue, Maywood, IL 60153, USA

Correspondence should be addressed to Gerard V. Aranha; garanha@lumc.edu

Academic Editor: Harald Schrem

Introduction. Several histopathologic features of periampullary tumors have been shown to be correlated with prognosis. We evaluated their association with mortality at multiple time points. *Methods.* A retrospective chart review identified 207 patients with periampullary adenocarcinomas who underwent pancreaticoduodenectomy between January 1, 2001 and December 31, 2009. Clinicopathologic features were assessed, and the data were analyzed using univariate and multivariate methods. *Results.* In univariate analysis, perineural invasion had a strong association with 1-year mortality (OR 3.03, CI 1.42–6.47), and one lymph node (LN) increase in the LN ratio (LNR) equated with a 5-fold increase in mortality. In contrast, LN status (OR 6.42, CI 3.32–12.41) and perineural invasion (OR 5.44, CI 2.81–10.52) had the strongest associations with mortality at 3 years. Using Cox proportional hazards, perineural invasion (HR 2.61, CI 1.77–3.85) and LN status (HR 2.69, CI 1.84–3.95) had robust associations with overall mortality. Recursive partitioning analysis identified LNR as the most important risk factor for mortality at 1 and 3 years. *Conclusions.* Overall mortality was closely related to the LNR within the first year, while longer follow-up periods demonstrated a stronger association with perineural invasion and overall LN status. Therefore, the current staging for periampullary tumors may need to be updated to include the LNR.

1. Introduction

Several histopathologic features of periampullary adenocarcinoma tumors correlate with survival following resection, including lymph node (LN) status, perineural infiltration, lymphovascular invasion, and lymph node ratio (LNR). Both perineural infiltration and lymphovascular invasion in pancreaticoduodenectomy specimens were found to be associated with a decreased 5-year survival [1]. Perineural invasion alone has also been shown to be a strong predictor of survival in patients with periampullary, duodenal, and ampullary adenocarcinomas [2–4]. Talamini et al. identified a higher resectability rate and better prognosis in patients with ampulla of Vater tumors and emphasized that the LN status likely influenced survival outcomes [5]. More recently,

the utility of the LNR, defined here as the number of positive LN divided by the total number of LN assessed in a surgical specimen, has been highlighted as a potential factor in predicting mortality [6, 7].

For nonperiampullary tumors, the LNR has also been correlated with prognosis, including gastric cancer [8], esophageal squamous cell carcinoma [9], small bowel adenocarcinoma [10], colorectal cancer [11], breast cancer [12], and melanoma [13]. Notably, the LNR was an independent prognostic indicator for overall survival in patients undergoing curative gastrectomy for gastric cancer, but it did not prove to be superior to standard pN staging [14]. In contrast, the LNR in patients with node-positive breast cancer was able to further subdivide patients across all pN groups, suggesting that the LNR may add prognostic value to the traditional TNM classification [15]. Furthermore, the LNR may be a more precise predictor of survival than traditional pN staging in some patients with colon cancer [16, 17]. In patients with cholangiocarcinoma, LN metastasis serves as a major prognostic factor, while the number of LN resected and the LNR also yield high prognostic value [18, 19]. Considering this, the LNR has been proposed as a superior prognostic variable for numerous types of tumors.

As such, the association between the LNR and periampullary tumors has also been investigated. Following curative resection for ampulla of Vater carcinoma, the LNR and a minimum of 16 evaluated nodes were identified as robust prognostic factors for disease-specific survival [20]. In contrast, retrospective evaluations of pancreatic cancer and ampullary carcinoma demonstrated that the number of metastatic nodes, but not LNR, was one of the most important prognostic factors [21, 22]. However, a significant association between the LNR and survival for patients with pancreatic cancer was identified in separate studies [6, 23–25]. Furthermore, using data from patients undergoing pancreaticoduodenectomy for pancreatic adenocarcinoma, the LNR has been shown to be one of the most powerful predictors of short- and long-term survival [25] and has been suggested as a new tool for stratifying patients in future trials [6]. Thus, beyond the qualitative LN status (positive or negative nodes), the LNR may provide a quantitative tool that improves the current classification system for periampullary tumors [7, 26].

Although most of the aforementioned studies evaluated the association between various histopathologic features and prognosis, they were unable to instigate significant changes in the staging classification for periampullary tumors. This outcome was likely attributable to the fact that their focus was often seeking only one variable as the best predictor of their outcome, as opposed to utilizing several criteria similar to the current TNM staging to better classify periampullary tumors. Therefore, we aim to evaluate the association between mortality and several histopathologic features of periampullary adenocarcinoma tumors, including the LNR, at multiple time points in order to better predict patient prognosis.

2. Methods

We performed a retrospective review to assess the correlation between several histopathologic features of periampullary adenocarcinoma tumors and mortality following surgical intervention. We identified 207 patients with periampullary adenocarcinoma tumors who underwent attempted curative resection (pancreaticoduodenectomy, R0 or R1 resection completed) between January 1, 2001 and December 31, 2009. Patients with concurrent malignancies, a history of periampullary adenocarcinoma (or other pancreatic cancers), or perioperative mortalities (i.e., patients dying within 30 days of surgery) were excluded. The Social Security Death Index was utilized to determine current living status (last updated at April 27, 2012). Clinical and histopathologic features were assessed from the medical record, and overall survival at 1 year, 3 years, and to date was determined. Although pathology and operative reports were available for all patients, more

detailed records were not routinely uploaded into our electronic medical record until 2006, which limited the collection and utilization of some clinical parameters. The variables considered in our study were the most consistently reported. Disease-free survival was unable to be calculated due to the limited follow-up at our institution. This study was approved by the Loyola University Health Systems Institutional Review Board.

2.1. Statistical Analysis. Statistical analyses were conducted using Stata 10.0 (StataCorp, College Station, TX). Categorical variables were analyzed using Chi-squared (χ^2) tests, and continuous variables were analyzed using Mann-Whitney U tests. Statistical significance was defined as $P \leq 0.05$ (2-sided). Univariate and multivariable logistic regression were performed to assess clinicopathologic characteristics associated with 1- and 3-year mortality following surgical resection (odds ratios and 95% confidence intervals reported). The selection of variables for the multivariate analyses was based upon the results of the univariate analyses. Similarly, univariate and multivariate Cox proportional hazard model analyses were performed to evaluate the relationship of these features with all mortality to date (hazard ratios and 95% confidence intervals reported). The variables were selected based upon the results of the logistic regression analyses.

Classification and Regression Trees (CART 6.0; Salford Systems, San Diego, CA) were used to analyze the interactions between 11 different risk factors and the outcomes of interest and 1- and 3-year mortality. The risk factors included age, gender, subtype of periampullary tumor, tumor size, pathologic margin status, LN status, total number of LN removed, number of positive LN, LNR (number of positive LN/total number of LN removed), perineural infiltration, and lymphovascular invasion. CART analysis was used to grow a decision tree using the Gini splitting criteria with a minimum number of 10 parent node cases and a minimum number of cases for the child nodes of 1. Given the limited size of the data set ($n = 207$), the tree's classification accuracy was determined by way of a cross-validation method. To do this, the data were allotted (i.e., jackknifed) into five segments. One segment was successfully held out while the remaining segments were used to grow a tree, and the classification accuracy of the holdout segment was recorded. The overall cross-validation accuracy was determined by summing the results across all of the jackknifed segments.

3. Results

Of the 207 patients identified, there were 106 males and 101 females with a median age of 69 years (range 28–87 years). There were 17–28 surgeries performed annually (median 23 surgeries) between 2001 and 2009. Most tumors were pancreatic in origin (56% versus 23% ampullary, 12% duodenum, and 9% distal common bile duct). Similar proportions were noted in a cohort of patients from the SEER cancer registry who underwent pancreaticoduodenectomy between 1993 and 2003: 62.5% pancreatic, 18.9% ampullary, 7% duodenal, and 11.6% distal bile duct [27]. The median tumor size was

TABLE 1: Clinicopathologic characteristics stratified by survival at one and three years.

Covariate	1 year				3 years			
	Overall	Alive	Dead	P	Overall	Alive	Dead	P
Age (years)								
Median	69	68	71	0.014	69	67.5	70	0.064
Range	28–87	28–87	30–87		28–87	28–87	30–87	
Gender								
Male	106	82	24	0.143	97	42	55	0.279
Female	101	69	32		90	32	58	
Tumor size (cm)								
Median	2.75	2.5	3.2	0.001	2.75	2.3	3	<0.001
Range	0.4–8.5	0.4–6.5	1–8.5		0.4–8.5	0.4–5.2	0.8–8.5	
Margins								
Negative	146	116	30	0.001	130	64	66	<0.001
Positive	61	35	26		57	10	47	
Lymphovascular invasion								
Negative	101	81	20	0.022	93	53	40	<0.001
Positive	106	70	36		94	21	73	
Perineural invasion								
Negative	70	60	10	0.003	62	41	21	<0.001
Positive	137	91	46		125	33	92	
Overall LN status								
Negative	74	63	11	0.003	67	45	22	<0.001
Positive	133	88	45		120	29	91	
Positive LN								
Median	1	1	3	<0.001	1	0	2	<0.001
Range	0–21	0–18	0–21		0–21	0–11	0–21	
Total LN assessed								
Median	19	19	19	0.598	19	18.5	19	0.656
Range	1–45	1–45	4–41		1–45	4–45	1–41	
LNR								
Median	0.077	0.056	0.141	<0.001	0.077	0	0.118	<0.001
Range	0-1	0-1	0–0.75		0-1	0–0.733	0-1	

LN: lymph nodes; LNR (lymph node ratio) = (number of positive LN)/(total LN removed) $*$ 100.

2.75 cm, and an R0 resection was achieved in 70.5% of patients (n = 146). Lymphovascular invasion was noted in 51% of cases (n = 106), and perineural infiltration was reported in 66% (n = 137). The median number of LN identified in the surgical specimen was 19 LN. At least one LN was positive in 64% of patients (n = 133), and the median number of positive LN was one. The median LNR was 7.7%. While 207 patients were followed up for at least 1 year, only 187 had been followed up for at least 3 years at the time of analysis. At 1-year follow-up, significant differences between survivors and nonsurvivors were noted for 8 clinicopathologic features (age, tumor size, margin status, lymphovascular invasion, perineural invasion, overall LN status, number of positive LN, and LNR; Table 1). Excluding age, similar differences were observed between the two groups at 3-year follow-up (Table 1). The median overall follow-up was 1.9 years, while it was 5.6 years for survivors alone and 1.7 years for

nonsurvivors alone. The crude overall survival was 31% at the end of the follow-up period. Overall survival at 1 year was 73% and dropped to 40% by 3 years after surgery.

Using univariate logistic regression, 1-year mortality was independently associated with 7 clinicopathologic characteristics: age, tumor size, margin status, lymphovascular invasion, perineural infiltration, LN status, and LNR (data not shown). More specifically, perineural invasion had the strongest association with 1-year mortality (OR 3.03, CI 1.42–6.47), although LN status (OR 2.93, CI 1.41–6.1) and margin status (OR 2.87, CI 1.5–5.49) were quite similar. Additionally, an increase in the LNR by 1% increased the odds of mortality by 1.03-fold. However, the average number of LN removed was 20; thus, a change by 1 LN would equate with a 5% change in the LNR and thus a 1.16-fold increase in the odds of mortality. Multivariate analysis also revealed a significant association between 1-year mortality and the LNR

TABLE 2: Multivariate logistic regression analyses between clinicopathologic features and one- and three-year mortality following surgical resection.

Covariate	1-year mortality				3-year mortality			
	Odds ratio	95% CI	P	Pseudo R^2	Odds ratio	95% CI	P	Pseudo R^2
Model A								
Age	1.04	1–1.08	0.027		1.02	0.99–1.05	0.225	
Tumor size	1.51	1.17–1.95	0.001	0.108	1.56	1.19–2.04	0.001	0.129
Margin status	2.64	1.34–5.2	0.005		4.14	1.89–9.08	<0.001	
Model B								
Age	1.04	1.01–1.08	0.022		1.02	0.99–1.06	0.144	
Tumor size	1.53	1.18–1.98	0.001	0.123	1.6	1.21–2.12	0.001	0.206
Margin status	2.32	1.16–4.65	0.017		3.3	1.44–7.55	0.005	
Lymphovascular invasion	1.91	0.96–3.82	0.066		4.51	2.24–9.07	<0.001	
Model C								
Age	1.04	1–1.08	0.026		1.02	0.99–1.05	0.168	
Tumor size	1.49	1.15–1.93	0.003	0.122	1.62	1.21–2.16	0.001	0.195
Margin status	2.06	1–4.25	0.052		2.5	1.08–5.81	0.032	
Perineural invasion	2.09	0.91–4.84	0.083		4.37	2.09–9.13	<0.001	
Model D								
Age	1.04	1.01–1.08	0.022		1.02	0.99–1.05	0.18	
Tumor size	1.45	1.11–1.88	0.006	0.129	1.5	1.12–2	0.006	0.225
Margin status	2.24	1.12–4.5	0.023		3.39	1.46–7.89	0.005	
LN status	2.39	1.07–5.35	0.034		5.51	2.71–11.2	<0.001	
Model E								
Age	1.04	1.01–1.08	0.017		1.02	0.99–1.05	0.236	
Tumor size	1.45	1.12–1.88	0.005	0.133	1.43	1.09–1.89	0.011	0.202
Margin status	2.21	1.09–4.46	0.028		3.31	1.44–7.61	0.005	
LNR (%)	1.02	1–1.04	0.017		1.07	1.03–1.11	0.001	

LN: lymph nodes; LNR (lymph node ratio) = (number of positive LN)/(total LN removed) ∗ 100.

(OR 1.02, CI 1–1.04; Table 2). Notably, the model adjusting for the LNR (model E) accounts for 13.3% of the variability (adjusted R^2) in 1-year mortality, while the other models account for 10.8–12.9% (Table 2).

For 3-year mortality, univariate logistic regression analyses revealed independent associations with 6 clinicopathologic characteristics: tumor size, margin status, lymphovascular invasion, perineural infiltration, LN status, and LNR (data not shown). In contrast to 1-year mortality where perineural invasion was strongest, at 3 years the overall LN status (positive or negative) had the strongest association (OR 6.42, CI 3.32–12.41). However, perineural invasion remained a strong predictor (OR 5.44, CI 2.81–10.52). Similar to 1-year mortality, an increase in the LNR by 1% increased the odds of mortality by 1.08-fold. Thus, a change by 1 LN would equate with a 5% change in the LNR (assuming 20 LN were assessed) and consequently a 1.47-fold increase in the odds of mortality. Therefore, qualitative LN status and perineural invasion appear to be stronger predictors than LNR in predicting 3-year mortality. This is further supported by multivariate analyses where the model adjusting for overall LN status (model D) accounts for 22.5% of the variability in 3-year mortality (adjusted R^2), while the other models account for 12.9–20.6% (Table 2). Similar findings were noted using univariate Cox proportional hazards, where perineural

infiltration (HR 2.61, CI 1.77–3.85) and overall LN status (HR 2.69, CI 1.84–3.95) had strong associations with overall mortality (data not shown). In multivariate Cox analyses, all clinicopathologic characteristics included were significant independent predictors ($P < 0.05$) in all models (Table 3). More specifically, the presence of positive LN appeared to have the strongest crude association with overall mortality.

3.1. CART Analysis for 1- and 3-Year Mortality. To create the CART decision trees, 11 risk factors were entered into the software to classify survivor and nonsurvivor patients at 1- and 3-year follow-up. Variables included age (continuous), gender (male or female), tumor size (continuous), margin status (positive or negative), tumor subtype (pancreatic, distal common bile duct, ampullary, or duodenal), lymphovascular invasion (positive or negative), perineural invasion (positive or negative), LN status (positive or negative), number of positive LN (continuous), total number of LN removed (continuous), and LNR (continuous).

For 1-year mortality, the CART tree grown with the training data set contained 7 levels (Figure 1). The most important factor was the LNR as 84% with a LNR ≤ 0.1 were alive at 1 year ($n = 102$ of 122). Of patients with a LNR > 0.1, the next most important risk factor was tumor size, where 100% of patients with tumors ≤2.05 were alive at

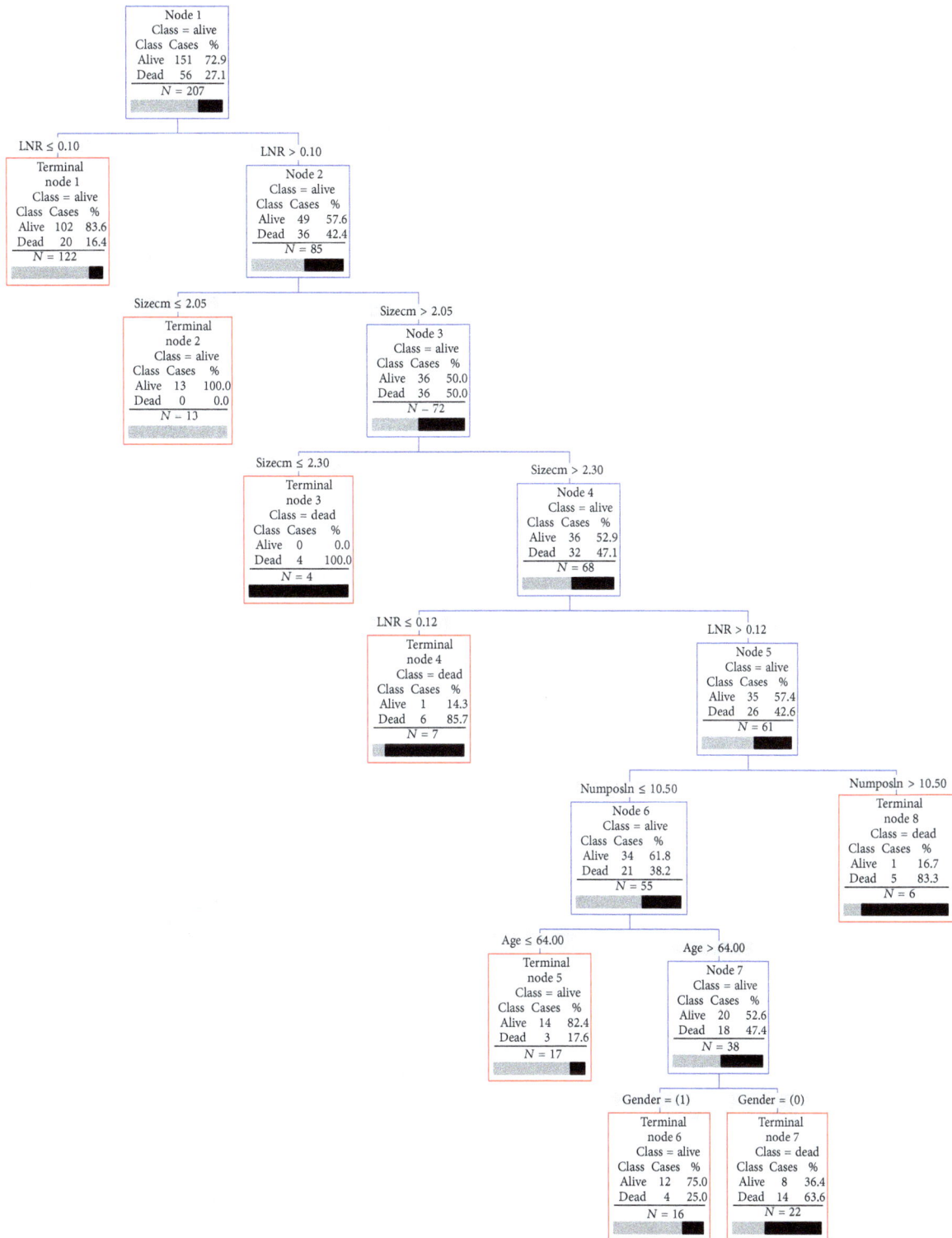

FIGURE 1: Results of recursive partitioning analysis to predict 1-year mortality. Numposln: number of positive lymph nodes; Sizecm: tumor size in centimeters; LNR: lymph node ratio.

TABLE 3: Cox regression multivariate analysis between pathologic features and overall survival.

Covariate	Number of patients	Hazard ratio	95% CI	P
Model A				
Age		1.02	1–1.04	0.019
Tumor size	206	1.31	1.16–1.48	<0.001
Margin status		2.12	1.5–3.01	<0.001
Model B				
Age		1.02	1–1.04	0.018
Tumor size	206	1.35	1.19–1.52	<0.001
Margin status		1.69	1.17–2.44	0.005
Lymphovascular invasion		1.96	1.37–2.82	<0.001
Model C				
Age		1.02	1–1.04	0.014
Tumor size	206	1.3	1.15–1.47	<0.001
Margin status		1.58	1.09–2.29	0.016
Perineural invasion		2.19	1.44–3.32	<0.001
Model D				
Age		1.02	1.01–1.04	0.008
Tumor size	206	1.27	1.12–1.43	<0.001
Margin status		1.75	1.23–2.5	0.002
LN status		2.44	1.64–3.64	<0.001
Model E				
Age		1.02	1–1.04	0.012
Tumor size	206	1.28	1.13–1.45	<0.001
Margin status		1.95	1.37–2.76	<0.001
LNR (%)		1.02	1.01–1.03	<0.001

LN: lymph nodes; LNR (lymph node ratio) = (number of positive LN)/(total LN removed) * 100.

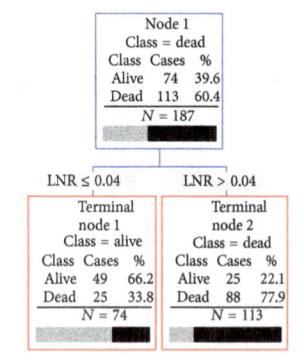

FIGURE 2: Results of recursive partitioning analysis to predict 3-year mortality.

1 year ($n = 13$) and 100% of those with tumors >2.05 but ≤2.3 died ($n = 4$). Further splits were developed, and the decision tree had an overall classification accuracy of 82% for the training data set. To validate these findings, a subset of the data was used to test the model, yielding a score of 74% overall accuracy (Table 4).

For 3-year mortality, the CART tree grown with the training data set contained only one level (Figure 2). The most important factor was again the LNR as 78% with a LNR > 0.04 were deceased at 3 years ($n = 88$ of 113) and 66% of those with a LNR ≤ 0.04 were alive ($n = 49$ of 74). This decision tree had an overall classification accuracy of 73% for the training data set, which was similar for the testing data set (overall accuracy 72%; Table 4).

4. Discussion

Based on a similar cohort of patients undergoing pancreaticoduodenectomies from 1998 to 2007 at our institution, we previously demonstrated an inverse relationship between the LNR and survival, which was strongest for pancreatic and ampullary tumors [7]. Here, we again demonstrate that a higher LNR is likely a significant risk factor for patients undergoing attempted curative resection of a periampullary adenocarcinoma tumor. Using multiple analytic methods, it proved to be a significant variable in univariate and multivariate regression analyses, as well as being identified as the best initial stratification variable in recursive partitioning analysis. More specifically, the CART analyses suggest that the two most important risk factors for determining 1-year mortality were the LNR and tumor size, while only the LNR was able to risk-stratify patients at 3 years. A focused, separate analysis of 246 patients with specifically pancreatic adenocarcinoma reported a significant prognostic value of the LNR for both short- and long-term survival after PD [25]. This was similarly confirmed in a recent study of 551 patients who underwent resection for periampullary tumors, and a LNR > 0.2 was identified as an independent prognostic factor for overall survival [28]. While our analyses included the LNR as a continuous variable, one of the original studies evaluating the association between the LNR and pancreatic cancer found a statistically significant difference only for patients with a ratio of 15% to 19% [29], which has subsequently been used as the categorical cutoff for other follow-up studies [7, 28]. The slight difference in cutoff values between the earlier report and the current investigation may be related to the inclusion of all periampullary tumors here.

In this study, we wished to determine whether LNR by itself or other risk factors influenced survival in all four periampullary adenocarcinoma tumors over a longer period of time. We demonstrated that several other histopathologic features appeared to be significantly associated with prognosis, including tumor size, margin status, qualitative LN status, perineural infiltration, and lymphovascular invasion. Data on tumor grade and adjuvant therapies were incomplete and, thus, not included in our analyses. Excluding the LNR, perineural invasion appeared to be most significantly associated with 1-year mortality, while overall LN status yielded a stronger correlation at 3-year follow-up, although both variables were significant at both time points. In a similar study of 346 patients undergoing resection for periampullary cancers, only nodal metastasis and neural invasion significantly predicated overall survival in multivariate analysis [30]. Nevertheless, as noted in a recent study of 1,147 patients over three decades, long-term survival has not significantly

TABLE 4: Classification accuracy of CART analysis for 1-year and 3-year mortality.

	Training set				Testing set			
	Total cases	Dead	Alive	% Accuracy	Total cases	Dead	Alive	% Accuracy
1-year mortality								
Actual class								
Dead	56	29	27	52%	56	17	39	30%
Alive	151	10	141	93%	151	15	136	90%
			Overall % Accuracy	82%			Overall % Accuracy	74%
3-year mortality								
Actual class								
Dead	113	88	25	78%	113	85	28	75%
Alive	74	25	49	66%	74	25	49	66%
			Overall % Accuracy	73%			Overall % Accuracy	72%

CART: Classification and Regression Trees.

improved for patients undergoing resection for pancreatic cancer [31], which highlights the importance of creating novel stratification systems to help develop targeted and more appropriate treatment regimens.

It has been proposed that the subtype of periampullary tumor also contributes to prognosis [32, 33]. Therefore, identification of biomarkers that aid in distinguishing the various subtypes may consequently correlate with survival. For example, recent investigations have demonstrated that hepatocyte nuclear factor 4-alpha (HNF4α) is an effective tool for identifying different ampullary cancer subtypes and is an independent predictor of a favorable prognosis [34]. Although limited by a relatively small sample size, subdividing our patient population by tumor subtype did not appear to influence patient stratification in our recursive partitioning analysis.

Others have suggested that a minimum number of LN need to be assessed in the surgical specimen in order to optimize prognostic accuracy and prevent stage migration errors. Using a cohort of 5,465 patients from the SEER cancer registry that underwent pancreaticoduodenectomy between 1993 and 2003, Gutierrez et al. demonstrated that a minimum of 10 LN should be examined in order to determine LN status [27]. Here, the mean number of LN assessed was 19.8, but there was one patient with only 1 LN identified in the surgical specimen (per report) and 17 patients with fewer than 10 LN reported. Of this patient subset, 1-year survival was 53% versus 74.7% for patients with $\geq$10 LN assessed (P = 0.053). By 3-year follow-up, this initially notable difference disappeared (3-year survival 41.2% for those with <10 LN versus 39.4% for those with $\geq$10 LN). Furthermore, there was no significant difference overall between 1- or 3-year survivors and nonsurvivors based on the total number of LN assessed (Table 1). These findings suggest that the total number of LN evaluated may be an early risk factor but likely becomes less important as time progresses.

One of this study's strengths and weaknesses is the inclusion of patients over a 9-year period. During this time, the analysis of the pathologic specimens likely evolved with the emerging data related to margin status. For example, a study by Verbeke et al. was one of the first to evaluate

the implementation of a standardized protocol for assessing resection margins in pancreatic head adenocarcinomas and found a significantly higher R1 rate with the newer protocol (R1 rate 85% with the standardized protocol versus 53% with the nonstandardized protocol) [35]. The R1 rates, however, were not significantly altered by the implementation of the standardized protocol for ampullary or distal bile duct cancers [35]. The R1 rates for all periampullary adenocarcinoma tumors in this study varied from 7% in 2008 to 56.5% in 2005, while the most recent rate in 2009 was 23% and the overall was 29%. Furthermore, the resection margin status was significantly associated with mortality in our regression analyses. Although it is clear that specimen dissection technique and standardization of the pathologic examination are crucial [36, 37], the advancements in imaging over recent years have also influenced the selection of patients appropriate for attempted surgical resection [38] and, thus, the overall margin status and ability to achieve an R0 resection.

In addition to the more traditional histopathologic features assessed in surgical specimens, current research is investigating other potential biomarkers that may better correlate with prognosis and/or potentially aid in early diagnosis. Cancer antigens CA19-9 and CA125 were some of the earlier biomarkers to be evaluated, but they lack sensitivity and specificity to be used for predicting prognosis [39]. Currently, serum CA19-9 levels are used primarily for diagnosis and/or following patients with active or a history of pancreatic cancer [39, 40]. In an attempt to find novel biomarkers of the disease, one study found that CD56 and certain mucins were associated with vascular and perineural invasion and together may serve as markers of prognosis in patients with periampullary tumors [41]. Cyclin D1 was also found to be independently associated with prognosis in some periampullary tumors [42, 43], while p16 protein has shown some correlation with perineural invasion and, thus, potentially prognosis [44]. Although some of these biomarkers show great promise, their exact utility in prognosticating outcomes has yet to be validated in routine clinical practice.

In contrast, the information needed to calculate the LNR of a surgical specimen is often readily available in most pathology reports. Furthermore, it has the potential to serve as an adjunct to traditional TNM staging and may have additive risk stratification capability, which may be particularly important early in the disease course when survival declines most rapidly. Our study systematically evaluated this and several other histopathologic features at multiple time points in order to adequately assess the ability of these variables to risk-stratify these tumors. In addition, our findings are supported by a unique and thorough analysis, which not only included traditional multivariate regression analyses, but also were further verified by another underutilized technique called recursive partitioning. The benefits of the latter method are its capacity to consider numerous variables simultaneously (even more than that typically recommended for multivariate analyses), its ability to consider one variable in the context of other variables, and the mathematical calculations performed to determine the best stratification variable for the specified outcome within a particular data set. While regression methods may be more useful when seeking to quantify the relative contribution of the explanatory variables, recursive partitioning often provides insight into the data structure and relationships between variables. This analytical method has been used previously for similar questions [45, 46], but our study is one of the first to apply this technique as a tool for risk-stratifying patients with periampullary tumors. As suggested by Cook and Goldman, this simple and intuitive type of analysis for classifying subjects has the potential to help identify novel and synergistic interactions among multiple variables and potentially aids in developing more practical risk stratification tools [47].

5. Conclusions

Overall mortality appears to be more closely related to the LNR within the first year following surgery. Longer follow-up periods, however, demonstrated a stronger association between overall mortality and the qualitative LN status and perineural invasion. Evidence suggests that the current staging paradigm for periampullary adenocarcinoma tumors may need to be updated to include the LNR. However, further investigations are required to fully evaluate the utility of the LNR as either a replacement or an adjunct to the standard pN staging. In addition, patients living beyond a certain time frame following curative resection may require reanalysis for determining their continued prognosis.

Acknowledgment

This study received funding from the Department of Surgery, Loyola University Health Systems, USA.

References

[1] J. W. C. Chen, M. Bhandari, D. S. Astill et al., "Predicting patient survival after pancreaticoduodenectomy for malignancy: histopathological criteria based on perineural infiltration and lymphovascular invasion," *HPB*, vol. 12, no. 2, pp. 101–108, 2010.

[2] S. Cecchini, C. Correa-Gallego, V. Desphande et al., "Superior prognostic importance of perineural invasion vs. lymph node involvement after curative resection of duodenal adenocarcinoma," *Journal of Gastrointestinal Surgery*, vol. 16, no. 1, pp. 113–120, 2012.

[3] J. H. Lee, K. G. Lee, H. Ryou et al., "Significance analysis of histologic type and perineural invasion as prognostic factors after curative resection of ampulla of vater carcinoma," *Hepato-Gastroenterology*, vol. 57, no. 99-100, pp. 646–652, 2010.

[4] M. H. van Roest, A. S. Gouw, P. M. Peeters et al., "Results of pancreaticoduodenectomy in patients with periampullary adenocarcinoma: perineural growth more important prognostic factor than tumor localization," *Annals of Surgery*, vol. 248, no. 1, pp. 97–103, 2008.

[5] M. A. Talamini, R. C. Moesinger, H. A. Pitt et al., "Adenocarcinoma of the ampulla of Vater: a 28-year experience," *Annals of Surgery*, vol. 225, no. 5, pp. 590–600, 1997.

[6] T. M. Pawlik, A. L. Gleisner, J. L. Cameron et al., "Prognostic relevance of lymph node ratio following pancreaticoduodenectomy for pancreatic cancer," *Surgery*, vol. 141, no. 5, pp. 610–618, 2007.

[7] M. G. Hurtuk, C. Hughes, M. Shoup, and G. V. Aranha, "Does lymph node ratio impact survival in resected periampullary malignancies?" *American Journal of Surgery*, vol. 197, no. 3, pp. 348–352, 2009.

[8] O. Asoglu, H. Karanlik, M. Parlak et al., "Metastatic lymph node ratio is an independent prognostic factor in gastric cancer," *Hepato-Gastroenterology*, vol. 56, no. 91-92, pp. 908–913, 2009.

[9] Y. P. Liu, L. Ma, S. J. Wang et al., "Prognostic value of lymph node metastases and lymph node ratio in esophageal squamous cell carcinoma," *European Journal of Surgical Oncology*, vol. 36, no. 2, pp. 155–159, 2010.

[10] M. J. Overman, C.-Y. Hu, R. A. Wolff, and G. J. Chang, "Prognostic value of lymph node evaluation in small bowel adenocarcinoma: analysis of the surveillance, epidemiology, and end results database," *Cancer*, vol. 116, no. 23, pp. 5374–5382, 2010.

[11] R. Rosenberg, J. Friederichs, T. Schuster et al., "Prognosis of patients with colorectal cancer Is associated with lymph node ratio a single-center analysis of 3026 patients over a 25-year time period," *Annals of Surgery*, vol. 248, no. 6, pp. 968–978, 2008.

[12] S. C. Schiffman, K. M. McMasters, C. R. Scoggins, R. C. Martin, and A. B. Chagpar, "Lymph node ratio: a proposed refinement of current axillary staging in breast cancer patients," *Journal of the American College of Surgeons*, vol. 213, no. 1, pp. 45–52, 2011.

[13] S. Mocellin, S. Pasquali, C. Riccardo Rossi, and D. Nitti, "Validation of the prognostic value of lymph node ratio in patients with cutaneous melanoma: a population-based study of 8,177 cases," *Surgery*, vol. 150, no. 1, pp. 83–90, 2011.

[14] A. Bilici, B. B. O. Ustaalioglu, M. Gumus et al., "Is metastatic lymph node ratio superior to the number of metastatic lymph nodes to assess outcome and survival of gastric cancer?" *Onkologie*, vol. 33, no. 3, pp. 101–105, 2010.

[15] M. E. Danko, K. M. Bennett, J. Zhai, J. R. Marks, and J. A. Olson Jr., "Improved staging in node-positive breast cancer patients using lymph node ratio: results in 1,788 patients with long-term follow-up," *Journal of the American College of Surgeons*, vol. 210, no. 5, pp. 797.e1–805.e1, 2010.

[16] E. A. Manilich, R. P. Kiran, T. Radivoyevitch, I. Lavery, V. W. Fazio, and F. H. Remzi, "A novel data-driven prognostic model for staging of colorectal cancer," *Journal of the American College of Surgeons*, vol. 213, no. 5, pp. 579.e2–588.e2, 2011.

[17] R. Rosenberg, J. Engel, C. Bruns et al., "The prognostic value of lymph node ratio in a population-based collective of colorectal cancer patients," *Annals of Surgery*, vol. 251, no. 6, pp. 1070–1078, 2010.

[18] Y. Oshiro, R. Sasaki, A. Kobayashi et al., "Prognostic relevance of the lymph node ratio in surgical patients with extrahepatic cholangiocarcinoma," *European Journal of Surgical Oncology*, vol. 37, no. 1, pp. 60–64, 2011.

[19] D. Tamandl, K. Kaczirek, B. Gruenberger et al., "Lymph node ratio after curative surgery for intrahepatic cholangiocarcinoma," *British Journal of Surgery*, vol. 96, no. 8, pp. 919–925, 2009.

[20] M. Falconi, S. Crippa, I. Domínguez et al., "Prognostic relevance of lymph node ratio and number of resected nodes after curative resection of ampulla of Vater carcinoma," *Annals of Surgical Oncology*, vol. 15, no. 11, pp. 3178–3186, 2008.

[21] Y. Murakami, K. Uemura, T. Sudo et al., "Number of metastatic lymph nodes, but not lymph node ratio, is an independent prognostic factor after resection of pancreatic carcinoma," *Journal of the American College of Surgeons*, vol. 211, no. 2, pp. 196–204, 2010.

[22] J. Sakata, Y. Shirai, T. Wakai, Y. Ajioka, K. Akazawa, and K. Hatakeyama, "Assessment of the nodal status in ampullary carcinoma: the number of positive lymph nodes versus the lymph node ratio," *World Journal of Surgery*, vol. 35, no. 9, pp. 2118–2124, 2011.

[23] M. B. Slidell, D. C. Chang, J. L. Cameron et al., "Impact of total lymph node count and lymph node ratio on staging and survival after pancreatectomy for pancreatic adenocarcinoma: a large, population-based analysis," *Annals of Surgical Oncology*, vol. 15, no. 1, pp. 165–174, 2008.

[24] T. N. Showalter, K. A. Winter, A. C. Berger et al., "The influence of total nodes examined, number of positive nodes, and lymph node ratio on survival after surgical resection and adjuvant chemoradiation for pancreatic cancer: a secondary analysis of RTOG 9704," *International Journal of Radiation Oncology, Biology and Physics*, vol. 81, no. 5, pp. 1328–1335, 2011.

[25] C. E. Weber, E. A. Bock, M. G. Hurtuk et al., "Clinical and pathologic features influencing survival in patients undergoing pancreaticoduodenectomy for pancreatic adenocarcinoma," *Journal of Gastrointestinal Surgery*, vol. 18, no. 2, pp. 340–347, 2014.

[26] M. La Torre, M. Cavallini, G. Ramacciato et al., "Role of the Lymph node ratio in pancreatic ductal adenocarcinoma. Impact on patient stratification and prognosis," *Journal of Surgical Oncology*, vol. 104, no. 6, pp. 629–633, 2011.

[27] J. C. Gutierrez, D. Franceschi, and L. G. Koniaris, "How many lymph nodes properly stage a periampullary malignancy?" *Journal of Gastrointestinal Surgery*, vol. 12, no. 1, pp. 77–85, 2008.

[28] S. G. Farid, G. A. Falk, D. Joyce et al., "Prognostic value of the lymph node ratio after resection of periampullary carcinomas," *HPB*, vol. 16, no. 6, pp. 582–591, 2014.

[29] M. Sierzega, T. Popiela, J. Kulig, and K. Nowak, "The ratio of metastatic/resected lymph nodes is an independent prognostic factor in patients with node-positive pancreatic head cancer," *Pancreas*, vol. 33, no. 3, pp. 240–245, 2006.

[30] I. Hatzaras, N. George, P. Muscarella, W. S. Melvin, E. C. Ellison, and M. Bloomston, "Predictors of survival in periampullary cancers following pancreaticoduodenectomy," *Annals of Surgical Oncology*, vol. 17, no. 4, pp. 991–997, 2010.

[31] J. M. Winter, M. F. Brennan, L. H. Tang et al., "Survival after resection of pancreatic adenocarcinoma: results from a single institution over three decades," *Annals of Surgical Oncology*, vol. 19, no. 1, pp. 169–175, 2012.

[32] T. S. Riall, J. L. Cameron, K. D. Lillemoe et al., "Resected periampullary adenocarcinoma: 5-year survivors and their 6- to 10-year follow-up," *Surgery*, vol. 140, no. 5, pp. 764–772, 2006.

[33] A. Westgaard, S. Tafjord, I. N. Farstad et al., "Pancreatobiliary versus intestinal histologic type of differentiation is an independent prognostic factor in resected periampullary adenocarcinoma," *BMC Cancer*, vol. 8, article 170, 2008.

[34] F. Ehehalt, P. Rümmele, S. Kersting et al., "Hepatocyte nuclear factor (HNF) 4α expression distinguishes ampullary cancer subtypes and prognosis after resection," *Annals of Surgery*, vol. 254, no. 2, pp. 302–310, 2011.

[35] C. S. Verbeke, D. Leitch, K. V. Menon, M. J. McMahon, P. J. Guillou, and A. Anthoney, "Redefining the R1 resection in pancreatic cancer," *British Journal of Surgery*, vol. 93, no. 10, pp. 1232–1237, 2006.

[36] C. S. Verbeke and I. P. Gladhaug, "Resection margin involvement and tumour origin in pancreatic head cancer," *British Journal of Surgery*, vol. 99, no. 8, pp. 1036–1049, 2012.

[37] B. M. Rau, K. Moritz, S. Schuschan, G. Alsfasser, F. Prall, and E. Klar, "R1 resection in pancreatic cancer has significant impact on long-term outcome in standardized pathology modified for routine use," *Surgery*, vol. 152, no. 3, supplement 1, pp. S103–S111, 2012.

[38] V. Chaudhary and S. Bano, "Imaging of the pancreas: recent advances," *Indian Journal of Endocrinology and Metabolism*, vol. 15, supplement 1, pp. S25–S32, 2011.

[39] L. C. Fry, K. Mönkemüller, and P. Malfertheiner, "Molecular markers of pancreatic cancer: development and clinical relevance," *Langenbeck's Archives of Surgery*, vol. 393, no. 6, pp. 883–890, 2008.

[40] G. Sandblom, S. Granroth, and I. C. Rasmussen, "TPS, CA 19-9, VEGF-A, and CEA as diagnostic and prognostic factors in patients with mass lesions in the pancreatic head," *Upsala Journal of Medical Sciences*, vol. 113, no. 1, pp. 57–64, 2008.

[41] M. M. Aloysius, A. M. Zaitoun, S. Awad, M. Ilyas, B. J. Rowlands, and D. N. Lobo, "Mucins and CD56 as markers of tumour invasion and prognosis in periampullary cancer," *British Journal of Surgery*, vol. 97, no. 8, pp. 1269–1278, 2010.

[42] M. C. Chang, Y. T. Chang, C. T. Sun, Y. F. Chiu, J. T. Lin, and Y. W. Tien, "Differential expressions of cyclin D1 associated with better prognosis of cancers of ampulla of vater," *World Journal of Surgery*, vol. 31, no. 5, pp. 1135–1141, 2007.

[43] A. Tomazic, V. Pegan, K. Ferlan-Marolt, A. Pleskovic, and B. Luzar, "Cyclin D1 and bax influence the prognosis after pancreatoduodenectomy for periampullary adenocarcinoma," *Hepato-Gastroenterology*, vol. 51, no. 60, pp. 1832–1837, 2004.

[44] E. Tuncer, N. Şen Türk, S. Arici, S. E. Düzcan, and N. Çalli Demirkan, "Expression of p16 protein and cyclin D1 in periampullary carcinomas," *Turk Patoloji Dergisi*, vol. 27, no. 1, pp. 17–22, 2011.

[45] M. Garzotto, T. M. Beer, R. G. Hudson et al., "Improved detection of prostate cancer using classification and regression

tree analysis," *Journal of Clinical Oncology*, vol. 23, no. 19, pp. 4322–4329, 2005.

[46] Y. Chang, L. Chen, K. Chung, and M. Lai, "Risk groups defined by Recursive Partitioning Analysis of patients with colorectal adenocarcinoma treated with colorectal resection," *BMC Medical Research Methodology*, vol. 12, article 2, 2012.

[47] E. F. Cook and L. Goldman, "Empiric comparison of multivariate analytic techniques: advantages and disadvantages of recurrence partitioning analysis," *Journal of Chronic Diseases*, vol. 37, no. 9-10, pp. 721–731, 1984.

10

C-Jun N-Terminal Kinase 2 Promotes Liver Injury via the Mitochondrial Permeability Transition after Hemorrhage and Resuscitation

Christoph Czerny,[1,2] **Tom P. Theruvath,**[1] **Eduardo N. Maldonado,**[1] **Mark Lehnert,**[2] **Ingo Marzi,**[2] **Zhi Zhong,**[1] **and John J. Lemasters**[1,3]

[1] *Center for Cell Death, Injury & Regeneration, Departments of Pharmaceutical & Biomedical Sciences,*
 Medical University of South Carolina, Charleston, SC 29425, USA
[2] *Departement of Trauma Surgery, J.W. Goethe University Frankfurt am Main, 60590 Frankfurt am Main, Germany*
[3] *Biochemistry & Molecular Biology, Medical University of South Carolina, MSC 140, Charleston, SC 29425, USA*

Correspondence should be addressed to John J. Lemasters, jjlemasters@musc.edu

Academic Editor: Peter Schemmer

Hemorrhagic shock leads to hepatic hypoperfusion and activation of mitogen-activated stress kinases (MAPK) like c-Jun N-terminal kinase (JNK) 1 and 2. Our aim was to determine whether mitochondrial dysfunction leading to hepatic necrosis and apoptosis after hemorrhage/resuscitation (H/R) was dependent on JNK2. Under pentobarbital anesthesia, wildtype (WT) and JNK2 deficient (KO) mice were hemorrhaged to 30 mm Hg for 3 h and then resuscitated with shed blood plus half the volume of lactated Ringer's solution. Serum alanine aminotransferase (ALT), necrosis, apoptosis and oxidative stress were assessed 6 h after resuscitation. Mitochondrial polarization was assessed by intravital microscopy. After H/R, ALT in WT-mice increased from 130 U/L to 4800 U/L. In KO-mice, ALT after H/R was blunted to 1800 U/l ($P < 0.05$). Necrosis, caspase-3 activity and ROS were all substantially decreased in KO compared to WT mice after H/R. After sham operation, intravital microscopy revealed punctate mitochondrial staining by rhodamine 123 (Rh123), indicating normal mitochondrial polarization. At 4 h after H/R, Rh123 staining became dim and diffuse in 58% of hepatocytes, indicating depolarization and onset of the mitochondrial permeability transition (MPT). By contrast, KO mice displayed less depolarization after H/R (23%, $P < 0.05$). In conclusion, JNK2 contributes to MPT-mediated liver injury after H/R.

1. Introduction

Multiple trauma is the principal cause of hemorrhagic shock and is typically the consequence of traffic accidents, falls, and, in time of war, casualties of combat [1, 2]. After hemorrhagic shock, resuscitation can lead to multiple organ dysfunction syndrome (MODS), which remains the most significant contributor to late mortality and intensive care unit resource utilization in critical care medicine [3, 4]. The liver is quite vulnerable to injury after ischemia and reperfusion (I/R). After I/R, hepatic necrosis is the predominant mode of cell death, whereas apoptosis is of less importance [5–7]. However, apoptosis and necrosis share common pathways, particularly the mitochondrial permeability transition (MPT) [8].

The MPT is caused by opening of high conductance MPT pores in the mitochondrial inner membrane, which leads to mitochondrial depolarization, uncoupling of oxidative phosphorylation, and large amplitude mitochondrial swelling [9]. The MPT plays a prominent role in the pathogenesis of cell death after I/R injury and a variety of other stresses [9–12]. After onset of the MPT, necrotic cell killing (oncosis) can occur as a consequence of ATP depletion, whereas swelling of mitochondria after the MPT leads to rupture of the outer membrane and release of proapoptotic proteins like cytochrome c. The extent of ATP depletion is crucial to whether necrosis or apoptosis occurs, since caspase-dependent apoptosis requires ATP, and necrosis does not occur until ATP is depleted by more than 85%.

c-Jun N-terminal kinase (JNK) is a stress-activated protein kinase that becomes activated after stresses like ultraviolet (UV) radiation, I/R and inflammation [13–16]. JNK-dependent phosphorylation of the transcription factor c-Jun/AP-1 promotes gene expression for an enhanced immune response [17]. JNK can also induce apoptosis via JNK-mediated phosphorylation of proapoptotic Bcl2 family proteins, such as Bim and Bmf, leading to mitochondrial outer membrane permeabilization, release of cytochrome c, and caspase activation [18, 19]. Moreover, translocation of activated JNK to mitochondria promotes the MPT [20, 21]. JNK becomes activated after experimental liver transplantation, warm hepatic I/R and hemorrhage/resuscitation (H/R), and pharmacological inhibition of JNK decreases liver injury, improves liver function, and increases survival in these settings [14, 15, 22–25]. Liver expresses two isoforms of JNK—JNK1 and JNK2 [26]. In models of acetaminophen hepatotoxicity, TNFα-dependent hepatic injury, warm I/R to liver and liver transplantation, JNK2 deficient mice are relatively protected against injury compared to wildtype mice [27–30].

Another organ vulnerable to injury during H/R is the gut. H/R compromises the barrier function of the gut, causing toxins and bacterial products like lipopolysaccharide (LPS) to enter the liver via the portal vein [31]. LPS and other gut-derived toxins entering the liver after H/R stimulate free radical generation and proinflammatory cytokine release by Kupffer cells to contribute to hepatic injury and increased cytokines in the blood stream [32–35]. Since JNK2 is also associated with the loss of barrier function of the gut [36, 37], we hypothesized that JNK2 is important for promotion of liver injury after H/R. Here, we test this hypothesis and show that liver injury decreases and hepatic function improves after H/R to JNK2 deficient mice in comparison to wildtype mice. These improvements are associated with improved mitochondrial function.

2. Materials and Methods

2.1. Chemicals and Reagents. Rhodamine 123 (Rh123) and other reagents were purchased from Sigma-Aldrich (St. Louis, MO, USA).

2.2. Animals. Experiments were performed using protocols approved by the Institutional Animal Care and Use Committee. C57BL/6 (wildtype) and JNK2-deficient (B6.129S2-Mapk9tm1Flv/J on a C57BL background) mice were obtained from Jackson Laboratory (Bar Harbor, ME). All mice used were males of 8 to 10 weeks of age and weighing 21–25 g.

2.3. Hemorrhagic Shock and Resuscitation. After an overnight fast, mice were anesthetized with sodium pentobarbital (80 mg/kg body weight). Under spontaneous breathing, the left and right femoral arteries were exposed and cannulated

with polyethylene-10 catheters (SIMS Portex), as described [15]. Before insertion, the catheters were flushed with normal saline containing heparin (100 IU/l). One catheter was connected via a transducer to a pressure analyzer (Micro-Med; Louisville, KY, USA), and blood was withdrawn over 5 min via the second catheter into a heparinized syringe (10 units) to a mean arterial pressure of 30 mm Hg. This pressure was maintained for 3 h by the reinfusion or withdrawal of shed blood. An animal temperature controller was used to maintain rectal temperature between 36.6 and 37.3°C. After 3 h, mice were resuscitated with the shed blood followed by lactated Ringer's solution corresponding to 50% of the shed blood volume infused with a syringe pump over 30 min. Adequacy of resuscitation was determined by the restoration of blood pressure to ~80 mm Hg. After resuscitation, the catheters were removed, the vessels were ligated, and the groin incisions were closed. Sham-operated animals underwent the same surgical procedures without hemorrhage. In sham-operated mice, pentobarbital anesthesia lasted up to 120 min before the animals began to awaken, and a second injection was required to continue the anesthesia. In mice undergoing H/R, a second injection of pentobarbital was not necessary to maintain anesthesia, most likely due to decreased pentobarbital metabolism by the hypoperfused liver. Over the course of the experiments, no mortality in any group occurred. For the determination of H/R-dependent liver damage, mice were anesthetized, and the two right dorsal liver lobes were snap frozen in liquid nitrogen. The remaining liver was flushed with saline through the portal vein, fixed by infusion of 4% buffered paraformaldehyde, and embedded in paraffin.

2.4. Alanine Aminotransferase (ALT). Blood samples to measure ALT were collected from the inferior vena cava 6 h after H/R for analysis using a kit (Sigma Chemical, St. Louis, MO, USA).

2.5. Histology. Necrosis was evaluated 6 h after H/R in 4-μm paraffin sections stained with hematoxylin and eosin (H&E). Necrosis was identified by standard morphologic criteria (e.g., loss of architecture, karyolysis, vacuolization, increased eosinophilia). Areas of necrosis were outlined in 10 random fields for each liver. Images were captured (Olympus BH-2 Microscope; Micropublisher 5.0 RTV, Center Valley, PA, USA), and the area percentage of necrosis was quantified using a computer program (BioQuant BQ Nova Prime 6.7, R&M Biometrics, Nashville, TN, USA).

2.6. Caspase-3. Liver tissue (~100 mg) was homogenized (Polytron PT-MR2100, Kinematica, Luzern, Switzerland) in 1 mL of lysis buffer containing 0.1% 3[(3-cholamidopropyl)dimethylammonio]-propanesulfonic acid, 5 mM DTT, 2 mM EDTA, 1 mM pefabloc, 10 ng/mL pepstatin A, 10 ng/mL aprotinin, 20 μg/mL leupeptin and 10 mM HEPES buffer, pH 7.4. After centrifugation at 15,000 rpm for 30 min, activity of caspase-3 in the supernatant was determined using a Caspase-3 Colorimetric Assay Kit (R&D Systems,

Minneapolis, MN) according to the manufacturer's instructions. Activity was normalized to protein concentration and expressed as fold increase compared to sham.

2.7. 4-Hydroxynonenal. Paraffin sections were deparaffinized, rehydrated, and incubated with polyclonal antibodies against 4-hydroxynonenal (4-HNE, Alpha Diagnostics; San Antonio, TX, USA) in PBS (pH 7.4) containing 1% Tween 20 and 1% bovine serum albumin. Peroxidase-linked secondary antibody and diaminobenzidine (Peroxidase Envision Kit, DAKO) were used to detect specific binding.

2.8. Intravital Microscopy. At 4 h after H/R, mice were anesthetized with pentobarbital (50 mg/kg, i.p.) and connected to a small animal ventilator via a tracheostomy and respiratory tube (22-gauge catheter), as described [29]. Laparotomy was performed, and a polyethylene-10 catheter was inserted into the distal right colic vein. Using a syringe pump, a membrane potential indicating fluorophore, Rh123 (1 μmol/mouse), was infused via the catheter over 10 min. After prone positioning of the mouse, the liver was gently withdrawn from the abdominal cavity and placed over a glass coverslip on the stage of an inverted microscope. Rh123 fluorescence was excited with 820 nm light from a Chameleon Ultra Ti-Sapphire pulsed laser (Coherent, Santa Clara, CA, USA) and imaged with a Zeiss LSM 510 NLO laser scanning confocal microscope using a 63 × 1.3 NA water-immersion objective lens. Green Rh123 fluorescence was collected through a 525 ± 25 nm band pass filter. During image acquisition, the respirator was turned off for ~5 sec to eliminate breathing movement artifacts. In 20 fields per liver, hepatocytes were scored for bright punctate Rh123 fluorescence signifying polarized mitochondria or a dimmer diffuse cytosolic fluorescence denoting depolarized mitochondria. Image analysis was performed in a blinded manner.

2.9. Statistical Analysis. Data are presented as means ± S.E., unless noted otherwise. Statistical analysis was performed by ANOVA with Student-Newman-Keuls test, as appropriate, using $P < 0.05$ as the criterion of significance.

3. Results

3.1. Decreased ALT Release and Liver Necrosis after Hemorrhage and Resuscitation of JNK2-Deficient Mice. After sham operation, serum ALT averaged 112 ± 15 U/L in wildtype and JNK2 deficient mice (Figure 1). After H/R, ALT increased to 4860 ± 538 U/L 6 h after resuscitation in wildtype mice compared to 1806 ± 126 U/L in JNK2-deficient mice ($P < 0.001$, Figure 1).

In sham-operated wildtype and JNK2-deficient mice, liver histology was normal and indistinguishable from untreated mice (Figure 2(a) and data not shown). At 6 h after H/R to wildtype mice, large areas of hepatic necrosis developed with a predominantly pericentral and midzonal distribution (Figure 2(b)). In JNK2-deficient mice, hepatic necrosis after H/R decreased from $24.5 \pm 1.5\%$ in wildtype mice to $6.6 \pm 1.5\%$ ($P < 0.05$, Figures 2(c) and 2(d)).

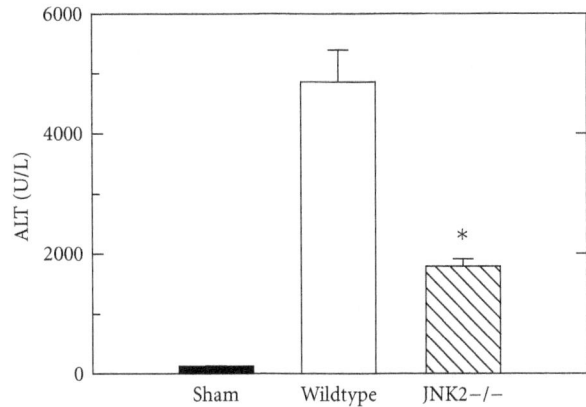

FIGURE 1: Decreased alanine aminotransferase (ALT) release after hemorrhage/resuscitation in JNK2-deficient mice. Wildtype and JNK2-deficient (JNK2−/−) mice were subjected to sham operation or bled to a mean arterial pressure of 30 mm Hg and resuscitated after 3 h, as described in Section 2. Blood was collected at 6 h after resuscitation for ALT measurement. Group sizes were 5-6 mice/group. *$P < 0.05$ versus wildtype. Average ALT values of wildtype and JNK2 deficient mice after sham operation were not statistically significantly different and are pooled.

Thus, hepatic necrosis in JNK2-deficient mice after H/R was decreased by more than two-thirds in comparison to wildtype mice (Figure 2(d)).

3.2. Decreased Apoptosis after Hemorrhage and Resuscitation of JNK2-Deficient Mice. Caspase 3 activity was measured in liver extracts at 6 h after H/R of wildtype- and JNK2-deficient mice in comparison to sham-operated mice. After sham operation, caspase 3 activity in the liver was nearly undetectable (Figure 3). After H/R of wildtype mice, caspase 3 activity increased significantly by 7.6-fold. By contrast after H/R of JNK2-deficient mice, hepatic caspase 3 activity increased only 2.6-fold ($P < 0.05$ versus wildtype, Figure 3).

3.3. Improved Mitochondrial Function In Vivo after Hemorrhage and Resuscitation of JNK2-Deficient Livers. Intravital multiphoton microscopy revealed bright fluorescence of Rh123 in hepatocytes at 4 h after sham operation. The punctate pattern denoted polarization of individual mitochondria. No differences in Rh123 fluorescence were observed between livers of wildtype- and JNK2-deficient mice (Figure 4(a) and data not shown). We then imaged Rh123 fluorescence at 4 h after H/R. This time point was selected because previous studies of liver transplantation after cold ischemic storage showed that 4 h after reperfusion was a time point where mitochondrial dysfunction could be detected prior to onset of cell death [38]. At 4 h after H/R in wildtype mice, Rh123 staining became diffuse and dim in many hepatocytes indicative of depolarized mitochondria (Figure 4(b)). By contrast, after H/R of JNK2-deficient mice, mitochondria depolarized in fewer hepatocytes than in wildtype mice (Figure 4(c)). Rather, most hepatocytes

(a)

(b)

(c)

(d)

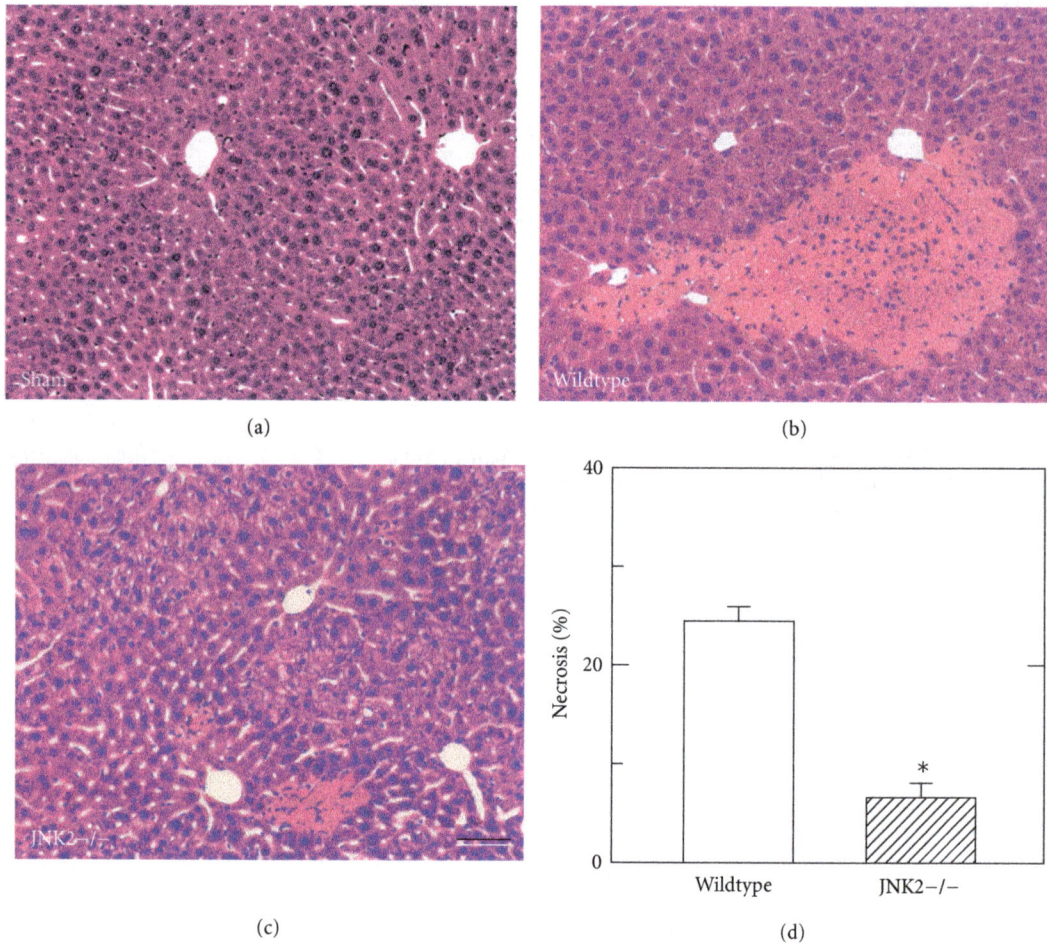

FIGURE 2: Decreased necrosis after hemorrhage and resuscitation in JNK2 deficient mice. At 6 h after resuscitation, necrosis was assessed by H&E in livers from sham-operated wildtype mice (a) and from wildtype- (b) and JNK2-deficient (c) mice after H/R. Bar is 50 μm. In (d), the percent area of necrosis is averaged from 5 livers per group. Necrosis was not present after sham operation of either wildtype- or JNK2 deficient mice and is not plotted. *$P < 0.05$.

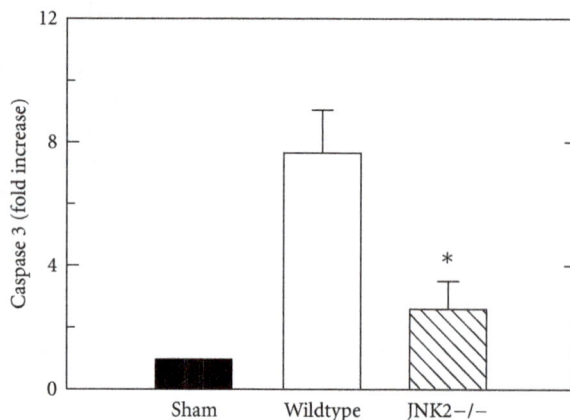

FIGURE 3: Decreased caspase 3 activation after hemorrhage and resuscitation of JNK2-deficient mice. At 6 h postoperatively, caspase 3 activity was assessed after sham operation and after H/R of wildtype and JNK2-deficient (JNK2−/−)mice, as described in Section 2. $P < 0.05$ versus wildtype, $n = 5$ per group.

exhibited bright, punctate staining by Rh123 in JNK2-deficient mice. In these experiments, hepatocytes were scored for Rh123 staining. In sham-operated mice, virtually no hepatocytes contained depolarized mitochondria. At 4 h after H/R of wildtype mice, 58% of hepatocytes contained depolarized mitochondria (Figure 4(d)). By contrast, at 4 h after H/R of JNK2-deficient mice, hepatocytes with depolarized mitochondria became 23%, less than half of that in wildtype mice ($P < 0.05$ versus wildtype, Figure 4(d)).

3.4. Decreased Oxidative Stress after Hemorrhage and Resuscitation of JNK2-Deficient Mice. We used 4-HNE immunohistochemistry to evaluate oxidative stress in mouse livers 6 h after H/R. 4-HNE is a product of lipid peroxidation that forms protein adducts that are recognized by anti-4-HNE antibodies. After sham operation, the brown reaction product of 4-HNE immunohistochemistry was virtually undetectable (Figure 5(a)). By contrast at 6 h after H/R of wildtype mice, wide confluent areas of HNE

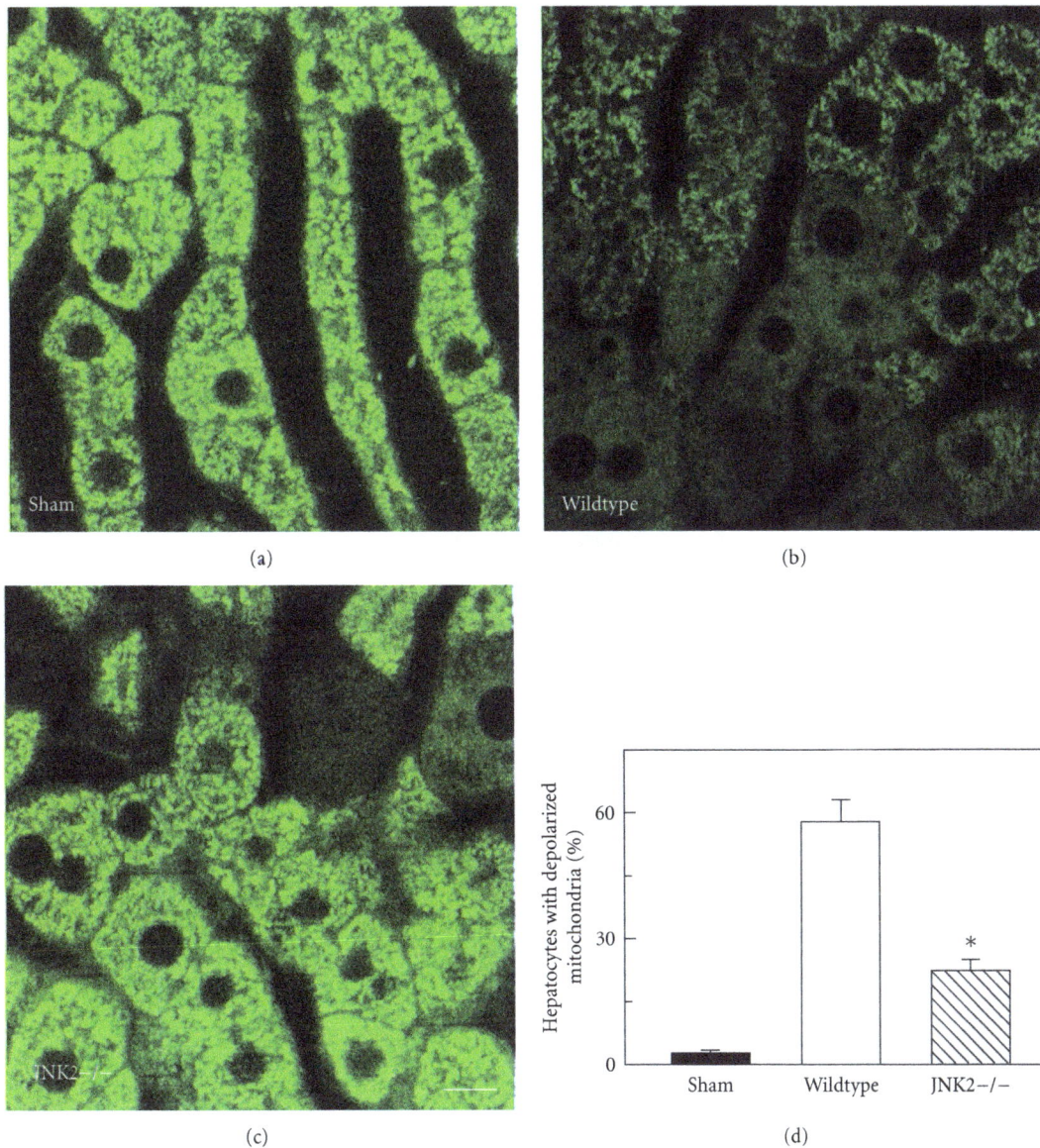

FIGURE 4: Decreased mitochondrial depolarization after hemorrhage and resuscitation of JNK2-deficient mice. Multiphoton imaging of hepatic Rh123 fluorescence was performed at 4 h after sham operation to wildtype mice (a) and H/R of wildtype- (b) and JNK2-deficient (c) mice, as described in Section 2. The percentage of hepatocytes per HPF with depolarized mitochondria is plotted in (d). Bar is 10 μm. $P < 0.05$ versus other groups; $n = 3$ per group.

immunoreactivity developed in pericentral and midzonal areas with relative sparing the periportal regions (Figure 5(b)). After H/R of JNK2-deficient mice, HNE immunoreactivity was substantially decreased and confined mostly to pericentral regions (Figure 5(c)).

4. Discussion

4.1. Decreased Liver Injury after Hemorrhagic Shock and Resuscitation of JNK2-Deficient Mice. Systemic inflammatory response syndrome (SIRS) and MODS following H/R are major problems after multiple trauma [3, 4]. H/R also causes hepatic necrosis and apoptosis [15, 23, 39]. The goal of this study was to evaluate the impact of JNK2 on

hepatic injury and mitochondrial dysfunction after H/R. Our findings show a specific role for JNK2 in liver injury after H/R, since JNK2-deficient mice had decreased hepatic injury and mitochondrial dysfunction after H/R in comparison to wildtype mice (Figures 1–4).

4.2. Reperfusion Injury after Hemorrhagic Shock and Resuscitation Induces Necrosis and Apoptosis through JNK2 Signaling. JNK becomes activated in various models of liver injury, and pharmacological inhibition of JNK decreases liver injury [14, 15, 22–24, 40–42]. In particular, JNK inhibition with the peptide inhibitor, DJNKI-1, decreases hepatic damage and inflammation after H/R [23]. However, JNK inhibitors are nonspecific with regards to the two isoforms of JNK, JNK1

(a)

(b)

(c)

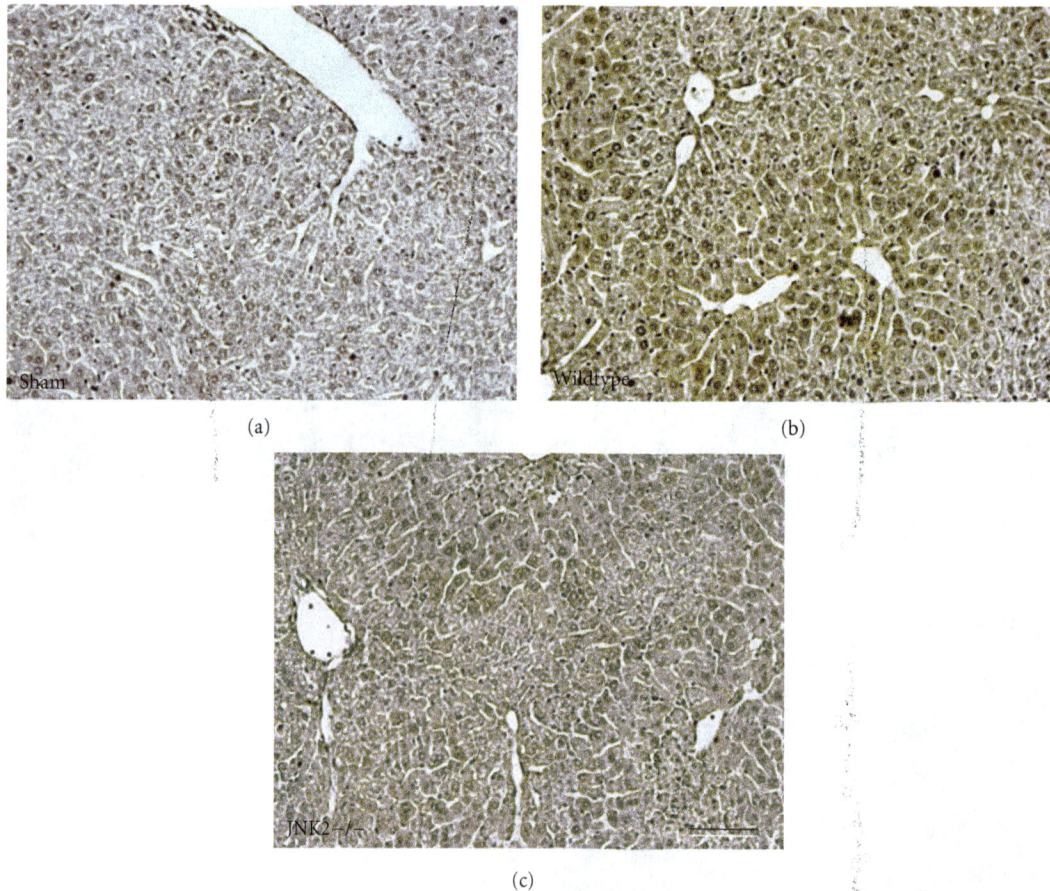

FIGURE 5: Decreased 4-hydroxynonenal immunostaining after hemorrhage and resuscitation of JNK2-deficient mice. ROS generation was assessed by 4-hydroxynonenal immunocytochemistry livers at 6 h after sham operation of wildtype mice (a) and after H/R to wildtype- (b) and JNK2-deficient (c) mice, as described in Section 2. Bar is 50 μm. $n = 5$ per group.

and JNK2, that are expressed in liver. Previous studies show that injury after orthotopic mouse liver transplantation and warm hepatic I/R decreases in JNK2-deficient livers compared to wildtype [29, 30]. In H/R, the specific roles of JNK isoforms are unknown. Therefore, we investigated the role of JNK2 by comparing JNK2-deficient mice and wildtype mice.

JNK2 deficiency decreased both necrosis and apoptosis in liver after H/R. Necrosis assessed by ALT and histology and apoptosis assessed by caspase 3 activity were decreased by 60% or more in JNK2-deficient mice compared to wildtype (Figures 1 and 2). Nonetheless, necrosis was the predominant mode of cell death after H/R. These results are in agreement with earlier results after liver transplantation and warm I/R [29, 30].

4.3. JNK2 Deficiency Attenuates Formation of Reactive Oxygen Species after Hemorrhage and Resuscitation. Reactive oxygen species (ROS) mediate, at least in part, liver injury after H/R, warm I/R, and storage/reperfusion injury occurring in liver transplantation. A consequence of ROS formation is peroxidation of polyunsaturated fatty acids, such as linoleic and arachidonic acids, which leads to 4-HNE generation and formation of 4-HNE-protein adducts. In the present study, hepatic 4-HNE immunostaining was marked after

H/R to wildtype mice but substantially diminished in JNK2-deficient mice (Figure 5). This indicates that JNK2 signaling has a role in promoting ROS generation after H/R. Such ROS can directly damage proteins, lipids, and DNA, as well as to help induce the MPT.

4.4. JNK2 Signaling after H/R Induces Mitochondrial Depolarization and Promotes Liver Injury. To test the hypothesis that the JNK2 isoform specifically promotes mitochondrial dysfunction after H/R, we used intravital multiphoton microscopy of Rh123 to assess mitochondrial polarization. This technique allows direct assessment of mitochondrial polarization in livers of living animals. Four hours after H/R of wildtype livers, mitochondrial depolarization occurred in more than 50% of hepatocytes. Mitochondrial depolarization occurred prior to cell death, since after 4 h few cells labeled with propidium iodide, a marker of nonviable cells (data not shown), as described previously [29]. After H/R of JNK2-deficient mice, mitochondrial depolarization was markedly decreased in comparison to wildtype mice (Figure 4). Minocycline and N-methyl-4-isoleucine cyclosporin are specific inhibitors of the MPT that prevent mitochondrial depolarization after I/R and orthotopic rat liver transplantation with no direct effect on mitochondrial respiration and oxidative phosphorylation [29]. Thus, mitochondrial depolarization visualized by intravital multiphoton microscopy, which was attenuated in JNK2-deficient mice, most likely represents onset of the MPT. Several studies indicate involvement of the MPT in acetaminophen hepatotoxicity [12, 20]. In acetaminophen hepatotoxicity, activated JNK translocates to mitochondria to induce MPT onset, which can be prevented by JNK inhibitors [20]. Thus, protection against mitochondrial depolarization in JNK2-deficient livers after H/R implies that JNK2 is directly involved in promoting the MPT in wildtype livers after H/R stress.

4.5. Other Mechanisms Promoting JNK2-Dependent Toxicity. H/R is also associated with a proinflammatory milieu in the gut lumen that promotes loss of barrier function [31]. Moreover, JNK2 mediates osmotic stress-induced tight junction disruption in the intestinal epithelium [36], although JNK1 is reported to mediate apical junction disassembly triggered by calcium depletion [37]. Impaired intestinal barrier function promoted by JNK during H/R may therefore also lead to portal vein endotoxemia, activation of TLR4 with phosphorylation of MAPKs, and increased production of inflammatory cytokines and ROS by hepatic Kupffer cells [34, 35, 43, 44]. Future studies will be needed to characterize how JNK2-dependent actions inside and outside hepatocytes contribute causally to liver injury, mitochondrial dysfunction, and development of MODS/SIRS after H/R.

4.6. Therapeutic Implications. An important implication of the present findings is that JNK2 represents a unique therapeutic target for treatment and prevention of hepatic injury and possibly SIRS and MODS after H/R. D-JNKI-1 and other existing JNK inhibitors are nonspecific and inhibit all JNK isoforms: JNK1, JNK2, and JNK3 [45]. JNK2 in our model of H/R plays a detrimental role, but JNK1 and/or JNK3 may have beneficial effects in liver and other tissues, especially since JNK1/JNK2 double knockout mice are not viable [46]. Thus, a specific JNK2 inhibitor might provide greater and more specific benefit after H/R and decrease the potential of toxicity by JNK1 and/or JNK3 inhibition, but such an inhibitor still awaits development.

List of Abbreviations

4-HNE: 4-hydroxynonenal
ALT: Alanine aminotransferase
H/R: Hemorrhage and resuscitation
H&E: Hematoxylin and eosin
HEPES: 4-(2-hydroxyethyl)-1-piperazineethanesulfonic acid
HPF: High-power field
MODS: Multiple organ dysfunction syndrome
MPT: Mitochondrial permeability transition
Rh123: Rhodamine 123
ROS: Reactive oxygen species
SIRS: Systemic inflammatory response syndrome.

Acknowledgments

This work was supported, in part, by Grants DK37034 and DK073336 from the National Institutes of Health and Grant W81XWH-09-1-0484 from the Department of Defense. Imaging facilities for this research were supported, in part, by Cancer Center Support Grant P30 CA138313 to the Hollings Cancer Center, Medical University of South Carolina. Portions of this work were presented at the International Shock Congress, Cologne, Germany, June 28–July 2, 2008 and at the Annual Meeting of the American Association for the Study of Liver Diseases, San Francisco, CA, USA, October 31–November 4, 2008.

References

[1] R. F. Bellamy, "The causes of death in conventional land warfare: implications for combat casualty care research," *Military Medicine*, vol. 149, no. 2, pp. 55–62, 1984.

[2] F. A. Moore, B. A. McKinley, and E. E. Moore, "The next generation in shock resuscitation," *The Lancet*, vol. 363, no. 9425, pp. 1988–1996, 2004.

[3] A. E. Baue, R. Durham, and E. Faist, "Systemic inflammatory response syndrome (SIRS), multiple organ dysfunction syndrome (MODS), multiple organ failure (MOF): are we winning the battle?" *Shock*, vol. 10, no. 2, pp. 79–89, 1998.

[4] D. Dewar, F. A. Moore, E. E. Moore, and Z. Balogh, "Postinjury multiple organ failure," *Injury*, vol. 40, no. 9, pp. 912–918, 2009.

[5] J. S. Gujral, T. J. Bucci, A. Farhood, and H. Jaeschke, "Mechanism of cell death during warm hepatic ischemia-reperfusion in rats: apoptosis or necrosis?" *Hepatology*, vol. 33, no. 2, pp. 397–405, 2001.

[6] H. Jaeschke and J. J. Lemasters, "Apoptosis versus oncotic necrosis in hepatic ischemia/reperfusion injury," *Gastroenterology*, vol. 125, no. 4, pp. 1246–1257, 2003.

[7] H. A. Rüdiger, R. Graf, and P. A. Clavien, "Liver ischemia: apoptosis as a central mechanism of injury," *Journal of Investigative Surgery*, vol. 16, no. 3, pp. 149–159, 2003.

[8] J. S. Kim, T. Qian, and J. J. Lemasters, "Mitochondrial permeability transition in the switch from necrotic to apoptotic cell death in ischemic rat hepatocytes," *Gastroenterology*, vol. 124, no. 2, pp. 494–503, 2003.

[9] J. J. Lemasters, T. P. Theruvath, Z. Zhong, and A. L. Nieminen, "Mitochondrial calcium and the permeability transition in cell death," *Biochimica et Biophysica Acta*, vol. 1787, no. 11, pp. 1395–1401, 2009.

[10] J. S. Kim, L. He, and J. J. Lemasters, "Mitochondrial permeability transition: a common pathway to necrosis and apoptosis," *Biochemical and Biophysical Research Communications*, vol. 304, no. 3, pp. 463–470, 2003.

[11] A. P. Halestrap, "Mitochondria and reperfusion injury of the heart-A holey death but not beyond salvation," *Journal of Bioenergetics and Biomembranes*, vol. 41, no. 2, pp. 113–121, 2009.

[12] K. Kon, J. S. Kim, H. Jaeschke, and J. J. Lemasters, "Mitochondrial permeability transition in acetaminophen-induced necrosis and apoptosis of cultured mouse hepatocytes," *Hepatology*, vol. 40, no. 5, pp. 1170–1179, 2004.

[13] C. Rosette and M. Karin, "Ultraviolet light and osmotic stress: activation of the JNK cascade through multiple growth factor and cytokine receptors," *Science*, vol. 274, no. 5290, pp. 1194–1197, 1996.

[14] C. A. Bradham, R. F. Stachlewitz, W. Gao et al., "Reperfusion after liver transplantation in rats differentially activates the mitogen-activated protein kinases," *Hepatology*, vol. 25, no. 5, pp. 1128–1135, 1997.

[15] M. Lehnert, T. Uehara, B. U. Bradford et al., "Lipopolysaccharide-binding protein modulates hepatic damage and the inflammatory response after hemorrhagic shock and resuscitation," *American Journal of Physiology*, vol. 291, no. 3, pp. G456–G463, 2006.

[16] H. Rensing, H. Jaeschke, I. Bauer et al., "Differential activation pattern of redox-sensitive transcription factors and stress-inducible dilator systems heme oxygenase-1 and inducible nitric oxide synthase in hemorrhagic and endotoxic shock," *Critical Care Medicine*, vol. 29, no. 10, pp. 1962–1971, 2001.

[17] M. Rincón and R. J. Davis, "Regulation of the immune response by stress-activated protein kinases," *Immunological Reviews*, vol. 228, no. 1, pp. 212–224, 2009.

[18] K. Lei and R. J. Davis, "JNK phosphorylation of Bim-related members of the Bcl2 family induces Bax-dependent apoptosis," *Proceedings of the National Academy of Sciences of the United States of America*, vol. 100, no. 5, pp. 2432–2437, 2003.

[19] C. Tournier, P. Hess, D. D. Yang et al., "Requirement of JNK for stress-induced activation of the cytochrome c- mediated death pathway," *Science*, vol. 288, no. 5467, pp. 870–874, 2000.

[20] N. Hanawa, M. Shinohara, B. Saberi, W. A. Gaarde, D. Han, and N. Kaplowitz, "Role of JNK translocation to mitochondria leading to inhibition of mitochondria bioenergetics in acetaminophen-induced liver injury," *The Journal of Biological Chemistry*, vol. 283, no. 20, pp. 13565–13577, 2008.

[21] S. Win, T. A. Than, D. Han, L. M. Petrovic, and N. Kaplowitz, "c-Jun N-terminal kinase (JNK)-dependent acute liver injury from acetaminophen or tumor necrosis factor (TNF) requires mitochondrial Sab protein expression in mice," *The Journal of Biological Chemistry*, vol. 286, pp. 37051–37058, 2011.

[22] T. Uehara, B. Bennett, S. T. Sakata et al., "JNK mediates hepatic ischemia reperfusion injury," *Journal of Hepatology*, vol. 42, no. 6, pp. 850–859, 2005.

[23] M. Lehnert, B. Relja, V. Sun-Young Lee et al., "A peptide inhibitor of C-JUN N-terminal kinase modulates hepatic damage and the inflammatory response after hemorrhagic shock and resuscitation," *Shock*, vol. 30, no. 2, pp. 159–165, 2008.

[24] T. Uehara, X. X. Peng, B. Bennett et al., "c-Jun N-terminal kinase mediates hepatic injury after rat liver transplantation," *Transplantation*, vol. 78, no. 3, pp. 324–332, 2004.

[25] L. A. King, A. H. Toledo, F. A. Rivera-Chavez, and L. H. Toledo-Pereyra, "Role of p38 and JNK in liver ischemia and reperfusion," *Journal of Hepato-Biliary-Pancreatic Surgery*, vol. 16, no. 6, pp. 763–770, 2009.

[26] M. A. Bogoyevitch, "The isoform-specific functions of the c-Jun N-terminal kinases (JNKs): differences revealed by gene targeting," *BioEssays*, vol. 28, no. 9, pp. 923–934, 2006.

[27] B. K. Gunawan, Z. X. Liu, D. Han, N. Hanawa, W. A. Gaarde, and N. Kaplowitz, "c-Jun N-terminal kinase plays a major role in murine acetaminophen hepatotoxicity," *Gastroenterology*, vol. 131, no. 1, pp. 165–178, 2006.

[28] Y. Wang, R. Singh, J. H. Lefkowitch, R. M. Rigoli, and M. J. Czaja, "Tumor necrosis factor-induced toxic liver injury results from JNK2-dependent activation of caspase-8 and the mitochondrial death pathway," *The Journal of Biological Chemistry*, vol. 281, no. 22, pp. 15258–15267, 2006.

[29] T. P. Theruvath, C. Czerny, V. K. Ramshesh, Z. Zhong, K. D. Chavin, and J. J. Lemasters, "C-Jun N-terminal kinase 2 promotes graft injury via the mitochondrial permeability transition after mouse liver transplantation," *American Journal of Transplantation*, vol. 8, no. 9, pp. 1819–1828, 2008.

[30] T. P. Theruvath, M. C. Snoddy, Z. Zhong, and J. J. Lemasters, "Mitochondrial permeability transition in liver ischemia and reperfusion: role of c-Jun N-terminal kinase 2," *Transplantation*, vol. 85, no. 10, pp. 1500–1504, 2008.

[31] B. F. Rush, A. J. Sori, T. F. Murphy, S. Smith, J. J. Flanagan, and G. W. Machiedo, "Endotoxemia and bacteremia during hemorrhagic shock. The link between trauma and sepsis?" *Annals of Surgery*, vol. 207, no. 5, pp. 549–554, 1988.

[32] R. Landmann, F. Scherer, R. Schumann, S. Link, S. Sansano, and W. Zimmerli, "LPS directly induces oxygen radical production in human monocytes via LPS binding protein and CD14," *Journal of Leukocyte Biology*, vol. 57, no. 3, pp. 440–449, 1995.

[33] J. M. Feng, J. Q. Shi, and Y. S. Liu, "The effect of lipopolysaccharides on the expression of CD14 and TLR4 in rat Kupffer cells," *Hepatobiliary and Pancreatic Diseases International*, vol. 2, no. 2, pp. 265–269, 2003.

[34] J. P. Hunt, C. T. Hunter, M. R. Brownstein et al., "Alteration in kupffer cell function after mild hemorrhagic shock," *Shock*, vol. 15, no. 5, pp. 403–407, 2001.

[35] T. Huynh, J. J. Lemasters, L. W. Bracey, and C. C. Baker, "Proinflammatory Kupffer cell alterations after femur fracture trauma and sepsis in rats," *Shock*, vol. 14, no. 5, pp. 555–560, 2000.

[36] G. Samak, T. Suzuki, A. Bhargava, and R. K. Rao, "c-Jun NH2-terminal kinase-2 mediates osmotic stress-induced tight junction disruption in the intestinal epithelium," *American Journal of Physiology*, vol. 299, no. 3, pp. G572–G584, 2010.

[37] N. G. Naydenov, A. M. Hopkins, and A. I. Ivanov, "c-Jun N-terminal kinase mediates disassembly of apical junctions in model intestinal epithelia," *Cell Cycle*, vol. 8, no. 13, pp. 2110–2121, 2009.

[38] T. P. Theruvath, Z. Zhong, P. Pediaditakis et al., "Minocycline and N-methyl-4-isoleucine cyclosporin (NIM811) mitigate storage/reperfusion injury after rat liver transplantation through suppression of the mitochondrial permeability transition," *Hepatology*, vol. 47, no. 1, pp. 236–246, 2008.

[39] M. Lehnert, G. E. Arteel, O. M. Smutney et al., "Dependence of liver injury after hemorrhage/resuscitation in mice on NADPH oxidase-derived superoxide," *Shock*, vol. 19, no. 4, pp. 345–351, 2003.

[40] Z. Zhong, R. F. Schwabe, Y. Kai et al., "Liver regeneration is suppressed in small-for-size liver grafts after transplantation: involvement of c-Jun N-terminal kinase, cyclin D1, and defective energy supply," *Transplantation*, vol. 82, no. 2, pp. 241–250, 2006.

[41] E. L. Marderstein, B. Bucher, Z. Guo, X. Feng, K. Reid, and D. A. Geller, "Protection of rat hepatocytes from apoptosis by inhibition of c-Jun N-terminal kinase," *Surgery*, vol. 134, no. 2, pp. 280–284, 2003.

[42] C. Saito, J. J. Lemasters, and H. Jaeschke, "C-Jun N-terminal kinase modulates oxidant stress and peroxynitrite formation independent of inducible nitric oxide synthase in acetaminophen hepatotoxicity," *Toxicology and Applied Pharmacology*, vol. 246, no. 1-2, pp. 8–17, 2010.

[43] Y. M. Yao, S. Bahrami, G. Leichtfried, H. Redl, and G. Schlag, "Pathogenesis of hemorrhage-induced bacteria/endotoxin translocation in rats: effects of recombinant bactericidal/permeability-increasing protein," *Annals of Surgery*, vol. 221, no. 4, pp. 398–405, 1995.

[44] B. M. Thobe, M. Frink, F. Hildebrand et al., "The role of MAPK in Kupffer cell Toll-like receptor (TLR) 2-, TLR4-, and

TLR9-mediated signaling following trauma-hemorrhage," *Journal of Cellular Physiology*, vol. 210, no. 3, pp. 667–675, 2007.

[45] R. F. Schwabe, H. Uchinami, T. Qian, B. L. Bennett, J. J. Lemasters, and D. A. Brenner, "Differential requirement for c-Jun NH2-terminal kinase in TNFalpha- and Fas-mediated apoptosis in hepatocytes," *The FASEB Journal*, vol. 18, no. 6, pp. 720–722, 2004.

[46] C. Y. Kuan, D. D. Yang, D. R. Samanta Roy, R. J. Davis, P. Rakic, and R. A. Flavell, "The Jnk1 and Jnk2 protein kinases are required for regional specific apoptosis during early brain development," *Neuron*, vol. 22, no. 4, pp. 667–676, 1999.

11

Reactive Lymphoid Hyperplasia of the Liver: A Clinicopathological Study of 7 Cases

Lei Yuan, Youlei Zhang, Yi Wang, Wenming Cong, and Mengchao Wu

Second Department of Hepatic Surgery, Eastern Hepatobiliary Surgery Hospital, Second Military Medical University, 225 Changhai Road, Shanghai 200438, China

Correspondence should be addressed to Yi Wang, wangyi-ehbh@163.com

Academic Editor: Giuliano Testa

Background. Reactive lymphoid hyperplasia (RLH) of the liver is a benign focal liver mass that may mimic a malignant liver tumor. Although rarely encountered in clinical practice, it often poses diagnostic and management dilemmas. *Methods*. Cases diagnosed as hepatic RLH between January 1996 and June 2011 were investigated in a retrospective study. Clinicopathological features as well as follow-up information of the cases were studied. *Results*. A total of seven cases of hepatic RLH were investigated, with a median age of 46 years (range: 33–76 years). Hepatic RLH was accompanied by concomitant diseases in some patients. The average size of hepatic lesions of our cases was 45 mm (range: 15–105 mm). All of the cases were not accurately diagnosed until confirmed by pathological findings, and surgical resections were performed for all. Postoperative course was uneventful for all of the patients during followup. *Conclusions*. RLH of the liver is a rare benign disease with a female predilection of unknown etiology. It is very difficult to correctly diagnose this disease without pathological results. Subtle differences on radiological findings of it may be helpful for differential diagnosis from other diseases. Curative resection of the lesion is suggested for the treatment of this disease.

1. Introduction

Reactive lymphoid hyperplasia (RLH), also termed as nodular lymphoid lesion [1, 2] or pseudolymphoma [3–8], is a rare benign condition which forms a liver mass typically infiltrated by massive heterogeneous mature lymphoid cells without prominent nuclear atypia, with formation of follicles and germinal centers. Up to now, there have been only scattered case reports about hepatic RLH [1–24]; the paucity of information about its clinicopathological features poses diagnostic and management dilemmas. Manifested as a focal liver mass, hepatic RLH may mimic a malignant liver tumor, often giving rise to misdiagnosis. Therefore, we reviewed our experience in a series of 7 patients with hepatic RLH who were treated by surgical resection. This was the largest series of cases of this disease so far, and a detailed evaluation of its clinical features, radiologic characteristics, and pathologic findings will assist in future diagnosis of this disease.

2. Methods

The data of all cases diagnosed as hepatic RLH or pseudolymphoma and treated by surgery in Eastern Hepatobiliary Surgery Hospital, a tertiary university hospital in China, between January 1996 and June 2011 were obtained from the computerized files. Results of imaging studies such as ultrasonography (US), computerized tomography (CT), and magnetic resonance imaging (MRI), the clinicopathological findings and the outcomes of followup of the patients were retrospectively reviewed.

All the patients underwent surgery with complete resection of lesion(s). The resected specimens were fixed in 4% buffered formalin, processed, and embedded in paraffin. Histologic sections were stained with hematoxylin and eosin. Immunohistochemistry of paraffin sections was carried out using EnVision system (a two-step staining technique) as described previously [25]. Negative control slides omitting

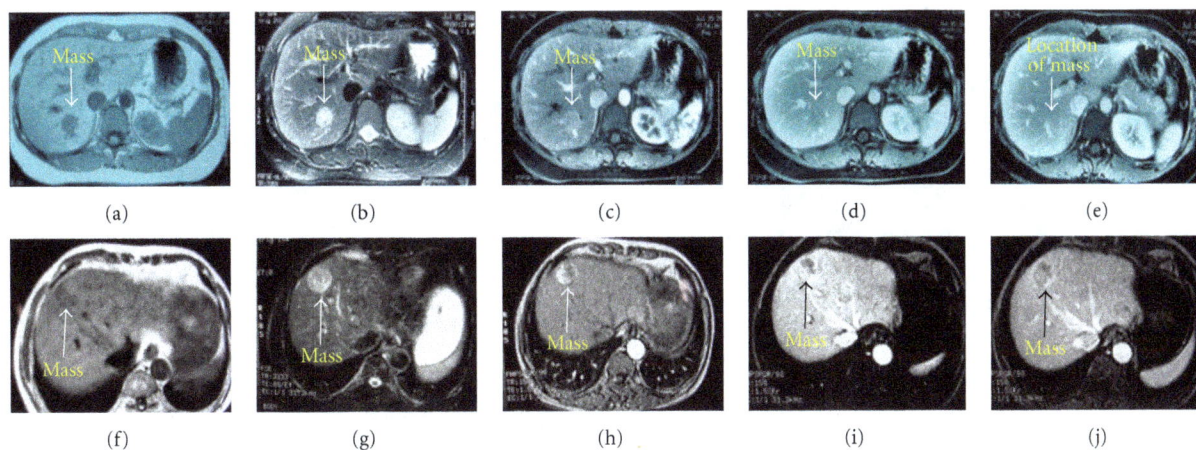

FIGURE 1: Comparison of appearances of hepatic RLH (a–e) with hepatocellular carcinoma (f–j) on fast spoiled gradient recalled echo (FSPGR) MRI. (a) On unenhanced T1-weighted image, the lesion is hypointense signal relative to normal liver parenchyma. (b) The lesion is hyperintense signal in the same location on T2-weighted image. (c) The lesion is enhanced in the arterial phase. (d) The lesion is hypodense in the portal phase. (e) The lesion is unclear in the delayed phase. (f) On plain T1-weighted imaging scan, the lesion is hypointense signal relative to normal liver parenchyma. (g) The lesion is hyperintense signal in the same location on T2-weighted image. (h) The lesion is significantly enhanced in the arterial phase. (i) The lesion is hypodense in the portal phase. (j) The lesion became more hypodense in the delayed phase.

the primary antibodies were included in all assays. The evaluation of the immunohistochemical findings was performed without any knowledge of the clinicopathologic data by two independent clinical pathologists.

After surgery, all the patients were monitored by serum-tumor markers, abdomen US, and chest X-ray every 1 to 3 months. If recurrence suspected, the patients underwent CT or MRI for further evaluation. The last followup was completed on December 31st, 2011 and the data were analyzed after the last followup.

3. Results

3.1. Patients' Demographics. From January 1996 to June 2011, a total of 45,000 patients with occupied lesion(s) in liver were admitted to our hospital for partial hepatectomy. In 7 of them, hepatic RLH was confirmed by pathological examination of resected specimens. There were 6 females and 1 male, with a median age of 46 years (range: 33–76 years). The patients were either asymptomatic or had mild nonspecific symptoms such as abdominal discomfort. Hepatitis B surface antigen was negative in 6 female patients, but positive in the male patient who was accompanied by cirrhosis. Hepatitis C virus antibody was negative in all the patients. Tumor markers including AFP, CEA, and CA19-9 were within normal range in all cases. Hepatic function tests and blood routine test were normal. Hemangiomas happened to occur simultaneously with RLH in two patients, and gall bladder calculi and fibroadenoma of breast are found in two female patients. In this series, the sizes of hepatic lesions varied from 13 × 15 mm to 105 × 65 mm on US scan, and the lesion of the male patient progressed during three years before operation (from 1.0 × 1.2 cm to 4.0 × 2.0 cm). Preoperatively, hepatocellular carcinoma (HCC)

was suspected in 6 patients and intrahepatic cholangiocellular carcinoma in the other one.

3.2. Surgical Outcomes. All the patients underwent curative local resections, and the postoperative course was uneventful in all cases. After surgery, no patient received subsequent therapy for hepatic RLH. Recurrence did not occur in any of our patients during a median followup of 68 months (range: 6–228 months).

3.3. Features on Imaging Studies. All the lesions of RLH were revealed as well-defined hypoechoic masses on US examination. The lesions were presented as hypodense masses on plain CT scan, slightly enhanced in the arterial phase, hypodense in the portal phase and the delayed phase as compared with liver parenchyma. MRI depicted hepatic RLH as nodular lesions with hypointense signal masses on T1-weighted imaging (Figure 1(a)), hyperintense signal on T2-weighted imaging (Figure 1(b)), and the lesions were moderately enhanced in the arterial phase (Figure 1(c)) followed by hypodense areas in the portal phase (Figure 1(d)) and unclear in the delayed phase (Figure 1(e)).

3.4. Pathologic and Immunohistochemical Analysis. On the cut sections, the lesions were grossly distinct firm nodules well demarcated from the surrounding liver tissue, sometimes encapsulated (5/7), with small areas of hemorrhage and necrosis (3/7) (Figure 2(a)). Histologic findings were similar for all the patients. Seen as a well-delineated nodular area microscopically, the lesions comprised a massive infiltration of heterogeneous mature lymphoid cells with no prominent nuclear atypia (Figure 2(c)), forming follicles (varied in size and shape) and germinal centers (Figure 2(b)), and there was no evidence of a monoclonal B cell population.

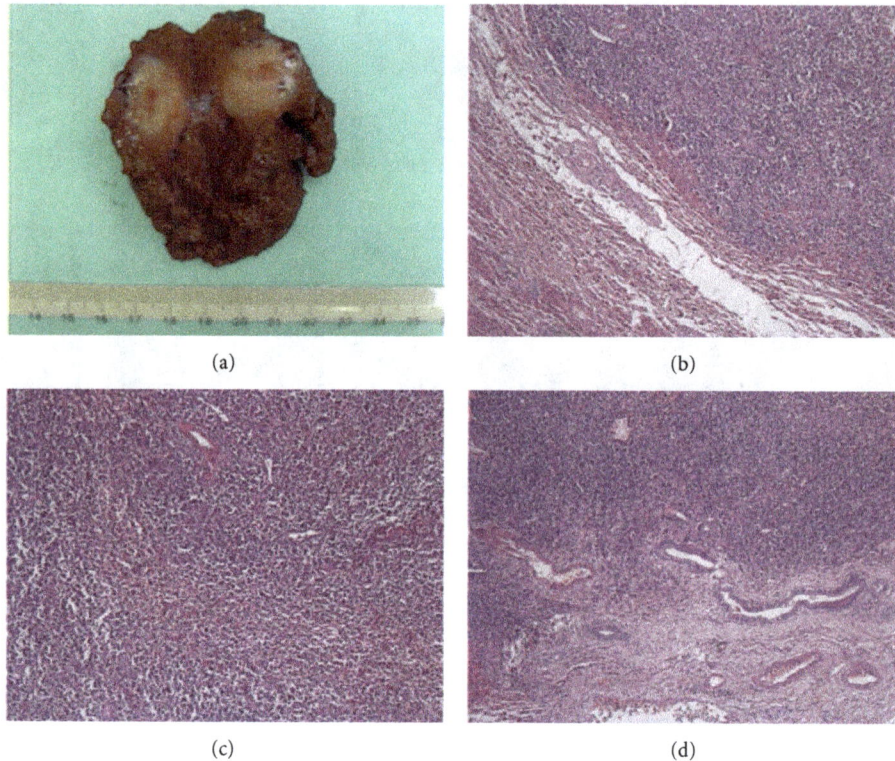

FIGURE 2: (a) Macroscopically, a cut section of the resected liver showed a well-circumscribed, encapsulated, yellow-white nodular lesion in segment 6, with small areas of hemorrhage and necrosis. (b) Microscopically, the lesion was well demarcated and encapsulated, and comprised a massive infiltration of mature lymphoid cells, forming follicles and germinal centers (H&E staining, 100x magnification). (c) The infiltrated lymphoid cells was mature and heterogeneous, with no nuclear atypia or polymorphism (H&E staining, 100x magnification). (d) Note the lymphocytic infiltration in the portal tracts around the lesion (H&E staining, 100x magnification).

In addition, fibrous materials aggregating in parts of the lesions (4/7), lymphocytic infiltration in the portal tracts around the nodular lesion (5/7) (Figure 3(d)), and bile ductules (2/7) were seen within the lesion. Germinal centers mainly comprised CD20 (+) and LCA (+) lymphocytes (Figures 3(a) and 3(b)), while lymphocytes in the interfollicular area and surrounding germinal centers were CD3 (+) and/or CD45RO (+) (Figures 3(c) and 3(d)). A polyclonal pattern of IgH (immunoglobulin heavy chain) and TCR-γ (T-cell receptor gamma) gene rearrangements of lymphocytes in the lesion was found in most patients.

4. Discussion

RLH is a benign condition that may occur, besides in liver, in the gastrointestinal tract [26], orbit [27], lung [28], skin [29], and thyroid [30]. Hepatic RLH was first reported by Snover et al. in 1981[8], and only 34 cases have been reported in the English literature until now [1–25, 31, 32]. We found 7 cases from 45,000 patients who underwent hepatectomy for liver masses, indicating the rarity of this disease. The incidence rate of hepatic RLH seems to be discovered increasing with time, as shown in Figure 4, perhaps for the advances in diagnostic imaging technologies and the accumulation of doctors' experience. However, the incidence rate might be

underestimated due to doctors' limited understanding of this disease.

At present, this is the largest case series review of hepatic RLH. In total, 41 cases of hepatic RLH are reported, including 36 females and 5 males (median age of 57 years; range, 15–85 years). All hepatic RLH patients were adults except for one 15-year-old female. A female predilection of this disease was obvious in both the present series (6/7) and when considering the sum of all cases (36/41). 6 cases have multiple hepatic lesion of RLH, and there were 49 hepatic lesions altogether. The average size (in greatest dimension) of hepatic lesions of our cases was 45.0 mm (range: 15–105 mm), which was bigger than that (15.6 mm in average; range: 4–60 mm) of the reported cases. The background data and the clinical characteristics of these 41 patients were summarized in Table 1.

The exact etiology of this disease remains unclear. An association between the development of hepatic RLH and some disease such as autoimmune diseases [1, 4–7, 9, 11] and malignant tumors [3, 6, 10, 13, 15, 20, 22, 31] has been suggested to be most likely involved in previous reviews. However, we believe this is not convincing because such concomitant diseases were not found in this series, and the reviews are independent, intermittent case reports.

It is very difficult to make a correct diagnosis of hepatic RLH before operation, as almost all of the cases including

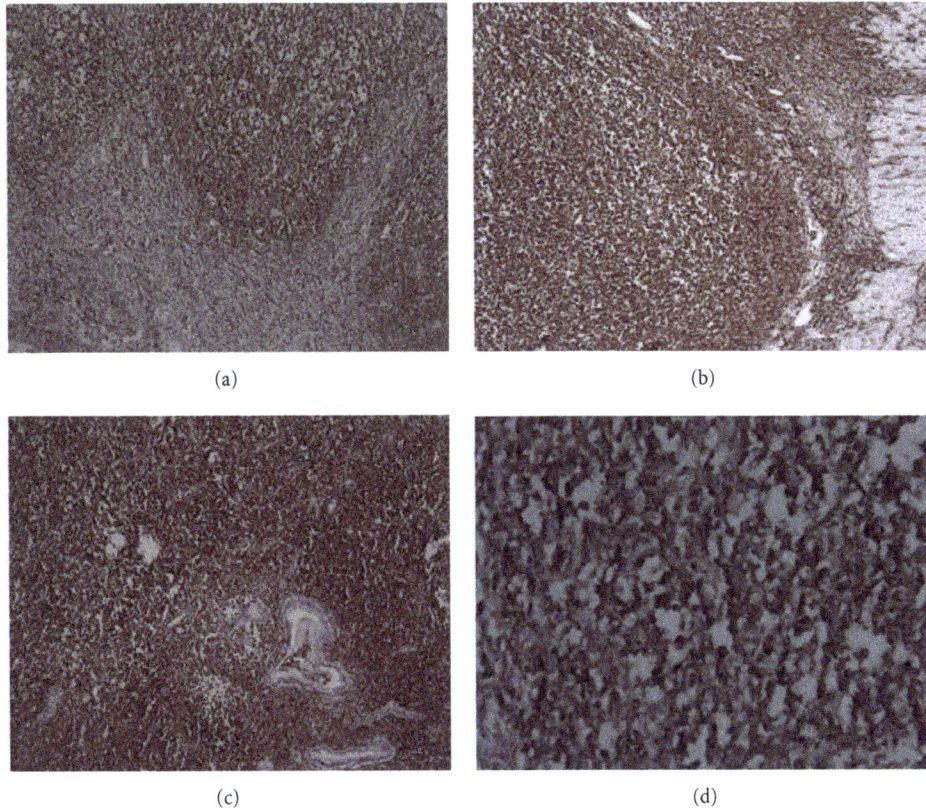

(a)

(b)

(c)

(d)

FIGURE 3: (a) Immuno.histochemistry showed that germinal centers mainly comprised CD20 (+) B lymphocytes (100x magnification) (b) Germinal centers mainly comprised LCA (+) lymphocytes (100x magnification) (c) T lymphocytes in interfollicular area and surrounding germinal centers were CD45RO (+) (100x magnification) (d) Germinal centers mainly comprised CD20 (+) B lymphocytes (400x magnification).

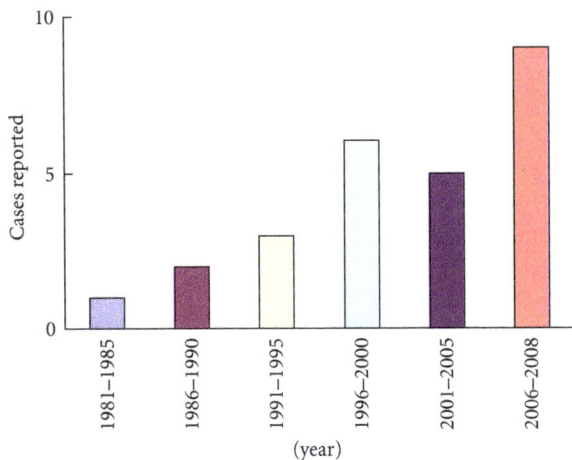

FIGURE 4: The incidence rate of this disorder seems to be increasing, calculated by the time when reported.

the reported have been misdiagnosed. Hepatic RLH has most frequently been misdiagnosed as HCC, as preoperative diagnosis are HCC (6/7) for our cases, while HCC (15/41) for all cases including the reported. Thus, differential diagnosis

between hepatic RLH and HCC is important but difficult, given their similarity on radiological appearances. However, in our cases, we found subtle differences in radiological findings between hepatic RLH and HCC. On MRI scan, hepatic RLH is always moderately enhanced in the arterial phase (Figure 1(c)), hypodense in the portal phase (Figure 1(d)) and unclear in the delayed phase (Figure 1(e)); while HCC is remarkably enhanced in the arterial phase (Figure 1(h)), prominently hypodense in the portal phase (Figure 1(i)) and more hypodense in the delayed phase (Figure 1(j)). The most characteristic radiological findng is that hepatic RLH becomes unclear in the delayed phase after injection of contrast agents. In addition, HCC is always accompanied by hepatitis virus infection and elevated level of AFP in China, which can be added to differential clues. From all the cases, we conclude the following radiological clues to help to diagnose hepatic RLH: (a) well-defined hypoechoic mass on the US images [4–7, 9–12, 14, 17–19, 23, 24, 32–34]; (b) low-density lesion in plain CT phase, mild enhancement in the arterial phase, hypodense areas in the portal phase [1–7, 9, 10, 12–18, 23, 24]; (c) hypointense signal on MRI T1-weighted imaging, hyperintense signal on T2-weighted imaging, moderately enhanced in the arterial phase, hypodense areas in the portal phase and unclear in the delayed

TABLE 1: Background data and clinical characteristics of all cases including the reported.

Background data and clinical characteristics	
Variables	Cases
Age (Y)	
15–30	1
31–60	21
60–85	19
Sex	
Female	36
Male	5
Concomitant disease	
Chronic hepatitis	7
Sjögren's syndrome	1
CREST syndrome	1
Autoimmune thyroiditis	5
Malignant tumor	12
Hepatic hemangioma/FNH	3
PBC	4
DM	2
Immunodeficiency	2
Size in the greatest dimension of lesions (cm)	
⩽4	37
>4	4
Number of lesions	
Solitary	35
Multiple	6
Location	
Rt. lobe	21
Lt. lobe	13
Lt. lobe and Rt. lobe	2
NA	5
Treatment	
Surgical resection	34
Transplantation	2
CNB and PEI	1
CNB and observation	3
Autopsy	1

Rt: right; Lt: left; Seg: segment NA: not available; PBC: primary biliary cirrhosis; FNH: focal nodular hyperplasia; DM: diabetes mellitus; PEI: percutaneous ethanol injections; CNB: core needle biopsy; NA: not available.

TABLE 2: Preoperative imaging findings of hepatic RLH of all cases including the reported.

Preoperative imaging findings	Cases
US	
Hypoechoic mass	7
CT	
Plain: hypodense	18
Arterial: significantly/slightly/peripherally enhanced	12
Parenchymal and portal: clearly/vaguely low	12
MRI	
Plain T1: low; T2: high	13
Arterial: highly/slightly enhanced	8
Portal and delayed: peripherally ring enhanced or clearly/vaguely hypointense	8
Angiography	
Hypervascularity	10

US: ultrasonographic; CT: computerized tomography; MRI: magnetic resonance imaging.

TABLE 3: Pathological characteristics of hepatic RLH of all cases including the reported.

Histological, immunohistochemical, and molecular findings	Cases
LIPTANL	22
Germinal center CD20/L26 (+)	26
Germinal center LCA (+)	6
Interfollicular area and surrounding germinal centers CD45RO/UCHL1 (+)	15
Area surrounding germinal centers CD3 (+)	11
Ductal structures at the periphery of the nodule CK7 (+)	5
Polyclonal in κ and λ light chain staining	26
Massive infiltration of heterogeneous mature lymphoid cells with no nuclear atypia, forming follicles and germinal centers	41

LIPTANL: lymphocytic infiltration in the portal tracts around the nodular lesion; NA: not available; L26 = CD20; UCHL1 = CD45RO.

phase [2, 3, 6, 10–15, 17, 18, 24]; (d) hypervascularity on angiography [11]. Preoperative imaging findings of the lesions of all the cases are listed in Table 2.

It is difficult to definitely recognize hepatic RLH by routine histologic evaluation alone. Common morphologic features include a well-demarcated region, hyperplastic lymphoid follicles with active germinal centers, hyalinized trabecular structures, and lymphocytic infiltration in the portal tracts around the nodular lesion [1, 5, 6, 9–15, 31, 35]. However, all of these appearances are not enough to distinguish hepatic RLH from inflammatory myofibroblastic

tumor and MALT lymphoma, given the similarity of morphologic features among them. Immunohistochemical and molecular genetic investigations are necessary to differentiate them [35]. In most hepatic RLH cases, germinal centers consist of polyclonal mature lymphocytes without cytologic atypia (mainly CD20 (+) and LCA (+)), and lymphocytes in the interfollicular area were predominantly CD3 (+) and/or CD45RO (+) (Table 3). In addition, polyclonal patterns of IgH and TCR-γ gene rearrangements of lymphocytes in the lesions were often observed (Table 3). However, in cases of primary hepatic MALT-type NHL [36–43], small B cells proliferating in lymphoid follicles displayed monoclonality. Although preoperative needle biopsy was applied in 5 reported cases [15, 17, 20, 35], it is not recommended because it cannot provide comprehensive details of results of immunohistochemical and molecular genetic studies. Also it is difficult to differentiate hepatic RLH from primary hepatic lymphoma only by needle biopsy [35].

Although hepatic RLH is generally thought to be benign, it might transform into malignant lymphoma [32], as reported in the lung [44] and stomach [45]. These early reports, however, were lack of the use of immunofluorescent and molecular techniques, and it is likely that these cases were in fact the early stage of primary lymphoma misdiagnosed as benign [46]. But evidence of progression from histologically benign, immunohistochemically polyclonal lymphoid infiltrates to malignant lymphoma in cutaneous pseudolymphoma has been reported in the literature [47]. Also we speculate hepatic RLH may grow with time, because the lesion of the male patient progressed during the three years before operation, similar to two reported cases [11, 18]. But different voices existed that hepatic RLH might have spontaneous regression, as in three cases [20, 35], diameter of the lesion had decreased during the followup without operation. However, it is not convincible because hepatic RLH was diagnosed by core needle biopsy in the three cases. Surgical resection is suggested both for treatment and for a definitive diagnosis of hepatic RLH even when pseudolymphoma is diagnosed preoperatively. Treatments for all the cases were surgical resection (7/7) in our series; while surgical resection (33/41), liver transplantation (2/41), percutaneous ethanol injection (1/41), core needle biopsy and observation (3/41) [20, 35], and unknown (2/41) in all cases including the reported. No complication related to surgical treatment happened. The prognosis of hepatic RLH is good, and all the patients treated by resection have shown no recurrence or progression to lymphoma.

In conclusion, hepatic RLH is a rare disease which mostly occurs in females, and the exact etiology of this disease is still unknown. Hepatic RLH has similar features with malignant liver tumors on radiological findings, but subtle differences such as "the lesion becomes unclear in the delayed phase on MRI scan with injection of contrast agents" can be found to be helpful for differential diagnosis. An accurate postoperative diagnosis of this disease depends not only on morphologic findings, but also on immunohistochemical analysis and molecular investigations. Given that hepatic RLH may grow with time or might even transform into malignant lymphoma, surgical resection is suggested, both for the safety and for good prognosis of the disease.

References

[1] S. Sharifi, M. Murphy, M. Loda, G. S. Pinkus, and U. Khettry, "Nodular lymphoid lesion of the liver: an immune-mediated disorder mimicking low-grade malignant lymphoma," *American Journal of Surgical Pathology*, vol. 23, no. 3, pp. 302–308, 1999.

[2] K. Willenbrock, S. Kriener, S. Oeschger, and M. L. Hansmann, "Nodular lymphoid lesion of the liver with simultaneous focal nodular hyperplasia and hemangioma: discrimination from primary hepatic MALT-type non-Hodgkin's lymphoma," *Virchows Archiv*, vol. 448, no. 2, pp. 223–227, 2006.

[3] V. Grouls, "Pseudolymphoma (inflammatory pseudotumor) of the liver," *Zentralblatt fur Allgemeine Pathologie und Pathologische Anatomie*, vol. 133, no. 6, pp. 565–568, 1987.

[4] T. Ohtsu, Y. Sasaki, H. Tanizaki et al., "Development of pseudolymphoma of liver following interferon-alpha therapy for chronic hepatitis B," *Internal Medicine*, vol. 33, no. 1, pp. 18–22, 1994.

[5] K. Katayanagi, T. Terada, Y. Nakanuma, and T. Ueno, "A case of pseudolymphoma of the liver," *Pathology International*, vol. 44, no. 9, pp. 704–711, 1994.

[6] S. R. Kim, Y. Hayashi, K. B. Kang et al., "A case of pseudolymphoma of the liver with chronic hepatitis C," *Journal of Hepatology*, vol. 26, no. 1, pp. 209–214, 1997.

[7] H. Okubo, H. Maekawa, K. Ogawa et al., "Pseudolymphoma of the liver associated with Sjögren's syndrome," *Scandinavian Journal of Rheumatology*, vol. 30, no. 2, pp. 117–119, 2001.

[8] D. C. Snover, A. H. Filipovich, L. P. Dehner, and W. Krivit, "'Pseudolymphoma'. A case associated with primary immunodeficiency disease and polyglandular failure syndrome," *Archives of Pathology and Laboratory Medicine*, vol. 105, no. 1, pp. 46–49, 1981.

[9] H. Isobe, S. Sakamoto, H. Sakai et al., "Reactive lymphoid hyperplasia of the liver," *Journal of Clinical Gastroenterology*, vol. 16, no. 3, pp. 240–244, 1993.

[10] H. Takahashi, H. Sawai, Y. Matsuo et al., "Reactive lymphoid hyperplasia of the liver in a patient with colon cancer: report of two cases," *BMC Gastroenterology*, vol. 6, article 25, 2006.

[11] K. Nagano, Y. Fukuda, I. Nakano et al., "Case report: reactive lymphoid hyperplasia of liver coexisting with chronic thyroiditis: radiographical characteristics of the disorder," *Journal of Gastroenterology and Hepatology*, vol. 14, no. 2, pp. 163–167, 1999.

[12] N. Maehara, K. Chijiiwa, I. Makino et al., "Segmentectomy for reactive lymphoid hyperplasia of the liver: report of a case," *Surgery Today*, vol. 36, no. 11, pp. 1019–1023, 2006.

[13] K. Sato, Y. Ueda, M. Yokoi, K. Hayashi, T. Kosaka, and S. Katsuda, "Reactive lymphoid hyperplasia of the liver in a patient with multiple carcinomas: a case report and brief review," *Journal of Clinical Pathology*, vol. 59, no. 9, pp. 990–992, 2006.

[14] T. Tanizawa, Y. Eishi, R. Kamiyama et al., "Reactive lymphoid hyperplasia of the liver characterized by an angiofollicular pattern mimicking Castleman's disease," *Pathology International*, vol. 46, no. 10, pp. 782–786, 1996.

[15] K. Shiozawa, H. Kinoshita, H. Tsuruta et al., "A case of pseudolymphoma of the liver diagnosed before operation," *Nipponn Syoukakibyou Gakkai Zassi*, vol. 101, no. 7, pp. 772–778, 2004.

[16] H. S. Park, K. Y. Jang, Y. K. Kim, H. C. Baik, and S. M. Woo, "Histiocyte-rich reactive lymphoid hyperplasia of the liver: unusual morphologic features," *Journal of Korean Medical Science*, vol. 23, no. 1, pp. 156–160, 2008.

[17] N. Matsumoto, M. Ogawa, M. Kawabata et al., "Pseudolymphoma of the liver: sonographic findings and review of the literature," *Journal of Clinical Ultrasound*, vol. 35, no. 5, pp. 284–288, 2007.

[18] T. Okada, H. Mibayashi, K. Hasatani et al., "Pseudolymphoma of the liver associated with primary biliary cirrhosis: a case report and review of literature," *World Journal of Gastroenterology*, vol. 15, no. 36, pp. 4587–4592, 2009.

[19] T. Machida, T. Takahashi, T. Itoh, M. Hirayama, T. Morita, and S. Horita, "Reactive lymphoid hyperplasia of the liver: a case report and review of literature," *World Journal of Gastroenterology*, vol. 13, no. 40, pp. 5403–5407, 2007.

[20] H. Ota, N. Isoda, F. Sunada et al., "A case of hepatic pseudolymphoma observed without surgical intervention," *Hepatology Research*, vol. 35, no. 4, pp. 296–301, 2006.

[21] R. Jiménez, A. Beguiristain, I. Ruiz-Montesinos, F. Garnateo, and M. Echenique Elizondo, "Nodular lymphoid hyperplasia of the liver. Pseudolymphoma," *Revista Española de Enfermedades Digestivas*, vol. 99, no. 10, pp. 299–306, 2007.

[22] E. Lin, "Reactive lymphoid hyperplasia of the liver identified by FDG PET," *Clinical Nuclear Medicine*, vol. 33, no. 6, pp. 419–420, 2008.

[23] K. Yoshikawa, M. Konisi, T. Kinoshita et al., "Reactive lymphoid hyperplasia of the liver: literature review and 3 case reports," *Hepato-Gastroenterology*, vol. 58, no. 109, pp. 1349–1353, 2011.

[24] J. Tuckett, M. Hudson, S. White, and J. Scott, "Reactive lymphoid hyperplasia of the liver: a case report and review of imaging characteristics," *European Journal of Radiology Extra*, vol. 79, no. 1, pp. e11–e14, 2011.

[25] E. Sabattini, K. Bisgaard, S. Ascani et al., "The EnVision++ system: a new immunohistochemical method for diagnostics and research. Critical comparison with the APAAP, ChemMate(TM), CSA, LABC, and SABC techniques," *Journal of Clinical Pathology*, vol. 51, no. 7, pp. 506–511, 1998.

[26] S. L. Abbondanzo and L. H. Sobin, "Gastric "pseudolymphoma": a retrospective morphologic and immunophenotypic study of 97 cases," *Cancer*, vol. 79, no. 9, pp. 1656–1663, 1997.

[27] D. M. Knowles, F. A. Jakobiec, L. McNally, and J. S. Burke, "Lymphoid hyperplasia and malignant lymphoma occurring in the ocular adnexa (orbit, conjunctiva, and eyelids): a prospective multiparametric analysis of 108 cases during 1977 to 1987," *Human Pathology*, vol. 21, no. 9, pp. 959–973, 1990.

[28] S. L. Abbondanzo, W. Rush, K. E. Bijwaard, and M. N. Koss, "Nodular lymphoid hyperplasia of the lung: a clinicopathologic study of 14 cases," *American Journal of Surgical Pathology*, vol. 24, no. 4, pp. 587–597, 2000.

[29] M. F. Baldassano, E. M. Bailey, J. A. Ferry, N. L. Harris, and L. M. Duncan, "Cutaneous lymphoid hyperplasia and cutaneous marginal zone lymphoma: comparison of morphologic and immunophenotypic features," *American Journal of Surgical Pathology*, vol. 23, no. 1, pp. 88–96, 1999.

[30] Y. Mizukami, N. Ikuta, T. Hashimoto et al., "Pseudolymphoma of the thyroid," *Acta Pathologica Japonica*, vol. 38, no. 10, pp. 1329–1336, 1988.

[31] L. Pantanowitz, P. F. Saldinger, and M. E. Kadin, "Pathologic quiz case: hepatic mass in a patient with renal cell carcinoma," *Archives of Pathology and Laboratory Medicine*, vol. 125, no. 4, pp. 577–578, 2001.

[32] S. I. Sato, T. Masuda, H. Oikawa et al., "Primary hepatic lymphoma associated with primary biliary cirrhosis," *American Journal of Gastroenterology*, vol. 94, no. 6, pp. 1669–1673, 1999.

[33] A. Nonomura, H. Minato, K. Shimizu et al., "Pseudolymphoma (reactive lymphoid hyperplasia) of the liver containing epithelioid cell granulomas and Schaumann's bodies in giant cells: a case report," *International Journal of Surgical Pathology*, vol. 6, no. 2, pp. 101–108, 1998.

[34] R. Jiménez, A. Beguiristain, I. Ruiz-Montesinos et al., "Image of the month: reactive lymphoid hyperplasia," *Archives of Surgery*, vol. 143, no. 8, pp. 805–806, 2008.

[35] Y. Zen, T. Fujii, and Y. Nakanuma, "Hepatic pseudolymphoma: a clinicopathological study of five cases and review of the literature," *Modern Pathology*, vol. 23, no. 2, pp. 244–250, 2010.

[36] C. J. Story, A. A. Morley, D. R. Turner, and R. Seshadri, "Diagnostic use of immunoglobulin and T-cell receptor gene rearrangements in lymphoproliferative disease," *Australian and New Zealand Journal of Medicine*, vol. 17, no. 1, pp. 1–8, 1987.

[37] P. G. Isaacson, P. M. Banks, P. V. Best, S. P. McLure, H. K. Muller-Hermelink, and J. I. Wyatt, "Primary low-grade hepatic B-cell lymphoma of mucosa-associated lymphoid tissue (MALT)-type," *American Journal of Surgical Pathology*, vol. 19, no. 5, pp. 571–575, 1995.

[38] J. P. Bronowicki, C. Bineau, P. Feugier et al., "Primary lymphoma of the liver: clinical-pathological features and relationship with HCV infection in French patients," *Hepatology*, vol. 37, no. 4, pp. 781–787, 2003.

[39] C. M. Kirk, D. Lewin, and J. Lazarchick, "Primary hepatic B-cell lymphoma of mucosa-associated lymphoid tissue," *Archives of Pathology and Laboratory Medicine*, vol. 123, no. 8, pp. 716–719, 1999.

[40] M. Maes, C. Depardieu, J. L. Dargent et al., "Primary low-grade B-cell lymphoma of malt-type occurring in the liver: a study of two cases," *Journal of Hepatology*, vol. 27, no. 5, pp. 922–927, 1997.

[41] R. M. Prabhu, L. J. Medeiros, D. Kumar et al., "Primary hepatic low-grade B-cell lymphoma mucosa-associated lymphoid tissue (MALT) associated with primary biliary cirrhosis," *Modern Pathology*, vol. 11, no. 4, pp. 404–410, 1998.

[42] M. Q. Ye, A. Suriawinata, C. Black, A. D. Min, J. Strauchen, and S. N. Thung, "Primary hepatic marginal zone B-cell lymphoma of mucosa-associated lymphoid tissue type in a patient with primary biliary cirrhosis," *Archives of Pathology and Laboratory Medicine*, vol. 124, no. 4, pp. 604–608, 2000.

[43] E. Zucca, A. Conconi, E. Pedrinis et al., "Nongastric marginal zone B-cell lymphoma of mucosa-associated lymphoid tissue," *Blood*, vol. 101, no. 7, pp. 2489–2495, 2003.

[44] M. N. Koss, L. Hochholzer, and P. W. Nichols, "Primary non-Hodgkin's lymphoma and pseudolymphoma of lung: a study of 161 patients," *Human Pathology*, vol. 14, no. 12, pp. 1024–1038, 1983.

[45] J. J. Brooks and H. T. Enterline, "Gastric pseudolymphoma. Its three subtypes and relation to lymphoma," *Cancer*, vol. 51, no. 3, pp. 476–486, 1983.

[46] E. A. Holland, G. G. Ghahremani, W. A. Fry, and T. A. Victor, "Evolution of pulmonary pseudolymphomas: clinical and radiologic manifestations," *Journal of Thoracic Imaging*, vol. 6, no. 4, pp. 74–80, 1991.

[47] B. F. Kulow, H. Cualing, P. Steele et al., "Progression of cutaneous B-cell pseudolymphoma to cutaneous B-cell lymphoma," *Journal of Cutaneous Medicine and Surgery*, vol. 6, no. 6, pp. 519–528, 2002.

12

"Incidentaloma" of the Liver: Management of a Diagnostic and Therapeutic Dilemma

Denis Ehrl,[1] Katharina Rothaug,[1] Peter Herzog,[2] Bernhard Hofer,[1] and Horst-Günter Rau[1]

[1] *Department of Visceral, Thoracic und Vascular Surgery, Clinic of Dachau, 85221 Dachau, Germany*
[2] *Department of Radiology, Clinic of Dachau, Krankenhausstrare 15, 85221 Dachau, Germany*

Correspondence should be addressed to Denis Ehrl, denis.ehrl@amperkliniken.de

Academic Editor: Alfred Königsrainer

The continuous development of highly sensitive clinical imaging increased the detection of focal lesions of the liver. These accidentally detected liver tumors without liver-specific symptoms such as cholestasis have been named "incidentalomas." Diagnostic tools such as sonography, computed tomography, or magnetic resonance imaging are used increasingly in asymptomatic individuals without defined suspected diagnoses in the setting of general prevention or followup after a history of malignancy. But despite continuous improvement of diagnostics, some doubt regarding the benign or malign behavior of a tumor remains. In case an asymptomatic hemangioma or FNH can be preoperatively detected with certainty, the indication for surgery must be very strict. In case of symptomatic liver lesions surgical resection should only be indicated with tumor-specific symptoms. In the remaining cases of benign lesions of the liver, a "watch and wait" strategy is recommended. In case of uncertain diagnosis, especially in patients with positive history of a malignant tumor or the suspected diagnosis of hepatocellular adenoma, surgical resection is indicated. Due to the continuous improvement of surgical techniques, liver resection should be done in the laparoscopic technique. Laparoscopic surgery has lower morbidity and shorter hospitalization than open technique.

1. Introduction

In recent years the rapid development of highly sensitive clinical imaging has led to the detection of focal lesions of the liver more frequently. In addition, diagnostic tools are used increasingly in asymptomatic individuals without defined suspected diagnoses in the setting of general prevention or followup after a history of malignancy [1–4]. Unfortunately, the histological nature of a hepatic tumor is rarely proven by one method of imaging, and even sophisticated technologies some doubt regarding the benign or malign behavior of a tumor remain in 10–40% [5, 6]. These accidentally detected liver tumors without liver-specific symptoms such as cholestasis or portal hypertension have been named "incidentalomas" [4]; the reported incidence of these findings ranges from 10.2 to 52% [7, 8]. Autopsy studies have demonstrated up to 52% benign liver lesions in the western population [9, 10]. Other authors could demonstrate an incidence of incidentalomas of 10.2–14.3% of CT scans [7–9]. Generally, these tumors can be true benign or malign neoplasms or so-called tumor-like lesions [3]. Malignant

tumors of the liver become usually only in stages of an advanced disease symptomatic. In case of metastases usually a primary tumor is known from the patient's history or can be diagnosed by endoscopy and thoracical and abdominal CT scans [2, 3].

Currently, there are no evidence-based guidelines regarding the appropriate approach to diagnosis, interpretation of imaging and laboratory findings, and the indication for surgical resection. Prospective, sufficiently powered, randomized controlled trials on the elective resection of benign liver lesions are lacking. Most recommendations are based on retrospective data with fewer than 60 patients or casuistic reports [1, 10, 11]. We want to add our personal experience and results to the upcoming discussion.

Generally a primarily conservative approach is considered to be the method of first choice in the treatment of proven benign liver tumors [1, 3, 5, 10, 11]. In total for about 5% of newly diagnosed benign liver tumors, surgery is warranted [10]. Despite the continuous improvement of the radiological and nuclear medical diagnostics, surgery is often just indicated because of the possibility of

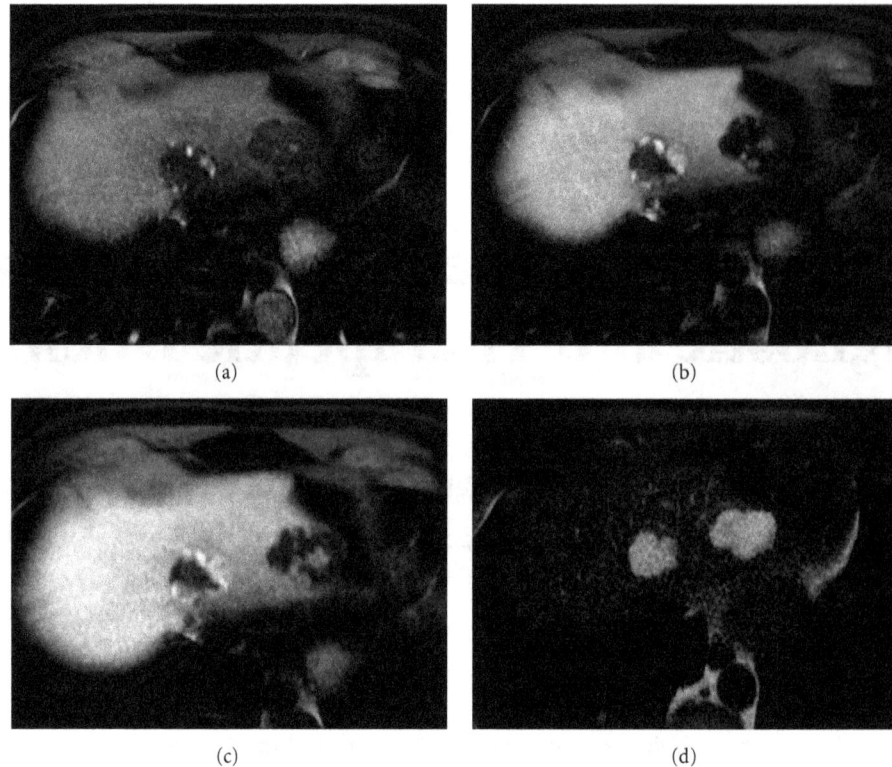

(a)   (b)

(c)   (d)

FIGURE 1: Two hemangiomas in gadolinium enhanced MRI (contrast medium: gadoxetic acid; disodium salt (Primovist, Eurokontrast GmbH, Heidelberg), scanner: GE Signa HDxt 1,5T (General Electric Company, USA)): peripheral nodular enhancement in T1 FS early arterial contrast phase (upper left): (T1 LAVA FS dynamic FA80, TR 185 TE 4,2), progressive centripetal enhancement in T1 FS late arterial (upper right): (T1 LAVA FS dynamic FA80, TR 185 TE 4,2) and portal-venous phase (lower left): (T1 LAVA FS dynamic FA80, TR 185 TE 4,2). Typical ill-shaped intermediate (less than in cysts) hyperintensity in T2 (lower right): (T2 FRFSE FS FA 90 TR 2500 TE 94,16). Lesion in left lobe is partially clotted with thrombosis and shows less enhancement.

a primary or secondary malignant tumor in the liver [12–15]. Other common indications for surgical resection include abdominal discomfort, tumor growth, history of adenoma, and rarely the desperate request of the patient [10, 11, 13]. An accepted emergency indication is acute bleeding of a benign liver lesion [16, 17]. This may occur as a free rupture with haemoperitoneum, as prolonged intrahepatic haemorrhage or hemobilia leading to gastrointestinal bleeding, the latter being considerably difficult to diagnose [16, 17]. In spite of the low morbidity and minimal mortality of liver resections in specialized institutions, surgical treatment of benign liver lesion is only justified in the above indications and requires precise criterions [3–5].

The cavernous and capillary hepatic hemangiomas, the focal nodular hyperplasia (FNH), and the hepatocellular adenoma are the most common benign lesions of the liver [1, 3, 11] and are presented below.

1.1. Hemangioma (Figure 1). These are usually diagnosed as asymptomatic incidental findings. In addition to nonspecific symptoms, hemangiomas also (rarely) rupture spontaneously or by trauma and then lead to acute hemorrhagic shock with upper abdominal pain [1, 10, 18]. In the worldwide literature a total of only 97 cases with a rupture of a hemangioma have been published, whereas a spontaneous rupture only happened in 47.4% of cases (46) [19]. Further

investigation showed that these spontaneously ruptured hemangiomas had a mean size of 11.2 cm [19]. In an acute situation, the immediate restitution of coagulation factors and rarely TAE are methods of choice [1, 10, 11, 18]. TAE teatment of a hemangioma is difficult and due to the aberrant collateral arterial circulation making almost improbable to stop the multiple inflow from different feeding arteries especially through the periphery of the hemangiomas. Despite therapy, in these situations the mortality rate is 30–40% [10].

Hemangiomas rarely occur in association with clinical syndromes. These include most of all the Kasabach-Merritt syndrome and the Blumgart-Bornman-Terblanche syndrome. The Kasabach-Merritt syndrome is characterized by a hemangioma bleeding, thrombocytopenia, and coagulopathy [1, 10]. The Blumgart-Bornman-Terblanche syndrome is accompanied by fever and abdominal pain [1, 20]. These syndromes can evoke minor and major complications and should be treated surgically [1].

Hemangiomas generally have no growth tendency. In the literature, however, cases of hemangioma growth during pregnancy or after estrogen administration are described [1, 10]. Hemangiomas <10 cm should generally not be treated, even before a pregnancy. In case of a planned pregnancy and a size >10 cm, due to the risk of a possible rupture, a definitive treatment should be discussed [1, 10]. Several studies have concluded that a spontaneous rupture of a hemangioma (even while pregnancy) [10, 19] occurs only very rarely, and therefore a prophylactic resection should only be conducted under special conditions and especially with a size of the hemangioma >11 cm [10]. In case of hemangiomas with high growth trend (>3 cm in 12 months), with symptomatic compression symptoms or recurrent pain, which may correlate with hemorrhage into the lesion, surgical intervention should be indicated [18, 19]. Because of hypotension, unexplained anemia, or diagnosis difficulties of the liver lesion, surgical intervention can be rarely necessary. In exceptional cases, individual patient factors, such as an extreme carcinogenicity phobia or high risk of rupture due to a patients career, sometimes require a resection of the lesion [18]. Overall, the indication for surgical intervention should be found cautiously [21, 22].

Treatment of choice is the parenchyma-saving enucleation or the sparing liver resection [10, 11, 18, 21]. In giant centrally located hemangioma a total vascular exclusion of the liver is a useful technical maneuver to save blood while dissecting it. Only in case of an extensive involvement of a liver lobe or central location, an anatomical resection is indicated [11]. In exceptional cases of giant hemangiomas and less functional parenchyma reserve, in the medical literature as a rarity a liver transplant is described [10].

1.2. Focal-Nodular Hyperplasia (FNH) (Figure 2). 10–20% of FNHs occur multifocally [1, 3, 10] and in 5–20% of cases these are diagnosed in combination with a hemangioma of the liver [10]. Clinical symptoms and complications are rare [11]. In case of newly diagnosed FNH, setting of oral contraceptives is currently not recommended [10]. The FNH has no malignant degeneration risk [1]. In the medical literature after initial diagnosis of FNH, a "wait and see" strategy is recommended [1, 10, 11]. For followup after 6 to 12 months, an imaging control investigation to identify a possible tendency of growth should be done [10]. Radiological long-term observations are not necessary.

In case of a FNH, there is primarily no indication for surgical intervention [1]. Surgical therapy can be discussed, especially for large expansive growing FNH nodes [5, 10]. This is especially for women wishing to have children clinically relevant. During pregnancy due to hormonal influences, a progressive growth of FNH could occur [10]. In case of an unambiguous preoperative diagnosis and indication for surgical intervention, the atypical resection is the treatment of choice [3, 5, 10, 11]. Often several liver segments are involved, resulting in an extension of the surgical procedure [11]. The literature describes no recurrence after resection [10].

1.3. Hepatocellular Adenoma (Figure 3). This lesion of the liver is often diagnosed as an incidental finding in asymptomatic patients. In association with an adenoma often right-sided upper abdominal pain (80%) with normal liver function values occurs [1, 3, 23, 24]. Rupture and subsequent acute bleeding event of a previously unknown adenoma occur at 10–30% of cases [1, 10, 23]. This spontaneous

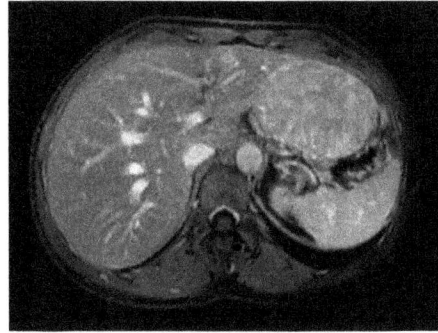

FIGURE 2: Focal nodular hyperplasia in gadolinium-enhanced MRI (contrast medium: gadoxetic acid; disodium salt (Primovist, Eurokontrast GmbH, Heidelberg), scanner: GE Signa HDxt 1,5T (General Electric Company, USA)): inhomogeneous hyperintensity on T1 FS in portal-venous contrast phase (T1 FSPGR FS FA12, TR 4,24 TE 2,04, TI 7).

rupture happens almost exclusively in adenomas >5 cm and is associated with a mortality of 8% [1, 23].

Beside the risk of acute bleeding complications, hepatocellular adenomas have a malignant degeneration risk from 4.2 to 10%, especially in inflammatory adenomas on MRI and/or the possibility of beta-catenin expression [1, 3, 10, 23, 24]. Generally adenomas of liver healthy patients arising by hormonal stimulation should be differentiated from those that arise due to a preexisting disease of the liver (like liver cirrhosis) and can degenerate into a HCC [24, 25]. Risk factors for malignant transformation are size of the adenoma (usually >5 cm), androgen or steroid use, male gender, and glycogen storage disease [24, 25].

The adenomatosis, with more than 10 adenomas in an otherwise normal liver, is a special form. This is gender unspecific and has no association with the use of hormones [26, 27].

The diagnostic differentiation from hemangioma is straightforward [3, 11]. The differential diagnosis of FNH is sometimes difficult [11, 24]. Grazioli et al. showed that gadoxetic acid-enhanced MRI (Primovist) facilitates the differentiation of hepatocellular adenoma and FNH [28]. The gadoxetic acid-enhanced MRI distinguishes between adenomas and FNH with sensitivity of 92% and specificity of 91% [28]. The differentiation to (highly) differentiated hepatocellular carcinoma (HCC), especially for the fibrolamellar type (FLC) of HCC is often problematic [29, 30]. For this reason, hepatic resection should be performed according to oncologic criteria of a simple atypical resection up to the extended hemihepatectomy [11, 24, 29, 30]. In nonhemorrhagic, hemorrhagic and especially in inflammatory adenomas on MRI and the possibility of beta catenin expression, the indication for surgery should be clear irrespective of size. Over 45% of adenomas demonstrate a progressive growth, so up to 25% of the operated patients require another surgical intervention [10, 24, 30]. After resection, the mortality is <1% [24, 29, 30]. In order to detect malignant transformation of adenomas in patients after resection, a strict followup is needed, containing annual imaging and regular AFP determination [10]. The liver

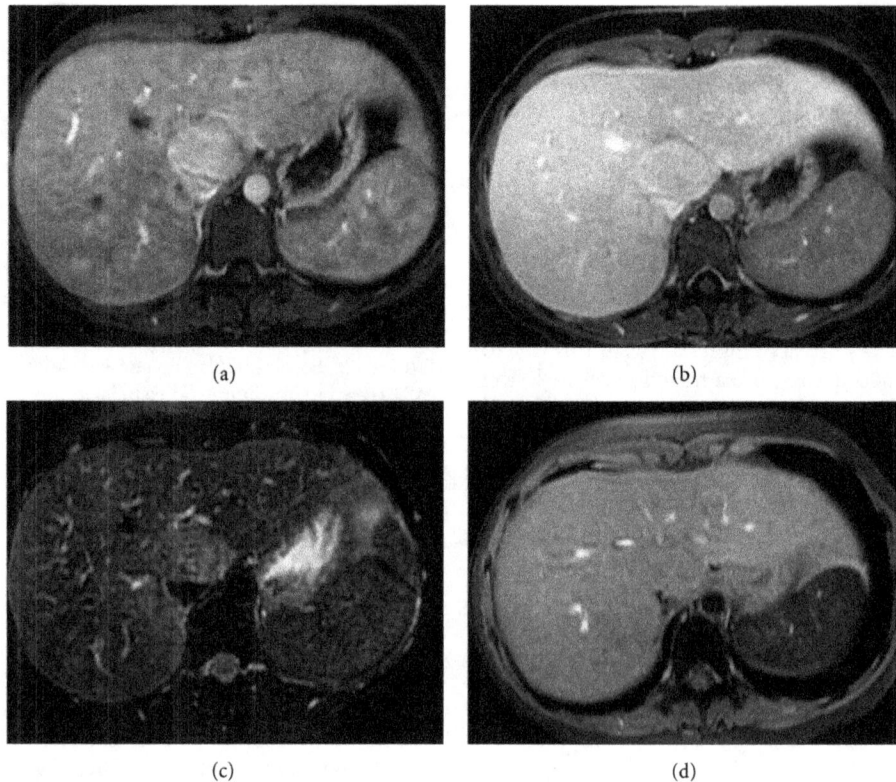

(a)   (b)

(c)   (d)

FIGURE 3: Segment 1 adenoma in gadolinium-enhanced MRI (contrast medium: gadoxetic acid; disodium salt (Primovist, Eurokontrast GmbH, Heidelberg), scanner: GE Signa HDxt 1,5T (General Electric Company, USA)): hyperintens. in T1 FS arterial contrast phase (upper left): (T1 LAVA FS dynamic FA80, TR 185 TE 4,2), partial equilibration to liver isointensity in T1 FS late portal-venous phase (upper right): (T1 FSPGR FS FA12, TR 4,24 TE 2,04, TI 7), slight hyperintensity on T2 FS (lower left): (T2 FRFSE FS FA 90 TR 2500 TE 94,16), and isointensity in unenhanced T1 fat sat. (lower right): (T1 LAVA FS dynamic FA80, TR 185 TE 4,2).

transplant is considered to be the ultima ratio in case of solid, very large, unresectable, symptomatic adenomas, in distinct adenomatosis of the liver with AFP increase or in case of multiple, progressive growing recurrence adenomas [10, 24].

1.4. Tumors of Unknown Dignity. Atypical tumors of the liver, such as the angiolipoma or cystadenoma, often have an inhomogeneous structure that usually a precise preoperative classification of a benign or a malignant tumor is impossible. This is the reason why in case of these tumors oncologic resections with appropriate security clearance are recommended [1, 11].

2. Patients and Methods

2.1. Tumor Entities. The conservative and surgical treatment of benign lesions of the liver includes several regenerative or real-neoplastic tumor entities. Depending on their origin, these tumors are divided in hepatocellular, endothelial, biliary, mesenchymal, and connective tissue tumors [11] (Table 1).

The benign lesions of the liver can be divided in solid tumors, in tumors with solid areas, or cystic tumors. They are uni- or multilocular [31, 32].

As illustrated in Table 2 (for the three most common benign liver tumors), with detailed history and clinical findings, first conclusions regarding the dignity of the tumor can be drawn. In addition tumor-associated demographic data, possible characteristics, and further diagnostic measures are listed in Table 2.

2.2. Tumor Diagnostics. Clinical symptoms of the patient are crucial for the extent and type of diagnostic measures to be executed. If the patient is burdened by severe symptoms of the tumor, resection is indicated and further diagnostic workup is dispensable. On the other hand, with an asymptomatic tumor and nonspecific findings, every attempt has to be made to ensure the diagnosis. The contrast medium- (CM-) based computed tomography (CT) (multiphase spiral CT) and magnetic resonance imaging (MRI), especially when using liver-specific CM (e.g., gadoxetic acid (Primovist)), are the methods of choice in the diagnosis of benign liver tumors [33, 34].

In clinical routine, sonography is primarily used as screening method. Through the use of CM and technical enhancements, such as tissue harmonic imaging, the importance of sonography in the diagnosis of benign liver lesions has greatly increased. The disadvantage of this method of investigation is the investigator dependency [35, 36].

TABLE 1: Surgically relevant tumor entities [37].

	Pseudotumors*	Benign neoplasia
Hepatocellular tumors	Focal nodular hyperplasia (FNH)	Hepatocellular adenoma
Endothelial tumors		Hemangioma
Biliary tumors	Von Meyenburg complex	Biliary cystadenoma
		Biliary duct adenoma
Mesenchymal tumors	Hamartoma	
Connective tissue tumors	Lipoma, angiolipoma, fibroma, leiomyoma	
Mixed-cellular tumors		Teratoma

*Regenerative and real-neoplastic tumors.

TABLE 2: Tumour-associated demographics [1, 3, 10, 11, 18].

	Prevalence	Age	F:M	Location	Size	Specialties
Hemangioma	5–20%	35–65	2–6:1	Subcapsular 90% unifocal	<5–30 cm	Synchronic hemangioma in skin, lung, or brain (10–15%); partly pregnancy associated increase of size; with partial thrombosis often acute pain; rarely DIC (Kasabach-Merritt syndrome)
FNH	2-3%	30–50	8:1	Subcapsular 80% unifocal	<5–15 cm	Growing: association with OC; rarely clin. symptoms
Adenoma	Rare (incidence: 0,3:100000 pat. pera*)	25–45	10:1	Subcapsular often unifocal	5–15 cm rare up to 30 cm	Arise and growth: association with OC (>5 years), diabetes mellitus, androgen or steroid use, male gender, glycogen storage disease, often symptomatic

* a: year, OC: oral contraceptive, DIC: disseminated intravascular coagulopathy.

Even nuclear medical procedures, such as the erythrocyte pool scintigraphy with 99Tc or hepatobiliary scintigraphy under the utilization of tumor-specific characteristics without precise morphological mapping of the lesion, can achieve a high sensitivity in diagnostics. Relatively high costs and limited availability preclude nuclear medicine procedures from more extensive use despite their proven diagnostic value [11, 38]. Table 3 summarizes the usual imaging procedures and the respective performance of the three most common benign liver lesions.

In medical literature there are only few publications with larger numbers of cases that match radiological diagnosis with the corresponding histopathologic findings after surgical resection. Grimm et al. showed, in 26 cases of histological confirmed benign liver tumors, that the multiphase CT or MRI examination only in 54% of the cases produced the correct preoperative diagnosis [39].

For the highest diagnostic "security" preoperatively, at least one imaging procedure should be performed using a suitable, liver-specific CM in combination with a nuclear medicine examination [11, 12]. As a result of this method, in only about 10% of liver tumors the dignity remains preoperatively unclear [10]. With these diagnostic possibilities, a hemangioma or FNH can be diagnosed with a specificity of <95% and a sensitivity of >80% [1, 11].

In addition to liver enzymes, bilirubin, and cholestasis, the laboratory testing should include the determination of the tumor markers AFP, CA 19-9, and CEA to distinguish it from malignant tumors of the liver [1, 3, 4, 10]. The integrity

of liver synthesis can be estimated by serum cholinesterase levels and the quick value. These parameters in combination with the morphological assessment of cirrhosis status and volume rendering of the planned resection allow a reasonable prediction of functional outcome [1, 3, 4].

In case of a symptomatic tumor, determinants of resectability such as size, location, relationship to the hilum, and the blood vessels are in the focus. Thereby a minimum of diagnostics, such as a sectional imaging, is sufficient. If in case of an asymptomatic neoplasia surgery is necessary, a graduated diagnostic procedure should be performed to determine the exact type of tumor and the subsequent appropriate therapy [4, 11].

In the literature, the performance of a percutaneous fine-needle biopsy (FNB) is controversially discussed. Because of the insufficient validity and often missing therapeutic consequences, the FNB should not be performed [12, 40–42]. Only 34–40% of FNB histologies are consistent with the histology of the surgical preparation [4, 10]. The puncture of the liver has a morbidity of 0.5% and a mortality of 0.05% [1, 4, 10]. Another nonnegligible risk is the possible seeding of malignant cells through the puncture of hepatocellular carcinoma (HCC). Huang et al. and Smith showed, through the puncture of the liver in up to 2% of cases, seeding of malignant cells in the needle tract occurs [43, 44].

In clinical practice preoperatively, the exact morphology of a tumor in up to 35–45% of cases is not clearly determined by radiological investigations. With the suspected diagnosis of a possible malignancy in these cases, often and completely

TABLE 3: Morphology of the most common benign lesions in imaging techniques [1, 3, 10, 11, 18, 33–35].

	Ultrasonography	Triphasic CT	MRI	18F-FDG PET scan	CT angiography
Hemangioma (Figure 1)	More often: cavernous (high flow): heterogeneous, hypoechoic, sometimes calcifying. More rare: capillary (low flow): homogeneous, hyperechoic, sharp limited, no halo. Doppler: low flow, low index, absence of spectral broadening	Early phase: iridic diaphragm phenomenon with peripheral nodular enhancement. Late phase: CM-enhancement rise, determination of the size	Peripheral enhancement, centripetal progression, T1: hypo intense T2: hyperintense Sensitivity >95% Specificity 95% 10% atypically	No uptake or photopenic defect compared to liver baseline	Cotton wool pooling of contrast, normal vessels without AV shunt, persistent enhancement
FNH (Figure 2)	Homogeneous, iso-, hypo- or hyperechoic, Central hyper echoic area Central aterial signal (50–70%: central scar) Doppler: high flow, spokes phenomenon, spectral broadening	Isodense with liver, Central low density Scar Arterial phase: homogeneous strongly enhance	Native: isodense T1: isodense T2: isodense hyper intense scar sensitivity >95% specificity >95%	No uptake	Hypervascular 70%; centrifugal supply
Adenoma (Figure 3)	Unspecific, Hypo- or hyper echoic Hemorrhage or necrosis: heterogeneous, anechoic center Doppler: variable flow, spectral broadening	Homogenous > heterogeneous Peripheral feeders filling in from periphery	T1 Gd: hyperintense T2: hyperintense (intralesional fat) capsule necrosis: T1: hypointense T2: hyperintense bleeding: T1 + T2: hyperintense	No uptake uptake If transformation to HCC in 30% of the cases	Hypervascular; large peripheral vessels; central scar if hemorrhage

CT: computed tomography, MRI: magnetic resonance imaging, FNH: focal-nodular hyperplasia CM: contrast medium, HCC: hepatocellular carcinoma.

understandable surgical resection of the lesion is indicated [11].

In case of a suspected adenoma due to the possible risk of malignant transformation or occult malignancy, surgical resection should be done initially or rarely after transarterial embolization (TAE). In acute bleeding with hemorrhagic shock, the extent of the diagnosis depends on the one hand on the urgency of the operation and on the other if the entity of tumor is previously known. In case of a known hemorrhagic hemangioma instead of a risky emergency surgery, a therapeutic TAE could be tried [45, 46]. In case of a nonhemorrhagic adenoma, TAE is not useful.

2.3. Indication. Because of preventive checkups, followup, and screening examinations, increasingly more asymptomatic liver lesions, especially in patients with a positive history of malignant tumor, are newly diagnosed. This has led to a shift in the spectrum of indications for surgery from symptomatic to asymptomatic patients. Depending on the tumor localization, specific symptoms such as a laboratory chemical cholestasis or portal hypertension are possible [1, 3, 10, 11]. Often nonspecific symptoms such as feeling some pain in the right upper abdomen, a feeling of fullness, or a vague dyspnea occur [42, 47]. Only because of a nonspecific pain syndrome, the indication for surgery should be avoided. D'Halluin et al. showed that up to 100% of nonspecific

symptoms with conservative therapy are to relieve, especially after finishing oral contraception [48].

The indication for surgery should be primary found in relation to the symptoms and the suspected diagnosis. In descending order in cases of an acute symptomatology such as bleeding, the suspicion of an adenoma or a lesion of unknown dignity, in particular with positive tumor history, a tumor-induced symptomatology, the progression of size, some nonspecific symptoms, or eventually also in case of a cancerophobia of the patient liver resection should be indicated [10–15].

In case of a prior history of hemangioma, if a spontaneous or traumatic rupture happens, the indications are entirely provided for the conservative approach, eventually after successful TAE [11, 18]. TAE treatment of hemangioma is very difficult and for this reason a treatment of second line.

2.4. Surgery. The recommendations for surgical management of benign liver lesions are based on the results of retrospective analysis or case reports with fewer than 60 patients (medical evidence 3-4) [10].

If the indication for surgery was found, parenchyma sparing techniques for operation should be preferred. If the diagnoses of hemangioma or FNH are proven, enucleation is the method of choice. With the enucleation the loss of functional liver parenchyma and, at the same time, blood loss and the risk of bile leaks can be reduced [4, 42, 49].

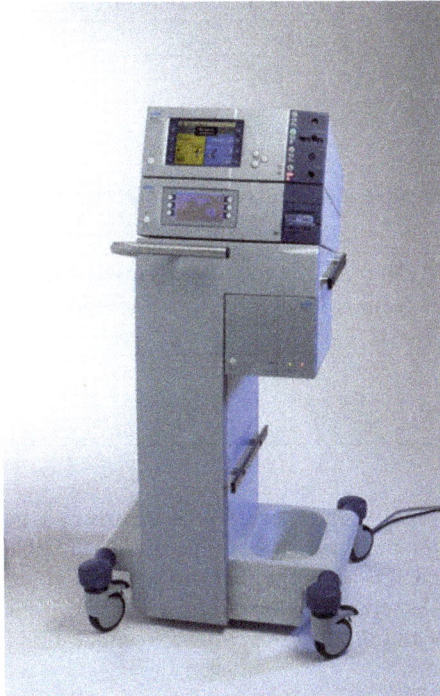

FIGURE 4: Waterjet dissector (Helix Hydro-Jet; Erbe Elektromedizin GmbH, Tübingen, Germany).

This leads to a significantly decreased perioperative morbidity and mortality [49]. Peripheral and/or smaller tumors should be resected in minimally invasive laparoscopic technique [10, 50, 51]. In our experience the waterjet dissection offers specific advantages (Figure 4). Compared to resections with the Cavitron ultrasonic surgical aspirator (CUSA) or by blunt dissection of the liver, the intraoperative blood loss and the time for resection can be significantly reduced [4, 51, 52]. In addition, bile ducts can be clearly visualized and closed by a clipping device, thereby avoiding postoperative bilioma. A Pringle maneuver for temporary vascular occlusion is not advocated when using water-jet dissection, because blood loss is minimal even without such measures and reperfusion damage to the residual liver can be significant [52]. The resection surface is meticulously inspected for venous and bile leakage, which can be closed by monofilamentous, resorbable sutures (Monosyn), and the whole plane is sealed by fibrin (TachoSil) [4, 51]. Anesthesiologic management of fluid intake is crucial; to minimize the blood loss at surgery, during resection the lowest possible PEEP and CVP pressures should be observed [11]. As previously noted in case of hemangiomas usually the enucleation (peripheral location), rarer a resection (central location, extensive tumor), is method of choice. In peripheral position of a FNH, the atypical liver resection is method of choice. Adenomas and tumors of unknown dignity should be resected for oncologic criteria (atypical resection to extended hemihepatectomy) [1, 4, 10, 11, 45].

2.5. Patient Population. This study only mentioned patients with one of the three most popular benign liver lesions, the

TABLE 4: Mean age in years of the subjects of our own collective and the literature.

	Dachau	Zülke et al. [11]	Charny et al. [47]	Weimann et al. [42]
Hemangioma	54.9	49.5	52	47.6
FNH	54.3	36	38	35.3
Adenoma	52.3	40	34	34

hemangioma, the hepatocellular adenoma, and the FNH. Not for all patients of our cohort, every diagnostic possibility, named in Table 3, was exhausted. Reasons for this approach were on the one hand often patients with a positive history of cancer (non-hepatogenous origin)—almost 50%—and on the other hand a unambiguously "malignancy-suspicious" liver lesion in one method of imaging. From 2004 till 2011, 40 patients (men and women) with one of these most common benign lesions of the liver underwent surgically treatment in the clinic of Dachau, Germany. The extent of surgical treatment ranged from atypical liver resection to extended hemihepatectomy. The liver resections were performed in laparoscopic and open technique. During surgical resection for all surgical specimens, a frozen section analyses was performed. Depending on the result of this examination, the extent of liver resection was determined. In our clinic generally parenchychma sparing techniques for surgical resection are preferred. For final histological results, all surgically resected liver tumors were examined in the Institute of Pathology, Rotkreuz hospital, Munich, Germany.

3. Results

3.1. Age and Gender Distribution. At the time of the liver resection, the age of the subjects in our series ranged from 23 to 72 years with a mean of 52.8 years. The ratio of men to females was 1.7 : 1. Tables 4 and 5 show the relevant important demographic information, age, and gender distribution divided into the three most common benign lesions of the liver, of our own patients collective compared to the literature. These tables show a higher mean age of patients in our collective and a less pronounced gender distribution. Reasons for these results are on the one hand the high number of patients with a history of cancer (non-hepatogenous origin) and on the other hand the lower number of patients in our collective compared to the literature. For instance, patients with an adenoma of the liver and a positive history of cancer would not be considered, the median age for patients with a adenoma totally was 42.1 years, and the gender distribution was 4 : 1. A similar pattern holds for the FNH and hemangioma.

3.2. Indication of Treatment. In patients with asymptomatic liver lesions, surgical intervention was mainly indicated since a primary or secondary malignancy could not be excluded with certainty. In case of symptomatic liver lesions, the indication for surgery was conducted on the one hand because of clinical symptoms, but on the other because a primary or secondary malignancy could not be preoperatively

TABLE 5: Gender distribution (females: men) of the subjects of our own collective and the literature.

	Dachau	Zülke et al. [11]	Charny et al. [47]	Weimann et al. [42]	Skalický et al. [5]
Hemangioma	1.6 : 1	1.2 : 1	3 : 1	2.9 : 1	2.3 : 1
FNH	2 : 1	2.5 : 1	9.5 : 1	11.5 : 1	2.1 : 1
Adenoma	1.3 : 1	2.4 : 1	5 : 1	3.9 : 1	1 : 2

TABLE 6: Indications for surgery of the three most common benign liver tumors (multiple answers in our own collective and Charny et al. [47]).

	Number of patients (n)			Health complaints (%)			Moot malignancy (%)		
	Dachau	Zülke et al. [11]	Charny et al. [47]	Dachau	Zülke et al. [11]	Charny et al. [47]	Dachau	Zülke et al. [11]	Charny et al. [47]
Hemangioma	21	12	39	29	58	59	71	25	33
FNH	12	21	18	17	42	44	92	33	61
Adenoma	7	15	8	88	33	37	57	67	75

excluded with certainty by means of morphological imaging. Most often patients of our series complained about right upper abdominal pain. Our patients also reported about indigestion, loss of appetite, and icterus. Table 6 compares the results of our own collective with those of the literature regarding the indication for elective surgical procedures. 81.3% of patients having health complaints had no history for carcinoma.

3.3. Types of Surgery. Beside the clinical and radiological diagnosis, the tumor location and size determine the extent and type of surgery. Table 7 shows the distribution of the respective surgical procedure for benign liver lesions of our own subjects in comparison to the literature.

The distribution of the respective applied surgical procedure shows in our collective of subjects as well as the collective of the reference centers a selected group. Therefore, these results do not reflect the expected approach in the surgical treatment of benign liver lesions. Normally in the vast majority of cases, atypical resections or enucleations would be expected and less segmental resections, resections of more than one segment, or hemihepatectomies.

Table 8 presents the size of operations for the three most common and atypical benign liver tumor entities of our patient cohort. With regard to hemangioma or FNH in more than 75% of all cases, an atypical or one segment resection was conducted. Larger and especially central hemangioma and FNH should be treated with a resection of more than one segment of the liver or even with a hemihepatectomy. Depending on the tumor size and location more than 70% of adenomas were oncologically treated with a segmental resection or with a resection of more than one segment.

3.4. Morbidity and Mortality. The low mortality rates result from the generally good preoperative liver morphology and function in patients with benign liver lesions. The rate of postoperative complications (minor) in our collective amounts in total for more than 15%. These results emphasize the need of a strict indication for liver resection, especially in primary asymptomatic patients (Table 9). The rate of surgical revision in our cohort was 0%.

The mortality and morbidity of laparoscopic liver resections in our own collective are presented in Table 10. The results are divided into the three most common benign liver lesions and show on the one hand a shorter hospitalization of patients and on the other a lower complication rate than open surgery.

3.5. Patients with a History of Malignant Tumor. Table 11 shows the number of subjects in our own collective where in the context of a history of cancer (non-hepatogenous origin) a lesion of the liver was noticed. In these cases a hepatic metastasis could not be radiologically excluded with certainty. Therefore the indication for resection of the liver lesion was set wider with regard to these subjects. Aim of this approach was on the one hand to get a definitive histology of "malignancy-suspicious" lesion and if needed to deliver an additional treatment such as chemotherapy or radiotherapy without loss of time, but also on the other to reach primarily a definitive treatment. In total, form 2004 to 2011, 185 patients with a history of cancer (non-hepatogenous origin) and a suspicion of liver metastasis were surgically treated in the Clinic of Dachau, Germany. After final histological examination, 15 (8.1%) of these "malignancy-suspicious" liver lesions revealed a benign result.

3.6. Compliance of Suspected Diagnosis and Operation-Histology. Table 12 presents the results of postoperative histological examination in comparison to the original diagnosis.

In 12% of cases a lesion of the liver was not known preoperatively and noticed during a laparoscopic cholecystectomy. In order to get histology, this incidental findings were completely laparoscopically, atypically resected. The subsequent histological examination showed uniformly the diagnosis of a hemangioma. In patients with a positive history of malignant disease, every intrahepatic mass of uncertain dignity was resected. Our high rate of 56% preoperative misdiagnosis for the hemangioma is therefore the result of including patients without a preoperative diagnosis and patients with limited preoperative imaging. If patients with a history of carcinoma or incidental perioperative findings are not considered in the analysis, there is an acceptable

TABLE 7: Distribution of surgical procedures.

	Dachau	Zülke et al. [11]	Charny et al. [47]	Weimann et al. [42]
	n (%)	n (%)	n (%)	n (%)
Atypical resection	20 (46)	15 (28)	33 (48)	84 (50)
Segmental resection, resection of more than one segment	19 (44)	32 (60)	12 (18)	38 (22)
Hemihepatectomy	4 (9)	6 (11)	23 (34)	47 (28)
Total	43	53	68	169

TABLE 8: Distribution of tumor-specific surgical procedure in our collective of subjects.

	Atypical resection	Segmental resection	Resection of more than one segment	Hemihepatectomy	Total
Hemangioma	11	6	2	2	21
FNH	6	3	1	2	12
Adenoma	2	4	1	0	7
Others	1	1	1	0	3

agreement of 76% of the results. With regard to FHN and adenoma, preoperative diagnosis was primarily uncertain or unreliable, this being particularly relevant for FNH with 58% and for adenoma with 72% when taking into account the patients with a history of cancer.

4. Discussion

The continuous development of imaging techniques enables to diagnose asymptomatic liver lesions with an increasingly high sensitivity and specificity [11, 18, 32–36, 38]. Based on the morphological and functional behavior of the various imaging procedures, the dignity of these lesions may partly be determined unambiguously [1–4, 18, 32–36, 38]. This assignment and classification is more difficult for patients with a positive malignant, non-hepatogenous history of tumor (especially in case of a colorectal and breast carcinoma).

In patients without history of malignant tumor, the FNH and the hemangioma are relatively straightforward to diagnose [3]. In the diagnosis of a hemangioma, the CM sonography, CT, or MRI is approximately equally effective [1, 3, 11, 18, 32–35]. With an MRI, a hemangioma can be diagnosed with a sensitivity of >95% and a specificity of 95% [1, 3, 11, 18, 32–35]. Method of choice in diagnosis of FNH is the MRI with liver-specific CM (e.g., gadoxetic acid; disodium salt (Primovist)). The sensitivity is >95%; the specificity is >95% [3, 11, 18, 32–35]. The diagnosis of an adenoma is often difficult. Method of choice is the MRI with liver-specific CM (e.g., gadoxetic acid; disodium salt (Primovist)) [1, 5, 11, 18, 32–35]. The diagnosis of a hepatocellular adenoma is only in premenopausal women with noncirrhotic liver, in case of the "classical" steroid-associated solitary adenoma, quite trivial to make [5]. Sometimes a hepatocellular adenoma and a FNH cannot be clearly differentiated [5]. Gradzioli et al. exposed in their study that gadoxetic acid-enhanced MRI (Primovist) facilitates the differentiation of hepatocellular adenoma and FNH with a sensitivity of 92% and specificity of 91% [28]. In the arterial phase the gadoxetic acid contrast enhancement of FNH (mean 94.3% ± 33.2) was significantly higher than

that of adenomas (mean 59.3% ± 28.1) ($P < .0001$) [28]. In the hepatobiliary phase, the lesion to liver contrast of hepatocellular adenomas showed strong negative values (mean −0.67 ± 0.24) and of FNH demonstrated minimally positive values (mean 0.05 ± 0.01) ($P < .0001$) [28]. Belghiti et al. [12] offered in their study with the aim of distinguishing FNH/adenoma, which in 83% of cases adenomas could be diagnosed preoperatively correctly (ultrasonography and CT). It was also apparent that all preoperative suspected diagnoses (ultrasound and CT) of FNH (18 cases) could be confirmed postoperatively, histologically (sensitivity 100%). But the histological analysis of 18 other cases also showed the diagnosis of FNH. In these patients preoperatively no unambiguous diagnosis (ultrasonography and CT) was possible (specificity 50%). Particularly problematic is the fact that postoperative, histological examination offered three HCC which were preoperative under the presumptive diagnosis of benign lesion of the liver [12]. These results emphasize the diagnostic difficulties in unclear, often asymptomatic liver lesions. Despite extensive diagnostics, the dignity of an asymptomatic liver lesion ultimately remains unclear in 10–40% of cases till surgical intervention and subsequent histology [5, 6, 11]. These points mentioned the problems in the treatment of asymptomatic liver lesions. On the one hand, an unnecessary operation with potential morbidity and mortality should be avoided; on the other often preoperatively malignancy could not be clearly excluded [5–9, 11] or a transformation into a malignancy (HCC) is feared [1, 3, 10, 23–30]. In the treatment of liver lesions, especially in case of an asymptomatic tumor, a gradual adapted approach is necessary [4, 11]. Especially with regard to questionable dignity, a critical assessment of the individual benefit-risk should be conducted [1, 4, 10, 11] (Figure 5). In our cohort despite the gradual adapted approach, often surgery was indicated by one malignancy suspect imaging. Reasons for this procedure were the high numbers of cases; the dignity of the lesion remains unclear despite extended diagnostics, to safe cost and especially the high number of patients without history for carcinoma having health complaints. In cases of asymptomatic lesions of the liver a gradual adapted approach was elected in our cohort.

TABLE 9: Mortality and morbidity of our subjects after resection of benign liver tumors in comparison to the literature.

	Mortality	Morbidity*	Revision	Hospitalization**
Weimann et al. [42]	0.6% (1/173)	24.9% (43/173)	—	—
Charny et al. [47]	0% (0/68)	20.6% (14/68)	—	8.5 d
Petri et al. [53]	0.9% (1/113)	27.4% (31/113)	—	—
Zülke et al. [11]	0% (0/55)	18.5% (10/55)	<5%	10 d
Dachau	0% (0/43)	16.3% (7/43)	0%	11 d

*Major and minor complications, **mean (laparoscopic and open resection).

TABLE 10: Mortality, morbidity, and hospitalization after resection of benign liver tumors during laparoscopic liver resections in our collective and share of laparoscopic procedures in relation to the total number of liver resections.

	Mortality	Morbidity*	Hospitalization**	Distribution***
Hemangioma	0% (0/7)	14.3% (1/7)	7 d	33.3%
FNH	0% (0/8)	0% (0/8)	11 d	66.7%
Adenoma	0% (0/4)	0% (0/4)	9 d	57.1%
Total	0% (0/19)	5% (1/19)	9 d	47.5%

*Major and minor complications, **mean (laparoscopic resection), ***percentage distribution of laparoscopic to open resections of the liver.

TABLE 11: Number of patients with a history of malignant tumor disease where hepatic resection was performed.

	Positive history for carcinoma	Radiological, no safe exclusion of a metastasis
Hemangioma	13	12
FNH	4	3
Adenoma	2	1

TABLE 12: Consistency of the preoperative diagnosis with the final postoperative histology.

	Dachau	Charny et al. [47]	Zülke et al. [11]
Hemangioma	7/16 (44)	27/39 (69)	9/12 (75)
FNH	4/12 (33)	7/18 (39)	10/21 (48)
Adenoma	3/7 (43)	6/8 (75)	5/16 (31)
Preoperatively unknown	5	—	—

Initially often close monitoring of liver lesions occurs without any major risk to the patient [4, 54]. In medical literature a correlation between tumor size and the occurrence of possible clinical symptoms is offered [11, 47]. In patients with unspecific symptoms primarily, a conservative therapy should be carried out. D'Halluin et al. showed that up to 100% of nonspecific symptoms are to relieve with conservative therapy, especially after finishing oral contraception [48]. Studies found out that only a total of about 5% of liver lesions is primarily treated surgically [1, 3, 5, 11].

The recommendations for surgical management of benign liver lesions are based on the results of retrospective analysis or case reports with fewer than 60 patients (medical evidence 3-4) [10].

At diagnosis of hepatocellular adenoma, surgical resection is indicated, because of the potential risk of malignant transformation and a possible life-threatening bleeding complication, even in case of a definite tumor regression and discontinuation of oral contraceptives [11, 55, 56] as well as absence of clinical symptoms [11, 55]. This indication should be regardless of the size of the adenoma [1, 11, 55, 56], especially in inflammatory adenomas on MRI and the possibility of beta catenin expression. In our cohort patients having a hepatocellular adenoma had health complaints in 86%. Only in 14% of cases surgery was indicated because of asymptomatic, preoperatively known adenoma.

Necrosis, hemorrhage, and thrombosis of benign lesions of the liver may often complicate the diagnosis [57, 58]. In such cases only the complete resection of the lesion can reach a definitive diagnosis.

The implementation of a percutaneous fine-needle biopsy (FNB) is discussed controversially in the literature. Due to the low expressiveness and lack of therapeutic consequences in most cases, FNB should not be performed [12, 40–42]. Only 34–40% of FNB histologies are consistent with the histology of the surgical preparation [4, 10]. In addition to a morbidity of 0.5% and a mortality of 0.05% [1, 4, 10], the FNB contains the risk of possible seeding of malignant cells through the puncture of a possible hepatocellular carcinoma (HCC). Studies have demonstrated that in case of a puncture of a liver lesion up to 2% seeding of malignant cells in the needle tract can occur [43, 44]. In accordance to these facts in our cohort, no FNB had been performed.

Asymptomatic hemangiomas do not require therapy [1, 3, 5, 10, 11]. In the current literature, there is disagreement whether asymptomatic hemangiomas depending on the size should be surgically treated. None of our patients had an acute rupture of the hemangioma, and also in the world literature, only a total of 97 cases of hemangioma rupture were published and only in 47.4% of cases (46) a spontaneous, life-threatening hemangioma rupture occurred [19]. Further investigation showed that these spontaneously ruptured hemangiomas had a mean size of 11.2 cm [19].

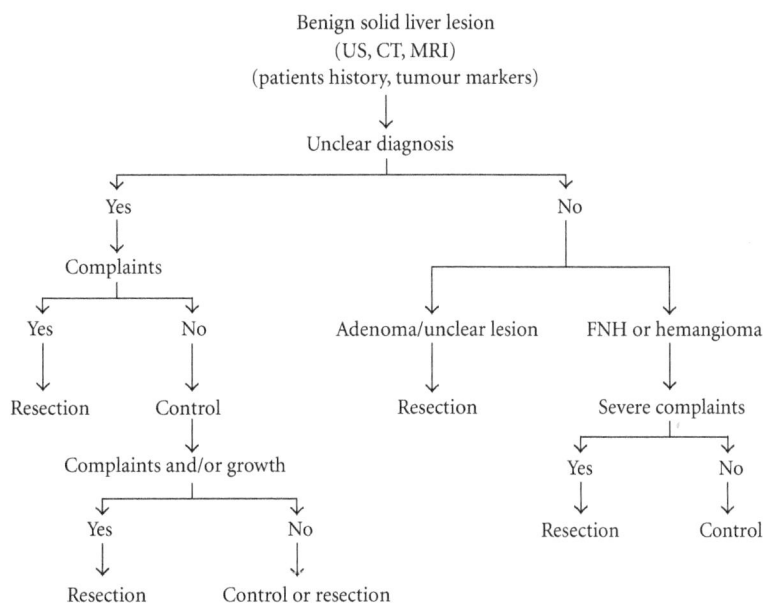

FIGURE 5: Algorithm for management of solid liver lesions (mod. from Terkivatan et al. [54]).

These studies reached the conclusion that a spontaneous rupture of a hemangioma occurs only very rarely and a prophylactic resection should only be done in case of specific requirements and especially for a size of the hemangioma >11 cm [1, 10, 19, 41]. For example, in patients with a large hemangioma (>11 cm) before a scheduled pregnancy, a definitive treatment should be discussed [10, 19]. Methods of choice in an acute hemangioma rupture are the immediate optimization of coagulation and sometimes a TAE [1, 10, 11, 18]. TAE treatment of a hemangioma is difficult and due to the aberrant collateral arterial circulation making almost improbable to stop the multiple inflow from different feeding arteries. The indication for surgical intervention should be provided in case of a high growth trend (>3 cm in 12 months), in symptomatic compression symptoms, or recurrent pain, which may correlate with hemorrhage into the lesion [18, 19]. Method of choice is the enucleation with minimal loss of parenchyma or a sparingly liver resection [10, 11, 18, 21]. In giant centrally located hemangioma a total vascular exclusion of the liver is a useful technical maneuver to save blood while dissecting it. The second key point to significantly lower the blood losses is reducing the surgically resection time [10, 18, 21]. None of our patients had an acute bleeding complication or rupture of the hemangioma. Patients of our cohort with a postoperatively ensured hemangioma had preoperatively rarely health complaints (29%), but often a moot malignancy (71%) and often a positive history for carcinoma (62%). In case of moot malignancy and history for carcinoma, extended surgical resections (liver segment resection) were performed in our clinic. Main reason for this approach was to remove a possible malignant tumor with sufficient safety distance. In case of a preoperatively know clinical symptomatic hemangioma and no history of carcinoma, always a parenchyma sparing technique was performed.

At the diagnosis of FNH, primarily no surgical intervention is indicated [1]. Large, displacing growing FNH nodes may require surgical treatment [5, 10]. This is particularly important for women wishing to have children. During pregnancy, it can lead to a progressive growth of the FNH because of hormone influences [10]. In case of an unambiguous preoperative diagnosis and indication for surgical intervention, the atypical resection is the treatment of choice [3, 5, 10, 11]. Often, the preoperative differential diagnosis of adenoma cannot be excluded with certainty. Gadoxetic acid-enhanced MRI enables the differentiation of FNH from adenoma best [28]. In these cases a surgical resection is indicated [11, 24]. In patients with a prior history of carcinoma (especially colorectal cancers and breast cancers, etc.), within a cancer followup a lesion in the liver was noticed, and hepatic metastasis could radiologically not be excluded; the indication for resection of the liver lesion should be set wider [10, 11, 24, 29, 30]. One aim of this approach is to get a definitive histology of the "malignancy-suspicious" lesion and if needed to deliver an additional treatment such as chemotherapy or radiotherapy without loss of time, but also to reach primarily a definitive therapy [1, 11, 29, 30]. Because of the high number of patients of our cohort with a positive history of cancer (47.5%) and radiologically not safe metastasis exclusion (84.2%), this approach was also chosen among these patients.

Requirements for a surgical intervention of benign lesions [4] are as follows:

(i) low surgical mortality (<1%),

(ii) low morbidity,

(iii) avoidance of blood transfusion,

(iv) good long-term results.

Our study and the current literature revealed that these conditions are fulfilled (see Section 3) and an elective liver resection currently can be considered to be safe and effective [4, 12]. The mortality of our cohort and in the literature was 0–0.9% [11, 42, 47, 53]. In contrast, the mortality in event of an emergency surgical intervention for acute bleeding adenoma in the literature is stated 5–10% [40, 42].

The postoperative morbidity in our collective in total was 16.3%, whereas no major complications occurred and no revision surgery had to be performed. This result of the morbidity for liver resections at benign liver lesions is generally equivalent to medical literature (7–28%) [11, 42, 47, 53]. Typical postoperative complications are a right-sided serothorax, a biliary leakage, a biloma, a postoperative bleeding, a subphrenic seroma/abscess, or a liver failure [5, 59]. To avoid such complications, a careful approach should be chosen for the liver resection. As already illustrated, for the lowest possible intraoperative blood loss the liver resection can be performed, for example, with the waterjet [4, 51, 52]. For this reason liver resection with the waterjet is standard in our clinic. In addition, a thorough ligation of bile ducts should be ensued, a continuation of blood flow in the portal venous and arterial system of healthy liver parenchyma (selective liver occlusion) should be performed, intraoperative blood losses should be avoided, and a thorough sealing of resection surface should be done (e.g., local fibrin) [4, 51]. Infective complications can be reduced by perioperative administration of antibiotics [10].

In case of symptomatic benign tumors of the liver, surgical intervention in 80% of cases leads to a decrease of complaints [4, 54]. Rarely the preoperative symptoms persist and sometimes even new complaints occur because of the surgical intervention [4]. These points illustrate the strict obligation of indication for surgical intervention in case of benign liver lesions.

Medical literature offers a low postoperative complication rate, in laparoscopic and open liver resections [50, 60]. With appropriate selection, a laparoscopic liver resection should primarily be made, because shorter hospitalization and fewer minor complications, with identical major complications are recorded [4, 10, 50]. These results were also confirmed in our collective. The rate of complications (minor and major) for liver resection in open technique was 16.5% and 5% for laparoscopic technique. Also the hospitalisation was shorter in case of laparoscopic surgery (9 days versus 11 days). For these results it is critical to note that currently extended liver resections are more frequently, like in our collective, performed in an open technique and for these interventions are to be expected both higher morbidity and a longer hospitalisation. In the medical literature studies with larger numbers of subjects are missing, where extensive liver resections for benign lesions in laparoscopic and open technique relating to mortality, morbidity, and hospitalization are compared. Smaller studies have already shown that even hemihepatectomy can be safely performed laparoscopically [10, 61]. Currently, in the literature the implementation of extensive laparoscopic and laparoscopic assisted liver resection is critically discussed [3, 4, 11, 50, 61]. The laparoscopic liver resection has disadvantages primarily in case of extended, central findings in the exact three dimensional orientation of the surgeon,

such as the preparation of the great vessels. Bleeding complications are the most common reason for conversion to open liver resection [50, 61]. Other disadvantages of laparoscopic surgery are often a higher time exposure, the higher costs, and the dependence on the surgeon [4]. Nevertheless, in the future in case of a surgical treatment of a benign liver tumor, laparoscopic liver resection by experienced surgeons will be the gold standard [10].

5. Conclusion

Despite continuous improvement of diagnostic possibilities, the dignity for up to 40% of incidentally detected liver lesions cannot be determined reliably till the final postoperative histology. In case of uncertain diagnosis, especially in patients with positive history of a malignant tumor or the suspected diagnosis of hepatocellular adenoma, surgical resection is indicated. In case an asymptomatic hemangioma or FNH can be preoperatively detected with certainty the indication for surgery must be very reluctant. In case of symptomatic liver lesions, surgical resection should only be indicated with tumor-specific symptoms. In the remaining cases of benign lesions of the liver, a "watch and wait" strategy is recommended. Due to the continuous improvement of surgical techniques, liver resection should also be done in the laparoscopic technique in case of more than one liver-segment resection or hemihepatectomy. Laparoscopic surgery has lower morbidity and shorter hospitalization than open technique.

References

[1] N. Assy, G. Nasser, A. Djibre, Z. Beniashvii, S. Elias, and J. Zidan, "Characteristics of common solid liver lesions and recommendations for diagnostic workup," World Journal of Gastroenterology, vol. 15, no. 26, pp. 3217–3227, 2009.

[2] S. Delorme, "Radiologische diagnostik der leber," Radiologe, vol. 40, no. 10, pp. 904–915, 2000.

[3] M. Galanski, S. Jördens, and J. Weidemann, "Diagnosis and differential diagnosis of benign liver tumors and tumor-like lesions," Chirurg, vol. 79, no. 8, pp. 707–721, 2008.

[4] M. Loss, C. Zülke, A. Obed, O. Stöltzing, and H. J. Schlitt, "Surgical therapy of benign liver tumors," Chirurg, vol. 79, no. 8, pp. 722–728, 2008.

[5] T. Skalický, V. Třeška, A. Sutnar et al., "Surgical treatment of benign liver tumours—indications and results," Zentralblatt fur Chirurgie, vol. 134, no. 2, pp. 141–144, 2009.

[6] D. Strobel and T. Bernatik, "Diagnostik bei fokalen Leberläsionen-Stellenwert der Kontrastmittelsonografie," Deutsches Ärzteblatt, vol. 103, pp. 789–793, 2006.

[7] B. S. Kuszyk, D. A. Bluemke, B. A. Urban et al., "Portal-phase contrast-enhanced helical CT for the detection of malignant hepatic tumors: sensitivity based on comparison with intraoperative and pathologic findings," American Journal of Roentgenology, vol. 166, no. 1, pp. 91–95, 1996.

[8] L. H. Schwartz, E. J. Gandras, S. M. Colangelo, M. C. Ercolani, and D. M. Panicek, "Prevalence and importance of small hepatic lesions found at CT in patients with cancer," Radiology, vol. 210, no. 1, pp. 71–74, 1999.

[9] P. J. Karhunen, A. Penttila, and K. Liesto, "Benign bile duct tumours, non-parasitic liver cysts and liver damage in males," Journal of Hepatology, vol. 2, no. 1, pp. 89–99, 1986.

[10] K. Hoffmann and P. Schemmer, "Benigne solide Tumoren der Leber," *Allgemein- und Viszeralchirurgie Up2date*, vol. 5, pp. 135–146, 2011.

[11] C. Zülke, M. Loss, I. Iesalnieks et al., "Benign liver lesions: indication for surgery and postoperative results," *Viszeralchirurgie*, vol. 39, no. 2, pp. 86–97, 2004.

[12] J. Belghiti, D. Pateron, Y. Panis et al., "Resection of presumed benign liver tumours," *British Journal of Surgery*, vol. 80, no. 3, pp. 380–383, 1993.

[13] A. Blachar, M. P. Federle, J. V. Ferris et al., "Radiologists' performance in the diagnosis of liver tumors with central scars by using specific CT criteria," *Radiology*, vol. 223, no. 2, pp. 532–539, 2002.

[14] M. P. Federle and G. Brancatelli, "Imaging of benign hepatic masses," *Seminars in Liver Disease*, vol. 21, no. 2, pp. 237–249, 2001.

[15] A. M. Xu, H. Y. Cheng, D. Chen, Y. C. Jia, and M. C. Wu, "Plane and weighted tri-phase helical CT findings in the diagnosis of liver focal nodular hyperplasia," *Hepatobiliary and Pancreatic Diseases International*, vol. 1, no. 2, pp. 219–223, 2002.

[16] N. Corigliano, P. Mercantini, P. M. Amodio et al., "Hemoperitoneum from a spontaneous rupture of a giant hemangioma of the liver: report of a case," *Surgery Today*, vol. 33, no. 6, pp. 459–463, 2003.

[17] T. Terkivatan, J. H. W. de Wilt, R. A. de Man, R. R. van Rijn, H. W. Tilanus, and J. N. M. Ijzermans, "Treatment of ruptured hepatocellular adenoma," *British Journal of Surgery*, vol. 88, no. 2, pp. 207–209, 2001.

[18] H. J. Gassel, I. Klein, U. Steger, M. Simon, and A. Thiede, "Cavernous liver hemangioma: rational diagnostics and therapeutic approach," *Viszeralchirurgie*, vol. 40, no. 1, pp. 37–44, 2005.

[19] M. Donati, G. A. Stavrou, A. Donati, and K. J. Oldhafer, "The risk of spontaneous rupture of liver hemangiomas: a critical review of the literature," *Journal of Hepato-Biliary-Pancreatic Surgery*. In press.

[20] J. H. Sewell and K. Weiss, "Spontaneous rupture of hemangioma of the liver. A review of the literature and presentation of illustrative case," *Archives of Surgery*, vol. 83, pp. 729–733, 1961.

[21] S. I. Schwartz and W. C. Husser, "Cavernous hemangioma of the liver. A single institution report of 16 resections," *Annals of Surgery*, vol. 205, no. 5, pp. 456–465, 1987.

[22] O. Farges, S. Daradkeh, and H. Bismuth, "Cavernous hemangiomas of the liver: are there any indications for resection?" *World Journal of Surgery*, vol. 19, no. 1, pp. 19–24, 1995.

[23] D. Erdogan, O. R. C. Busch, O. M. van Delden, F. J. W. Ten Kate, D. J. Gouma, and T. M. van Gulik, "Management of spontaneous haemorrhage and rupture of hepatocellular adenomas. A single centre experience," *Liver International*, vol. 26, no. 4, pp. 433–438, 2006.

[24] J. H. B. M. Stoot, R. J. S. Coelen, M. C. de Jong, and C. H. Dejong, "Malignant transformation of hepatocellular adenomas into hepatocellular carcinomas: a systematic review including more than 1600 adenoma cases," *HPB*, vol. 12, no. 8, pp. 509–522, 2010.

[25] P. Flemming, U. Lehmann, D. Steinemann, H. Kreipe, and L. Wilkens, "Leberzelladenom. Entartungspotenzial und abgrenzung vom HCC," *Pathologe*, vol. 27, no. 4, pp. 238–243, 2006.

[26] L. Chiche, T. Dao, E. Salamé et al., "Liver adenomatosis: reappraisal, diagnosis, and surgical managemen: 8 new cases and review of the literature," *Annals of Surgery*, vol. 231, no. 1, pp. 74–81, 2000.

[27] L. Grazioli, M. P. Federle, T. Ichikawa, E. Balzano, M. Nalesnik, and J. Madariaga, "Liver adenomatosis: clinical, histopathologic, and imaging findings in 15 patients," *Radiology*, vol. 216, no. 2, pp. 395–402, 2000.

[28] L. Grazioli, M. P. Bondioni, H. Haradome et al., "Hepatocellular adenoma and focal nodular hyperplasia: value of gadoxetic acid-enhanced MR imaging in differential diagnosis," *Radiology*, vol. 262, no. 2, pp. 520–529, 2012.

[29] J. Neuberger, B. Portmann, H. B. Nunnerley, M. Davis, J. W. Laws, and R. Williams, "Oral-contraceptive-associated liver tumours: occurrence of malignancy and difficulties in diagnosis," *The Lancet*, vol. 1, no. 8163, pp. 273–276, 1980.

[30] L. C. Tao, "Oral contraceptive-associated liver cell adenoma and hepatocellular carcinoma: cytomorphology and mechanism of malignant transformation," *Cancer*, vol. 68, no. 2, pp. 341–347, 1991.

[31] B. Y. Choi and M. H. Nguyen, "The diagnosis and management of benign hepatic tumors," *Journal of Clinical Gastroenterology*, vol. 39, no. 5, pp. 401–412, 2005.

[32] C. Zülke and H. J. Schlitt, "Incidentalomas of the liver and gallbladder : evaluation and therapeutic procedure," *Chirurg*, vol. 78, no. 8, pp. 698–712, 2007.

[33] P. J. Mergo, J. D. Engelken, T. Helmberger, and P. R. Ros, "MRI in focal liver disease: a comparison of small and ultrasmall superparamagnetic iron oxide as hepatic contrast agents," *Journal of Magnetic Resonance Imaging*, vol. 8, no. 5, pp. 1073–1078, 1998.

[34] A. J. Ruppert-Kohlmayr, M. M. Uggowitzer, C. Kugler, D. Zebedin, G. Schaffler, and G. S. Ruppert, "Focal nodular hyperplasia and hepatocellular adenoma of the liver: differentiation with multiphasic helical CT," *American Journal of Roentgenology*, vol. 176, no. 6, pp. 1493–1498, 2001.

[35] T. Isozaki, K. Numata, T. Kiba et al., "Differential diagnosis of hepatic tumors by using contrast enhancement patterns at US," *Radiology*, vol. 229, no. 3, pp. 798–805, 2003.

[36] D. Strobel, S. Raeker, P. Martus, E. G. Hahn, and D. Becker, "Phase inversion harmonic imaging versus contrast-enhanced power Doppler sonography for the characterization of local liver lesions," *International Journal of Colorectal Disease*, vol. 18, no. 1, pp. 63–72, 2003.

[37] D. G. D. Wight, *Atlas of Liver Pathology*, Kluwer Academic Publishers, Dordrecht, The Netherlands, 2nd edition, 1993.

[38] K. F. Gratz and A. Weimann, "Diagnosis of liver tumors—when is scintigraphy of value?" *Zentralbl Chir*, vol. 123, pp. 111–118, 1998.

[39] J. Grimm, S. Müller-Hülsbeck, J. Blume, J. Biederer, and M. Heller, "Comparison of biphasic spiral CT and MnDPDP-enhanced MRI in the detection and characterization of liver lesions," *Rofo Fortschr Geb Rontgenstr Neuen Bildgeb Verfahr*, vol. 173, pp. 266–272, 2001.

[40] P. Herman, V. Pugliese, M. A. C. Machado et al., "Hepatic adenoma and focal nodular hyperplasia: differential diagnosis and treatment," *World Journal of Surgery*, vol. 24, no. 3, pp. 372–376, 2000.

[41] S. Shimizu, T. Takayama, T. Kosuge et al., "Benign tumors of the liver resected because of a diagnosis of malignancy," *Surgery Gynecology and Obstetrics*, vol. 174, no. 5, pp. 403–407, 1992.

[42] A. Weimann, B. Ringe, J. Klempnauer et al., "Benign liver tumors: differential diagnosis and indications for surgery," *World Journal of Surgery*, vol. 21, no. 9, pp. 983–991, 1997.

[43] G. T. Huang, J. C. Sheu, P. M. Yang, H. S. Lee, T. H. Wang, and D. S. Chen, "Ultrasound-guided cutting biopsy for the diagnosis of hepatocellular carcinoma—a study based on 420

patients," *Journal of Hepatology*, vol. 25, no. 3, pp. 334–338, 1996.

[44] E. H. Smith, "Complications of percutaneous abdominal fine-needle biopsy: review," *Radiology*, vol. 178, no. 1, pp. 253–258, 1991.

[45] N. Corigliano, P. Mercantini, P. M. Amodio et al., "Hemoperitoneum from a spontaneous rupture of a giant hemangioma of the liver: report of a case," *Surgery Today*, vol. 33, no. 6, pp. 459–463, 2003.

[46] T. Terkivatan, J. H. de Wilt, R. A. de Man et al., "Indications and long-term outcome of treatment for benign hepatic tumors: a critical appraisal," *Archives of Surgery*, vol. 136, no. 9, pp. 1033–1038, 2001.

[47] C. K. Charny, W. R. Jarnagin, L. H. Schwartz et al., "Management of 155 patients with benign liver tumours," *British Journal of Surgery*, vol. 88, no. 6, pp. 808–813, 2001.

[48] V. D'Halluin, V. Vilgrain, G. Pelletier et al., "Natural history of focal nodular hyperplasia. A retrospective study of 44 cases," *Gastroenterologie Clinique et Biologique*, vol. 25, no. 11, pp. 1008–1010, 2001.

[49] R. Gedaly, J. J. Pomposelli, E. A. Pomfret, W. D. Lewis, and R. L. Jenkins, "Cavernous hemangioma of the liver: anatomic resection versus enucleation," *Archives of Surgery*, vol. 134, no. 4, pp. 407–411, 1999.

[50] B. Descottes, D. Glineur, F. Lachachi et al., "Laparoscopic liver resection of benign liver tumors: results of a multicenter European experience," *Surgical Endoscopy and Other Interventional Techniques*, vol. 17, no. 1, pp. 23–30, 2003.

[51] H. G. Rau, E. Buttler, G. Meyer, H. M. Schardey, and F. W. Schildberg, "Laparoscopic liver resection compared with conventional partial hepatectomy—a prospective analysis," *Hepatogastroenterology*, vol. 45, no. 24, pp. 2333–2338, 1998.

[52] H. G. Rau, A. Zimmermann, C. Wardemann, and F. W. Schildberg, "Standards of surgical techniques in liver metastases," *Chirurgische Gastroenterologie Interdisziplinar*, vol. 19, no. 4, pp. 333–339, 2003.

[53] A. Petri, J. Höhn, A. Wolfárd et al., "Surgery of benign liver tumors: indications for treatment. Personal experience and review of the literature," *Magyar Onkologia*, vol. 47, no. 4, pp. 391–395, 2003.

[54] T. Terkivatan, J. H. de Wilt, R. A. de Man et al., "Indications and long-term outcome of treatment for benign hepatic tumors: a critical appraisal," *Archives of Surgery*, vol. 136, no. 9, pp. 1033–1038, 2001.

[55] S. C. Gordon, K. J. Reddy, and A. S. Livingstone, "Resolution of a contraceptive-steroid-induced hepatic adenoma with subsequent evolution into hepatocellular carcinoma," *Annals of Internal Medicine*, vol. 105, no. 4, pp. 547–549, 1986.

[56] H. Tesluk and J. Lawrie, "Hepatocellular adenoma. Its transformation to carcinoma in a user of oral contraceptives," *Archives of Pathology and Laboratory Medicine*, vol. 105, no. 6, pp. 296–299, 1981.

[57] N. Ren, L. X. Qin, Z. Y. Tang, Z. Q. Wu, and J. Fan, "Diagnosis and treatment of hepatic angiomyolipoma in 26 cases," *World Journal of Gastroenterology*, vol. 9, no. 8, pp. 1856–1858, 2003.

[58] C. N. Yeh, M. F. Chen, C. F. Hung, T. C. Chen, and T. C. Chao, "Angiomyolipoma of the liver," *Journal of Surgical Oncology*, vol. 77, no. 3, pp. 195–200, 2001.

[59] O. Katsuhisa, O. Kazuo, Y. Kadokawa et al., "Comparison of the grade evaluated by "Liver damage" of Liver Cancer Study Group of Japan and Child-Pugh classification in patients with hepatocellular carcinoma," *Hepatology Research*, vol. 34, no. 4, pp. 266–272, 2006.

[60] J. I. Tsao, J. P. Loftus, D. M. Nagomey, M. A. Adson, and D. M. Ilstrup, "Trends in morbidity and mortality of hepatic resection for malignancy: a matched comparative analysis," *Annals of Surgery*, vol. 220, no. 2, pp. 199–205, 1994.

[61] M. Abu Hilal, A. Badran, F. di Fabio, and N. W. Pearce, "Pure laparoscopic en bloc left hemihepatectomy and caudate lobe resection in patients with intrahepatic cholangiocarcinoma," *Journal of Laparoendoscopic and Advanced Surgical Techniques A*, vol. 21, no. 9, pp. 845–849, 2011.

13

Hepatocellular Carcinoma in the Pediatric Population: A Population Based Clinical Outcomes Study Involving 257 Patients from the Surveillance, Epidemiology, and End Result (SEER) Database (1973–2011)

Christine S. M. Lau,[1,2] Krishnaraj Mahendraraj,[1] and Ronald S. Chamberlain[1,2,3]

[1]Department of Surgery, Saint Barnabas Medical Center, Livingston, NJ 07039, USA
[2]Saint George's University School of Medicine, True Blue, Grenada
[3]Department of Surgery, New Jersey Medical School, Rutgers University, Newark, NJ 07103, USA

Correspondence should be addressed to Ronald S. Chamberlain; rchamberlain@barnabashealth.org

Academic Editor: Piotr Kalicinski

Introduction. Hepatocellular carcinoma (HCC) is a rare pediatric cancer accounting for 0.5% of all pediatric malignancies. This study examines a large cohort of HCC patients in an effort to define the factors impacting clinical outcomes in pediatric HCC patients compared to adults. *Methods*. Demographic and clinical data on 63,771 HCC patients (257 pediatric patients ≤ 19 and 63,514 adult patients age ≥ 20) were abstracted from the SEER database (1973–2011). *Results*. HCC was more common among males (59.5% pediatric and 75.1% adults) and Caucasians (50.4% and 50.5%), $p < 0.05$. Children more often presented with fibrolamellar variant HCC (24.1% versus 0.3%, $p = 0.71$) and advanced HCC, including distant disease (33.1% versus 20.8%, $p < 0.001$), and tumors > 4 cm in size (79.6% versus 62.0%, $p = 0.02$). Pediatric HCC patients undergoing surgery (13.107 versus 8.324 years, $p < 0.001$) had longer survival than adult HCC patients. Overall mortality was lower (65.8% versus 82.0%, $p < 0.001$) in the pediatric HCC group. *Conclusion*. HCC is a rare pediatric malignancy that presents most often as an advanced tumor, >4 cm in Caucasian males. Children with HCC achieve significantly longer mean overall survival compared to adults with HCC, primarily attributable to the more favorable fibrolamellar histologic variant, and more aggressive surgical intervention, which significantly improves survival.

1. Introduction

Primary liver neoplasms in childhood are rare and constitute 1-2% of all pediatric tumors [1]. Hepatocellular carcinoma (HCC) is the second most common primary hepatic malignancy in children following hepatoblastoma and accounts for approximately one-third of all primary hepatic malignancies in children and approximately 0.5% of all pediatric malignancies [2]. The age-standardized rates of HCC range from approximately 7.5 per 100,000 men in North America to as high as 20 per 100,000 men in Eastern and Southeastern Asia [3, 4]. HCC in children is much rarer, with an age-adjusted incidence rate of 0.7 per 1,000,000 in the USA [5]. The incidence of HCC is significantly greater in Eastern and Southeastern Asia and in Africa, where hepatitis B infection is

endemic [3]. HCC has also been observed in young children with inherited metabolic disorders and in older children with maternal transmission of hepatitis B infection [5–8].

While surgery remains the mainstream of treatment for patients with HCC, survival rates are poor [9]. In a series of 218 pediatric HCC cases, Allan et al. reported an overall 5-year survival of 24% and a 20-year survival of only 8% [10].

HCC in the pediatric population is much less prevalent than in adults. Current knowledge regarding pediatric HCC is limited, and very few studies have examined treatment approaches and outcomes in children with HCC. This study sought to examine a large cohort of adult and pediatric HCC from the Surveillance, Epidemiology, and End Results (SEER) database, in an effort to identify demographic, clinical, and treatment strategies which impact clinical outcomes and potentially guide therapeutic decision-making and assist in clinical trial development and appropriate accrual.

2. Methods

Data for the current study was extracted from the Surveillance, Epidemiology, and End Result (SEER) database provided by the National Cancer Institute between 1973 and 2011. SEER Stat software version 8.0.4 was utilized to extract data from 18 SEER registries (Alaska Native Tumor Registry, Arizona Indians, Cherokee Nation, Connecticut, Detroit, Georgia Center for Cancer Statistics, Greater Bay Area Cancer Registry, Greater California, Hawaii, Iowa, Kentucky, Los Angeles, Louisiana, New Jersey, New Mexico, Seattle-Puget Sound, and Utah).

63,771 patients with histologically confirmed hepatocellular carcinoma were identified and exported to IBM SPSS v20.2. Patients with a primary diagnosis of HCC were identified to form the final study cohort, using the SEER International Classification of Disease for Oncology (ICD-O-3) codes 8170/3, 8171/3, 8172/3, 8173/3, 8174/3, and 8175/3. Demographic and clinical data extracted included age, gender, race, tumor morphology, stage, grade, size, and type of treatment received (surgery, radiation, both or no treatment). The 63,771 patients included in this study were grouped into pediatric patients (defined as age $\leq$ 19 years) and adult patients (defined as age $\geq$ 20 years). Patients with *in situ* cancers, those with nonspecific site of tumor origin, and those in whom histologic confirmation of their cancer was not available were excluded from the final study cohort. Endpoints examined included 1-, 2-, and 5-year overall survival, mortality, and cancer-specific mortality. Categorical variables were compared using the Chi-Square test, and continuous variables were compared using Student's t-test and analysis of variance (ANOVA). Multivariate analysis using the "backward Wald" method was performed to calculate odds ratios (OR) and determine independent factors affecting survival. Missing and unknown data were excluded from the multivariate analysis. Kaplan-Meier analysis was used to compare long term actuarial survival between groups. Statistical significance was accepted at the level of $p < 0.05$.

3. Results

3.1. Demographic Data. 63,771 cases of HCC were reported in the SEER database between 1973 and 2011. The mean age at diagnosis was 64 ± 13 years. There were significantly more adult patients than pediatric patients (99.6% versus 0.4%). 99.6% of cases ($N = 63,514$) occurred in adults with a mean age at diagnosis of 64 ± 12 years, while only 0.4% of cases ($N = 257$) occurred in pediatric patients with a mean age at diagnosis of 13 ± 5 years (Table 1).

The majority of HCC diagnoses occurred in Caucasians ($N = 32,130$; 50.5%), followed by Asian, Pacific Islander or Native Americans ($N = 13,347$; 21.0%), Hispanics ($N = 10,285$; 16.2%), and African Americans ($N = 7,829$; 12.3%), $p < 0.05$. HCC was more common among Caucasians in both the pediatric and adult population groups (50.4% and 50.5%, $p = 0.03$); however, pediatric HCC was significantly

more common among Hispanics (19.3% versus 16.2%, $p = 0.03$) and less common among African Americans (11.4% versus 12.3%, $p = 0.02$) and Asian/Pacific Islander/Native Americans (18.9% versus 21.0%, $p = 0.03$), compared to adult HCC.

Among all 63,771 HCC patients, 75.1% were male ($N = 47,862$), and 24.9% were female ($N = 15,909$), resulting in a male to female ratio of 3.01 : 1, $p < 0.001$. HCC was more common among males in both the pediatric and adult populations (59.5% and 75.1%). Among the 257 pediatric HCC patients, 59.5% were males ($N = 153$) and 40.5% were females ($N = 104$), resulting in a male to female ratio of 1.47 : 1, $p < 0.001$. Among the 63,514 adult HCC patients, 75.1% were males ($N = 47,709$) and 24.9% were females ($N = 15,805$), resulting in a male to female ratio of 3.02 : 1, $p < 0.001$.

3.2. Tumor Characteristics. Among pediatric patients, 24.1% ($N = 62$) had fibrolamellar HCC (fHCC), 1.2% ($N = 3$) had clear cell HCC, and the remaining 74.7% ($N = 192$) had HCC NOS (Table 2). Morphology was more varied among adult HCC patients. 0.5% ($N = 336$) had clear cell HCC, 0.3% ($N = 212$) had fHCC, 0.1% ($N = 66$) had scirrhous HCC, 0.1% ($N = 36$) had spindle cell HCC, <0.1% ($N = 17$) had pleomorphic HCC, and 98.9% ($N = 62,847$) had HCC NOS. The fHCC variant was far more common among pediatric patients, compared to adult patients (24.1% versus 0.3%, $p = 0.71$).

47.9% ($N = 25,755$) of HCC cases presented with localized disease, 31.2% ($N = 16,777$) had regional involvement, and 20.8% ($N = 11,193$) had metastatic spread at the time of diagnosis, $p < 0.001$. Pediatric patients had a higher rate of regional disease (38.8% versus 31.2%, $p < 0.001$) and distant disease (33.1% versus 20.8%, $p < 0.001$) and a lower rate of localized disease (28.1% versus 48.0%, $p < 0.001$), compared to adult patients.

62.0% ($N = 24,255$) of HCC were >4 cm, 30.0% ($N = 11,720$) were 2–4 cm, 7.9% ($N = 3,071$) were <2 cm, and 0.1% ($N = 45$) were microscopic lesions, $p < 0.05$. A greater percentage of pediatric patients had a tumor size greater than 4 cm (79.6% versus 62.0%, $p = 0.02$) compared to adult patients.

Overall, 38.0% ($N = 8,467$) of HCC were moderately differentiated, 35.1% ($N = 7,813$) were well differentiated, and 23.9% ($N = 5,317$) were poorly differentiated, $p < 0.05$. 3.0% ($N = 672$) were undifferentiated, $p = 0.06$. Pediatric patients more often presented with well differentiated tumors (35.8% versus 35.1%, $p = 0.02$) and less often with moderately (34.7% versus 38.0%, $p = 0.01$) or poorly differentiated tumors (23.2% versus 23.9%, $p = 0.01$).

3.3. Treatment. 20.9% ($N = 12,769$) of all HCC patients were treated with surgery alone while 4.0% ($N = 2,459$) of patients received radiation alone, and 0.5% ($N = 330$) of patients were treated with both surgery and radiation. 74.5% ($N = 45,558$) of patients received no treatment, $p < 0.005$ (Table 3). Pediatric patients were more likely to receive treatment (52.6% versus 25.3%, $p < 0.005$) compared to adult patients. Among those receiving treatment, surgical

TABLE 1: Demographic profiles of 63,514 adults and 257 pediatric patients with hepatocellular carcinoma from the Surveillance, Epidemiology, and End Results (SEER) database, 1973–2011.

Variables	Overall	Pediatric patients	Adult patients	p value
N (%)	63,771	257 (0.4%)	63,514 (99.6%)	—
Age, (Mean ± SD)	64 ± 13	13 ± 5	64 ± 12	<0.001
Mean overall survival (years)	2.833 ± 0.076	7.988 ± 0.845	2.781 ± 0.075	<0.001
Gender, N (%)				
Male	47,862 (75.1%)	153 (59.5%)	47,709 (75.1%)	<0.001
Female	15,909 (24.9%)	104 (40.5%)	15,805 (24.9%)	<0.001
Race, N (%)[**]				
Caucasian	32,130 (50.5%)	128 (50.4%)	32,002 (50.5%)	0.03
African American	7,829 (12.3%)	29 (11.4%)	7,800 (12.3%)	0.02
Hispanic	10,285 (16.2%)	49 (19.3%)	10,239 (16.2%)	0.03
Asian/Pacific Islander/Native Americans	13,347 (21.0%)	48 (18.9%)	13,299 (21.0%)	0.03

N = number; SD = standard deviation; [**]data presented for patients with available information only.

TABLE 2: Tumor characteristics of 63,514 adults and 257 pediatric patients with hepatocellular carcinoma from the Surveillance, Epidemiology, and End Results (SEER) database, 1973–2011.

Variables	Overall	Pediatric patients	Adult patients	p value
N (%)	63,771	257 (0.4%)	63,514 (99.6)	—
Morphology, N (%)				
Pleomorphic	17 (<0.0%)	0 (0.0%)	17 (<0.0%)	0.63
Clear cell	339 (0.5%)	3 (1.2%)	336 (0.5%)	0.16
Spindle cell	36 (0.1%)	0 (0.0%)	36 (0.1%)	0.81
Scirrhous	66 (0.1%)	0 (0.0%)	66 (0.1%)	0.77
Fibrolamellar	274 (0.4%)	62 (24.1%)	212 (0.3%)	0.71
NOS	63,039 (98.9%)	192 (74.7%)	62,847 (98.9%)	0.09
Grade, N (%)[**]				
Well differentiated	7,813 (35.1%)	34 (35.8%)	7,779 (35.1%)	0.02
Moderately diff.	8,467 (38.0%)	33 (34.7%)	8,434 (38.0%)	0.01
Poorly diff.	5,317 (23.9%)	22 (23.2%)	5,295 (23.9%)	0.01
Undifferentiated	672 (3.0%)	6 (6.3%)	666 (3.0%)	0.06
Stage, N (%)[**]				
Localized	25,755 (47.9%)	68 (28.1%)	25,687 (48.0%)	<0.001
Regional	16,777 (31.2%)	94 (38.8%)	16,683 (31.2%)	<0.001
Distant	11,193 (20.8%)	80 (33.1%)	11,113 (20.8%)	<0.001
Tumor size, N (%)[**]				
Microscopic	45 (0.1%)	0 (0.0%)	45 (0.1%)	0.01
Under 2 cm	3,071 (7.9%)	16 (9.9%)	3,055 (7.8%)	0.02
2 to 4 cm	11,720 (30.0%)	17 (10.5%)	11,703 (30.1%)	0.02
Over 4 cm	24,255 (62.0%)	129 (79.6%)	24,126 (62.0%)	0.02

cm = centimeters; diff. = differentiated; N = number; NOS = not otherwise specified; SD = standard deviation; [**]data presented for patients with available information only.

resection alone was the most common treatment modality in both pediatric and adult patients (92.4% and 82.0%). More pediatric patients received surgery as primary treatment (48.6% versus 20.8%, $p < 0.001$).

Patients who received surgery as the primary modality of treatment experienced significant survival benefit (mean survival 8.560 ± 0.297 years), compared to those who received a combination of surgery and radiation (3.649 ± 0.499 years), primary radiation only (1.190 ± 0.064 years), or no

treatment (1.253 ± 0.046 years), $p < 0.005$. Pediatric patients who received surgery (13.107±1.306 years versus 8.324±0.302 years, $p < 0.001$) or a combination of both surgery and radiation (13.667±13.500 years versus 3.287±0.387 years, $p < 0.005$) had significantly longer survivals than adult patients. Pediatric HCC patients who received combination surgery and radiation had similar survival compared to surgery alone (13.667 ± 13.500 years versus 13.107 ± 1.306 years). In contrast, adult HCC patients who received combination

TABLE 3: Treatment and survival outcomes of 63,514 adults and 257 pediatric patients with hepatocellular carcinoma from the Surveillance, Epidemiology, and End Results (SEER) database, 1973–2011.

Variables	Overall	Pediatric patients	Adult patients	p value
N (%)	63,771	257 (0.4%)	63,514 (99.6%)	—
Mean overall survival (years ± SD)	2.833 ± 0.076	7.988 ± 0.845	2.781 ± 0.075	<0.001
Treatment, N (%)**				
No treatment	45,558 (74.5%)	118 (47.4%)	45,440 (74.7%)	<0.005
Surgery only	12,769 (20.9%)	121 (48.6%)	12,648 (20.8%)	<0.001
Radiation only	2,459 (4.0%)	8 (3.2%)	2,451 (4.0%)	<0.005
Both surgery and radiation	330 (0.5%)	2 (0.8%)	328 (0.5%)	<0.005
Actuarial survival by treatment (years ± SD)**				
No treatment	1.253 ± 0.046	2.072 ± 0.598	1.243 ± 0.046	<0.005
Surgery only	8.560 ± 0.297	13.107 ± 1.306	8.324 ± 0.302	<0.001
Radiation only	1.190 ± 0.064	1.807 ± 0.447	1.189 ± 0.064	<0.001
Both surgery and radiation	3.649 ± 0.499	13.667 ± 13.500	3.287 ± 0.387	<0.005
Actuarial survival by morphology (years ± SD)**				
Pleomorphic	1.591 ± 0.653	—	1.591 ± 0.653	—
Clear cell	2.526 ± 0.215	1.833 ± 1.090	2.526 ± 0.215	0.832
Spindle cell	0.628 ± 0.149	—	0.628 ± 0.149	—
Scirrhous	2.228 ± 0.362	—	2.228 ± 0.362	—
Fibrolamellar	6.905 ± 0.617	9.110 ± 1.204	6.016 ± 0.653	0.002
NOS	2.688 ± 0.072	6.529 ± 0.881	2.650 ± 0.072	<0.001
Overall mortality, N (%)				
Alive	11,538 (18.1%)	88 (34.2%)	11,450 (18.0%)	<0.001
Dead	52,233 (81.9%)	169 (65.8%)	52,064 (82.0%)	<0.001
Cancer specific mortality, N (%)				
Alive	11,538 (18.1%)	88 (34.2%)	11,450 (18.0%)	<0.001
Cancer death	39,999 (62.7%)	156 (60.7%)	39,843 (62.7%)	<0.001
Noncancer death	12,234 (19.2%)	13 (5.1%)	12,221 (19.3%)	<0.001
Cumulative survival (%)				
1-year		61%	34%	<0.001
2-year		47%	23%	<0.001
5-year		30%	12%	<0.001

N = number; SD = standard deviation; **data presented for patients with available information only.

surgery and radiation had worse survival than those receiving surgery alone (3.287 ± 0.387 years versus 8.324 ± 0.302 years). Survival was slightly better among pediatric patients receiving radiation only (1.807 ± 0.447 years versus 1.189 ± 0.064 years, $p < 0.001$) or no treatment (2.072 ± 0.598 years versus 1.243±0.046 years, $p < 0.005$), compared to their adult counterparts.

Overall, the fHCC variant was associated with the greatest survival (6.905±0.617 years). Pediatric fHCC experienced significant longer survival than adult fHCC (9.110 ± 1.204 years versus 6.016 ± 0.653 years, $p = 0.002$).

3.4. Outcomes. The mean actuarial survival for pediatric patients was significantly higher than adult patients (7.988 ± 0.845 years versus 2.781 ± 0.075 years, $p < 0.001$). For all HCC patients, the overall and cancer specific mortality were found to be 81.9% and 62.7%, respectively, $p < 0.001$ (Table 3). Overall and cancer-specific mortality among the pediatric patients (65.8% and 60.7%) were significantly lower

compared with adult patients (82.0% and 62.7%), $p < 0.001$. Cumulative 1-, 2- and 5-year survival rates were significantly higher amongst the pediatric patients (61%, 47%, and 30%) as compared to adult patients (34%, 23%, and 12%), $p < 0.001$. Kaplan-Meier curve illustrates significantly better 40-year actuarial survival for pediatric HCC patients compared to adults (Figure 1).

3.5. Fibrolamellar versus Nonfibrolamellar Hepatocellular Carcinoma. 274 cases of fHCC were reported, with a mean age of 64 ± 12 years, representing 0.4% of all HCC cases. 22.6% of fHCC cases ($N = 62$) were pediatric patients, while 77.4% ($N = 212$) were adults. 24.1% of pediatric patients had fHCC, compared to 0.3% of adults. fHCC was more common among males in both pediatric and adult populations with a male to female ratio of 1.21 : 1 among pediatric patients and 1.59 : 1 among adults (Table 4). Non-fHCC had a much higher prevalence among males, with male-to-female ratios of 1.57 : 1 among pediatric patients and 3.03 : 1 among adults, $p < 0.001$.

TABLE 4: Demographic profiles of fibrolamellar and nonfibrolamellar hepatocellular carcinoma for 63,514 adults and 257 pediatric patients from the Surveillance, Epidemiology, and End Results (SEER) database, 1973–2011.

	Total		Pediatrics		Adults		p value
	fHCC	Non-fHCC	fHCC	Non-fHCC	fHCC	Non-fHCC	
N (%)	274 (0.4%)	63,497 (99.6%)	62 (24.1%)	195 (75.9%)	212 (0.3%)	63,302 (99.7%)	—
Age, (mean ± SD)	64 ± 12	63 ± 12	14 ± 4	13 ± 4	64 ± 12	63 ± 12	—
Gender, N (%)							
Male	164 (59.9%)	47,698 (75.1%)	34 (54.8%)	119 (61.0%)	130 (61.3%)	47,579 (75.2%)	<0.001
Female	110 (40.1%)	15,799 (24.9%)	28 (45.2%)	76 (39.0%)	82 (38.7%)	15,723 (24.8%)	<0.001
Race, N (%)**							
Caucasian	175 (64.1%)	31,955 (50.5%)	35 (56.5%)	93 (48.4%)	140 (66.4%)	31,862 (50.5%)	NS
African American	32 (11.7%)	7,797 (12.3%)	9 (14.5%)	20 (10.4%)	23 (10.9%)	7,777 (12.3%)	NS
Hispanic	40 (14.7%)	10,245 (16.2%)	15 (24.2%)	34 (17.7%)	25 (11.8%)	10,211 (16.2%)	NS
Asian/Pacific Islander/Native Americans	26 (9.5%)	13,321 (21.0%)	3 (4.8%)	45 (23.4%)	23 (10.9%)	13,276 (21.0%)	NS

fHCC = fibrolamellar hepatocellular carcinoma; N = number; NS = not statistically significant with p value > 0.05; SD = standard deviation; ** data presented for patients with available information only.

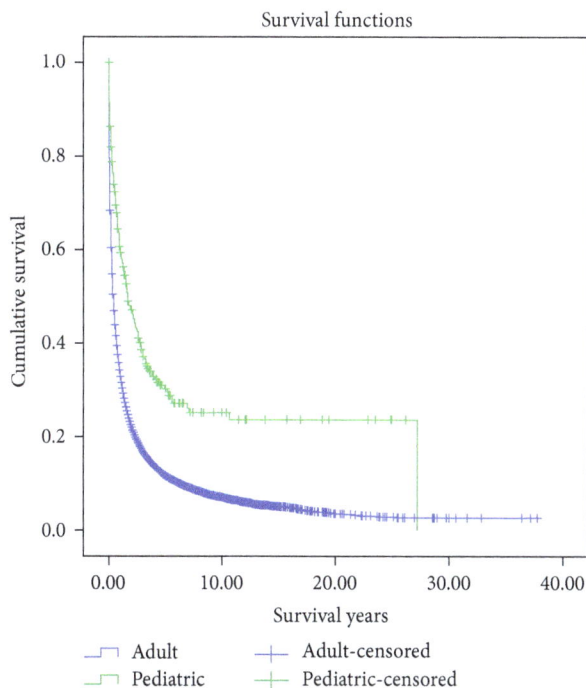

FIGURE 1. Kaplan-Meier curves illustrating actuarial survival for pediatric and adult patients with hepatocellular carcinoma from the Surveillance, Epidemiology, and End Results (SEER) database, 1973–2011.

37.2% (N = 96) of fHCC cases presented as localized disease, 33.3% (N = 86) had regional disease, and 29.5% (N = 76) had distant disease (Table 5). fHCC had a higher rate of regional disease (33.3% versus 31.2%, p < 0.001) and distant disease (29.5% versus 20.8%, p < 0.001) and a lower rate of localized disease (37.2% versus 48.0%, p < 0.001), compared to non-fHCC. Most fHCC were moderately differentiated tumors (50.0%; N = 41), while 26.8% (N = 22) were well differentiated, and 23.2% (N = 19) were poorly differentiated. fHCC had higher rates of moderately differentiated tumors

(50.0% versus 38.0%, p > 0.05) and similar rates of poorly differentiated tumors (23.2% versus 23.9%, p > 0.05), but lower rates of well differentiated tumors (26.8% versus 35.1%, p = NS). A greater proportion of fHCC had tumors > 4 cm (86.8% versus 61.9%, p > 0.05). 90.9% of pediatric fHCC presented with tumors > 4 cm, while 85.3% of adult fHCC presented with tumors > 4 cm.

A greater proportion of fHCC patients received treatment (54.9% versus 25.3%, p < 0.001), compared to non-fHCC (Table 6). Surgery was the most common treatment modality utilized in both fHCC and non-fHCC; however, significantly more fHCC patients received surgery alone (49.6% versus 20.8%) or combination of surgery and radiation (2.6% versus 0.5%, p < 0.001), compared to non-fHCC. A greater proportion of fHCC received surgical resection alone in both pediatric (66.1% versus 42.8%, p < 0.001) and adult populations (44.7% versus 20.7%, p < 0.001), compared to non-fHCC.

Patients with fHCC treated with surgery (mean survival 11.325 ± 0.966 years) and combination of surgery and radiation (7.393 ± 2.937 years) experienced significant survival benefit, compared to those who received radiation only (1.111 ± 0.348 years) or no treatment (1.916 ± 0.464 years), p < 0.001 (Table 7). Patients with fHCC treated with surgery (11.325 ± 0.966 years versus 8.345 ± 0.296 years) and combination surgery and radiation (7.393 ± 2.937 years versus 3.475 ± 0.489 years) had longer survivals than patients with non-fHCC, p < 0.001.

Overall (66.1% versus 82.0%, p < 0.001) and cancer-specific mortality (56.2% versus 62.8%, p < 0.001) were lower among fHCC patients, compared to non-fHCC. fHCC had a higher mean overall survival in both pediatric patients (9.110 ± 1.1204 years versus 6.424 ± 0.866 years) and adult patients (6.016 ± 0.653 years versus 2.657 ± 0.072 years), compared to non-fHCC. Patients with fHCC also had longer 1-year, 2-year, and 5-year cumulative survival (67%, 50%, 31%) compared to non-fHCC (34%, 23%, 12%). Kaplan-Meier curve illustrates significantly better 20-year actuarial survival for fHCC compared to non-fHCC (Figure 2).

TABLE 5: Tumor characteristics of fibrolamellar and nonfibrolamellar hepatocellular carcinoma for 63,514 adults and 257 pediatric patients from the Surveillance, Epidemiology, and End Results (SEER) database, 1973–2011.

	Total		Pediatrics		Adults		p value
	fHCC	Non-fHCC	fHCC	Non-fHCC	fHCC	Non-fHCC	
N (%)	274 (0.4%)	63,497 (99.6%)	62 (24.1%)	195 (75.9%)	212 (0.3%)	63,302 (99.7%)	—
Grade, N (%)**							
Well differentiated	22 (26.8%)	7,791 (35.1%)	6 (37.5%)	28 (35.4%)	16 (24.2%)	7,763 (35.1%)	NS
Moderately diff.	41 (50.0%)	8,426 (38.0%)	8 (50.0%)	25 (31.6%)	33 (50.0%)	8,401 (38.0%)	NS
Poorly diff.	19 (23.2%)	5,298 (23.9%)	2 (12.5%)	20 (25.3%)	17 (25.8%)	5,278 (23.9%)	NS
Undifferentiated	0 (0.0%)	672 (3.0%)	0 (0.0%)	6 (7.6%)	0 (0.0%)	666 (3.0%)	NS
Stage, N (%)**							
Localized	96 (37.2%)	25,659 (48.0%)	15 (25.0%)	53 (29.1%)	81 (40.9%)	25,606 (48.1%)	<0.001
Regional	86 (33.3%)	16,691 (31.2%)	24 (40.0%)	70 (38.5%)	62 (31.3%)	16,621 (31.2%)	<0.001
Distant	76 (29.5%)	11,117 (20.8%)	21 (35.0%)	59 (32.4%)	55 (27.8%)	11,058 (20.8%)	<0.001
Size, N (%)**							
Microscopic	0 (0.0%)	45 (0.1%)	0 (0.0%)	0 (0.0%)	0 (0.0%)	45 (0.1%)	NS
Under 2 cm	4 (2.0%)	3,067 (7.9%)	1 (1.8%)	15 (14.0%)	3 (2.0%)	3,052 (7.9%)	NS
2 to 4 cm	23 (11.2%)	11,697 (30.1%)	4 (7.3%)	13 (12.1%)	19 (12.7%)	11,684 (30.1%)	NS
Over 4 cm	178 (86.8%)	24,077 (61.9%)	50 (90.9%)	79 (73.8%)	128 (85.3%)	23,998 (61.9%)	NS

cm = centimeters; diff. = differentiated; fHCC = fibrolamellar hepatocellular carcinoma; N = number; NS = not statistically significant with p value > 0.05; NOS = not otherwise specified; SD = standard deviation; **data presented for patients with available information only.

TABLE 6: Treatment and survival outcomes of fibrolamellar and nonfibrolamellar hepatocellular carcinoma for 63,514 adults and 257 pediatric patients from the Surveillance, Epidemiology, and End Results (SEER) database, 1973–2011.

	Total		Pediatrics		Adults		p value
	fHCC	Non-fHCC	fHCC	Non-fHCC	fHCC	Non-fHCC	
N (%)	274 (0.4%)	63,497 (99.6%)	62 (24.1%)	195 (75.9%)	212 (0.3%)	63,302 (99.7%)	—
Treatment, N (%)**							
No treatment	121 (45.1%)	45,437 (74.7%)	19 (30.6%)	99 (52.9%)	102 (49.5%)	45,338 (74.7%)	<0.001
Surgery only	133 (49.6%)	12,636 (20.8%)	41 (66.1%)	80 (42.8%)	92 (44.7%)	12,556 (20.7%)	<0.001
Radiation only	7 (2.6%)	2,452 (4.0%)	2 (3.2%)	6 (3.2%)	5 (2.4%)	2446 (4.0%)	<0.001
Both surgery and radiation	7 (2.6%)	323 (0.5%)	0 (0.0%)	2 (1.1%)	7 (3.4%)	321 (0.5%)	<0.001
Mean overall survival, (years ± SD)			9.110 ± 1.204	6.424 ± 0.866	6.016 ± 0653	2.657 ± 0.072	<0.001
Overall mortality, N (%)							
Alive	93 (33.9%)	11,445 (18.0%)	32 (51.6%)	56 (28.7%)	61 (28.8%)	11,389 (18.0%)	<0.001
Dead	181 (66.1%)	52,052 (82.0%)	30 (48.4%)	139 (71.3%)	151 (71.2%)	51,913 (82.0%)	<0.001
Cancer specific mortality, N (%)							
Alive	93 (33.9%)	11,445 (18.0%)	32 (51.6%)	56 (28.7%)	61 (28.8%)	11,389 (18.0%)	<0.001
Cancer death	154 (56.2%)	39,845 (62.8%)	30 (48.4%)	126 (64.6%)	124 (58.5%)	39,719 (62.7%)	<0.001
Noncancer death	27 (9.9%)	12,207 (19.2%)	0 (0.0%)	13 (7.7%)	27 (12.7%)	12,194 (19.3%)	<0.001

fHCC = fibrolamellar hepatocellular carcinoma; N = number; NS = not statistically significant with p value > 0.05; SD = standard deviation; **data presented for patients with available information only.

3.6. Multivariate Analysis. Multivariate analysis identified regional disease (OR 1.9, CI = 1.1–3.1), distant disease (OR 4.5, CI = 2.3–8.8), and tumor size > 4 cm (OR 4.5, CI = 1.7–9.8) as being independently associated with increased mortality in the pediatric population, $p < 0.005$. Similarly, adults with distant disease (OR 6.5, CI = 4.3–9.1), poorly or undifferentiated disease (OR 7.5, CI = 5.3–9.6), and tumor size > 4 cm (OR 8.1, CI = 5.3–11.6) were found to have the highest odds of mortality on multivariate analysis, $p < 0.005$. fHCC was not found to be favorable in either pediatric, adult,

or overall populations, $p > 0.05$. For the pediatric population with fHCC disease, distant disease (OR 3.2, CI = 2.2–5.7) and tumor size > 4 cm (OR 1.6, CI = 1.0–2.2) were independently associated with increased mortality, $p < 0.001$.

4. Discussion

The development of HCC is associated with multiple etiologies, high incidence rates, and high mortality [2]. The overall incidence of HCC varies from approximately 10 per 100,000

TABLE 7: Comparing survival outcomes of fibrolamellar and nonfibrolamellar hepatocellular carcinoma from the Surveillance, Epidemiology, and End Results (SEER) database, 1973–2011.

	fHCC	Non-fHCC	p value
N (%)	274 (0.4%)	63,497 (99.6%)	—
Survival by treatment, (years ± SD)**			
No treatment	1.916 ± 0.464	1.246 ± 0.046	<0.001
Surgery only	11.325 ± 0.966	8.345 ± 0.296	<0.001
Radiation only	1.111 ± 0.348	1.190 ± 0.064	<0.001
Both surgery and radiation	7.393 ± 2.937	3.475 ± 0.489	<0.001
Cumulative survival (%)**			
1-year	67%	34%	<0.001
2-year	50%	23%	<0.001
5-year	31%	12%	<0.001

fHCC = fibrolamellar hepatocellular carcinoma; N = number; SD = standard deviation; **data presented for patients with available information only.

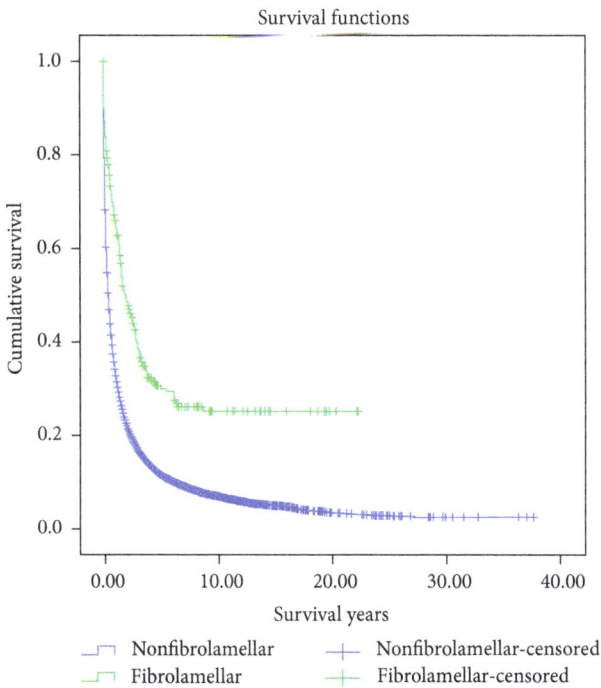

FIGURE 2: Kaplan-Meier curves illustrating actuarial survival for patients with fibrolamellar and nonfibrolamellar hepatocellular carcinoma from the Surveillance, Epidemiology, and End Results (SEER) database, 1973–2011.

in North America to as high as 20 per 100,000 in countries where hepatitis B is endemic, such as Southeastern Asia [3, 4]. Based on previous studies, the incidence of pediatric HCC in the United States has remained relatively stable, with some authors documenting reduction in HCC rates of >10% following immunization against hepatitis B in endemic countries [10–13]. While adult HCC is often associated with chronic hepatitis B infection and liver cirrhosis, most pediatric HCC are *de novo* tumors and are not related to cirrhosis [14, 15]. In cases where pediatric HCC is associated with cirrhosis, it is most often in the context of biliary atresia, Fanconi's syndrome, and hepatitis B [6, 7, 14]. Pediatric HCC

is also associated with metabolic diseases such as hereditary tyrosinemia and glycogen storage disease type IA [6, 7, 14].

Despite being the second most common primary pediatric liver malignancy following hepatoblastoma, HCC is rare in children and adolescents under the age of 20 and accounts for less than 1% of all HCC cases [14]. Similar to previously published data, this study identified a higher male HCC incidence rate for both pediatric and adult populations (59.5% and 75.1%) as well as finding that HCC was more prevalent among Caucasians in both populations [2, 5, 10, 15]. Interestingly, a higher percentage of pediatric HCC occurred among Hispanic patients, while much lower percentage of African Americans were affected. These results are consistent with previous retrospective studies conducted by McAteer et al. and Allan et al., in which over 60% of pediatric HCC occurred in Caucasians [2, 10]. These results suggest that Caucasian males in the pediatric population are at highest risk for HCC, and pediatricians should maintain a higher degree of suspicion for HCC when these patients present with suspicious or nonspecific signs and symptoms.

This study identified that pediatric patients present with more advanced disease and larger tumor sizes compared to adult HCC patients. Pediatric patients also exhibited higher rates of regional and distant disease, and lower rates of localized disease compared to adults. A greater percentage of pediatric patients had tumors larger than 4 cm compared to adults. These results are similar to the findings of Allan et al., which reported that 35% of pediatric patients had regional disease, 34% had distant disease, and only 27% had local disease [10]. The remaining 4% were unstaged [10]. Conversely, McAteer et al. reported that most children affected with HCC presented with localized and regional disease (45.6% and 35.4% resp.), compared to distant disease (19.0%) [2]. This disparity can be partly explained by the difficulty in diagnosing HCC in children. Most patients are asymptomatic until the tumor grows sufficiently large enough to cause abdominal symptoms or a palpable abdominal mass [1, 14, 16, 17]. The vague symptoms associated with HCC usually do not result in limitations in daily activities or signs of hepatic insufficiency, contributing to a delay in diagnosis and likely accounting for its more advanced stages and larger size [16]. This study identified that fHCC was more likely to present with larger tumors as well as regional and distant disease. fHCC is the most common histology among pediatric patients, which could also account for the larger and less favorable stage distribution among pediatric HCC. Eggert et al. have previously reported on 47,040 HCC patients, including 183 fHCC patients, and also reported on greater proportions of fHCC presented with tumors > 5 cm (63% versus 34%) and distant disease (33% versus 13%), compared to non-fHCC, p < 0.0001 [18].

Surgical resection is the gold standard therapy for HCC [2, 14]. In this study, pediatric patients were far more likely to be treated with surgical resection than adults, even though surgical resection was associated with a significantly improved survival in all patients. While complete excision of the HCC tumor remains the only chance for cure and prolonged survival, rates of complete excision remain low [16]. Improved survival and high resectability rates in pediatric patients are at least in part due to a higher prevalence of the indolent fHCC variant among younger patients [18]. The significantly larger percentage of pediatric patients with fHCC observed in this study is consistent with a prior SEER study in which fHCC variant was the most common variant found in the pediatric population and accounted for 41.3% of surgically treated pediatric HCC and 25.4% of nonsurgically treated pediatric HCC [2]. In a retrospective SEER study by Allan et al. involving 218 patients (55 fHCC and 160 non-fHCC), fHCC was more likely to be treated with surgery (69% versus 46%, p = 0.003) and was associated with significantly improved survival, compared to non-fHCC [10]. Surgically resected fHCC was associated with significantly higher 10-year survival rates compared to non-fHCC (59% versus 37%, p = 0.002) [10].

Nonsurgical and adjuvant treatments for HCC, including chemoembolization, ethanol injection, and radiofrequency ablation, are often utilized when surgery is not possible or as a bridge to surgery with the goal of tumor shrinkage or for palliation in unresectable cancer [14]. Radiation treatment alone is rarely used for the treatment of HCC, and only 4% of patients in this study received radiation alone. Chemotherapy for HCC is limited, and HCC remains one of the most chemoresistant tumors [15]. Czauderna et al. studied 42 patients and reported that while 49% of patients obtained a partial response to chemotherapy, survival improved by less than 5% among responders [15]. These authors also reported a 5-year survival of 28% and event-free-survival (EFS) of 17% [15]. Zhang et al. studied 45 pediatric HCC patients and reported a median survival of 6 months [19]. Patients who had surgical resection had a significantly longer survival (median survival of 28.6 months) compared to those who received chemotherapy (4 months) or no treatment (5 months), p < 0.001 [19].

Although surgery is the primary therapy for all HCC, approximately 80% of HCC patients present with unresectable tumors, either due to large tumor burden, underlying hepatic dysfunction or metastatic disease [20]. Surgery is most beneficial in patients with good hepatic function and the absence of cirrhosis but is typically contraindicated in patients with extensive cirrhosis for when transplant may play

a more critical role [20, 21]. Multiple studies have demonstrated that liver transplant confers both a significant survival advantage and a lower risk of recurrence versus surgical resection alone [22–24]. Very limited data is available on liver transplant for pediatric HCC; however, it also appears to improve overall survival in comparison to surgical resection [25–29]. Austin et al. studied 196 patients (41 patients with HCC and 135 patients with hepatoblastoma) from the United Network for Organ Sharing (UNOS) database and reported that the overall actuarial 1-, 5-, and 10-year survival for pediatric HCC liver recipients < 18 years of age were 86%, 63%, and 58%, which were similar to survival rates for pediatric liver transplants for hepatoblastoma (79%, 69%, 66%), p = 0.73 [25]. Metastatic or recurrent disease accounted for 86% of HCC deaths [25]. Despite the successes shown with liver transplantation, its use is substantially limited by organ availability.

Although HCC remain an aggressive malignancy typically associated with poor overall and cancer-specific survival, affected pediatric patients fare far better than their adult counterparts, with significantly improved mean overall survival as well as 1-, 2-, and 5-year cumulative survival. This is particularly interesting since pediatric patients typically present with more advanced disease and larger tumors. Prolonged survival among pediatric patients is likely at least partly a reflection of a much higher prevalence of the fHCC variant as well as lower rates of cirrhosis in affected children.

As with nearly all cancers, advanced stage at presentation makes it difficult to achieve total surgical resection and is therefore associated with poor prognosis [10, 14]. In the current study, distant disease and tumor sizes > 4 cm were associated with increased mortality in both children and adults, which is consistent with prior reports [2, 10].

Despite presenting with larger tumors and more advanced disease, fHCC was associated with significantly prolonged survival compared to non-fHCC in both the pediatric and adult population. The slow progressive, indolent disease course of fHCC accounts for the difficulty in diagnosing fHCC until later stages, as well as the prolonged survival [18]. Furthermore, fHCC patients are more likely to receive initial treatment with radiofrequency ablation, surgical resection, or transplantation. Similar results have been published in prior studies [10, 18]. Eggert et al. studied 47,040 HCC patients, including 183 fHCC patients, and reported that fHCC was associated with higher 5-year survival compared to non-fHCC (33.6% versus 16.1%) [18]. Allan et al. studied 218 pediatric HCC patients and reported significantly greater overall survival for fHCC compared to non-fHCC as demonstrated by 5-year Kaplan Meier curves (p = 0.002) [10]. Conversely, the Childhood Liver Tumor Strategy Group (SIOPEL) reported on 62 HCC patients (24 with fHCC and 38 with non-fHCC) and reported no significant difference in EFS at 3-year follow-up (22% versus 28%, p = 0.30) or 3-year overall survival (42% versus 33%, p = 0.24) between fHCC and non-fHCC [30]. They also reported that 42% of patients with non-fHCC died within 1 year, whereas only 2% of fHCC patients died [30].

There are several limitations of this study which should be taken into account. First, the SEER database did not accurately code for important clinical factors such as socioeconomic status, geography, tumor depth, method of diagnostic confirmation, hepatitis B vaccination status, liver transplantation information, and comorbidities such as hepatitis B infection and liver cirrhosis, which may have had an influence on survival. Second, information on diagnostic imaging and follow-up was lacking. Data on surgical and radiation therapy utilized was available in the SEER database; however information on surgical resection margins and chemotherapy received was not, and this limits the study's ability to comment on the impact of adjuvant or neoadjuvant therapy. There may also be an element of selection bias in this data set, since SEER registries are more likely to sample from urban rather than rural areas. Despite these limitations, the SEER database contains data from 26% of the United States population, and these findings can be generalized to the overall population.

5. Conclusion

Despite being the second most common primary hepatic malignancy in children, HCC remains a rare disease among pediatric patients, accounting for approximately 0.5% of all new pediatric malignancies, with a world-wide age-adjusted incidence of approximately 2 per 100,000 persons. Similar to adults, HCC occurs most commonly among Caucasian male children; however, more Hispanics and less African American children are affected. Given the rarity of pediatric HCC and the vague nonspecific presentation, diagnosing pediatric HCC is often delayed, resulting in more advanced disease and larger tumors. Despite this fact, a significantly greater proportion of pediatric patients are affected with the indolent fHCC histologic variant, which is more amenable to surgery. Surgery is the preferred treatment and significantly prolongs survival in affected patients. Although radiation is associated with poorer outcomes in the adult population, adjuvant radiation may prolong survival in the pediatric population. Given the limited number of patients who received radiotherapy in the current study, as well as the grim prognosis of pediatric HCC and the high overall and cancer-specific mortality associated with this disease, additional studies investigating the role of radiation in pediatric HCC treatment are required to more precisely identify its role in the treatment of these patients.

References

[1] R. L. Meyers, "Tumors of the liver in children," *Surgical Oncology*, vol. 16, no. 3, pp. 195–203, 2007.

[2] J. P. McAteer, A. B. Goldin, P. J. Healey, and K. W. Gow, "Surgical treatment of primary liver tumors in children: outcomes analysis of resection and transplantation in the SEER database," *Pediatric Transplantation*, vol. 17, no. 8, pp. 744–750, 2013.

[3] C. Bosetti, F. Turati, and C. La Vecchia, "Hepatocellular carcinoma epidemiology," *Best Practice & Research Clinical Gastroenterology*, vol. 28, no. 5, pp. 753–770, 2014.

[4] J. Ferlay, H.-R. Shin, F. Bray, D. Forman, C. Mathers, and D. M. Parkin, "Estimates of worldwide burden of cancer in 2008: GLOBOCAN 2008," *International Journal of Cancer*, vol. 127, no. 12, pp. 2893–2917, 2010.

[5] A. Darbari, K. M. Sabin, C. N. Shapiro, and K. B. Schwarz, "Epidemiology of primary hepatic malignancies in U.S. children," *Hepatology*, vol. 38, no. 3, pp. 560–566, 2003.

[6] F. J. van Spronsen, C. M. A. Bijleveld, B. T. van Maldegem, and F. A. Wijburg, "Hepatocellular carcinoma in hereditary tyrosinemia type I despite 2-(2 nitro-4-3 trifluoro- methylbenzoyl)-1, 3-cyclohexanedione treatment," *Journal of Pediatric Gastroenterology and Nutrition*, vol. 40, no. 1, pp. 90–93, 2005.

[7] L. M. Franco, V. Krishnamurthy, D. Bali et al., "Hepatocellular carcinoma in glycogen storage disease type Ia: a case series," *Journal of Inherited Metabolic Disease*, vol. 28, no. 2, pp. 153–162, 2005.

[8] N. Hadzic, A. Quaglia, and G. Mieli-Vergani, "Hepatocellular carcinoma in a 12-year-old child with piZZ α1-antitrypsin deficiency," *Hepatology*, vol. 43, no. 1, article 194, 2006.

[9] E. P. Tagge, D. U. Tagge, J. Reyes et al., "Resection, including transplantation, for hepatoblastoma and hepatocellular carcinoma: impact on survival," *Journal of Pediatric Surgery*, vol. 27, no. 3, pp. 292–297, 1992.

[10] B. J. Allan, B. Wang, J. S. Davis et al., "A review of 218 pediatric cases of hepatocellular carcinoma," *Journal of Pediatric Surgery*, vol. 49, no. 1, pp. 166–171, 2014.

[11] M.-H. Chang, "Cancer prevention by vaccination against hepatitis B," *Recent Results in Cancer Research*, vol. 181, pp. 85–94, 2009.

[12] M.-H. Chang, S.-L. You, C.-J. Chen et al., "Decreased incidence of hepatocellular carcinoma in hepatitis B vaccinees: a 20-year follow-up study," *Journal of the National Cancer Institute*, vol. 101, no. 19, pp. 1348–1355, 2009.

[13] H. Tajiri, H. Tanaka, S. Brooks, and T. Takano, "Reduction of hepatocellular carcinoma in childhood after introduction of selective vaccination against hepatitis B virus for infants born to HBV carrier mothers," *Cancer Causes and Control*, vol. 22, no. 3, pp. 523–527, 2011.

[14] S. Emre and G. J. McKenna, "Liver tumors in children," *Pediatric Transplantation*, vol. 8, no. 6, pp. 632–638, 2004.

[15] P. Czauderna, G. Mackinlay, G. Perilongo et al., "Hepatocellular carcinoma in children: results of the first prospective study of the International Society of Pediatric Oncology group," *Journal of Clinical Oncology*, vol. 20, no. 12, pp. 2798–2804, 2002.

[16] J.-C. Chen, C.-C. Chen, W.-J. Chen, H.-S. Lai, W.-T. Hung, and P.-H. Lee, "Hepatocellular carcinoma in children: clinical review and comparison with adult cases," *Journal of Pediatric Surgery*, vol. 33, no. 9, pp. 1350–1354, 1998.

[17] Y.-H. Ni, M.-H. Chang, H.-Y. Hsu et al., "Hepatocellular carcinoma in childhood. Clinical manifestations and prognosis," *Cancer*, vol. 68, no. 8, pp. 1737–1741, 1991.

[18] T. Eggert, K. A. McGlynn, A. Duffy, M. P. Manns, T. F. Greten, and S. F. Altekruse, "Fibrolamellar hepatocellular carcinoma in the USA, 2000-2010: a detailed report on frequency, treatment and outcome based on the surveillance, epidemiology, and end results database," *United European Gastroenterology Journal*, vol. 1, no. 5, pp. 351–357, 2013.

[19] X.-F. Zhang, X.-M. Liu, T. Wei et al., "Clinical characteristics and outcome of hepatocellular carcinoma in children and adolescents," *Pediatric Surgery International*, vol. 29, no. 8, pp. 763–770, 2013.

[20] A. Zarrinpar, F. Kaldas, and R. W. Busuttil, "Liver transplantation for hepatocellular carcinoma: an update," *Hepatobiliary and Pancreatic Diseases International*, vol. 10, no. 3, pp. 234–242, 2011.

[21] M. B. Thomas, D. Jaffe, M. M. Choti et al., "Hepatocellular carcinoma: consensus recommendations of the National Cancer Institute Clinical Trials Planning Meeting," *Journal of Clinical Oncology*, vol. 28, no. 25, pp. 3994–4005, 2010.

[22] K. K. Lee, D. G. Kim, I. S. Moon, M. D. Lee, and J. H. Park, "Liver transplantation versus liver resection for the treatment of hepatocellular carcinoma," *Journal of Surgical Oncology*, vol. 101, no. 1, pp. 47–53, 2010.

[23] J. Zhou, Z. Wang, S.-J. Qiu et al., "Surgical treatment for early hepatocellular carcinoma: comparison of resection and liver transplantation," *Journal of Cancer Research and Clinical Oncology*, vol. 136, no. 9, pp. 1453–1460, 2010.

[24] S. Mikhail, D. Cosgrove, and A. Zeidan, "Hepatocellular carcinoma: systemic therapies and future perspectives," *Expert Review of Anticancer Therapy*, vol. 14, no. 10, pp. 1205–1218, 2014.

[25] M. T. Austin, C. M. Leys, I. D. Feurer et al., "Liver transplantation for childhood hepatic malignancy: a review of the United Network for Organ Sharing (UNOS) database," *Journal of Pediatric Surgery*, vol. 41, no. 1, pp. 182–186, 2006.

[26] C. Arikan, M. Kilic, D. Nart et al., "Hepatocellular carcinoma in children and effect of living-donor liver transplantation on outcome," *Pediatric Transplantation*, vol. 10, no. 1, pp. 42–47, 2006.

[27] S. Kosola, J. Lauronen, H. Sairanen, M. Heikinheimo, H. Jalanko, and M. Pakarinen, "High survival rates after liver transplantation for hepatoblastoma and hepatocellular carcinoma," *Pediatric Transplantation*, vol. 14, no. 5, pp. 646–650, 2010.

[28] J. D. Reyes, B. Carr, I. Dvorchik et al., "Liver transplantation and chemotherapy for hepatoblastoma and hepatocellular cancer in childhood and adolescence," *Journal of Pediatrics*, vol. 136, no. 6, pp. 795–804, 2000.

[29] H. Ismail, D. Broniszczak, P. Kaliciński et al., "Liver transplantation in children with hepatocellular carcinoma. Do Milan criteria apply to pediatric patients?" *Pediatric Transplantation*, vol. 13, no. 6, pp. 682–692, 2009.

[30] V. B. Weeda, M. Murawski, A. J. McCabe et al., "Fibrolamellar variant of hepatocellular carcinoma does not have a better survival than conventional hepatocellular carcinoma—results and treatment recommendations from the Childhood Liver Tumour Strategy Group (SIOPEL) experience," *European Journal of Cancer*, vol. 49, no. 12, pp. 2698–2704, 2013.

14

Hepatocellular Adenoma: Evaluation with Contrast-Enhanced Ultrasound and MRI and Correlation with Pathologic and Phenotypic Classification in 26 Lesions

Anne-Frédérique Manichon,[1] Brigitte Bancel,[2] Marion Durieux-Millon,[1] Christian Ducerf,[3] Jean-Yves Mabrut,[3] Marie-Annick Lepogam,[4] and Agnès Rode[1]

[1] *Department of Radiology, Croix Rousse Hospital, Grande rue de la Croix-Rousse, 69004 Lyon Cedex 04, France*
[2] *Department of Pathology, Croix Rousse Hospital, 103 Grande rue de la Croix-Rousse, 69004 Lyon Cedex 04, France*
[3] *Department of Digestive Surgery, Croix Rousse Hospital, 103 Grande rue de la Croix-Rousse, 69004 Lyon Cedex 04, France*
[4] *Site Laccasagne, 162 Avenue Laccassagne, 69424 Lyon, France*

Correspondence should be addressed to Anne-Frédérique Manichon, afmanichon@gmail.com

Academic Editor: Giuliano Testa

Purpose. To review the contrast-enhanced ultrasonographic (CEUS) and magnetic resonance (MR) imaging findings in 25 patients with 26 hepatocellular adenomas (HCAs) and to compare imaging features with histopathologic results from resected specimen considering the new immunophenotypical classification. *Material and Methods.* Two abdominal radiologists reviewed retrospectively CEUS cineloops and MR images in 26 HCA. All pathological specimens were reviewed and classified into four subgroups (steatotic or HNF 1α mutated, inflammatory, atypical or β-catenin mutated, and unspecified). Inflammatory infiltrates were scored, steatosis, and telangiectasia semiquantitatively evaluated. *Results.* CEUS and MRI features are well correlated: among the 16 inflammatory HCA, 7/16 presented typical imaging features: hypersignal T2, strong arterial enhancement with a centripetal filling, persistent on delayed phase. 6 HCA were classified as steatotic with typical imaging features: a drop out signal, slight arterial enhancement, vanishing on late phase. Four HCA were classified as atypical with an HCC developed in one. Five lesions displayed important steatosis (>50%) without belonging to the HNF1α group. *Conclusion.* In half cases, inflammatory HCA have specific imaging features well correlated with the amount of telangiectasia and inflammatory infiltrates. An HCA with important amount of steatosis noticed on chemical shift images does not always belong to the HNF1α group.

1. Introduction

Hepatocellular adenomas (HCAs) are uncommon primary benign tumours, usually found in young and middle-aged women, typically encountered in the presence of a long history of oral contraceptive use (OCs) [1]. HCAs can be solitary and are monoclonal tumours. They are considered now as a heterogeneous entity. Several pathomolecular features have recently been described [2, 3]. Based on two molecular criteria (HNF1α mutations and β-catenin mutations) and an additional histological criterion, four subgroups can be defined: HNF1α mutated adenomas, β-catenin mutated adenomas, and inflammatory and/or telangiectatic adenomas; the fourth group has no particular morphological and molecular features.

Each HCA subtype is potentially associated with different evolutionary risk factors. β-catenin mutated HCAs are more frequently associated with the development of hepatocellular carcinoma (HCC) whereas inflammatory/telangiectatic HCAs have a significant risk of haemorrhage and also a slight risk of degeneration [4].

The noninvasive differentiation of HCA from other benign tumours (especially with focal nodular hyperplasia) has remained a challenge because of their highly variable appearance. Magnetic resonance imaging (MRI) has been considered as the most comprehensive imaging workup for

(a)

(b)

(c)

(d)

(e)

(f)

(g)

(h)

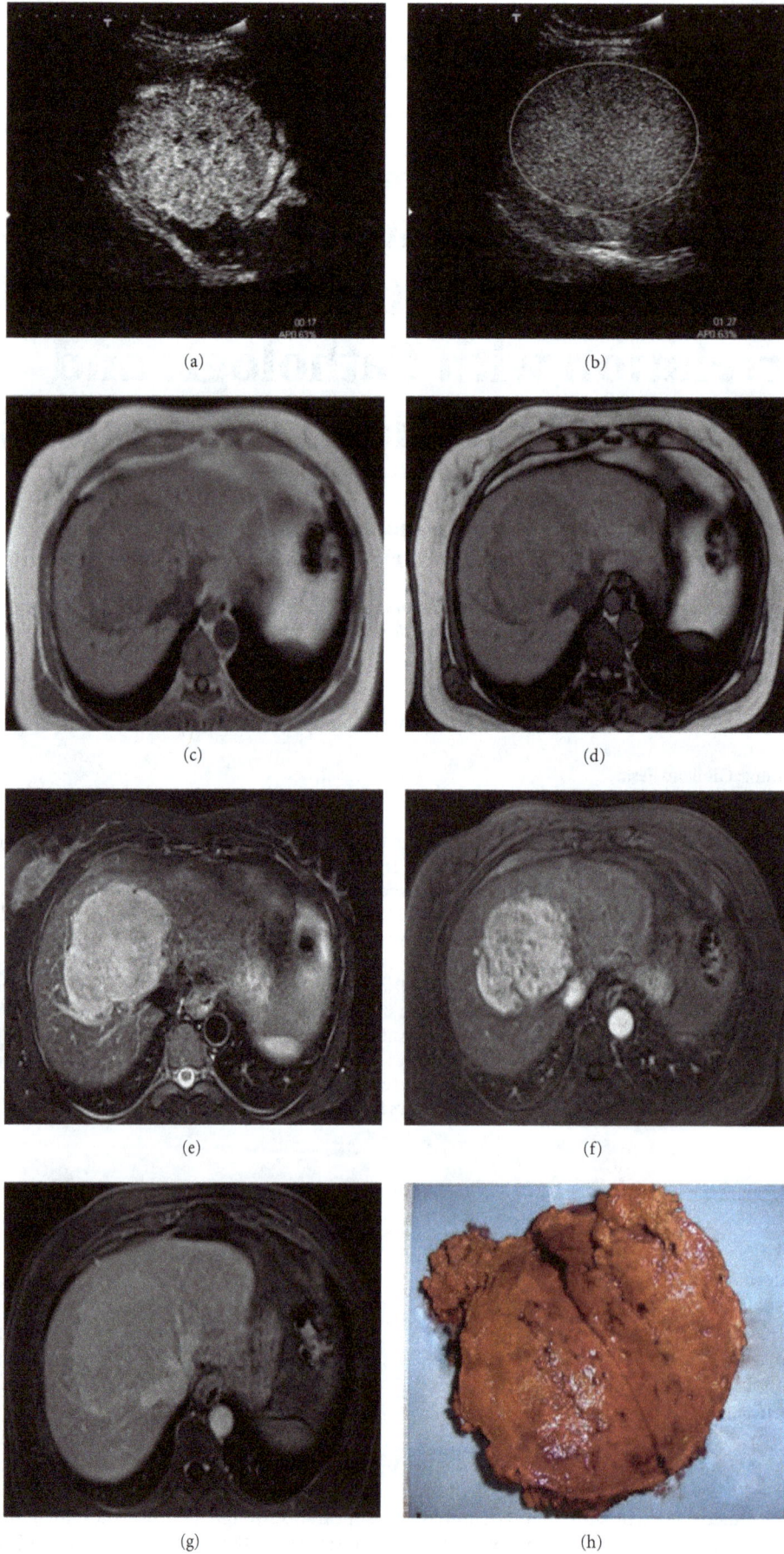

FIGURE 1: Continued.

(i)

(j)

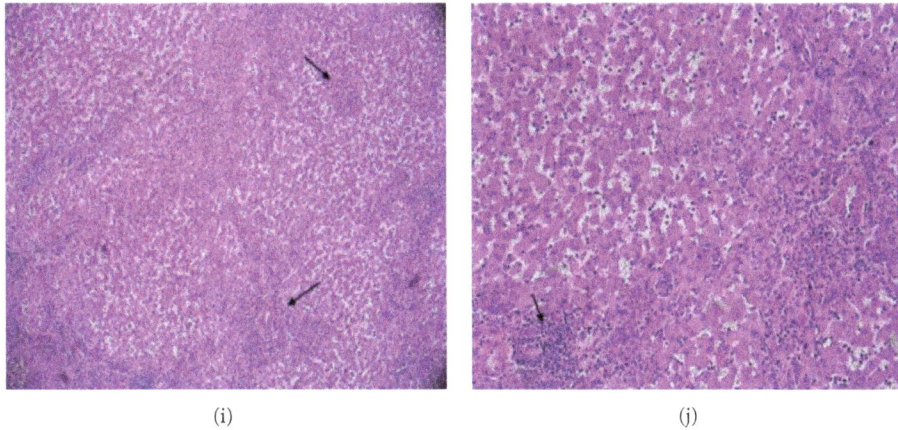

FIGURE 1: Inflammatory HCA (with typical imaging features): (a) The 10 cm lesion located in segments VIII and IV shows a marked hypervascularity after contrast injection on CEUS, (b) which is persistent in the delayed phase. (c) It is slightly hypointense with the surrounding parenchyma on T1W images with (d) no signal drop-out on the chemical shift sequence and (e) a high signal intensity on T2W fat-suppressed images. (f) It has a strong arterial enhancement after gadolinium administration, (g) which is persistent in the delayed phase. (h) Photograph of the resected specimen revealing a well-circumscribed brown mass with some vessels cut in a transverse plane. (i, j) It shows typical aspects with obvious telangiectasia (70%) and inflammatory infiltrates (grade 3) (black arrows) around thick arteries.

HCA diagnosis [5]. Contrast-enhanced ultrasound (CEUS) has been found to have a good sensitivity and specificity to characterise a focal liver lesion due to a major advantage: continuous imaging over the whole enhancement period [6].

We, therefore, performed a retrospective analysis of 26 HCAs in 25 patients with the aim of identifying MRI and CEUS features specifically associated with each subtype which have not been well described in the radiological literature. The originality of this study is the correlation between imaging features and pathological semiquantitative evaluation of inflammatory infiltrates, steatosis, and telangiectasias specifically according to their immunophenotypical classification.

2. Patients and Methods

Among the 48 HCA patients undergoing surgery at our institution hospital (from 2003 to 2010), we identified 23 patients in which liver MRI scans, CEUS, and suitable pathological materials were available. The other 25 patients were excluded from this study due to a lack of complete MRI data ($n = 7$) or contrast-enhanced US data ($n = 18$). The mean time between contrast-enhanced US and MRI was 6 weeks (0 day–9 months). Surgery was performed in a mean time of one month after imaging (0 day–7 months).

We also followed another two HCA patients with available liver biopsies, appropriate MRI and contrast-enhanced US data.

We, therefore, included a total of 25 patients (26 HCAs) in the series.

This study was conducted in agreement with French law (March 4, 2002) and the Declaration of Helsinki, and patient consent was not required.

Clinical information was collected including sex, age, circumstances of diagnosis, body mass index, oral contraceptive or anabolic use, and presence of diabetes. Biological test results such as CRP level, liver function tests, and fibrinogen were also collected.

2.1. Pathologic Analysis. All cases (24 resection and 2 biopsy) were reviewed retrospectively by one pathologist (B. Bancel) with expertise in hepatic pathology. Pathological analysis was performed on paraffin-tissue sections stained with hematoxylin-eosin, Masson's trichrome, and reticulin staining. Tumour characteristics, including size, number of nodules, and presence of haemorrhage were reported.

The extent of steatosis and sinusoidal dilatation/ telangiectasia in the HCA was arbitrarily defined as a percentage of involvement at low magnification as absent (less than 5%; grade 0), mild (5% to 29%; grade 1), moderate (30% to 50%; grade 2), or severe (more than 50%; grade 3). Inflammatory infiltrates were scored as absent (grade 0), a few inflammatory infiltrates without any foci (grade 1), one lymphocytic foci/per 10 high power fields (HPF, grade 2), or 2 and more lymphocytic foci/ per 10 HPF (grade 3). Cytologic atypia, acinar pattern, or monomorphism of the cells was recorded. In the nontumoural liver, we evaluated the fibrosis, the steatosis, and the presence of undetected nodules. If lesions were multiple, we only included nodules in which CEUS was performed and could be correlated with the resected lesion.

According to the recent classification [7], our cases were classified into four subtypes based on morphological criteria: (1) inflammatory HCA characterised by sinusoidal dilatation, abortive portal tracts, a more or less obvious ductular reaction inflammation and naked arteries; (2) steatotic HCA, lacking sinusoidal dilatation/telangiectasia and inflammation, is characterised by diffuse steatosis (>50%); (3) atypical HCA identified as those displaying some cellular monomorphism and a few acinar structures, features that by themselves are not sufficient to support a diagnosis of malignancy; (4) nodules without any of

(a)

(b)

(c)

(d)

(e)

(f)

(g)

(h)

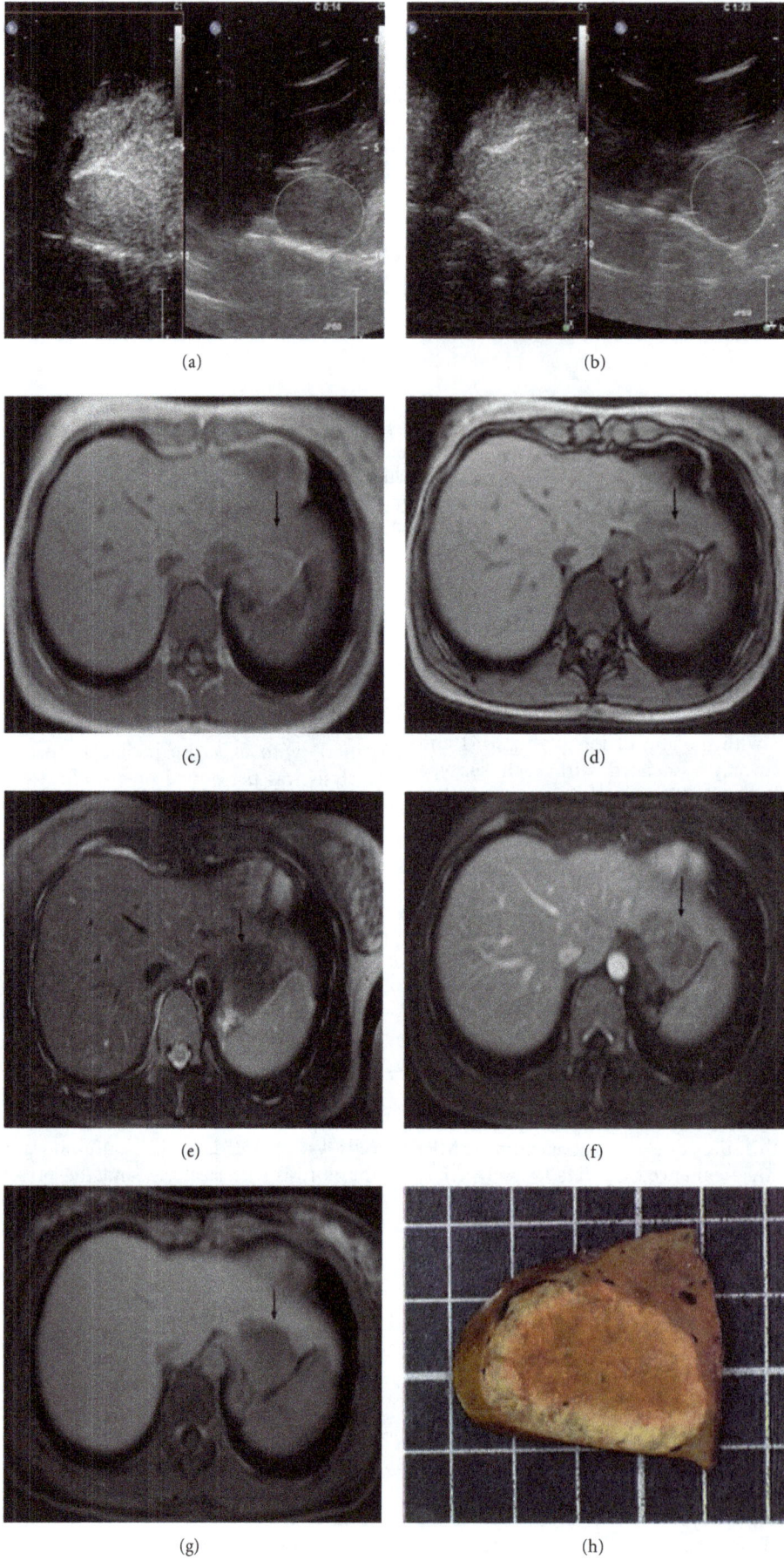

FIGURE 2: Continued.

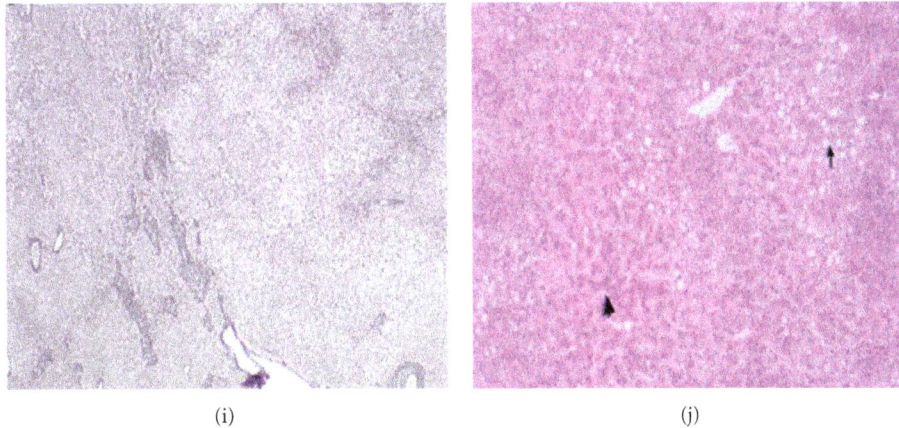

(i)   (j)

FIGURE 2: Inflammatory HCA (with less typical imaging features): (a) the 5 cm lesion has slight and homogeneous enhancement after microbubble contrast agent injection and (b) becomes isoechoic relative to the adjacent liver parenchyma. (c) The lesion (black arrow) located in segment II is isointense on T1W images with (d) a drop-out signal on chemical shift images and (e) hypointense on T2 fat-suppressed images. (f) The arterial enhancement is slight (g) with a wash out in the delayed phase. (h) Macroscopic picture: well-limited, nonencapsulated tan-colour lesion without haemorrhagic changes. (i, j) The tumour shows moderate telangiectasia (30%, arrow head) mixed with steatotic hepatocytes (40%, black arrow).

these above mentioned characteristics were reported as unclassified HCAs.

Immunohistochemical analysis was performed on 4 μm-thick formalin-fixed and paraffin-embedded sections using antibodies against liver fatty acid binding protein (LFABP Novocastra Labs, dilution 1 : 20), antiserum amyloid A (SAA Novocastra Labs, dilution 1 : 20), β-catenin (Novocastra Labs, dilution 1 : 20), and glutamine synthetase (Novocastra Labs, dilution 1 : 20). Full immunophenotypic characterisation was performed in only 11 cases.

2.2. Imaging Protocols. All 25 patients underwent MR and CEUS before surgery.

All MR imaging examinations were performed with 1.5 T system; 12 in our hospital with Magnetom Avanto or Symphony Siemens Medical System and 13 in others imaging centres. The 12 patients underwent a preoperative MRI examination in our hospital with a dedicated phase-array coil for signal reception. The following sequences were acquired and analysed: axial breath-hold T1-weighted fast field-echo pulse sequence; axial in-phase and out-phase chemical shift GRE T1-weighted images; (repetition time/echo time 129/2,38 and 4,76 msec; flip angle, 70°; field of view, 380 mm; matrix, 158 × 256; number of sections, 30; section thickness, 6 mm; gap, 15%; two signals acquired), a respiratory-triggered, fat-suppressed, T2-weighted fast spin-echo pulse sequence (repetition time/echo time, 2100/84 msec; flip angle, 150°; field of view, 350 mm; matrix, 207 × 384; number of sections, 30; section thickness, 6 mm; gap, 10%; one signal acquired), and a fat suppressed dynamic gadolinium-enhanced T1W gradient echo sequences during the arterial phase, portal venous phase, and delayed phase, with administration of gadolinium-based contrast medium (repetition time/echo time, 3,89/1,51 msec; flip angle, 25°; field of view, 420 mm; matrix, 144 × 384; number of sections, 52; section thickness, 3 mm; gap, 20%; one signal acquired).

For the 13 patients who underwent initial MRI examination elsewhere, the inclusion criteria were the ability of at least five sequences from 1.5 T magnetic resonance machine, including in-phase and out-of-phase chemical shift GRE T1W images, fat-suppressed T2W images, and fat-suppressed gadolinium-enhanced T1W sequences during arterial, portal venous, and delayed phases.

All 25 sonographic studies were performed by one of our abdominal radiologists using Philips IU 22, Siemens Elegra or Aplio XG Toshiba. First, a baseline investigation of the liver in B-mode, using greyscales, was performed with a 3.5 MHz curvilinear-array transducer. The lesion was measured routinely. Subsequently, dynamic real-time contrast-enhanced sonography was performed using contrast-coherent imaging, with the same curvilinear-array transducer, with a focus in the area of interest. A low mechanical index (<0.2) was selected to avoid microbubble disruption. Contrast-enhanced sonographic studies were performed immediately after the administration of 2.4 mL of sulfur hexafluoride–filled micro bubbles (BR 1, SonoVue, Bracco) as a bolus with a 20 gauge peripheral IV cannula followed by 10 mL of saline and the chronometer was started. A second injection of Sonovue was performed when judged necessary or to explore a second lesion.

The entire examination was tape recorded to allow later review.

2.3. Imaging Analysis. All images were interpreted retrospectively and separately in consensus by two abdominal radiologists (A. Rode, M. Durieux-Millon; 17 and 7 years of experience, resp.) with knowledge of the diagnosis of HCA but without knowledge of the pathological subgroup; a consensus was obtained in cases of difference. MRI and CEUS obtained in each patient were reviewed separately (Figures 1, 2, and 3).

(a)

(b)

(c)

(d)

(e)

(f)

(g)

(h)

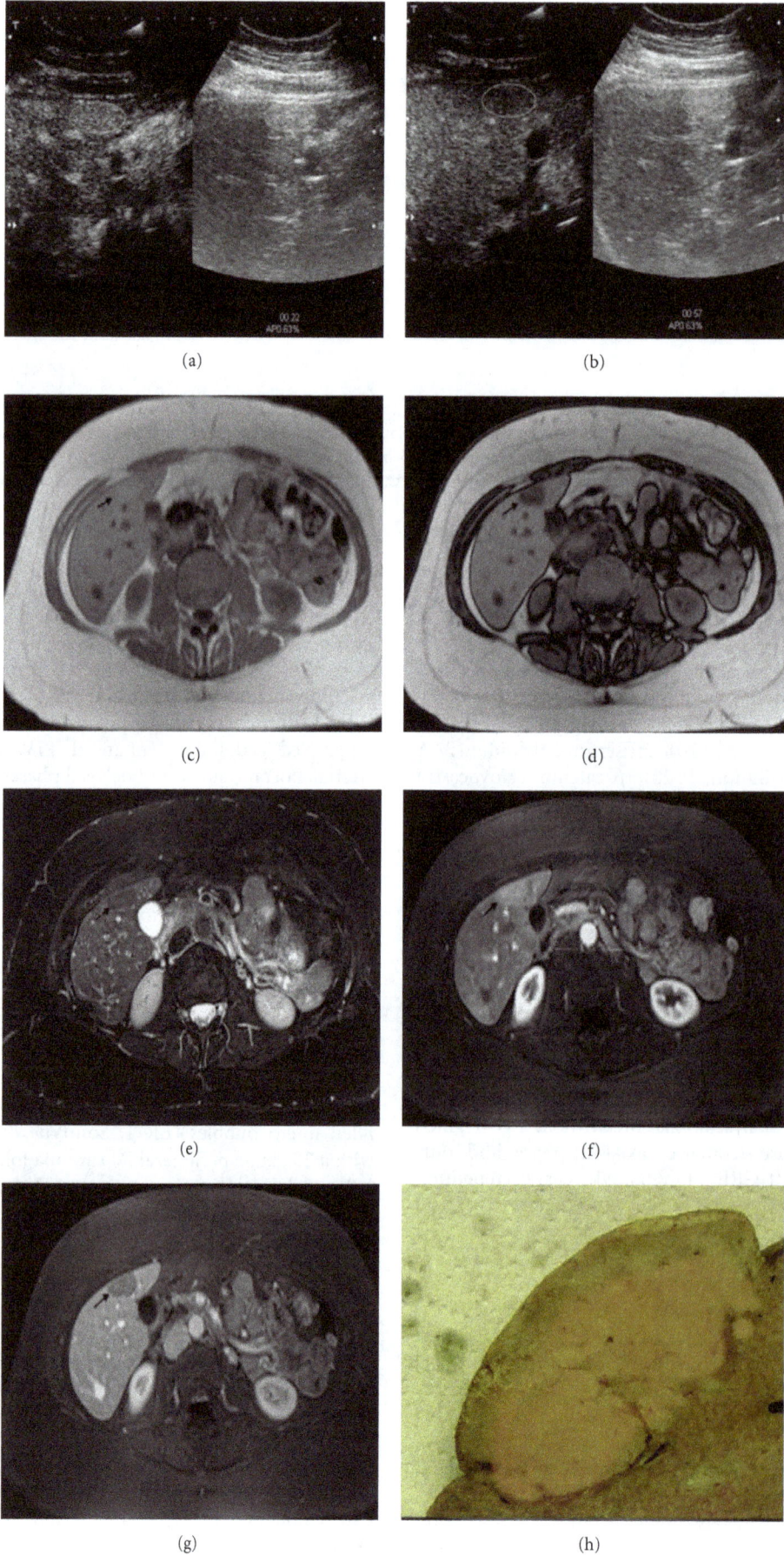

Figure 3: Continued.

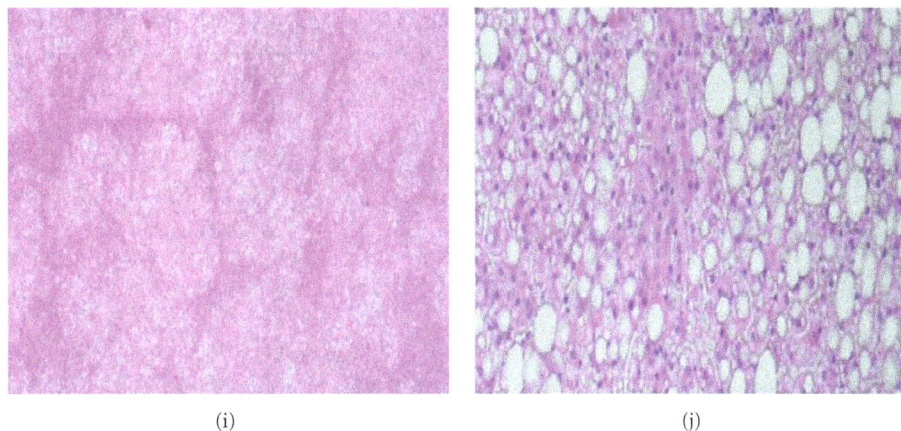

(i)	(j)

FIGURE 3: Steatotic HCA. (a) The 2.2 cm lesion, hyperechoic in B mode, has a very slight arterial enhancement, (b) which becomes isoechoic in the delayed phase after microbubble contrast agent injection. (c) The lesion (black arrow) appears isointense on T1W images with (d) an important drop-out signal on the chemical shift sequence, and (e) is hypointense on T2W images with (f) a slight arterial enhancement and (g) an apparent wash out in delayed phases. (h) Macroscopic picture shows a well limited tan-colour lesion. (i, j) Pathologic examination shows important proliferation of hepatocytes with extensive macro- and microvesicular steatosis.

The U.S. patterns were analysed: in B-mode, the echogenicity (classified as hypo echoic, iso echoic, or hyper echoic to the adjacent liver parenchyma); after Sonovue injection: the enhancement pattern in arterial, portal-venous, and late phase (none, slightly, moderately or intense); the homogeneity of enhancement (homogeneous or non-homogeneous), the direction of enhancement (centripetal, centrifugal or diffuse).

The following criteria were analysed on MRI: signal intensity of the lesion on unenhanced T1- and T2-weighted images compared to the adjacent parenchyma (hypo, iso, hyper intense); presence or not of a drop-out signal on chemical shift sequence, presence of haemorrhage within the lesion, the enhancement pattern in arterial, portal venous and late phase (none, slighly intense, moderately intense, intense), and the homogeneity of the enhancement.

2.4. Statistical Analysis. Statistical analysis was carried out using SAS software v 9.1. Qualitative variables and adenoma subtypes were compared with each other in contingency tables using a chi-square or Fisher's exact test. For quantitative variables, data were expressed as median and its minimal and maximal value. The differences between quantitative variables were evaluated with the Wilcoxon test (as a nonparametric test). All reported P values were 2-tailed; a P value of less than 0.05 was considered statistically significant. The P values reported in Table 2 were calculated using 3 subtypes of adenoma (inflammatory, steatotic, and atypical) and 4 subtypes (inflammatory with typical imaging features, inflammatory with less typical imaging features, steatotic and atypical). Kappa statistics were calculated to assess interobserver agreement in each assessed finding. Agreement was graduated as $\kappa < 0.20$, poor; 0.20–0.39, fair; 0.40–0.59, moderate; 0.60–0.79, substantial; or 0.80–1.00, almost perfect [8].

3. Results

3.1. Clinical Findings. Clinical and biological findings are resumed in Table 1.

Among the 25 patients, 23 patients were women (mean age 37 years; age range 21–52) and 2 were men (39 and 45 years old). Fifteen patients (60%) were asymptomatic and 10 (40%) had abdominal pain, with discovery of a liver haematoma in 2 (one inflammatory and one atypical HCA) cases. Sixteen patients (69.6%) had used oral contraceptives for a long period (more than two years). Three patients (12%) had type 2 diabetes (due to obesity) (with 2 inflammatory HCAs). No familial diabetes was found. Six women (24%) were overweight and had a BMI > 25, including 4 obese with a BMI > 30 (with 5 inflammatory HCAs and one with an atypical HCA).

3.2. Pathological Findings. The results are summarised in Table 2.

Among the 26 nodules, 16 (62%) in 15 patients were telangiectatic/inflammatory HCAs. The extent of inflammatory infiltrate and telangiectasia varied from case to case. Telangiectasia and inflammatory infiltrate were both marked in 8 cases (50%). Steatosis was diffuse in 2, and focal in one. A haemorrhagic component was found in 2 lesions and one case had an intraparenchymal haematoma (1.3 cm). No cytological abnormalities or acinar structures were seen.

Six *HCAs* (23% of HCAs) in 6 patients were classified as *steatotic*. They displayed moderate to marked steatosis and lacked sinusoidal dilatation or inflammatory infiltrate. Steatosis was diffuse in all but one case, in which it was irregularly distributed. Two cases (diameters of 6.5 and 9 cm) had microscopic haemorrhages.

Four *HCAs* were classified as *atypical*. They did not show any inflammation. One case had a marked steatosis (50%) and one had some steatotic foci and a central haemorrhage.

TABLE 1: Main clinical and biological data considering HCA subtype.

	Inflammatory HCA patients ($n = 15$) lesions ($n = 16$)	Steatotic HCA patients ($n = 6$) lesions ($n = 6$)	Atypical HCA patients ($n = 4$) lesions ($n = 4$)
Age median {min-max}	37 {23–50}	33,5 {26–52}	44,5 {21–47}
Sex	$F = 14\ M = 1$	$F = 5\ M = 1$	$F = 4\ M = 0$
OP (or anabolic) use >2 years	10	2	4
BMI > 25 kg/m^2	5	0	1
Diabetes	2	0	1
Inflammatory Sd (CRP or fibrinogen)	6	0	2
Cholestasis	7	0	2
Circumstances of diagnosis	by chance: 8 abdominal pain: 7	by chance: 5 abdominal pain: 1	by chance: 2 abdominal pain: 2
Solitary HCA	8	2	2
Multiple HCA <10	2	0	1
Multiple HCA ≥10	5	4	1

OP: oestroprogestative.
BMI: body mass index.
CRP: C-reactive protein.

TABLE 2: Main pathological data considering HCA subtype.

	Inflammatory HCA $n = 16$		Steatotic HCA $n = 6$	Atypical HCA $n = 4$
	Inflammatory HCA with typical imaging features $n = 7$	Inflammatory HCA with less typical imaging features $n = 9$		
Size of the nodule analyzed {min-max} (cm)	7,6 {4,2–13}	5,5 {3,5–9}	3,75 {2,2–9}	8,25 {2,5–11}
Steatosis				
grade 0 (<5%)	4	5	0	2
grade 1 (5–29%)	3	1	0	1
grade 2 (30–49%)	0	1	0	1
grade 3 (≥50%)	0	2	6	0
Telangiectasia				
grade 0 (<5%)	0	0	6	4
grade 1 (5–29%)	0	3	0	0
grade 2 (30–49%)	2	4	0	0
grade 3 (≥50%)	5	2	0	0
Inflammatory Infiltrates				
grade 0	0	1	1	2
grade 1	0	4	5	2
grade 2	4	0	0	0
grade 3	3	4	0	0

In one patient (3.8%), a well-differentiated HCC arose as distinct nodules within an atypical HCA (11 cm) without any vascular invasion. Demonstration of nuclear and/or cytoplasmic β-catenin expression was positive in only this latter case, in both areas of HCA and hepatocellular carcinoma.

No lesion was classified in the unspecified group.

The nontumoural liver was nonfibrous, F0-1 according to Metavir in all cases.

Immunohistochemistry showed an abnormal expression of β-catenin and glutamine synthetase in only one case (the HCA with malignant transformation). None of the telangiectatic/inflammatory HCAs tested had an abnormal expression of β-catenin, but they displayed an over-expression of SAA.

3.3. General Imaging Findings. All the imaging results are summarised in Table 3 (with *P* values). Substantial to almost perfect interobserver agreement ($\kappa > 0.60$) was achieved for all the imaging criteria.

3.3.1. Inflammatory Group. Two subgroups could be distinguished on imaging: one, homogeneous, with typical imaging features (7 lesions/16 IHCA) and another one, more heterogeneous, with less typical imaging features (9 lesions/16 IHCA).

The typical imaging features observed in inflammatory HCA are as follows:

(i) with CEUS, a fast arterial centripetal filling and a persistent enhancement in the portal and delayed phases;

(ii) with MRI: a strong hyper intense signal on T2W images and a strong arterial enhancement, associated with a persistent enhancement on portal and delayed phase. Six inflammatory HCAs (and none in other group) showed a hyper intense signal on T1W sequence.

In the remaining group of lesions, with less typical imaging presentation: 4 are not hyper intense on T2W sequence, 3 have a drop-out signal on chemical shift sequence.

3.3.2. Steatotic HCA. Three major MRI features were found to be significantly associated with this group.

(i) First the signal drop-out on chemical shift MRI sequences was found in all 6 steatotic HCAs, diffuse in 5 and focal in 1.

(ii) Secondly, arterial enhancement was always considered to be slight or moderate.

(iii) Finally, all lesions presented a washout on portal or delayed phase.

The atypical group did not have any imaging features considered to be significantly associated with it. Our case of histologically confirmed malignant transformation within an otherwise atypical adenoma (11 cm) was not suspected based on the usual radiological criteria for HCC. It appeared heterogeneous, mostly hypointense on T1W with a slight drop-out signal on chemical shift sequence, hyperintense on T2W. It showed a strong arterial enhancement on CEUS and MRI, persistent on delayed phase.

3.4. Correlation between Imaging Features and Pathological Findings. The two subgroups within the inflammatory group based on imaging features are correlated with pathological findings: all the HCA with typical imaging features displayed an important amount of telangiectasia (grade ≥ 2)

associated with an inflammation infiltrates quoted ≥ 2 on our four grade scale; whereas in the remaining group of lesions, only one out of 9 displayed both criteria (telangiectasia grade ≥ 2 and inflammation ≥ 2), the other 8 had either important telangiectasia or marked inflammation.

The drop-out signal on chemical shift MRI sequences is well correlated with the fat repartition within the lesion. The steatotic HCA with a patchy signal drop-out on chemical shift sequences had an irregular fat repartition on pathological analysis. The five lesions with a drop-out signal on chemical shift sequence without belonging to the steatotic HCA showed an amount of steatosis $\geq 30\%$.

4. Discussion

The current study retrospectively investigated imaging features with MRI and CEUS, in solitary or multiple HCAs, in relation to clinicopathological characteristics, including histological subtype.

Most *inflammatory HCAs* occur in overweight or obese patients in a context of long OP use and are often associated with a biological inflammatory syndrome [9, 10]. In our study, inflammatory HCAs are characterised by their vascular changes. But in contrast to previous studies [10–12], the diagnostic circumstances of our cases were fortuitous and never due to acute bleeding, with only 2 cases of liver haematoma of less than 10 cm in diameter. A malignant transformation is also possible even in the absence of β-catenin mutation [9]. In this context, the radiological identification of such lesions may be useful.

We demonstrate, for the first time, that two distinct subgroups of inflammatory HCAs can be recognised on imaging, closely correlated with severity of telangiectasias and inflammatory infiltrates. The typical imaging features, as previously described [5], are the hyperintense signal on the T2W sequence, a strong and homogeneous arterial enhancement on MRI, and persistent enhancement in the delayed phase on MRI. In addition, we find persistent enhancement in the delayed phase with CEUS confirming a good correspondence between the two imaging techniques. These typical imaging features are associated with marked telangiectasias (grade ≥ 2) and inflammatory infiltrates (quoted as ≥ 2). The other subgroup of inflammatory HCAs has a less typical imaging presentation: not always hyperintense on the T2W sequence, some cases with a wash out at delayed phase or a drop-out signal on the chemical shift sequence, with significant steatosis. These mixed (steatotic and peliotic) HCAs, according to Lewin et al. [13], should not be misinterpreted as steatotic HCAs.

A hyperintense signal on T1W is another typical characteristic of this inflammatory group. This does not reflect sinusoidal dilatation [14] as 3 other nodules with more than 60% of telangiectasias are hypointense on the T1W sequence. The explanation of the hypersignal T1W already seen in others lesions such as some cirrhotic nodules is unknown; bleeding, fatty degeneration, and a large amount of Cu^{2+} can play a paramagnetic role in tissue and determine this hyperintensity pattern [15].

TABLE 3: Radiological (CEUS and MRI) features considering HCA subtype.

			Inflammatory HCA (typical on imaging) $n = 7$	Inflammatory HCA (less typical on imaging) $n = 9$	Steatotic HCA $n = 6$	Atypical HCA $n = 4$	P values*
CEUS	B mode	HypoE	3 (43%)	5 (56%)	0	1 (25%)	
		IsoE	2 (29%)	1 (11%)	1 (17%)	1 (25%)	0,2958
		HyperE	2 (29%)	3 (33%)	5 (83%) (1 heterogeneous)	2 (50%)	
	Arterial enhancement	None	0	0	1 (17%)	0	
		Slight	0	3 (33%)	2 (33%)	2 (50%)	0,1514
		Moderate	3 (43%)	3 (33%)	3 (50%)	0	
		Intense	4 (57%)	3 (33%)	0	2 (50%)	
	Delayed enhancement	Persistent	6 (86%)	0	0	2 (50%)	
		IsoE	1 (14%)	6 (67%)	3 (50%)	1 (25%)	0,0019
		HypoE	0	3 (33%)	3 (50%)	1 (25%)	
	Homogeneousness enhancement	Homogeneous	7 (100%)	5 (56%)	5 (83%)	2 (50%)	0,0517
		Heterogeneous	0	4 (44%)	1 had no enhancement	2 (50%)	
	Filling direction	Centripetal	6 (86%)	7 (78%)	1 (17%)	2 (50%)	0,1012
		Indifferent	1 (14%)	2 (22%)	4 (67%)1 had no enhancement	2 (50%)	0,0273**
MRI	T1	HypoS	1 (14%)	3 (33%)	3 (50%)	1 (25%)	
		IsoS	4 (57%)	2 (22%)	3 (50%)	3 (75%)	0,2253
		HyperS	2 (29%)	4 (33%)	0	0	
	IN/OUT	No drop out	7 (100%)	6 (67%)	0	2 (50%)	1,79E−04
		Drop out	0	3 (44%)	6 (100%) included 1 heterogeneous	2 (50%) included 1 heterogeneous	
	T2	HypoS	7 (100%)	3 (33%)	3 (50%)	1 (25%)	
		IsoS	0	1 (11%)	1 (17%)	2 (50%)	0,1012
		HyperS	0	5 (56%)	2 (33%)	1 (25%)	
	Arterial enhancement	None	0	0	1 (17%)	1 (25%)	
		Slight	0	2 (22%)	3 (50%)	0	0,0026
		Moderate	0	2 (22%)	2 (33%)	2 (50%)	
		Intense	7 (100%)	5 (56%)	0	1 (25%)	
	Delayed phase	Persistent	6 (86%)	3 (33%)	0	2 (50%)	
		IsoS	1 (14%)	1 (11%)	0	0	0,005
		HypoS	0	5 (56%)	6 (100%)	2 (50%)	

* Test made with 4 categories of HCAs (inflammatory typical on imaging, inflamm less typical on imaging, steatotic and atypic),
**Test made with 3 categories of HCAs (inflammatory, steatotic and atypic).

Previously, before recent pathologic and molecular studies, inflammatory HCAs were categorised with focal nodular hyperplasia. CEUS is useful to appreciate the direction of filling of the lesion and enables us to clear up the situation if a FNH is suspected. It appears that almost all of inflammatory HCA have a centripetal filling at the arterial time of injection (P = 0.0273), and also a persistent enhancement at the late phase. This persistent enhancement at late phase is a discriminant sign not only for focal nodular hyperplasia, but also for other HCA subgroups.

Steatotic HCA is histologically considered as a homogeneous group of tumours. They are characterised by prominent steatosis without any other specific features. It is necessary to underline that these two tumourigenic pathways, HNF1-α inactivation, and β-catenin mutations, are mutually exclusive [5], so this group of steatotic HCAs is less exposed to the risk of malignant transformation.

The homogeneity of the signal drop-out is well correlated with the diffuse repartition of fat within the lesion in pathological findings, unlike hepatocellular carcinoma, which usually has a focal steatosis. The arterial enhancement is never strong on either MRI or CEUS, and vanished in the delayed phase. The slight arterial enhancement on CEUS and MRI can be explained by a focal compression of the sinusoids due to steatosis and a less important blood flow [16]. The marked hypointensity in the MRI delayed phase is related to the slight previous enhancement and the persistent gradient of signal between the liver and the nodule due to the fat saturation.

However, the drop-out signal on chemical shift is not specific for the steatotic HCA group: in our study, we also found 3 inflammatory HCAs and 3 atypical HCAs with drop-out signals, explained by an important amount of fat on pathologic examination. Thus, in contrast to Laumonier's study [5], a steatotic lesion, after either pathologic analysis or radiologic examination, does not systematically belong to the group of HCAs with HNF1-α mutations.

Atypical HCA is associated with cytological abnormalities and an increased risk of malignant transformation. One out of 26 had evidence of well-differentiated HCC without vascular invasion within an atypical adenoma on pathology. The occurrence of HCC appears in different series in about 5–10% of cases [17], In a recent study [4], the risk of malignant transformation was 4% in women and 47% in men. It is observed in tumours greater than 8 cm in diameter [18]. However, the clinical relevance of β-catenin is poor for predicting malignant transformation as staining is focal. Only 20% of malignant HCAs in the series of Dokmak et al. [11] were mutated, a rate similar to that of Zucman-Rossi's study [19], whereas in Farges's study [4], 2/3 of HCAs with malignant transformation were β-catenin activated and 1/3 displayed cell atypias.

Our patients with adenomatosis had the same final pathological classification and imaging features as the group of solitary adenomas. As discussed by previous authors [11, 20], adenomatosis is probably not a specific entity of HCA as thought until now [21], and the number does not constitute a determining factor in its evolution [22]. Multiple HCAs in the same patient belong to the same pathological group (because they are monoclonal tumours), and pathological features most "at risk" determine the final classification.

Our study has three major limitations. First, the number of patients is small. Large multi-institutional studies are needed to corroborate our findings. The frequency of complications in our study does not represent the real percentage described in the previous studies. Secondly, this is a retrospective study and blind reading was carried out in cases with a confirmed diagnosis of adenoma. Thirdly, most of our cases did not have a immunohistochemistry analysis

for subtyping HCA. But the pathological features of the subgroups are well recognised, some of these immunostains are not routinely available. The pathologist's conclusion was mostly based on the morphological analysis gold standard as it has been proved in different studies [11] and because there is a good agreement between morphological analysis and immunophenotypical classification.

In conclusion , differentiating inflammatory HCA from FNH and other HCA subgroups is important as it significantly affects treatment decisions. Because of a significant incidence of complications (haemorrhage and malignancy), it may be useful to recognise different subgroups of HCAs. Using imaging (MRI and CEUS), some telangiectatic HCAs can be detected because of characteristic specific features: a hyperintense signal on T2W, a spontaneous hyperintense signal on T1W and a strong arterial enhancement on MRI, which is persistent in the delayed phase. This particular profile of enhancement on MRI is also well correlated with that on CEUS.

A diffuse drop-out signal on chemical shift sequence and a slight arterial enhancement is very suggestive of a steatotic HCA corresponding to the HNF1 subgroup, but the presence of a marked steatosis is not specific to this aetiology and can also be recognised in inflammatory or atypical (corresponding to the -catenin mutated group) HCAs.

If we are able to recognise imaging features associated with these different subgroups of HCAs, liver biopsy is probably no longer useful to confirm the diagnosis prior to resection.

References

[1] L. Giannitrapani, M. Soresi, E. La Spada, M. Cervello, N. D'Alessandro, and G. Montalto, "Sex hormones and risk of liver tumor," *Annals of the New York Academy of Sciences*, vol. 1089, pp. 228–236, 2006.

[2] S. Rebouissou, P. Bioulac-Sage, and J. Zucman-Rossi, "Molecular pathogenesis of focal nodular hyperplasia and hepatocellular adenoma," *Journal of Hepatology*, vol. 48, no. 1, pp. 163–170, 2008.

[3] P. Bioulac-Sage, J. Frédéric Blanc, S. Rebouissou, C. Balabaud, and J. Zucman-Rossi, "Genotype phenotype classification of hepatocellular adenoma," *World Journal of Gastroenterology*, vol. 13, no. 19, pp. 2649–2654, 2007.

[4] O. Farges, N. Ferreira, S. Dokmak, J. Belghiti, P. Bedossa, and V. Paradis, "Changing trends in malignant transformation of hepatocellular adenoma," *Gut*, vol. 60, no. 1, pp. 85–89, 2011.

[5] H. Laumonier, P. Bioulac-Sage, C. Laurent, J. Zucman-Rossi, C. Balabaud, and H. Trillaud, "Hepatocellular adenomas: magnetic resonance imaging features as a function of molecular pathological classification," *Hepatology*, vol. 48, no. 3, pp. 808–818, 2008.

[6] H. Trillaud, J. M. Bruel, P. J. Valette et al., "Characterization of focal liver lesions with SonoVue-enhanced sonography: international multicenter-study in comparison to CT and MRI," *World Journal of Gastroenterology*, vol. 15, no. 30, pp. 3748–3756, 2009.

[7] P. Bioulac-Sage, "Les tumeurs hepato-cellulaires benignes, donnees morphologiques et moleculaires: une nouvelle classification," *Acta Endoscopica*, vol. 36, no. 3, pp. 335–340, 2006.

[8] J. R. Landis and G. G. Koch, "The measurement of observer agreement for categorical data," *Biometrics*, vol. 33, no. 1, pp. 159–174, 1977.

[9] V. Paradis, A. Champault, M. Ronot et al., "Telangiectatic adenoma: an entity associated with increased body mass index and inflammation," *Hepatology*, vol. 46, no. 1, pp. 140–146, 2007.

[10] P. Bioulac-Sage, H. Laumonier, G. Couchy et al., "Hepatocellular adenoma management and phenotypic classification: the Bordeaux experience," *Hepatology*, vol. 50, no. 2, pp. 481–489, 2009.

[11] S. Dokmak, V. Paradis, V. Vilgrain et al., "A single-center surgical experience of 122 patients with single and multiple hepatocellular adenomas," *Gastroenterology*, vol. 137, no. 5, pp. 1698–1705, 2009.

[12] L. Barthelmes and I. S. Tait, "Liver cell adenoma and liver cell adenomatosis," *HPB*, vol. 7, no. 3, pp. 186–196, 2005.

[13] M. Lewin, A. Handra-Luca, L. Arrivé et al., "Liver adenomatosis: classification of MR imaging features and comparison with pathologic findings," *Radiology*, vol. 241, no. 2, pp. 433–440, 2006.

[14] H. Honda, K. Kaneko, T. Maeda et al., "Small hepatocellular carcinoma on magnetic resonance imaging: relation of signal intensity to angiographic and clinicopathologic findings," *Investigative Radiology*, vol. 32, no. 3, pp. 161–168, 1997.

[15] P. Attal, V. Vilgrain, G. Brancatelli et al., "Telangiectatic focal nodular hyperplasia: US, CT, and MR imaging findings with histopathologic correlation in 13 cases," *Radiology*, vol. 228, no. 2, pp. 465–472, 2003.

[16] E. A. Psatha, R. C. Semelka, D. Armao, J. T. Woosley, Z. Firat, and G. Schneider, "Hepatocellular adenomas in men: MRI findings in four patients," *Journal of Magnetic Resonance Imaging*, vol. 22, no. 2, pp. 258–264, 2005.

[17] O. Farges and S. Dokmak, "Malignant transformation of liver adenoma: an analysis of the literature," *Digestive Surgery*, vol. 27, no. 1, pp. 32–38, 2010.

[18] J. L. Deneve, T. M. Pawlik, S. Cunningham et al., "Liver cell adenoma: a multicenter analysis of risk factors for rupture and malignancy," *Annals of Surgical Oncology*, vol. 16, no. 3, pp. 640–648, 2009.

[19] J. Zucman-Rossi, E. Jeannot, J. T. van Nhieu et al., "Genotype-phenotype correlation in hepatocellular adenoma: new classification and relationship with HCC," *Hepatology*, vol. 43, no. 3, pp. 515–524, 2006.

[20] S. M. Hussain, I. C. van den Bos, R. S. Dwarkasing, J. W. Kuiper, and J. den Hollander, "Hepatocellular adenoma: findings at state-of-the-art magnetic resonance imaging, ultrasound, computed tomography and pathologic analysis," *European Radiology*, vol. 16, no. 9, pp. 1873–1886, 2006.

[21] L. Grazioli, M. P. Federle, T. Ichikawa, E. Balzano, M. Nalesnik, and J. Madariaga, "Liver adenomatosis: clinical, histopathologic, and imaging findings in 15 patients," *Radiology*, vol. 216, no. 2, pp. 395–402, 2000.

[22] R. Veteläinen, D. Erdogan, W. de Graaf et al., "Liver adenomatosis: re-evaluation of aetiology and management," *Liver International*, vol. 28, no. 4, pp. 499–508, 2008.

15

Risk Factors Associated with Reoperation for Bleeding following Liver Transplantation

Maxwell A. Thompson,[1] David T. Redden,[2] Lindsey Glueckert,[1] A. Blair Smith,[3] Jack H. Crawford,[3] Keith A. Jones,[3] Devin E. Eckhoff,[4] Stephen H. Gray,[4] Jared A. White,[4] Joseph Bloomer,[5] and Derek A. DuBay[4]

[1] University of Alabama at Birmingham, Birmingham, AL 35294, USA
[2] Biostatistics Division, School of Public Health, University of Alabama at Birmingham, Birmingham, AL 35294, USA
[3] Department of Anesthesia, University of Alabama at Birmingham, Birmingham, AL 35294, USA
[4] Liver Transplant and Hepatobiliary Surgery, University of Alabama at Birmingham, 701 ZRB, 1530 3rd Avenue South, Birmingham, AL 35294-0007, USA
[5] Transplant Hepatology, University of Alabama at Birmingham, Birmingham, AL 35294, USA

Correspondence should be addressed to Derek A. DuBay; ddubay@uabmc.edu

Academic Editor: Uta Dahmen

Introduction. This study's objective was to identify risk factors associated with reoperation for bleeding following liver transplantation (LTx). *Methods.* A retrospective study was performed at a single institution between 2001 and 2012. Operative reports were used to identify patients who underwent reoperation for bleeding within 2 weeks following LTx (operations for nonbleeding etiologies were excluded). *Results.* Reoperation for bleeding was observed in 101/928 (10.8%) of LTx patients. The following characteristics were associated with reoperation on multivariable analysis: recipient MELD score (OR 1.06/MELD unit, 95% CI 1.03, 1.09), number of platelets transfused (OR 0.73/platelet unit, 95% CI 0.58, 0.91), and aminocaproic acid utilization (OR 0.46, 95% CI 0.27, 0.80). LTx patients who underwent reoperation for bleeding had a longer ICU stay (5 days ± 7 versus 2 days ± 3, $P < 0.001$) and hospitalization (18 days ± 9 versus 10 days ± 18, $P < 0.001$). The risk of death increased in patients who underwent reoperation for bleeding (HR 1.89, 95% CI 1.26, 2.85). *Conclusion.* Reoperation for bleeding following LTx was associated with increased resource utilization and recipient mortality. A lower threshold for intraoperative platelet transfusion and antifibrinolytics, especially in patients with high lab-MELD score, may decrease the incidence of reoperation for bleeding following LTx.

1. Introduction

Approaches to the perioperative management for liver transplantation have been adapted over time. Early experience with liver transplantation focused on the management of coagulopathy and involved extraordinary utilization of blood component therapy [1, 2]. Despite advances in anesthesia and surgical techniques manifesting in lower overall transfusion requirements [3, 4], bleeding is still the most frequent serious early complication following liver transplantation, occurring in approximately 20% of patients [5]. Coagulopathy management thus remains a major concern during orthotopic liver

transplantation. Several recent and historic studies clearly demonstrate an association between intraoperative blood transfusion and mortality [6–9]. Interestingly, much variability exists between institutions with regard to coagulopathy management suggesting the need for more evidence to guide practice [2, 10, 11].

Postoperative bleeding can be life-threatening and requires reoperation in 10–15% of patients [5, 12] for hemorrhage control and/or hematoma evacuation. Reoperation for bleeding contributes to the overall mortality [13] and financial burden [14, 15] of liver transplantation. Many studies have attempted to identify risk factors associated with reoperation following liver transplantation; both donor and recipient variables have been reported [16, 17]. Previous research has identified that intraoperative estimated blood loss [18], increased intraoperative packed red blood cell (pRBC) transfusion [12, 18, 19], and total number of intraoperative blood products transfused are associated with reoperation following liver transplantation. In addition to massive transfusion, the UCLA group [20] found that recipient intraoperative vasopressor utilization, use of extended criteria donors, and recipient intraoperative glucose variability were also associated with reoperation for bleeding following liver transplantation. The problem with these sets of data is that they do little to help to predict, either before or during liver transplantation, the patients who are at increased risk for posttransplant bleeding. Identifying patients at increased risk of bleeding is important so a more aggressive approach to intraoperative coagulopathy management can be utilized. Furthermore, other than aggressive intraoperative glucose management, these studies did not identify modifiable risk factors associated with increased incidence of reoperation for bleeding.

The primary goal of this study was to identify risk factors associated with reoperation for bleeding following liver transplantation that may inform intraoperative coagulopathy management. Elucidation of such risk factors would aid in liver transplant coagulopathy planning by identifying patients in whom preemptive interventions are most appropriate.

2. Methods

2.1. Definition of Groups. Ethics approval for this study was obtained from the University of Alabama Institutional Review Board Protocol number X100310006. The requirement for written informed consent was waived by the Institutional Review Board.

A retrospective chart review was performed on all patients over 19 years of age who received a liver transplant at the University of Alabama at Birmingham between 2001 and 2012. Patients were identified from an internal transplant database that is used for clinical purposes. Patients were grouped based on whether or not a reoperation was performed for bleeding within 2 weeks of liver transplantation. The reoperation for bleeding group included any patient who required an unplanned exploratory laparotomy for either surgical management of active hemorrhage or evacuation of a hematoma. Operative notes were examined for the indication "hemoperitoneum, evacuation of hematoma, surgical management of active hemorrhage, or abdominal washout." Other indications for reoperation such as bile leaks, vascular thrombosis, acute graft failure, or septicemia were excluded from the postoperative bleeding group.

2.2. Data Collected. Recipient demographics, comorbidities, selected laboratory values, operative details, and pertinent postoperative data were collected. Baseline demographics included age, gender, race, etiology of liver disease, lab-MELD scores, body mass index (BMI), and whether or not the patients were in the intensive care unit (ICU) immediately

prior to transplant. Recipient comorbidities included the presence of diabetes, hypertension, dyslipidemia, chronic renal insufficiency, and coronary artery disease. Immediate pretransplant laboratory values included hematocrit, platelet count, and international normalized ratio (INR). Operative details included operative length, cold and warm ischemia time, blood products administered (red blood cells, fresh frozen plasma, platelets, and cryoglobulin), procoagulants administered (aminocaproic acid, Hospira, Lake Forest, IL, USA, and conjugated estrogens, Pfizer Canada, Kirkland, QC, Canada), epigastric surgical history (defined as a nonlaparoscopic, noncholecystectomy foregut intervention), vascular reconstruction (arterial conduit and/or mesenteric venous bypass), and retransplantation. Postoperative variables included intensive care unit length of stay, total posttransplant hospital length of stay, number of readmissions following transplant, graft failure, survival, and cause of death. Donor characteristics were summarized via the donor risk index (DRI) [21] which is a risk estimate of time to graft failure; variables included donor age, donor race, donor height, donor cause of death, type of donation (partial/split or whole), donor locations (regional, national, or local share), and donation after cardiac death.

2.3. Intraoperative Coagulopathy Management. The UAB liver transplant anesthesia utilizes both the thromboelastogram (TEG) functional assessment clot formation as well as INR, PTT, and platelet counts to manage intraoperative coagulopathy. The TEG assay is serially performed at the start of the transplant, during the anhepatic phase, and following reperfusion. If the R time is prolonged during the hepatectomy phase, conjugated estrogens are given at 1 mg/kg. Estrogens have been demonstrated to increase platelet adhesiveness [22, 23]. If the R time is within normal limits during the hepatectomy stage, then estrogens are given after reperfusion if the R time becomes prolonged then. Fresh frozen plasma (FFP) is used if estrogens fail to correct the R time. If FFP fails to adequately correct TEG parameters, hypofibrinogenemia exists, and surgical bleeding continues, cryoprecipitate is administered. Platelets (1 pheresed Unit) are administered if the platelet count is less than 50,000 and the surgical assessment is that of nonsurgical bleeding or if the maximum amplitude of the TEG is decreased. Epsilon aminocaproic acid (Amicar 2.5 gram iv) is used during the neohepatic stage (early reperfusion) if the TEG shows fibrinolysis.

2.4. Intensive Care Unit Posttransplant Coagulopathy Management. The UAB Surgical Intensive Care Unit utilizes a combination of the surgical drain effluent characteristics, INR, PTT, platelet counts, and thromboelastogram (TEG) functional assessment clot formation to manage posttransplant coagulopathy. In general, platelets and clotting factors are only administered in the setting of active bleeding, sanguineous drain output, a decreasing hematocrit, or extreme laboratory values.

2.5. Statistical Analysis. Descriptive statistics (sample means and variances) for continuous variables (age, body mass index, MELD score, and donor risk index) were calculated to provide measures of central location and variability around the mean. For categorical variables (race, comorbidities, etc.), sample proportions falling within each category were calculated. To test the primary hypothesis that long-term survival varied by reoperation for bleeding, Log-Rank tests were used, and Kaplan-Maier curves were constructed to examine/compare liver transplant survival distributions. Multivariable Cox regression analyses were performed to control for potentially confounding variables. Demographics and comorbidities were compared between groups (reoperation for bleeding versus control group) using Chi-Square tests for categorical variables and two-sample t-tests for continuous variables. To examine which demographics and factors were associated with odds of reoperation for bleeding, multivariable logistic regression models were developed. All analyses were conducted using SAS 9.3 (Cary NC) and statistical significance was defined as a P value less than or equal to 0.05.

3. Results

3.1. Baseline Demographics (Table 1). The reoperation for bleeding group consisted of 101/928 (10.8%) of liver transplant patients. The mean age, race, BMI, and etiology of liver disease were not statistically significant between the reoperation for bleeding group and control group. There was a trend towards fewer males in the reoperation for bleeding group, but this did not reach statistical significance. The average lab-MELD score at the time of transplantation was significantly higher in the reoperation for bleeding group compared to the control group (23.8 ± 8.1 versus 20.4 ± 7.9, $P < 0.001$). Similarly, a significantly higher percentage of the patients from the reoperation for bleeding group had been in the ICU at the time of transplantation compared to the control group (23.2% versus 12.9%, $P = 0.005$). The immediate pretransplant hematocrit (26.0 ± 8.0 versus 25.8 ± 8.9, $P = 0.80$) and platelet counts (88.8 versus 79.9, $P = 0.14$) were similar between groups whereas the INR was elevated in the patients from the reoperation for bleeding group compared to the control group (2.1 ± 0.9 versus 1.9 ± 0.9, $P = 0.04$).

The reoperation for bleeding was performed within 1 week in 79/101 (78%) of the patients and after 1 week in the remaining 22/101 (22%). An active bleeding source was identified in 27/101 (27%) patients whereas in the remaining 74/101 (73%) patients the bleeding etiology was diagnosed as coagulopathic bleeding. Identifying an active bleeding source was more common when the reoperation for bleeding was performed within 48 hours after transplant (<48 hr 41% versus >48 hr 12%, $P = 0.002$).

3.2. Donor and Operative Characteristics. There were no differences in donor age, donor race, donor cause of death, or donor height between groups. The only difference between groups was a significantly higher percentage of organ grafts from regional donor in the reoperation for bleeding versus control group (31.0% versus 18.8%, $P = 0.0025$). Despite the difference in utilization of regional donors, there was no significant difference in the donor risk index (DRI) between

TABLE 1: Baseline demographics.

Variable	Reoperation for bleeding	Control group	P value
Group	$n = 101$	$n = 827$	
Age (years)	51.7 ± 11.9	53.5 ± 9.7	0.16
Male (%)	54.5	63.4	0.08
Race			
Caucasian %	81.2	85.9	0.43
African-American %	14.9	10.8	
BMI	29.6 ± 6.3	29.0 ± 6.4	0.43
Etiology of liver disease (%)			
Hepatitis C	44.6	36.4	0.11
NASH/cryptogenic	15.8	20.6	0.26
Laennec's	9.0	12.7	0.28
Cholestatic (PBC, PSC)	9.9	11.9	0.55
Other[a]	8.9	9.0	0.98
MELD Score	23.8 ± 8.1	20.4 ± 7.9	<0.001
ICU prior to liver transplant (%)	23.2	12.9	0.005
Comorbidities			
Dyslipidemia	12.9	13.6	0.85
Diabetes	21.8	26.3	0.33
CAD	5.0	3.5	0.47
CRI	10.9	7.5	0.24
Hypertension	51.5	47.3	0.42
Baseline lab values			
Platelet count ($\times 10^9$/L)	88.8	79.9	0.14
Hematocrit	26.0 ± 8.0	25.8 ± 8.9	0.80
INR	2.1 ± 0.9	1.9 ± 0.9	0.04
Split liver transplant (%)	1.0	0.25	0.30

Data presented as percent or mean ± standard deviation.
[a]Other diagnoses include autoimmune hepatitis, alpha 1 antitrypsin deficiency, hemochromatosis, fulminant liver failure, Budd-Chiari syndrome, Wilson's disease, polycystic liver disease, nonhepatocellular carcinoma neoplastic disease, sarcoidosis, secondary biliary cirrhosis, Caroli's disease, and cystinosis.
NASH: nonalcoholic steatohepatitis; PBC: primary biliary cirrhosis; PSC: primary sclerosing cholangitis; MELD: Model for End-Stage Liver Disease; BMI: body mass index; CAD: coronary artery disease; CRI: chronic renal insufficiency; INR: International normalized ratio.

reoperations for bleeding versus control group (1.6 ± 0.4 versus 1.5 ± 0.4, $P = 0.61$).

There were no differences in operation length, cold ischemia time, or warm ischemia time between groups (Table 2). The number of units of platelets transfused intraoperatively was significantly lower in the reoperation for bleeding group compared to the control group (1.1 ± 1.4 versus 1.9 ± 3.7, $P < 0.001$). There were no statistical differences in units of red blood cells transfused between groups when analyzing as a continuous variable (4.3 ± 4.2 versus 3.7 ± 3.5, $P = 0.19$). Because mass red blood cell transfusion has been indicated as a risk factor for reoperation in previous studies [12, 16–20], we further analyzed red blood cells transfusion by categorizing units of red blood cells

TABLE 2: Characteristics of the liver transplant operation.

Variable	Reoperation for bleeding	Control group	P value
Operation length (min)	269.8 ± 119.6	278.2 ± 104.9	0.50
Cold ischemia time (min)	405.5 ± 166.9	390.8 ± 174.4	0.41
Warm ischemia time (min)	49.3 ± 45.7	47.9 ± 18.4	0.46
Transfusion[a]			
Red blood cells (units)	4.3 ± 4.2	3.7 ± 3.5	0.19
Fresh frozen plasma (units)	1.8 ± 2.6	1.5 ± 1.8	0.19
Platelets (units)	1.1 ± 1.4	1.9 ± 3.7	<0.001
Cryo administered (%)	4.49	1.33	0.05
Last fibrinogen level	151.8 ± 107.4	124.6 ± 49.6	0.22
Estrogen administered (%)	26.97	35.37	0.11
Amicar administered (%)	20.22	30.19	0.05
Epigastric surgical history (%)	24.8	24.2	0.91
Vascular reconstruction[b] (%)	1.0	4.4	0.17
Retransplant (%)	5.0	4.3	0.80

Data presented as percent or mean ± standard deviation.
[a]Blood products transfused only during the liver transplant operation do not include data on reoperation for bleeding.
[b]Includes both arterial conduits and mesenteric venous bypass grafts.

transfused into quartiles and comparing these groups but again demonstrated no association with reoperation ($P = 0.31$). Similarly, there were no differences in units of fresh frozen plasma transfused between groups when analyzing as a continuous variable (1.8 ± 2.6 versus 1.5 ± 1.8, $P = 0.19$) or as a quartile categorical variable ($P = 0.28$). Cryoprecipitate was used infrequently but statistically more often in the reoperation for bleeding group compared to the control group (4.5% versus 1.3%, $P = 0.05$). There was a trend toward less estrogen usage in the reoperation for bleeding group, although this did not reach statistical significance (27.0% versus 35.4%, $P = 0.11$). Aminocaproic acid was administered less often in the reoperation for bleeding group compared to the control group (20.2% versus 30.2%, $P = 0.05$). The frequency of epigastric surgical history, venous or arterial reconstruction, and retransplant rates was similar in both groups (Table 2).

The platelet count immediately following liver transplantation was not statistically different between groups (77.98 ± 33.21 versus 80.74 ± 41.33, $P = 0.63$). The platelet count was significantly lower in the reoperation for bleeding group by 24 hours (72.69 ± 30.52 versus 83.76 ± 45.59, $P = 0.01$) and by 96 hours (52.85 ± 24.30 versus 65.83 ± 44.65, $P = 0.001$) following liver transplantation. There were no differences in INR immediately postoperatively or at 24 or 48 hours. The median time to INR <2 was 2 days in both groups.

3.3. Analysis of Factors Associated with Reoperation for Bleeding (Table 3). A univariate and multivariable analysis of factors associated with reoperation for bleeding following liver transplant was performed. On univariate analysis, the following variables were associated with reoperation for bleeding following liver transplant: lab-MELD score (OR

1.05/point, 95% CI 1.03, 1.08, $P < 0.0001$), ICU immediately prior to transplant (OR 2.05, 95% CI 1.23, 3.15, $P = 0.0057$), platelets transfused during transplantation (OR 0.87/unit, 95% CI 0.76, 0.99, $P = 0.0373$), and utilization of aminocaproic acid (OR 0.59, 95% CI 0.34, 0.99, $P = 0.05$). A multivariable model was fitted to determine the association with reoperation for bleeding (Table 3). All variables statistically significant on the univariate analysis as well as the following clinically important variables were entered into the model: surgeon, recipient history of epigastric surgery, donor risk index, warm ischemia time, duration of the operation, units pRBC transfused, and units FFP transfused. Recipient lab-MELD score (OR 1.06/MELD unit, 95% CI 1.03–1.09, $P < 0.0001$), number of platelets transfused (OR 0.73/platelet unit, 95% CI 0.58–0.91, $P = 0.004$), and utilization of aminocaproic acid (OR 0.46, 95% CI 0.27, 0.80, $P = 0.006$) were statistically associated with reoperation for bleeding following liver transplant. Figure 1(a) illustrates the risk of reoperation as a function of platelets transfused including the mean number of platelets before transplant, immediately after transplant, and 24 hours after transplant. Figure 1(b) illustrates the risk of reoperation for bleeding as a function of lab-MELD score quartiles.

3.4. Outcome Characteristics (Figure 2). The risk of death was increased in liver transplant recipients who underwent reoperation for bleeding versus those that did not (HR 1.89, 95% CI 1.26–2.85). The survival curves continue to separate until about 9 months postoperatively, at which time the difference in survival becomes relatively constant. Death prior to discharge was observed in 4.95% of the patients reoperated for bleeding versus 2.54% of the control group ($P = 0.17$). There was significantly higher mortality rates within 12 months of transplantation observed in the reoperation for bleeding group (15.84% versus 7.78%, $P = 0.007$). The causes of death in each group are presented in Table 4.

There were no differences in 1-, 3-, or 5-year survival based upon platelet transfusion (no platelets transfused, $n = 301$: 93%, 87%, 81% versus 1 or more units of platelets transfused, $n = 627$: 90%, 84%, 78%, $P = 0.26$). Liver transplant patients who underwent reoperation for bleeding had a longer total ICU stay (5 days ± 7 versus 2 days ± 3, $P < 0.001$) and hospitalization (18 days ± 9 versus 10 days ± 18, $P < 0.001$) (data expressed as median ± interquartile range). There were no statistical differences in the number of readmissions between the reoperations for bleeding and control group.

4. Discussion

There is need for more clinical studies to guide intraoperative management of coagulopathy during liver transplantation [2, 10, 11]. Approaches vary from preventive practices that involve decision-making based on laboratory values and some type of "recipe" for product administration associated with each unit of blood transfused, to the other extreme of not even addressing the coagulopathy until the new liver is reperfused. Even when there is a clear-cut coagulopathy present, it is often not obvious what to administer to

TABLE 3: Univariate and multivariable analysis of factors associated with reoperation for bleeding following liver transplantation.

Variable	Univariate analysis			Multivariable analysis		
	Odds ratio	95% CI	P value	Odds ratio	95% CI	P value
Lab-MELD	1.05	1.03, 1.08	<0.0001	1.06	1.03, 1.09	<0.0001
Surgical history	0.93	0.42, 2.10	0.87			
ICU Pre-LTx	2.05	1.23, 3.15	0.006			
WIT (Min)	1.00	0.99, 1.01	0.48			
OR length	0.99	0.98, 1.00	0.13			
DRI	0.85	0.48, 1.52	0.58			
pRBC	1.04	0.99, 1.10	0.13			
FFP	1.09	0.99, 1.20	0.08			
PLT	0.87	0.76, 0.99	0.04	0.73	0.58, 0.91	0.004
Estrogen	0.67	0.41, 1.10	0.12			
Aminocaproic acid	0.59	0.34, 0.99	0.05	0.46	0.27, 0.80	0.006

MELD: Model for End-Stage Liver Disease; ICU: intensive care unit; LTx: liver transplantation; WIT: warm ischemia time; OR: operating room; DRI: donor risk index; pRBC: packed red blood cells; FFP: fresh frozen plasma; PLT: platelet; LTx: liver transplantation.

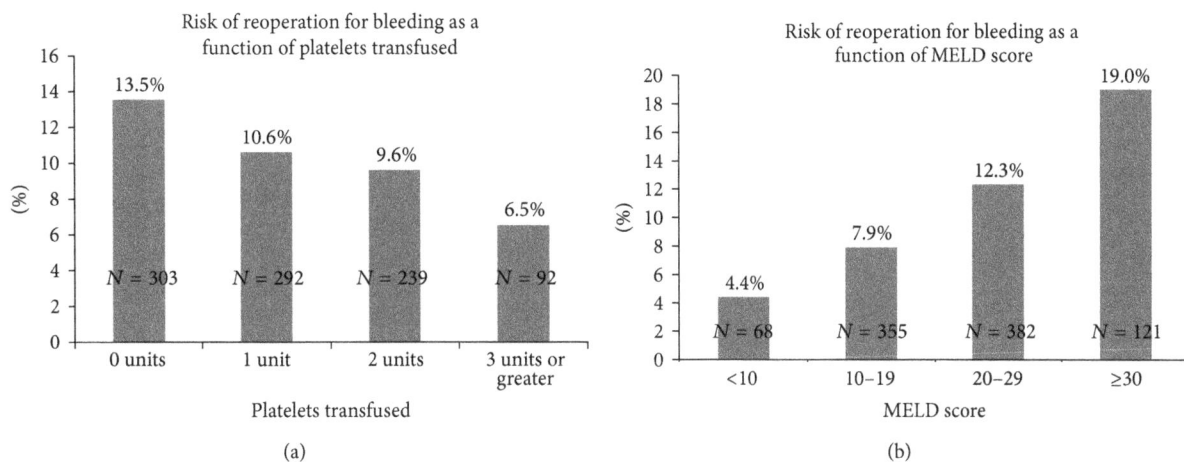

FIGURE 1: (a) Risk of reoperation as a function of platelets transfused. The risk of reoperation was highest in the group of liver transplant recipients that did not receive platelet transfusion during the transplant operation (13.7% risk estimate). Conversely, the lowest risk of reoperation for bleeding was observed in the group of patients that received the highest number of platelets transfused (5.9% risk estimate). (b) Risk of reoperation for bleeding as a function of lab-MELD score. There was a stepwise increase in the risk of reoperation for bleeding as recipient lab-MELD score increased. The lowest risk estimate was for a lab-MELD ≤10 (5.4% estimate) whereas the highest risk estimate was for a lab-MELD >30 (19.4% estimate).

ameliorate nonsurgical bleeding. Is it the best approach to treat an INR and platelet count or base decisions on a functional TEG assay? What threshold values should be treated? The holy grail of liver transplant coagulopathy is what to administer, when, and how much? A brief discussion with a group of transplant anesthesiologists/surgeons will quickly reveal the disparity in coagulopathy approaches with a lot of "based upon my training" or "in my experience" anecdotes, variability well described in the literature [10].

The goal of treating coagulopathy is preventing bleeding, especially postoperative bleeding requiring a second laparotomy. Reoperation is a (negative) quality measure tracked and reported by UNOS that is associated with significantly increased resource utilization [14, 15]. Previous studies examining risk factors for reoperation for bleeding following liver transplant essentially report that difficult liver transplant

operations associated with high blood product transfusion rates are associated with increased rates of reoperation [12, 13, 20]. This study, to the best of our knowledge, is the first to demonstrate a stepwise association between rising lab-MELD score and likelihood of reoperation for bleeding (Figure 1(b)). The odds of a reoperation for bleeding increased 1.06 per MELD point. The univariate analysis also suggested an association between ICU status and risk of reoperation for bleeding as well as regional donors and reoperation for bleeding. These associations, however, were not significant on multivariable analysis, probably because these variables are correlated with recipient high lab-MELD scores. The association of high lab-MELD score with reoperation for bleeding may be used to help to risk-stratify coagulopathy approaches prior to the transplant operation. For example, a more aggressive approach to perioperative coagulopathy

TABLE 4: Cause of death.

Variable	Reoperation for bleeding	Control group
Number of deaths	28 (27.7%)	137 (16.5%)
Cause of death[a]		
Infection	35.7%	25.6%
Cancer	3.6%	19.0%
Cardiac disease	3.6%	10.2%
Recurrent HCV	21.4%	9.5%
Other[b]	35.7%	35.8%
Death prior to discharge	4.95%	2.54%
Death within 12 months of LTx	15.84%	7.78%

[a] Proportions for cause of death are calculated on the subset of 165 individuals (137 with no hemorrhage, 28 with hemorrhage) that died within 60 months of transplant. All other proportions are based on total sample size.
[b] Other causes of death include chronic rejection, cerebrovascular accident, gastrointestinal bleeding, chronic renal failure, graft versus host disease, suicide, and recurrent Budd-Chiari syndrome.
HCV: hepatitis c virus; LTx: liver transplantation.

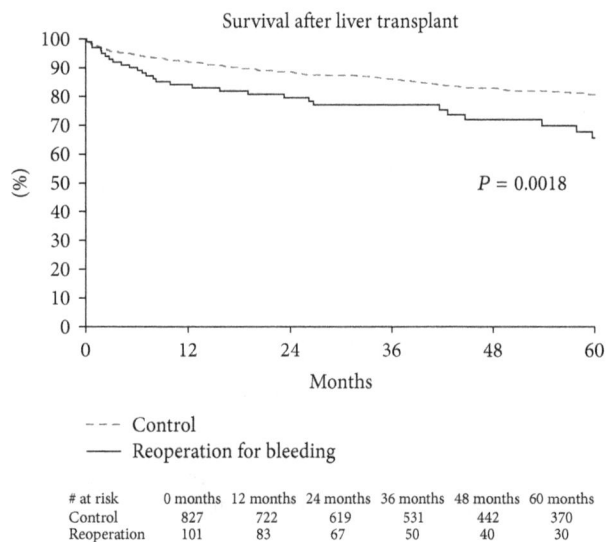

# at risk	0 months	12 months	24 months	36 months	48 months	60 months
Control	827	722	619	531	442	370
Reoperation	101	83	67	50	40	30

FIGURE 2: Survival after liver transplant stratified by reoperation for bleeding. Decreased survival was observed in the group of liver transplant recipients that underwent reoperation for bleeding ($P = 0.0018$).

management may be indicated including the prophylactic use of antifibrinolytics [24] and lower thresholds to administer blood products and concentrated factors [25].

Perhaps the most interesting finding of this study is that intraoperative platelet administration was associated with a significantly lower likelihood of reoperation for bleeding following liver transplantation. For each unit of platelets transfused, the odds of reoperation for bleeding decreased by 0.73. Figure 1(a) demonstrates that the highest risk of reoperation for bleeding was observed in the group that received no platelet transfusion, a liver transplant group that may have been predicted to be uncomplicated operations as

evidenced by the lack of perceived need for platelet transfusion. However, this group was associated with the highest rates of reoperation for bleeding. Conversely, those patients that received more than 1 unit of platelets may have been subjected to operations in which the surgeon was struggling to "dry up the field." Somewhat, surprisingly, there was no statistical association between plasma administration and decreased reoperation for bleeding, similar to that reported by Massicotte and the Montreal Liver Transplant group [26]. This observation is also similar to findings by Giannini et al. who reported that invasive procedure-related bleeding in cirrhotics listed for liver transplant was only observed in patients with severe thrombocytopenia, whereas significant coagulopathy was not associated [27].

Nonutilization of aminocaproic acid also was an independent risk factor predicting reoperation for bleeding. The decision to not administer antifibrinolytics can best be described as a practice variable amongst surgeons and anesthesiologists which is supported by reports associating thromboembolic events with antifibrinolytic administration [28]. However, the use of antifibrinolytics is generally considered safe and supported by multiple studies showing prophylactic or therapeutic administration decreases bleeding and reduces blood product administration [29–33]. Here we expand on these studies by demonstrating an association between decreased reoperation for bleeding and aminocaproic acid administration as a new finding.

Administration of blood products is not a benign intervention, however. There are reports that platelet transfusions are associated with decreased survival following liver transplantation [34, 35]. The Netherlands liver transplant group reported a higher hazard of death in transplant recipients that received platelets (HR 1.37/unit of platelets) compared to those patients that did not receive any platelets [35]. Our data did not demonstrate a similar relationship between platelet administration and mortality. In contrast, this study demonstrates that reoperation is the main factor associated with increased mortality after liver transplant. The increased hazard of death was 1.89 in liver transplant recipients who underwent reoperation for bleeding. These sets of data suggest that interventions that may decrease reoperations for bleeding may decrease posttransplant mortality, even if these interventions involve administering blood products. Another interesting finding is that the risk of death in patients that underwent reoperation for bleeding persisted for 1 year after transplant. Deaths due to infection and recurrent hepatitis C were numerically higher in the reoperation for bleeding group compared to the control group.

This study is limited by the fact that it is a single center study consisting of the results of a dedicated 4-member liver transplant anesthesia team and only 4 transplant surgeons. The results are influenced by the internal practice patterns by the liver transplant anesthesia and surgical team, which may limit generalizability. For example, the beneficial effect of platelets or aminocaproic acid may not be as important in programs with a more liberal approach to managing intraoperative coagulopathy. Finally, this study does not identify threshold values for platelet administration and the data do not suggest optimal timing of platelet administration.

In conclusion, this study demonstrates that reoperation for bleeding following liver transplantation is associated with significant resource utilization and increased postoperative mortality. The only modifiable risk factors associated with decreased risk of reoperation for bleeding were intraoperative platelet administration and aminocaproic acid utilization. Our data suggests that adequate platelet administration and use of antifibrinolytics may be key interventions in the management of liver transplant associated coagulopathy, especially in recipients with a high lab-MELD score. Utilization of this knowledge may be helpful for liver transplant anesthesia protocols designed to minimizing the incidence and impact of reoperation for bleeding following liver transplantation.

Acknowledgments

This research was funded by National Institute of Health, Grants nos. T35 HL007473 (Thompson and Gleuckert) and 1 K23 DK091514-01A1 (DuBay). The data from this paper was presented at the 2014 AHPBA Conference.

References

[1] Y. Ozier and M.-Y. Tsou, "Changing trends in transfusion practice in liver transplantation," *Current Opinion in Organ Transplantation*, vol. 13, no. 3, pp. 304–309, 2008.

[2] A. Walia and R. Schumann, "The evolution of liver transplantation practices," *Current Opinion in Organ Transplantation*, vol. 13, no. 3, pp. 275–279, 2008.

[3] Z. G. Hevesi, S. Y. Lapukhin, J. D. Mezrich, A.-C. Andrel, and M. Lee, "Designated liver transplant anesthesia team reduces blood transfusion, need for mechanical ventilation, and duration of intensive care," *Liver Transplantation*, vol. 15, no. 5, pp. 460–465, 2009.

[4] A. Walia, M. S. Mandell, N. Mercaldo et al., "Anesthesia for liver transplantation in US academic centers: institutional structure and perioperative care," *Liver Transplantation*, vol. 18, no. 6, pp. 737–743, 2012.

[5] R. Moreno and M. Berenguer, "Post-liver transplantation medical complications," *Annals of Hepatology*, vol. 5, no. 2, pp. 77–85, 2006.

[6] A. Rana, H. Petrowsky, J. C. Hong et al., "Blood transfusion requirement during liver transplantation is an important risk factor for mortality," *Journal of the American College of Surgeons*, vol. 216, no. 5, pp. 902–907, 2013.

[7] I. F. S. F. Boin, M. I. Leonardi, A. C. M. Luzo, A. R. Cardoso, C. A. Caruy, and L. S. Leonardi, "Intraoperative massive transfusion decreases survival after liver transplantation," *Transplantation Proceedings*, vol. 40, no. 3, pp. 789–791, 2008.

[8] E. Mor, L. Jennings, T. A. Gonwa et al., "The impact of operative bleeding on outcome in transplantation of the liver," *Surgery Gynecology and Obstetrics*, vol. 176, no. 3, pp. 219–227, 1993.

[9] M. E. Gamil, J. Pirenne, H. van Malenstein et al., "Risk factors for bleeding and clinical implications in patients undergoing liver transplantation," *Transplantation Proceedings*, vol. 44, no. 9, pp. 2857–2860, 2012.

[10] Y. Ozier, F. Pessione, E. Samain et al., "Institutional variability in transfusion practice for liver transplantation," *Anesthesia and Analgesia*, vol. 97, no. 3, pp. 671–679, 2003.

[11] R. Schumann, "Intraoperative resource utilization in anesthesia for liver transplantation in the united states: a survey," *Anesthesia and Analgesia*, vol. 97, no. 1, pp. 21–28, 2003.

[12] H. G. D. Hendriks, J. van der Meer, J. T. M. de Wolf et al., "Intraoperative blood transfusion requirement is the main determinant of early surgical re-intervention after orthotopic liver transplantation," *Transplant International*, vol. 17, no. 11, pp. 673–679, 2005.

[13] T. B. Liang, X. L. Bai, D. L. Li, J. J. Li, and S. S. Zheng, "Early postoperative hemorrhage requiring urgent surgical reintervention after orthotopic liver transplantation," *Transplantation Proceedings*, vol. 39, no. 5, pp. 1549–1553, 2007.

[14] D. Azoulay, D. Samuel, R. Adam et al., "Paul Brousse liver transplantation: the first 1,500 cases," *Clinical Transplants*, pp. 273–280, 2000.

[15] R. S. Brown Jr., N. L. Ascher, J. R. Lake et al., "The impact of surgical complications after liver transplantation on resource utilization," *Archives of Surgery*, vol. 132, no. 10, pp. 1098–1103, 1997.

[16] A. Rana, M. A. Hardy, K. J. Halazun et al., "Survival Outcomes Following Liver Transplantation (SOFT) score: a novel method to predict patient survival following liver transplantation," *American Journal of Transplantation*, vol. 8, no. 12, pp. 2537–2546, 2008.

[17] R. Wiesner, E. Edwards, R. Freeman et al., "Model for end-stage liver disease (MELD) and allocation of donor livers," *Gastroenterology*, vol. 124, no. 1, pp. 91–96, 2003.

[18] S. F. Kappa, D. L. Gorden, M. A. Davidson, J. K. Wright, and O. D. Guillamondegui, "Intraoperative blood loss predicts hemorrhage-related reoperation after orthotopic liver transplantation," *American Surgeon*, vol. 76, no. 9, pp. 969–973, 2010.

[19] A. Koffron and J. A. Stein, "Liver transplantation: indications, pretransplant evaluation, surgery, and posttransplant complications," *The Medical Clinics of North America*, vol. 92, no. 4, pp. 861–888, 2008.

[20] C. Park, M. Huh, R. H. Steadman et al., "Extended criteria donor and severe intraoperative glucose variability: association with reoperation for hemorrhage in liver transplantation," *Transplantation Proceedings*, vol. 42, no. 5, pp. 1738–1743, 2010.

[21] S. Feng, N. P. Goodrich, J. L. Bragg-Gresham et al., "Characteristics associated with liver graft failure: the concept of a donor risk index," *The American Journal of Transplantation*, vol. 6, no. 4, pp. 783–790, 2006.

[22] L. Frenette, J. Cox, P. McArdle, D. Eckhoff, and S. Bynon, "Conjugated estrogen reduces transfusion and coagulation factor requirements in orthotopic liver transplantation," *Anesthesia and Analgesia*, vol. 86, no. 6, pp. 1183–1186, 1998.

[23] M. Livio, P. M. Mannucci, G. Vigano et al., "Conjugated estrogens for the management of bleeding associated with renal failure," *The New England Journal of Medicine*, vol. 315, no. 12, pp. 731–735, 1986.

[24] I. Q. Molenaar, N. Warnaar, H. Groen, E. M. TenVergert, M. J. H. Slooff, and R. J. Porte, "Efficacy and safety of antifibrinolytic drugs in liver transplantation: a systematic review and meta-analysis," *American Journal of Transplantation*, vol. 7, no. 1, pp. 185–194, 2007.

[25] C. U. Niemann, M. Behrends, D. Quan et al., "Recombinant factor VIIa reduces transfusion requirements in liver transplant patients with high MELD scores," *Transfusion Medicine*, vol. 16, no. 2, pp. 93–100, 2006.

[26] L. Massicotte, D. Beaulieu, L. Thibeault et al., "Coagulation defects do not predict blood product requirements during liver transplantation," *Transplantation*, vol. 85, no. 7, pp. 956–962, 2008.

[27] E. G. Giannini, A. Greco, S. Marenco, E. Andorno, U. Valente, and V. Savarino, "Incidence of bleeding following invasive procedures in patients with thrombocytopenia and advanced liver disease," *Clinical Gastroenterology and Hepatology*, vol. 8, no. 10, pp. 899–902, 2010.

[28] R. J. Porte, "Antifibrinolytics in liver transplantation: they are effective, but what about the risk-benefit ratio?" *Liver Transplantation*, vol. 10, no. 2, pp. 285–288, 2004.

[29] J. F. Boylan, J. R. Klinck, A. N. Sandler et al., "Tranexamic acid reduces blood loss, transfusion requirements, and coagulation factor use in primary orthotopic liver transplantation," *Anesthesiology*, vol. 85, no. 5, pp. 1043–1048, 1996.

[30] R. J. Marcel, W. C. Stegall, C. Tracy Suit et al., "Continuous small-dose aprotinin controls fibrinolysis during orthotopic liver transplantation," *Anesthesia and Analgesia*, vol. 82, no. 6, pp. 1122–1125, 1996.

[31] M. Kaspar, M. A. Ramsay, A.-T. Nguyen, M. Cogswell, G. Hurst, and K. J. Ramsay, "Continuous small-dose tranexamic acid reduces fibrinolysis but not transfusion requirements during orthotopic liver transplantation," *Anesthesia & Analgesia*, vol. 85, no. 2, pp. 281–285, 1997.

[32] A. Dalmau, A. Sabaté, M. Koo et al., "The prophylactic use of tranexamic acid and aprotinin in orthotopic liver transplantation: a comparative study," *Liver Transplantation*, vol. 10, no. 2, pp. 279–284, 2004.

[33] A. Dalmau, A. Sabaté, F. Acosta et al., "Tranexamic acid reduces red cell transfusion better than ε-aminocaproic acid or placebo in liver transplantation," *Anesthesia and Analgesia*, vol. 91, no. 1, pp. 29–34, 2000.

[34] I. T. A. Pereboom, M. T. de Boer, E. B. Haagsma, H. G. D. Hendriks, T. Lisman, and R. J. Porte, "Platelet transfusion during liver transplantation is associated with increased postoperative mortality due to acute lung injury," *Anesthesia and Analgesia*, vol. 108, no. 4, pp. 1083–1091, 2009.

[35] M. T. de Boer, M. C. Christensen, M. Asmussen et al., "The impact of intraoperative transfusion of platelets and red blood cells on survival after liver transplantation," *Anesthesia and Analgesia*, vol. 106, no. 1, pp. 32–44, 2008.

16

Selective Interarterial Radiation Therapy (SIRT) in Colorectal Liver Metastases: How Do We Monitor Response?

D. Hipps, F. Ausania, D. M. Manas, J. D. G. Rose, and J. J. French

Hepato-Pancreato-Biliary and Transplant Surgery Unit, Freeman Hospital, Newcastle Upon Tyne NE7 7DN, UK

Correspondence should be addressed to D. Hipps; dhipps@gmail.com

Academic Editor: Hobart W. Harris

Radioembolisation is a way of providing targeted radiotherapy to colorectal liver metastases. Results are encouraging but there is still no standard method of assessing the response to treatment. This paper aims to review the current experience assessing response following radioembolisation. A literature review was undertaken detailing radioembolisation in the treatment of colorectal liver metastases comparing staging methods, criteria, and response. A search was performed of electronic databases from 1980 to November 2011. Information acquired included year published, patient numbers, resection status, chemotherapy regimen, criteria used to stage disease and assess response to radioembolisation, tumour markers, and overall/progression free survival. Nineteen studies were analysed including randomised controlled trials, clinical trials, meta-analyses, and case series. There is no validated modality as the method of choice when assessing response to radioembolisation. CT at 3 months following radioembolisation is the most frequently modality used to assess response to treatment. PET-CT is increasingly being used as it measures functional and radiological aspects. RECIST is the most frequently used criteria. *Conclusion.* A validated modality to assess response to radioembolisation is needed. We suggest PET-CT and CEA pre- and postradioembolisation at 3 months using RECIST 1.1 criteria released in 2009, which includes criteria for PET-CT, cystic changes, and necrosis.

1. Introduction

Selective interarterial radiation therapy (radioembolisation) is a relatively new approach to treating colorectal liver metastases in the UK. It was initially used in Australasia in 1990 [1] and has been licensed for use in Europe since 2002 [2]. Radioembolisation is used not only when conventional treatment has failed but also as first line treatment [3, 4] and it uses microspheres 20–60 microns in diameter [2]. These can be either glass or resin and are embedded with the beta emitting isotope yttrium 90. This has a half-life of 64.1 hours and decays to the stable Zirconium 90 [5].

The spheres are deployed using interventional radiology techniques via a catheter into the hepatic artery. The spheres then become lodged in the microvasculature within the tumour. Due to the small nature of the spheres, they provide interstitial high dose radiotherapy and arterial microembolisation becoming lodged in the arterioles supplying the tumour [6]. In simple transarterial embolization, the antitumour effect is via terminal artery blockade using an embolising agent such as gel foam or polyvinyl alcohol [7]. Radioembolisation as a consequence is a much less embolic procedure targeting its embolic effect further down the arterial tree and closer to the tumour leaving the surrounding liver tissue relatively intact. Experimental trials have shown that that particles of 40 microns or less have a 6–12-fold increase in chance of becoming lodged in the tumour vasculature [7] as opposed to the large particles sizes used in bland tran-sarterial embolisation.

The spheres emit high dose beta radiation to a limited area involving the tumour for an extended period of time when compared with conventional radiotherapy. The maximum penetration depth is 11 mm and the average penetration is 2.5 mm. The half-life is 64.1 hours which means that at 11 days, 94% of the isotope has decayed to infinity leaving only background radiation of no therapeutic value [2]. The consequence of these properties is that the surrounding liver tissue vascular supply and integrity remains relatively intact. The targeted approach of radioembolisation therapy is dependent on the fact that liver malignancies derive the majority of their blood supply from the hepatic artery [8]. As a result, the spheres are carried preferentially to the tumour site where they deliver the radiotherapy dose. With reference to tumour vascularity using both CT and angiography it was found that there was no statistical difference in median survival for both hypervascular and hypovascular tumours when using radioembolisation as a treatment modality, thus, both tumours are amenable to treatment [9].

The median survival for nonsurgically treated colorectal metastasis ranges from 5.7 to 19 months [10, 11]. In patients receiving no treatment, average survival is just 7.4 months [10], whilst meta-analysis of radioembolisation therapy have reported an improved survival rate of 10.8–29.4 months [4]. A randomised trial comparing radioembolisation plus chemotherapy versus chemotherapy (Fluorouracil/Leucovorin) alone showed that survival in the chemotherapy only arm was shorter (12.8 months) than the radioembolisation plus chemotherapy arm (29.4 months) [12]. A recent meta-analysis of radioembolisation as a treatment option for colorectal cancer liver metastasis showed a high "any response rate" of approximately 80% using CT response assessment for patients who had progressed on from first line conventional therapy. Furthermore, a greater than 90% response rate has been observed when radioembolisation has been used as first line therapy, as neoadjuvant to chemotherapy [4]. Potentially curative hepatic resection following downstaging/sizing by radioembolisation has been described but has only been possible in a minority of colorectal metastases cases. In the studies reviewed, hepatic resection was possible in 4 patients and has also been recorded in two separate case reports [13–15]. Radiologic complete response is rare. The highest complete response rate was 11% as judged per CT and 58% using PET. Response rate in this paper was measured using the studies' own criteria [16]. Assessing response to delivered therapies (including radioembolisation) is a crucial part of the treatment algorithm. With reference to radioembolisation, at present, a number of modalities are currently used and various criteria within these modalities are described. There appears to be no well validated standard process to recommend.

Current NICE (National Institute for Clinical Excellence) guidelines support the use of radioembolisation with systemic chemotherapy using Fluorouracil and Leucovorin for treatment of patients with hepatic metastases secondary to colorectal cancer which are not suitable for resection or ablation [17]. The Radioembolisation Brachytherapy Oncology Consortium (REBOC) recommends that candidates for radioembolisation are patients with unresectable primary to metastatic hepatic disease with liver-dominant tumour burden and a life expectancy greater than 3 months [18]. They recommend the use of radioembolisation therapy alone after failure of first line chemotherapy with Floxuridine during first line therapy or during first or second line chemotherapy as part of a clinical trial.

The aim of this paper is to review the methods used to assess response following radioembolisation in patients with colorectal liver metastases in an attempt to aid the clinician in selecting the most appropriate follow-up method.

2. Methods

A search of electronic databases was performed, Medline (PubMed), the Cochrane Library, Embase, and the Latin American and Caribbean Literature on Health Sciences (LILACS) from 1980 and to November 2011. Search terms based on the MeSH keywords were used, Liver Neoplasms, Colorectal Neoplasms, Neoplasm Metastasis, Yttrium Radioisotopes, Radioembolisation, Radioembolization, and SIRT.

To avoid publication bias both published and unpublished trials were identified through a computer-based search of the PubMed database. The set included randomized clinical trials, clinical trials, meta-analyses, and case series. Case reports were excluded. Papers were restricted to English language.

The search was also guided by examination of original and review article reference lists. Abstracts were not included in the analysis. Previous author's publications on the topic were excluded and only the most recent work was included.

The following information was acquired from each report: year of publication, number of patients, gender, resection status, chemotherapy regimen, modality, and criteria used to stage disease and assess response to radioembolisation, tumour markers, and overall/progression free survival.

All studies where radiological response was reported were included; although different criteria were encountered. Different study criteria for assessing tumour response available are RECIST [19], WHO [19], and EASL [20]; these are listed in Table 1. Where studies have used their own response criteria; these have been listed in Table 2.

3. Results

Nineteen studies evaluated the radiological/tumour marker response to radioembolisation and were used in this analysis. The studies included two randomized clinical trials, fifteen clinical trials, and three case series. Patient numbers varied from small case series up to 208 patients in the paper by Kennedy et al. [24]. All of the papers reviewed used CT as a staging method; 5 papers also used PET scan in addition to CT. Three papers were discarded as more recent studies by the same author were available [1, 12, 25]. Papers that did not distinguish outcome for colorectal metastases and other liver malignancies were excluded [26, 27]. Papers which did not list radiological response were also excluded [28].

The range of patient numbers in each study showed large variability (7–208). The total number of patients was 875. Patients evaluated in the studies had typically failed other treatment lines and were deemed to have advanced metastatic tumours not suitable for resection or ablation. Inclusion of patients with extra hepatic disease was variable; however, some studies did opt to include patients with extra hepatic disease [5, 22, 29]. Radioembolisation was also used in treatment naive patients [3]. The most common use was in conjunction with chemotherapy both systemic and local via the hepatic artery. Typical regimes used in early studies were Floxuridine, Fluorouracil, and Leucovorin. In later trials,

TABLE 1: Response evaluation criteria in solid tumours (RECIST) [19], world health organisation (WHO) [19], and european association for study of the Liver (EASL) [20].

	RECIST change in sum of the longest diameters	WHO change in sum of products	EASL
Complete response (CR)	Disappearance of all target lesions at 4 weeks	Disappearance of all target lesions at 4 weeks	100% necrosis of target lesions and no new lesions
Partial response (PR)	30% decrease in the Longest Diameter (LD) of target lesions at 4 weeks	50% decrease confirmed at 4 weeks	50–99% increase in necrosis
Stable disease (SD)	Neither sufficient shrinkage to qualify for PR nor sufficient increase to qualify for PD	Neither sufficient shrinkage to qualify for PR nor sufficient increase to qualify for PD	<50% increase in necrosis
Progressive disease (PD)	At least a 20% increase in the LD of target lesions; no CR, PR, or SD documented before increase	25% increase; no CR, PR, or SD documented before increase	≥25% increase in ≥1 lesion or ≥1 new lesion

CR: complete response, PR: partial response, SD: stable disease, PD: progressive disease.

TABLE 2: Individual study response criteria.

Study	Complete response %	Partial response %	Stable disease %
Anderson et al. 1992 [21]	Not measured	Not measured	Up to 25% increase or decrease in the sum of largest perpendicular diameters
Stubbs et al. 2006 [22]	Response defined as definite reduction in size of index lesions no enlarging or new lesions		No definite increase or decrease of lesion no new lesions
Boppudi et al. 2006 [23]	Not measured	Not measured	Less than a 10% change in sum of products of perpendicular diameters

radioembolisation was also used in the salvage setting where oxaliplatin and irinotecan had failed [15, 24].

In 10 of the 19 studies, CT was carried out at 3 months following radioembolisation. In the remaining studies it ranged from 1.5 to 6 months. RECIST (response evaluation criteria in solid tumours) criteria were used in 11/19 studies, WHO in 6/19, and local criteria in 3/19. Complete response rate ranged from 0 to 58% and a complete response rate was often not seen. Complete resolution on CT was rare; however, complete resolution was more common when assessed with PET scan 58% [16], whilst partial response varied from 0 to 90%. Stable disease was observed in 5–86% of the cases. Median survival from therapy ranged from 4.5 to 17 months.

When radioembolisation was used in treatment naive patients, 50% were partial responders compared with 28% of those patients who previously had been treated with 5FU [3]. There were however only four treatment naive patients included in the Lim et al. study [3].

A survival advantage was seen in patients who had a radiological and tumour marker response, compared to those patients that did not respond [22]. In a RCT reported by Gray et al. patients had an improved 1, 2, 3, and 5 year survival when compared with the chemotherapy only arm [30]. More recent studies used radioembolisation in the salvage setting when chemotherapy including oxaliplatin and irinotecan had failed [15, 24]. There was a significant difference in survival between responders (CR + PR + SD) and nonresponders determined by RECIST. Median survival was 16 versus 8 months, $P = 0.0006$, and survival in the responder group was 79.2% at 1 year compared with just 20.2%. At 2 years no nonresponders were alive, compared to 40.3% of the responding group. A median survival advantage was also seen in those patients who at the time of entering trials did not have extrahepatic disease (17 months versus 6.7 [31] and 37.8 months versus 13.4 [32]). Survival advantage was also seen more in patients which had previously responded to cetuximab and bevacizumab than in nonresponders [31]. Other factors noted in one paper which enrolled 133 patients to show a survival advantage were male patients (11 months versus 8 months), fewer chemotherapy cycles, and colonic site of primary versus rectal [33].

Radiological response to radioembolisation is described in Table 3.

Only 12 studies reported serum CEA levels (Table 4). These showed that there was generally a response in reduction of CEA levels (57–100%) following radioembolisation. Those who had a decrease in CEA also showed a survival advantage over those who did not, 19.1 months versus 9.3 months in one trial [31].

4. Discussion

The most common modality to assess response to radioembolisation was a CT scan performed at 3 months after treatment. Initial studies used the WHO staging criteria but since the publication of RECIST in 2000, more recent papers used these criteria to assess response. Response rates varied across the studies and also depended on the criteria used to judge response. Boppudi et al. showed a partial response rate of 14.8% when using the WHO definition but when the study's own criteria were applied the response rate was shown to increase to 76% [23]. This study's own response criteria

TABLE 3: Radiological response.

Study	Number of patients	Extra hepatic disease allowed	Chemotherapy treatment	Radiologic staging method	Time to restaging CT (months)	Time to restaging PET (months)	Staging criteria	Complete response %	Partial response %	Stable disease %	Curative treatment %	Median survival (months)	Median survival From radioembolisation (months)
Anderson et al. [21]	7	No	Pretreatment >1 month since last course	CT	2	NA	OWN	0	0	86	NR	NR	11
Andrews et al. [34]	17	No	Pretreatment with 5FU or HAC FUDR	CT	4	NA	WHO	0	29	29	NR	NR	13.8
Gray et al. [30]	36	No	Concurrent HAC FUDR Nonprotocol also received	CT	3*	NA	WHO	6	44	28	NR	NR	17.0
Wong et al. [16]	8	Yes	Pretreatment with 5FU, LV, and Irinotecan	CT PET	3	3	WHO	CT 11 PET 58	CT 16 PET 37	CT 16 PET 5	NR	NR	NR
Lim et al. [3]	32	Yes#	Concurrent 5FU	CT	2	NA	RECIST	0	31	28	NR	NR	NR
Murthy et al. [29]	9	Yes	Variable pretreatment regimes	CT MR PET	NR	NR	RECIST	0	0	56	NR	24.6	4.5
Lewandowski et al. [35]	27	No	Pretreatment with capecitabine, 5FU, LV, irinotecan, or oxaliplatin	CT PET	3	3	WHO	0	CT 35 PET 83	CT 52	NR	NR	9.3
Mancini et al. [36]	35	NR	Pretreatment based on oxaliplatinor irinotecan	CT	1.5	NA	RECIST	0	12.5	75	NR	NR	NR
Kennedy et al. [24]	208	Yes#	Pretreatment based on oxaliplatinor irinotecan	CT PET	3	3	WHO	0	35	55	NR	NR	10.5
Stubbs et al. [22]	100	Yes	Concurrent HAC 5FU	CT	3	NA	OWN	1	73	20	NR	16.2	11
Boppudi et al. [23]	54	No+	Concurrent HAC 5FU	CT	3	NA	OWN WHO	9.3 1.9	76 14.8	NR	NR	NR	14.1
Jakobs et al. [37]	18	No+	NR	CT	2–4	NA	RECIST	0	76% any response	NR	NR	NR	NR
Sharma et al. [5]	20	Yes	Concurrent Folfox4	CT	3	NA	RECIST	0	90	10	10% (resection)	NR	9.3
van Hazel et al. [38]	23	Yes#	Concurrent Irinotecan	CT	3	NA	RECIST	0	48	39	13	12.2	NR
Hoffmann et al. [6]	21	No	Variable pretreatment regimes	CT	3	NA	RECIST	0	NR	NR	5% (RFA)	NR	NR
Cosimelli et al. [15]	50	Yes*	Pretreatment based on oxaliplatinor irinotecan	CT	1.5	NA	RECIST	2	22	24	4% (resection)	NM	12.6
Chua et al. [33]	140	Yes○	NR	CT	6	NA	RECIST	1	31	31	NR	9	NR

TABLE 3: Continued.

Study	Number of patients	Extra hepatic disease allowed	Chemotherapy treatment[†]	Radiologic staging method	Time to restaging CT (months)	Time to restaging PET (months)	Staging criteria	Complete response %	Partial response %	Stable disease %	Curative treatment %	Median survival (months)	Median survival From radioembolisation (months)
Nace et al. [31]	51	Yes[#]	Prior treatment with various regimes	CT PET	3	3	RECIST	0	13	64			10.2
Kosmider et al. [32]	19	Yes[⊗]	FOLFOX or 5FU	CT	2	NA	RECIST	11	74	5	5% disease free at 6 years	29.4	10.4

NA: not applicable, NR: not recorded, HAC: hepatic artery chemotherapy, FUDR: floxuridine, 5FU: 5-fluorouracil, LV: leucovorin, FOLFOX: 5-fluorouracil, leucovorin, oxaliplatin, FOLFOX4: oxaliplatin cycle 4–12, fluorouracil, leucovorin.
*Limited by government funding, #if liver dominant site of disease, +if present counted as relative contraindication, *if present counted as relative contraindication, †if liver dominant site of disease each, nodule <3 mm as assessed by a 64 slice ct [15], ⊗limited extrahepatic metastases at cn site such as a solitary pulmonary metastases, ⊗limited pulmonary nodules or abdominal lymphadenopathy.

TABLE 4: CEA responses to radioembolisation at 3 months.

Study	Number of patients	Definition of CEA reduction	Percentage of patients (%) with CEA reduction
Gray et al. 2001 [30]	36	≥50%	72
Wong et al. 2002 [16]	8	Statistically significant	75
Murthy et al. 2005 [29]	9	NR	57
Lewandowski et al. 2005 [35]	27	50%	38
		80%	19
Kennedy et al. 2006 [24]	208	NR	70
Stubbs et al. 2006 [22]	100	82%	96
Jakobs et al. 2007 [37]	18	NR	82
Boppudi et al. 2006 [23]	54	75%	70
Sharma et al. 2007 [5]	20	NR	100*
Nace et al. 2011 [31]	51 (41 patients' levels recorded)	≥50%	41%
Kosmider et al. 2011 [32]	19	Median reduction 35%	100

NR: not recorded, *at 6 months.
The 23 patients in the van Hazel et al. [38] publication from 2009 also had a reduced CEA. Median serum CEA decreased by 82% in this trial where radioembolisation was used in conjunction with irinotecan chemotherapy.

to stable disease was judged as less than a 10% increase or decrease in the sum of the products of the perpendicular diameters of the index lesion. Stable disease as judged by WHO would have a less than 50% decrease or less than a 25% increase in the sum of the products of the perpendicular diameters of the index lesion [23]. This study's criteria are more lenient in judging response, this accounts for the increase in partial responders when compared with WHO criteria. Evaluation methods using necrosis and combined evaluation had overall better response rates: 45% and 50%, respectively, compared with the WHO and RECIST values of 19% and 24% [39]. Stubbs et al. reject WHO criteria for significantly underestimating response rate due to the length of time it takes for maximum size resolution to occur [22]. Instead they opt for a more lenient definition of response as listed above.

The RECIST criteria were revised in 2009 (RECIST 1.1) and this included criteria for judging PET response. It also has guidance for judging cystic changes that occur following radioembolisation. CT as judged previously may have been inaccurate due to haemorrhage, cystic degeneration, and oedema surrounding the tumour sites [16]. The other major changes to the criteria are highlighted in Table 5.

RECIST criteria are the most used of the assessment criteria, particularly given the inclusion of PET-CT scanning and guidance on the analysis of cystic changes. We would recommend the use of RECIST 1.1. In this review, all the papers using the RECIST criteria used version 1.0. In terms of timing of follow-up assessment, there is variability of between 1.5 and 6 months. Ten papers reviewed their patients at 3 months.

There has been conflicting evidence on timings of best response. Cosimelli et al. suggest that maximum response on CT scan was seen at 1.5 months [15]. Andrews et al. suggest that the parenchymal changes are most pronounced at 2 months [34], whereas Lewandowski et al. suggest best response is seen at 3-4 months in a review of interarterial treatments for hepatic malignancy [7]. This is also supported by Kennedy et al. who suggest that maximal CT and PET response occurs at 3 months [24]. Kosmider et al. showed that the best response as judged on CT varied from 0.9–50.3 months; however, the median value was 4.4 months [32] again supporting Lewandowski et al.

Although response to chemotherapy and radiotherapy is conventionally judged by change in size, tumour markers give a greater response rate [22, 24]. When CEA levels have been compared in a RCT with radioembolisation and chemotherapy versus chemotherapy alone; they have been favourable for the combined treatment of radioembolisation and chemotherapy (72% vs 47%). This is also correlated with improved survival [30].

When resection or postmortem examination has occurred, this has enabled a histological examination of the tumour; the yttrium 90 microspheres appeared as clustered eosinophil target structures [14] and the histopathological examination of the liver metastasis showed intralesional necrosis, fibrosis, and dystrophic calcifications [5, 14]. Conventional CT imaging demonstrates a difference mainly in tumour enhancement [20] which is very difficult to correlate with the histological response due to few cases where tissue is available for examination.

Few studies have used MRI to grade tumours, in the studies reviewed data was not clearly highlighted relating to MRI as an assessment tool [16, 20, 24]. It was offered as an alternative to CT as a staging tool; however, there are a number of studies that have used PET-CT scans to judge response [16, 24, 26].

PET-CT shows higher rates of partial and complete response [16, 24, 35, 39]. Unlike CT or MRI, PET-CT examines the functional element of the tumour. CEA is also a marker of metabolic function of the tumour. In one paper, all 6 PET-CT responders had a reduced level of CEA. None

TABLE 5: RECIST 1.0 versus 1.1 [40].

	RECIST 1.0	RECIST 1.1
Measurable disease at BL	Required, MTLS	When required then MTLS patients with nonmeasurable disease only are allowed
Minimum target lesion size	≥10 mm (Spiral CT) ≥20 mm (Conventional CT, MRI) Lymph node: not mentioned ≥20 mm (clinical)	≥10 mm (CT + MRI) ≥15 mm lymph nodes ≥20 mm chest X-ray ≥10 mm (clinical)
No. of measurable lesions	1–10 (5 per organ)	1–5 (2 per organ)
Measurement	Unidimensional	Unidimensional Lymph nodes = short axis
PD	20% increase in SLD from Nadir	20% increase in SOD + min. 5 mm increase from Nadir
Confirmation of CR and PR	After at least 28 days CR lymph node not mentioned	Only required, if response is primary endpoint and not randomized
Nonmeasurable assessment	Unequivocal progression considered as PD	(i) substantial worsening, (ii) tumour burden has increased sufficiently
Lymph node measurements	None	Specific instructions ≥15 mm, 10–14 mm, <10 mm CR lymph nodes must be <10 mm short axis
PET	Not available	May be considered to support CT, for PD and confirmation of CR

MTLS: Minimum Target Lesion Size. The size a lesion needs to be selected as a measurable target lesion at Baseline. SLD: old RECIST 1.0 sum of longest diameters for all measured target lesions' diameters to be added up at each time point. SOD: new RECIST 1.1 sum of diameters which are the longest of nonnodal lesions plus the longest of the short axis diameters of lymph nodes for measured target lesions' diameters to be added up at each time point.

of these responders showed an anatomical response when measured with CT or MRI [16]. The correlation between CEA and PET-CT is also supported in another publication by Wong et al. [41]. The metabolic response is correlated with a reduction in tumour load and this is reflected by a reduced level of CEA [16]; PET-CT also proved to be more sensitive in detecting extra hepatic and hepatic lesions [16]. Where cystic changes may occur conventional cross sectional imaging such as MRI or CT may show an increase in tumour size. PET-CT however shows partial resolution and decreased activity [16, 35, 41]. Studies have shown that PET has a greater sensitivity when compared with CT in detecting recurrent disease within previously treated metastases [41]. PET-CT in one study failed to detect new lesions measuring 5–11 mm that were detected on CT scan and also in a separate study lesions detected on MRI measuring 0.5–15 mm [42]. It is reported that the sensitivity of PET is significantly lower for detection of lesions less than 1.5 cm [39]. Overall, PET shows a greater sensitivity in measuring response in direct comparison with CT; 11 lesions were deemed to have had resolution compared with just 2 on CT [16]. It correlates with the functional elements of the tumour and thus gives a better indication of tumour activity. As PET assesses the functional metastases, it can be used to assess and identify new disease, monitor response, identify residual disease, and provide the basis in terms of assessment for further salvage radiotherapy or chemotherapy as required.

With reference to PET, imaging results are based upon the measurement of SUV or standardised uptake values (SUV) which is a relative measure of [18] fluoro-D-glucose or FDG. SUV is used to account for the two most significant sources of variation that occur: patient size and the amount of FDG

injected [43]. The paper by Gulec et al. recommends the use of functional tumour volume (FTV) and total lesion glycolysis (TLG) when using PET scans to assess the response to radioembolisation [44]. FTV refers to the size of the tumour that have any FDG uptake above the surrounding normal tissue uptake and the TLG was defined as the product of the functional volume and mean or maximum tumour SUV [44].

Patients found to have FTV values below 200 cc at pretreatment scans and below 30 cc at 4-week posttreatment scan were shown to have a survival advantage of greater than 12 months compared to their counterparts. Similar responses were seen in measurement of TLG in pretreatment <600 g and post treatment <100 g.

This study concluded that FTV and TLG were more informative measures of metabolic response on PET scan and results could be seen as early as 4 weeks. These results could be used as early predictors of anatomic tumour changes and a reduction in viable tumour cell volume and not just metabolic suppression. The conclusion of this paper was that FTV and TLG can be used for quantitative criteria for patient selection and disease prognostication when liver directed therapy is considered [44].

CT response was found to be highly variable which may be due to the use of concurrent and previous chemotherapy regimens used across the papers. Partial response ranged from 0% in some cases up to 90% in one paper [5]. Response was most often judged using the RECIST criteria as listed above. However, three papers used their own criteria, two rejected the WHO criteria due to underestimations of response [22, 23] and instead used more favourable study criteria to measure response.

In relation to the early response demonstrated on PET scans, changes were seen at 30 days on CT scans rather than the 3-4 month mark. These changes were in an attenuation decrease of more than 15%, and were 84.2% sensitive and 83.3% specific in predicting evaluation of response on PET scan [45]. Changes in attenuation showed higher correlation with metabolic activity of the tumour than with changes in tumour size due to composition changes such as areas of necrosis, which would show low attenuation.

The role of attenuation is in early prediction of treatment response. This would allow CT to be used earlier and more accurately in predicting response to treatment when PET scanning is not available. This information could then be used to plan a second radioembolisation procedure where further metastases exist in the opposite lobe [45]. These procedures typically take place 30–60 days after the initial treatment.

When PET-CT scans results and CEA levels were measured, then both showed a response, however on CT where a paradoxical increase in the size of lesions due to haemorrhage, cystic degeneration, and oedema surrounding the tumour site [16] would show progressive disease.

CEA remains a useful tool to assess metabolic function of the tumour in additions to PET-CT. PET scan can recognise the change in metabolic function. CT although the most widely used method of assessing response does not give the greatest sensitivity in measuring response when in direct comparison with PET-CT.

With regards to treatment workup and avoidance of side effects due to pulmonary or gastrointestinal complications, the paper by Denecke et al. demonstrates a suitable algorithm. They suggest first restaging the patient using CT thorax and abdomen followed by PET scan or use of PET-CT instead of individual scans. In this study, MRI followed on from PET scanning and excluded a further patients identifying lesions 0.5–15 mm. Restaging of patients using these methods streamlined patients who would benefit from radioembolisation rather than local ablative therapy.

Criteria included metastases numbers/size, which prevented local ablation, MRI showing less than 60% tumour load, no diffuse infiltration of entire organ, and liver only or liver dominant disease (extra hepatic deposits allowed if nonprogressive or no increase in size over 2–4 months) [42].

Once patients had proceeded through restaging therapy planning was commenced. This consisted of angiography and planar scintigraphy or SPECT-CT when available. The use of angiography allowed identification of target vessels and likely shunts and where necessary protective coiling is to be carried out. SPECT-CT was more accurate than CTA in predicting the distribution of microspheres and enabled further review to assess adequacy of coiling and prevent unintentional extrahepatic flow of microspheres. Following the algorithm laid out in this paper of the 13 remaining patients form the original 22 experienced no gastrointestinal or pulmonary side effects commonly seen following radiotherapy [42].

Currently, there are two large-scale trials evaluating the use of radioembolisation with chemotherapy versus chemotherapy alone as first line therapy for patients with colorectal liver metastases. The SIRFLOX trial is a multicentre trial with participating centres in Australia, The EU, New Zealand, and America. It is a prospective open labelled randomised controlled trial and compares radioembolisation with FOLFOX versus FOLFOX alone (with or without bevacizumab) [46]. The FOXFIRE trial is the UK equivalent. It is an open labelled randomised phase III trial of 5-Fluorouracil, Oxaliplatin, and Folinic acid ± interventional radioembolisation as first line treatment for patients with unresectable liver-only or liver-predominant metastatic colorectal cancer [47]. It aims to recruit 490 patients. Its primary objective will be to measure overall survival. The FOXFIRE trial will use the RECIST 1.1 staging criteria.

5. Conclusions

CT has previously been the assessment of choice in judging the response to radioembolisation. Although PET-CT has been shown to have limitations in detecting small metastases, this review suggests that PET-CT is a more sensitive modality. CEA remains a useful tool in assessing the functional element of a tumour and can be used to monitor response to treatment. CEA has only been measured in limited trials but it correlates with PET-CT scan results and has a role to play in determining response.

The updated RECIST 1.1 guidelines that include guidance on PET-CT should be the staging criteria of choice. The most appropriate time for assessment seems to be 3 months for both PET-CT and CT. However, using alternative measurements then the likely response can be predicted earlier with regard to using FTV and TLG for PET-CT and attenuation changes on CT scans. This early prediction has a role in further treatment planning.

In terms of use of radioembolisation for unresectable colorectal liver metastases, the greatest response was seen when used in treatment naive patients in conjunction with chemotherapy [12]. The use of radioembolisation plus HAC as a first line treatment reserves systemic chemotherapy allowing the use of systemic chemotherapy for when there is systemic disease or failure of first line treatment [22]. To avoid pulmonary and gastrointestinal morbidity, we suggest following the algorithm constructed by Denecke et al. [42].

There is no validated method to assess response that has been correlated with patient survival. However, we would recommend PET-CT pre- and postradioembolisation at 3 months, with concurrent measurements of CEA. Best response has been seen in treatment naive patients with unresectable metastases with use of HAC. The use of radioembolisation in this manner is currently supported by NICE.

References

[1] B. N. Gray, J. E. Anderson, M. A. Burton et al., "Regression of liver metastases following treatment with yttrium-90 microspheres," *Australian and New Zealand Journal of Surgery*, vol. 62, no. 2, pp. 105–110, 1992.

[2] SIRTEX, "What are SIR-spheres microspheres?" 2011, http://www.sirtex.com/content.cfm?sec=world&MenuID=A040E9B4.

[3] L. Lim, P. Gibbs, D. Yip et al., "Prospective study of treatment with selective internal radiation therapy spheres in patients with unresectable primary or secondary hepatic malignancies," *Internal Medicine Journal*, vol. 35, no. 4, pp. 222–227, 2005.

[4] M. A. D. Vente, M. Wondergem, I. van der Tweel et al., "Yttrium-90 microsphere radioembolization for the treatment of liver malignancies: a structured meta-analysis," *European Radiology*, vol. 19, no. 4, pp. 951–959, 2009.

[5] R. A. Sharma, G. A. Van Hazel, B. Morgan et al., "Radioembolization of liver metastases from colorectal cancer using Yttrium-90 microspheres with concomitant systemic oxaliplatin, fluorouracil, and leucovorin chemotherapy," *Journal of Clinical Oncology*, vol. 25, no. 9, pp. 1099–1106, 2007.

[6] R. T. Hoffmann, T. F. Jakobs, C. H. Kubisch et al., "Radiofrequency ablation after selective internal radiation therapy with Yttrium90 microspheres in metastatic liver disease-Is it feasible?" *European Journal of Radiology*, vol. 74, no. 1, pp. 199–205, 2010.

[7] R. J. Lewandowski, J.-F. Geschwind, E. Liapi, and R. Salem, "Transcatheter intraarterial therapies: rationale and overview," *Radiology*, vol. 259, no. 3, pp. 641–657, 2011.

[8] H. R. Bierman, R. L. Byron Jr., K. H. Kelley, and A. Grady, "Studies on the blood supply of tumors in man. III. Vascular patterns of the liver by hepatic arteriography in vivo," *Journal of the National Cancer Institute*, vol. 12, no. 1, pp. 107–131, 1951.

[9] K. T. Sato, R. A. Omary, C. Takehana et al., "The role of tumor vascularity in predicting survival after Yttrium-90 radioembolization for liver metastases," *Journal of Vascular and Interventional Radiology*, vol. 20, no. 12, pp. 1564–1569, 2009.

[10] R. Stangl, A. Altendorf-Hofmann, R. M. Charnley, and J. Scheele, "Factors influencing the natural history of colorectal liver metastases," *The Lancet*, vol. 343, no. 8910, pp. 1405–1410, 1994.

[11] J. M. McLoughlin, E. H. Jensen, and M. Malafa, "Resection of colorectal liver metastases: current perspectives," *Cancer Control*, vol. 13, no. 1, pp. 32–41, 2006.

[12] G. Van Hazel, A. Blackwell, J. Anderson et al., "Randomised phase 2 trial of SIR-spheres plus fluorouracil/leucovorin chemotherapy versus fluorouracil/leucovorin chemotherapy alone in advanced colorectal cancer," *Journal of Surgical Oncology*, vol. 88, no. 2, pp. 78–85, 2004.

[13] S. Garrean, A. Muhs, J. T. Bui et al., "Complete eradication of hepatic metastasis from colorectal cancer by Yttrium-90 SIRT," *World Journal of Gastroenterology*, vol. 13, no. 21, pp. 3016–3019, 2007.

[14] S. Pini, C. Pinto, B. Angelelli et al., "Multimodal sequential approach in colorectal cancer liver metastases: hepatic resection after yttrium-90 selective internal radiation therapy and cetuximab rescue treatment," *Tumori*, vol. 96, no. 1, pp. 157–159, 2010.

[15] M. Cosimelli, R. Golfieri, P. P. Cagol et al., "Multi-centre phase II clinical trial of yttrium-90 resin microspheres alone in unresectable, chemotherapy refractory colorectal liver metastases," *British Journal of Cancer*, vol. 103, no. 3, pp. 324–331, 2010.

[16] C.-Y. Wong, R. Salem, S. Raman, V. L. Gates, and H. J. Dworkin, "Evaluating 90 Y-glass microsphere treatment response of unresectable colorectal liver metastases by [18F]FDG pet: a comparison with CT or MRI," *European Journal of Nuclear Medicine*, vol. 29, no. 6, pp. 815–820, 2002.

[17] Excellence, "TNIfHaC. Selective internal radiation therapy for non-resectable colorectal metastases in the liver: overview," The National Institute for Health and Clinical Excellence, 2011, http://www.nice.org.uk.

[18] A. Kennedy, S. Nag, R. Salem et al., "Recommendations for radioembolization of hepatic malignancies using Yttrium-90 microsphere brachytherapy: a consensus panel report from the radioembolization brachytherapy oncology consortium," *International Journal of Radiation Oncology Biology Physics*, vol. 68, no. 1, pp. 13–23, 2007.

[19] P. Therasse, S. G. Arbuck, E. A. Eisenhauer et al., "New guidelines to evaluate the response to treatment in solid tumors," *Journal of the National Cancer Institute*, vol. 92, no. 3, pp. 205–216, 2000.

[20] L. Bester, P. G. Hobbins, S.-C. Wang, and R. Salem, "Imaging characteristics following 90yttrium microsphere treatment for unresectable liver cancer," *Journal of Medical Imaging and Radiation Oncology*, vol. 55, no. 2, pp. 111–118, 2011.

[21] J. H. Anderson, J. A. Goldberg, R. G. Bessent et al., "Glass yttrium-90 microspheres for patients with colorectal liver metastases," *Radiotherapy and Oncology*, vol. 25, no. 2, pp. 137–139, 1992.

[22] R. S. Stubbs, I. O'Brien, and M. M. Correia, "Selective internal radiation therapy with 90Y microspheres for colorectal liver metastases: single-centre experience with 100 patients," *ANZ Journal of Surgery*, vol. 76, no. 8, pp. 696–703, 2006.

[23] S. Boppudi, S. K. Wickremesekera, M. Nowitz, and R. Stubbs, "Evaluation of the role of CT in the assessment of response to selective internal radiation therapy in patients with colorectal liver metastases," *Australasian Radiology*, vol. 50, no. 6, pp. 570–577, 2006.

[24] A. S. Kennedy, D. Coldwell, C. Nutting et al., "Resin 90Y-microsphere brachytherapy for unresectable colorectal liver metastases: modern USA experience," *International Journal of Radiation Oncology Biology Physics*, vol. 65, no. 2, pp. 412–425, 2006.

[25] R. S. Stubbs, R. J. Cannan, and A. W. Mitchell, "Selective internal radiation therapy with 90 Yttrium microspheres for extensive colorectal liver metastases," *Journal of Gastrointestinal Surgery*, vol. 5, no. 3, pp. 294–302, 2001.

[26] L. R. Jiao, T. Szyszko, A. Al-Nahhas et al., "Clinical and imaging experience with yttrium-90 microspheres in the management of unresectable liver tumours," *European Journal of Surgical Oncology*, vol. 33, no. 5, pp. 597–602, 2007.

[27] A. Omed, J. A. T. Lawrance, G. Murphy et al., "A retrospective analysis of selective internal radiation therapy (SIRT) with yttrium-90 microspheres in patients with unresectable hepatic malignancies," *Clinical Radiology*, vol. 65, no. 9, pp. 720–728, 2010.

[28] K. T. Sato, R. J. Lewandowski, M. F. Mulcahy et al., "Unresectable chemorefractory liver metastases: radioembolization with 90Y microspheres: safety, efficacy, and survival," *Radiology*, vol. 247, no. 2, pp. 507–515, 2008.

[29] R. Murthy, H. Xiong, R. Nunez et al., "Yttrium 90 resin microspheres for the treatment of unresectable colorectal hepatic metastases after failure of multiple chemotherapy regimens: preliminary results," *Journal of Vascular and Interventional Radiology*, vol. 16, no. 7, pp. 937–945, 2005.

[30] B. Gray, G. Van Hazel, M. Hope et al., "Randomised trial of SIR-Spheres plus chemotherapy versus chemotherapy alone for treating patients with liver metastases from primary large bowel cancer," *Annals of Oncology*, vol. 12, no. 12, pp. 1711–1720, 2001.

[31] G. W. Nace, J. L. Steel, N. Amesur, A. Zajko, B. E. Nastasi, J. Joyce et al., "Yttrium-90 radioembolization for colorectal cancer liver metastases: a single institution experience," *International Journal of Surgical Oncology*, vol. 2011, Article ID 571261, 9 pages, 2011.

[32] S. Kosmider, T. H. Tan, D. Yip, R. Dowling, M. Lichtenstein, and P. Gibbs, "Radioembolization in combination with systemic chemotherapy as first-line therapy for liver metastases from colorectal cancer," *Journal of Vascular and Interventional Radiology*, vol. 22, no. 6, pp. 780–786, 2011.

[33] T. C. Chua, L. Bester, A. Saxena, and D. L. Morris, "Radioembolization and systemic chemotherapy improves response and survival for unresectable colorectal liver metastases," *Journal of Cancer Research and Clinical Oncology*, vol. 137, no. 5, pp. 865–873, 2011.

[34] J. C. Andrews, S. C. Walker, R. J. Ackermann et al., "Hepatic radioembolization with yttrium-90 containing glass microspheres: preliminary results and clinical follow-up," *Journal of Nuclear Medicine*, vol. 35, no. 10, pp. 1637–1644, 1994.

[35] R. J. Lewandowski, K. G. Thurston, J. E. Goin et al., "90Y microsphere (TheraSphere) treatment for unresectable colorectal cancer metastases of the liver: response to treatment at targeted doses of 135-150 Gy as measured by [18F]fluorodeoxyglucose positron emission tomography and computed tomographic imaging," *Journal of Vascular and Interventional Radiology*, vol. 16, no. 12, pp. 1641–1651, 2005.

[36] R. Mancini, L. Carpanese, R. Sciuto et al., "A multicentric phase II clinical trial on intra-arterial hepatic radiotherapy with 90Yttrium SIR-spheres in unresectable, colorectal liver metastases refractory to i.v. chemotherapy: preliminary results on toxicity and response rates," *In Vivo*, vol. 20, no. 6, pp. 711–714, 2006.

[37] T. F. Jakobs, R.-T. Hoffmann, G. Poepperl et al., "Mid-term results in otherwise treatment refractory primary or secondary liver confined tumours treated with selective internal radiation therapy (SIRT) using 90Y ttrium resin-microspheres," *European Radiology*, vol. 17, no. 5, pp. 1320–1330, 2007.

[38] G. A. van Hazel, N. Pavlakis, D. Goldstein et al., "Treatment of fluorouracil-refractory patients with liver metastases from colorectal cancer by using yttrium-90 resin microspheres plus concomitant systemic irinotecan chemotherapy," *Journal of Clinical Oncology*, vol. 27, no. 25, pp. 4089–4095, 2009.

[39] F. H. Miller, A. L. Keppke, D. Reddy et al., "Response of liver metastases after treatment with yttrium-90 microspheres: role of size, necrosis, and PET," *The American Journal of Roentgenology*, vol. 188, no. 3, pp. 776–783, 2007.

[40] RECIST, "RECIST version 1.1 update RECIST in practice," 2009, http://www.recist.com/recist-in-practice/22.html.

[41] C.-Y. O. Wong, R. Salem, F. Qing et al., "Metabolic response after intraarterial 90Y-glass microsphere treatment for colorectal liver metastases: comparison of quantitative and visual analyses by 18F-FDG PET," *Journal of Nuclear Medicine*, vol. 45, no. 11, pp. 1892–1897, 2004.

[42] T. Denecke, R. Rühl, B. Hildebrandt et al., "Planning transarterial radioembolization of colorectal liver metastases with Yttrium 90 microspheres: evaluation of a sequential diagnostic approach using radiologic and nuclear medicine imaging techniques," *European Radiology*, vol. 18, no. 5, pp. 892–902, 2008.

[43] P. E. Kinahan and J. W. Fletcher, "Positron emission tomography-computed tomography standardized uptake values in clinical practice and assessing response to therapy," *Seminars in Ultrasound, CT and MRI*, vol. 31, no. 6, pp. 496–505, 2010.

[44] S. A. Gulec, R. R. Suthar, T. C. Barot, and K. Pennington, "The prognostic value of functional tumor volume and total lesion glycolysis in patients with colorectal cancer liver metastases undergoing 90Y selective internal radiation therapy plus chemotherapy," *European Journal of Nuclear Medicine and Molecular Imaging*, vol. 38, no. 7, pp. 1289–1295, 2011.

[45] S. M. Tochetto, P. Rezai, M. Rezvani et al., "Does multidetector CT attenuation change in colon cancer liver metastases treated with90Y help predict metabolic activity at FDG PET?" *Radiology*, vol. 255, no. 1, pp. 164–172, 2010.

[46] SIRTEX, "SIRflox trial 2011," http://www.sirflox.com.

[47] Oncology Clinical Trials Office, "FOXFIRE Trial," 2011, http://www.octo-oxford.org.uk/alltrials/trials/FOXFIRE.html.

17

A Single Centre Experience of First "One Hundred Laparoscopic Liver Resections"

S. Rehman,[1] S. K. P. John,[1] J. J. French,[1] D. M. Manas,[1,2] and S. A. White[1,2]

[1] *Department of Hepatobiliary and Transplantation Surgery, The Freeman Hospital, Newcastle upon Tyne NE7 7DN, UK*
[2] *The Liver Research Group, The University of Newcastle, Leech Building, Framlington Place, Newcastle upon Tyne NE1 7RP, UK*

Correspondence should be addressed to S. Rehman; srkhanswati75@yahoo.com

Academic Editor: Guy Maddern

Background. Laparoscopic liver resection (LLR) has emerged as an alternative procedure to open liver resection in selected patients. The purpose of this study was to describe our initial experience of 100 patients undergoing LLR. *Methods.* We analysed a prospectively maintained hepatobiliary database of 100 patients who underwent LLR between August 2007 and August 2012. Clinicopathological data were reviewed to evaluate surgical outcomes following LLR. *Results.* The median age was 64 and median BMI 27. Patients had a liver resection for either malignant lesions ($n = 74$) or benign lesions ($n = 26$). Commonly performed procedures were segmentectomy/metastectomy ($n = 55$), left lateral sectionectomy (LLS) ($n = 26$), or major hepatectomy ($n = 19$). Complete LLR was performed in 84 patients, 9 were converted to open and 7 hand-assisted. The most common indications were CRLM ($n = 62$), followed by hepatic adenoma ($n = 9$) or hepatocellular carcinoma ($n = 7$). The median operating time was 240 minutes and median blood loss was 250 mL. Major postoperative complications occurred in 9 patients. The median length of stay (LOS) was 5 days. One patient died within 30 days of liver resection. *Conclusions.* LLR is a safe and oncologically feasible procedure with comparable short-term perioperative outcomes to the open approach. However, further studies are necessary to determine long-term oncological outcomes.

1. Introduction

Since the initial report in 1992 by Gagner et al. laparoscopic liver resection (LLR) has evolved for treating benign and malignant tumours of the liver in selected patients [1–5]. As the technical innovations in the field of laparoscopic surgery continue to evolve more and more minimally invasive liver surgery is being carried out in specialised centres [4–15]. A review by Nguyen et al. in 2009 reported outcomes following LLR of 2804 patients citing reduced intraoperative blood loss reduced postoperative morbidity and mortality, and shorter in-patient hospital stay [3], albeit with slightly longer operating times [2]. Similar results have been reported by other centres [9–14]. In general the benefits of LLR are less surgical trauma associated with less postoperative pain, reduced analgesic requirements, and an early return to normal daily activities [13–18]. However, such findings have never been proved by a randomised controlled trial, and starting one now would be difficult as LLR has already become an established procedure in most specialist laparoscopic HPB units [13–18].

LLR for benign lesions gained acceptance relatively early on [1–5]; however, enthusiasm for laparoscopic resection of malignant lesions developed rather slowly [1–3, 5, 7–13], the major obstacles being oncologic inadequacy [10, 11] and concerns over seeding of tumour cells at the time of surgery and perhaps an increased risk of tumour recurrence [10–13]. Moreover, in its infancy LLR carried with it concerns regarding an increased risk of intraoperative bleeding and air embolism [10]. However, recent advances in the surgical techniques and development of more laparoscopic devices have largely overcome these problems to a certain extent [15–21]. Nevertheless, its long-term oncological outcome and added benefit of improving quality of life are still yet to be proven [10–14]. Perhaps for most enthusiasts in the field minor LLRs have obvious advantages although major hepatectomy is still very controversial.

The aim of this study was to evaluate the clinical and oncological outcomes of our first 100 LLRs performed in a supraregional HPB and liver transplant unit in North East England.

2. Methods

We analysed a prospectively maintained HPB database for patients undergoing LLR between August 2007 and August 2012. The primary outcome measure was short-term surgical outcome. The secondary end points were midterm overall and disease-free survival. Three surgeons (D. M. Manas, J. J. French, and S. A. White) have performed LLR in our unit since 2007 and make up 10–15% of all liver resections. Before surgery, each patient was individually evaluated in our weekly multidisciplinary team (MDT) meeting with surgeons, pathologists, oncologists, gastroenterologists, and radiologists. All patients had an abdominal CT scan and liver-specific double-contrast magnetic resonance imaging (MRI).

Patients with good performance status, resectable liver disease, absence of extrahepatic disease, and sufficient functional parenchyma were considered suitable for LLR. Patients with tumours within 1 cm of the portal vein bifurcation, the inferior vena cava, or hepatic vein confluence and tumours involving the common hepatic duct were found unsuitable for LLR. Moreover, large tumours (>10 cm) and the need for a portal lymphadenectomy were also considered to be contra-indications for a LLR in our early series.

Patient demographics, indications, type of liver resection, intraoperative blood loss, duration of surgery (time from start of skin incision to the end of wound closure), conversion to open or hand-assisted, length of intensive care unit (ICU) stay, postoperative length of stay (LOS), postoperative complications, and mortality (within 30 days from surgery) were evaluated. The histological reports were all reviewed to assess resection margin status.

The extent of hepatic resection was recorded according to the Brisbane 2000 terminology of liver anatomy and resections [9]. Operative results and postoperative variables were analysed for minor resections and major hepatectomies (e.g., removal of three or more segments, right hepatectomy, or left hepatectomy) where appropriate [3]. Postoperative complications were classified as per the Dindo et al. [16] classification. Margin status was defined as R_0 when microscopically negative for tumour or R_1 for microscopically positive for tumour existing within 1 mm of the margin.

3. Surgical Technique

3.1. Patient Positioning. For resections of the left lateral segment and tumours in the anterior segments, for example, IVb, V, and VI, we preferred a supine position with split legs with the surgeon standing between the legs and assistants on either side. Five ports (ENDO PATH Xcel, Ethicon Endo-Surgery, LLC, USA) including three 12 mm ports are positioned, one supraumbilical port, two in the right and left midclavicular line, and two 5 mm ports in the right and left anterior axillary

line as described previously [17], but there has been a decrease in the number of ports with more experience.

3.2. Pringle's Manoeuvre. We always perform a staging laparoscopy to rule out extrahepatic disease at the time of the LLR. As part of the protocol a laparoscopic ultrasound (7.5 MHz, Aloka Co. Ltd., Tokyo, Japan) is performed to define the vascular anatomy and to confirm the location of metastases. Although various techniques for retracting the liver have been used in our series, the authors prefer to divide the falciform ligament and then place an Endoloop (Autosuture, Tyco Healthcare Ltd.) around the free edge of the ligamentum teres. This can be retracted superiorly by bringing the suture through the anterior abdominal wall using an Endo Close (Autosuture, Tyco Healthcare UK Ltd.) device. The suture is then held in a haemostat thus holding the ligament against the anterior abdominal wall or laterally. The gall bladder can also be used for retraction but some patients may have already had this removed.

Once the liver has been retracted and the hepato-duodenal ligament has been lifted a tape can then be placed, acting as a tourniquet around the hepatoduodenal ligament using a "Gold finger" (Gold finger, blunt dissector, Ethicon Endo surgery, Johnson & Johnson, USA) as previously described [17]. A nylon tape is passed through the snare in the tip of the Gold finger (Ethicon Endo-Surgery, Johnson & Johnson, USA). The Gold finger can be safely introduced through a 10 mm working port in the right upper quadrant due to its blunt and atraumatic tip. The Gold finger is then advanced around the porta hepatis until the tip of the nylon tape can be visualised on the left side of the hepatoduodenal ligament. The tape is then grasped through the port placed in the left upper quadrant in the midclavicular line. The two ends are positioned through the port onto the anterior abdominal wall and placed through a "snugger" using tubing (Suction tubing 10 cm, 7 mm, Pennine Healthcare Ltd., UK). The port is removed and then replaced with the tape lying adjacent on the outside of the port. With increasing experience this step has sometimes not been required at all.

3.3. Hilar Dissection and Parenchymal Transection. All major structures at the hilum are divided extrahepatically except the hepatic bile duct which is divided within the liver parenchyma using a suitable stapling device. Vascular staplers with roticulators are used to manage major pedicles and vessels. For right hepatectomy the right hepatic artery (RHA) and the right portal vein (RPV) are approached either anteriorly or laterally, usually posterior to the bile duct using locking Weck Clips. The Glissonian approach as described by Launois and Jamieson [21] was never used. Parenchymal transection was performed using either a combination of the cavitational ultrasonic aspirator (CUSA) or bipolar sealing device Tissue Link, the Harmonic Scalpel ultrasonic activated shears (Harmonic ACE) or Ligasure device. Tissue sealants such as Tisseel or Evicel were applied to the cut surface of the liver to further control bleeding from the parenchymal transection margin. The specimen is retrieved in an Endo-2 catch bag through a Pfannenstiel incision in most cases or

TABLE 1: Patients characteristics and surgical outcome.

Variable	Frequency
Age (median in years, range)	64 (22–84)
Sex (female : male)	52 : 48
BMI (median)	27 (16–40)
ASA grade (median)	2
Laparoscopic	84
HALR	7
Converted	9

through the previous midline incision if the indication was colorectal liver metastases (CRLM).

3.4. Followup. After initial followup between 4 to 6 weeks, all patients were regularly reviewed thereafter at 3, 6, 12, 18, and 24 months and yearly thereafter for the first 5 years for patients with malignant tumours. Patients with benign liver tumours were followed appropriately depending on their underlying pathological condition. Survival status was determined by review of the patients' medical records and defined as the time interval from the date of initial operation to the date of last clinical encounter or date of death if known.

3.5. Statistical Analysis. All results are expressed as median and ranges. The Mann-Whitney U test was applied to compare nonparametric data and the chi-squared test or Fisher's exact test were applied for analysis of categorical variables. Overall and disease-free survival was analysed by the Kaplan-Meier method and their significance was assessed using the log-rank test. The level of statistical significance was set at $P < 0.05$.

4. Results

74 patients had LLR for malignant disease, whereas 26 patients had resections for benign disease. There were 52 female and 48 male patients. The median age of all patients was 64 years (range 23–84 years) and median BMI was 27 (range 16–40) (Table 1).

Indications for surgery in the malignancy group were CRLM ($n = 62$), hepatocellular carcinoma (HCC $n = 7$), intrahepatic cholangiocarcinoma ($n = 3$), lymphoma ($n = 1$), and metastases from breast cancer ($n = 1$). Among the benign conditions the most common indications were adenoma ($n = 9$), biliary/liver cyst ($n = 6$), haemangioma ($n = 5$) (4 of these patients had a primary colorectal tumour and were suspected CRLM; however, histology of the resected liver revealed haemangioma, whereas one other patient had underlying ovarian primary tumour and was found to have indeterminate liver lesion, liver resection revealing a haemangioma), focal nodular hyperplasia (FNH $n = 4$), and angiomyolipoma ($n = 2$) (Table 2). The patient with lymphoma had a previous primary colorectal tumour that was thought to be a solitary secondary metastasis.

TABLE 2: Histological results in LLR $n = 100$.

Malignant tumour	$n = 74$
Colorectal liver metastases	62
Hepatocellular carcinoma	7
Cholangiocarcinoma	3
Metastases from breast cancer	1
Lymphoma	1
Benign tumour	$n = 26$
Adenoma	9
Biliary/liver cyst	6
Haemangioma	5
Focal nodular hyperplasia (FNH)	4
Angiomyolipoma	2

TABLE 3: Type of liver resection.

Types of liver resection $n = 100$	
Anatomical liver resection (major)	19
Right hemihepatectomy	7
Left hemihepatectomy	6
Extended L hemihepatectomy	2
Trisegmentectomy	4
Nonanatomical liver resection	55
Left lateral sectionectomy (LLS)	26

TABLE 4: Location of tumours.

Segmental position of liver tumour	Frequency ($n = 81$)
II	3
LLS (II, III)	16
III	7
IV, IVB	8
IV, V	6
V	9
V, VI	7
VI	8
VI, VII	12
VII	3
VIII	2

Major hepatectomy ($n = 19$).

Major hepatectomies were performed in 19 patients (19%) and included 7 right hemihepatectomies, 6 left hemihepatectomies, 2 extended left hemihepatectomies, and 4 trisegmentectomies. Out of the 19 major hepatectomies, five patients were converted to an open procedure and two patients had hand-assisted liver resection (HALR) (Tables 5 and 7). In our series complete laparoscopic liver resection was performed in 84 patients (84/100), 9 were converted to an open procedure (Tables 3, 5, and 7) and 7 patients had a hand-assisted surgical resection (HALR) (Tables 1 and 7). For the hand-assisted technique a minilaparotomy in the right upper quadrant or insertion of a handport was used for completion of the parenchymal transection (Table 4).

TABLE 5: Reasons for conversion to an open procedure.

Reason	Frequency ($n = 9$)
Tumour in close proximity to large vessel and concern over margin status	4
Difficult/prolonged hilar dissection	2
Unable to locate the tumour	1
Large bulky tumour/bleeding	2

TABLE 6: Perioperative outcome following LLR.

Variable	Frequency
Size of tumour (mm)	35 (2–80)
Operation time (min)	240 (45–540)
Blood loss (mLs)	250 (30–1200)
Hospital stay (days)	5 (1–22)
Morbidity rate (%)	9 (9)
30-day mortality rate	1 (1%)

Median values.

TABLE 7: Major hepatectomy.

Variable	Major hepatectomy ($n = 19$)
Operation time (mins)	302 (252-353)
Blood loss (mls)	481 (282–689)
Hospital stay (days)	8 (3–23)
Open conversion	5
HALR	2

Median (range values).

TABLE 8: Postoperative complications.

Complications	Frequency	Management
Bile leak	3	Conservative management ($n = 2$) Biliary stent placement ($n = 1$)
Intra-abdominal collection/hematoma	3	2-laparoscopic washout ($n = 2$) Percutaneous radiological drainage
Small bowel obstruction	1	Required laparotomy, small bowel resection at day 27
Chest infections	2	Treated with antibiotic ($n = 2$) One required ITU admission

The median overall operative time was 240 minutes (range 45–540 minutes), with a median blood loss of 250 mL (range 30–1200 mL). The median length of stay was 5 days (range 1–23 days) with a median of 1 day in either the ITU or HDU (1–8 days) (Table 6). A blood transfusion was required in only 11 patients. The median postoperative opiate requirement was 40 mg (range 30–100 mg). Moreover, in patients undergoing a major hepatectomy, the median operating time was 302 minutes (252–540), the median blood loss was 481 mLs (range 282–689), and median length of stay was 8 days (range 3–23 days) (Table 7). For patients undergoing LLS the median operative time was 195 minutes (range 45–285 minutes), median blood loss was 175 mLs (range 100–450 mL), median duration of analgesia requirement was 34 hours (range 8–62 hours), and median duration of hospital stay was 3 days (range 1–14 days) (Table 6).

Significant postoperative complications (Clavien-Dindo III/IV) occurred in 9 cases (9%) (Table 8). A bile leak requiring conservative management or stent placement was the most common complication ($n = 3$). A laparoscopic wash out was needed in 2 patients, one for an intra-abdominal haematoma and a second for an infected fluid collection, whilst another patient having a right-sided subphrenic fluid collection underwent an insertion of percutaneous radiological drainage. Two patients developed chest infections postoperatively requiring intravenous antibiotics, oxygen therapy, and chest physiotherapy; however, one of them deteriorated further and was shifted to the high dependency unit. One patient was readmitted 4 weeks after liver resection with signs and symptoms of small bowel obstruction, a CT scan confirmed findings of small bowel obstruction and thickening around a previous anastomosis. However, at laparotomy recurrence of the primary tumour was found at the previous anastomosis not detectable on previous imaging; the tumour was resected completely (Table 8). In-patient mortality was 1%. This patient developed a large pulmonary embolism and died two days after the surgery. The patient was on prophylactic Tinzaparin while on the ward.

In a carefully selected subset of patients undergoing LLR for malignancy, complete surgical resection (R_0) was achieved in 89% ($n = 62$, R_1 resection = 7) CRLM patients and 72% ($n = 7$, R_1 resection = 2) for patients with HCC. The median follow-up period was 14 months for CRLM (0.2–50 months) and HCC (11–40 months), respectively. The median recurrence-free survival was 18 months (range 8–28 months) in CRLM and 32 months (range 8–51 months) in HCC patients. Overall 3-year survival for CRLM patients was 78% with a median survival of 47 months (38–56 months) (Figure 1). A total of 10 patients died in the follow-up period, 8 due to progression of underlying disease. One patient died due to a cardiovascular event (3 years after liver resection) and one patient developed sepsis from a pneumonia and died from multiorgan failure 4 months after the liver resection.

5. Discussion

LLR has been established as a favourable alternative to an open procedure to treat both benign and malignant diseases of the liver [1–6] and hepatobiliary surgeons around the world are increasingly performing LLR with greater confidence [7–13]. However, concerns still remain regarding parenchymal transection methods, controlling bleeding, bile leaks, and incomplete resection [3, 14–18]. This study suggests that LLR is a feasible and safe procedure in selected patients. Patient selection for LLR is still an issue and careful consideration must be given to the indications for LLR, particularly the position of the tumour, whether it is multifocal, and whether the patient can withstand a prolonged pneumoperitoneum. In our department each individual patient was discussed in

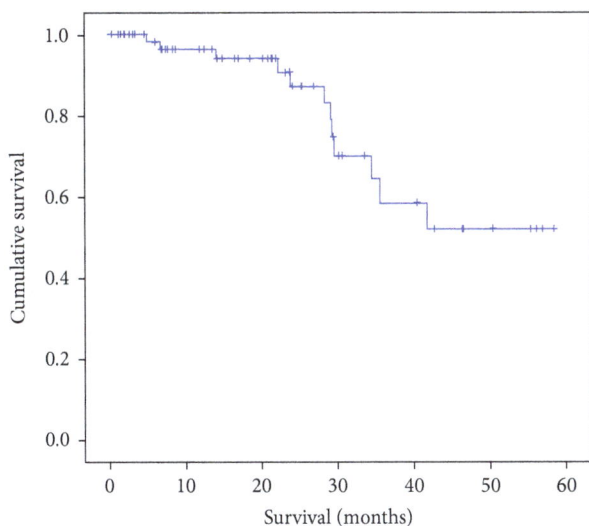

FIGURE 1: Overall survival for CRLM after LLR.

a multidisciplinary team meeting (MDT) comprising hepatobiliary surgeons, a radiologist, a pathologist, and gastroenterologists; the decision regarding LLR was mutually agreed. Generally patients with a large tumour (>10 cm) and those involving major vasculature, for example, inferior vena cava, or with invasion of other adjacent organs were found unsuitable for LLR but not exclusively.

LLS and wedge resections were the most frequently performed procedures. The Louisville Statement, 2008, has recommended LLS as a standard technique for resection of left-sided liver tumours [4] but in our experience we would advise not taking on these types of resections early on when tumours are close to the MHV/LHV confluence. In our series the majority of patients had either nonanatomical resections of segments (II, III, IVb, V, and VI) or LLS. Major hepatectomies were performed in 19 cases (19%). Major hepatectomy (right or left hepatectomy or trisegmentectomy) is a much more complex and technically demanding procedure [17, 18] and can be associated with increased intraoperative bleeding resulting in reduced exposure of the transection plane and potentially the tumour margins [17–20]. Abu Hilal et al. in their study of 133 patients undergoing LLR for liver malignancies presented data of 42 major hepatectomies [8]. Their results revealed major hepatectomies resulting in increased blood loss, increased operating time, and increased conversion rate [8]. Our results are similar to their findings. However, we maintained a low threshold for conversion to an open procedure if the tumour size was large and difficult to manipulate and mobilize or hemostasis was a major concern; sometimes these issues were overcome by using a hand-assisted procedure.

Our results have shown that the overall median operating time was 240 minutes (range 45–540 min) which is consistent with most previous reports [8–21]. Some individual reports comparing LLR to an open approach have reported shorter operating times for open hepatic resection [21]. However, a recent systematic review has found no significant difference between laparoscopic and open liver resection with regards to operating time [15]. Indeed with regards to LLS this is now quicker than an open approach in our centre.

One added benefit of LLR is less intraoperative blood loss and reduced blood transfusion requirements [2–10]. Our results revealed median intraoperative blood loss of 250 mL (range 30–1200 mL), similar to others [6, 12, 13, 20–28]. In our experience only 11 patients required a blood transfusion which is also similar to others [20–28]. We believe laparoscopic surgery provides better visualization of deep vascular structures with more precise and accurate surgery for tumours located in the left lateral and anterior segments. We used a combination of various devices for parenchymal transection to avoid excessive bleeding. These included a Cavitron ultrasonic surgical aspirator (CUSA), Ligasure and the Tissue link together facilitating excellent haemostasis and clear anatomy.

LLR causes less tissue trauma consequently reducing postoperative morbidity [3–9]. In our series only 9 patients developed clinically significant complications. Our results corroborate those of previous studies [7–11]. Another advantage of LLR is minimal scarring and potentially fewer adhesions thereby increasing the feasibility of a repeat liver resection [11]. Recent reports suggest no significant survival difference between primary and repeat liver resection [13–17].

Proponents of laparoscopic surgery claim shorter in-hospital stays for patients undergoing LLR [11–19]. Our results revealed an in-patient stay of 5 days (range 1–23 days). These results support the findings of previous reports in the literature [3–9]. Using our learning curve and enhanced recovery techniques LLS patients can be discharged home the next day or in most cases on the 2nd or 3rd postoperative day. Shorter hospital stay helps reduce cost for organisations during difficult economic circumstances [12]. However, overall cost effectiveness of the procedure is also dependent on theatre time and the cost of instruments, which critics believe is much higher in laparoscopic surgery [20]. Recent reports in the literature suggest equivalent cost for open and LLR [9, 13]. In addition, introduction of enhanced recovery programmes in hepatobiliary surgery may further increase the cost-effectiveness of LLR. However, only future studies looking specifically at economic evaluation of laparoscopic and open liver resection during the era of enhanced recovery programmes would be able to answer these questions.

Oncologic adequacy of LLR has frequently been reported in the literature [5–9, 13–17] and there is a trend amongst most hepatobiliary surgeons that LLR is a safe and an oncologically feasible procedure in carefully selected patients [3–14]. Our results have shown that of 74 patients undergoing LLR for malignant lesions complete surgical resection was achieved in 89% of patients with CRLM and 72% in patients with HCC. These results coincide well with previous reports [19–27]. Without any treatment the median survival of patients with CRLM is 6 to 9 months [26] but now long-term survival after liver resection has been reported to be up to 60% in some studies [2, 3, 7, 13–25]. Our results revealed a median disease-free survival of 18 months (range 8–28 months) in those with CRLM and 32 months (range 8–51 months) in those with HCC although numbers are far too small in the latter case to make any useful conclusion. Moreover, overall 3-year survival following laparoscopic liver resection for CRLM was 78%. Abu Hilal et al. in their study of 133 patients undergoing LLR for various hepatic malignancies reported a 78% overall 2-year survival and 64% disease-free survival for CRLM patients [8]. They have also reported a 77% overall 2-year survival in HCC patients [6]. Our survival data are comparable with various other series in the literature demonstrating feasible medium term survival following liver resection for malignant lesions [13–31].

Important limitations to our study are the relatively small sample size, yet it is still one of the largest series reported in Europe. Nonetheless, our results coincide with the majority of previously reported series [9–19]. Furthermore, in the absence of a randomised controlled trial, case series will continue to provide further evidence to our existing knowledge regarding LLR. Major obstacles to conducting a RCT would be patient selection and randomising to an "open resection" as LLR has already become the gold standard in some specialist centres.

Disclaimer

This study was presented in the ALSGBI 2013 conference, London UK, and was awarded the industry partners Top Free paper Abstract award.

References

[1] M. Gagner, M. Rheault, and J. Dubuc, "Laparoscopic partial hepatectomy for liver tumour," *Surgical Endoscopy*, vol. 6, p. 99, 1992.

[2] M. Gagner, T. Rogula, and D. Selzer, "Laparoscopic liver resection: benefits and controversies," *Surgical Clinics of North America*, vol. 84, no. 2, pp. 451–462, 2004.

[3] K. T. Nguyen, T. C. Gamblin, and D. A. Geller, "World review of laparoscopic liver resection-2804 patients," *Annals of Surgery*, vol. 250, no. 5, pp. 831–841, 2009.

[4] J. F. Buell, D. Cherqui, D. A. Geller et al., "The international position on laparoscopic liver surgery: The Louisville Statement, 2008," *Annals of Surgery*, vol. 250, no. 5, pp. 825–830, 2009.

[5] D. Cherqui, E. Husson, R. Hammoud et al., "Laparoscopic liver resections: a feasibility study in 30 patients," *Annals of Surgery*, vol. 232, no. 6, pp. 753–762, 2000.

[6] B. Topal, S. Fieuws, R. Aerts, H. Vandeweyer, and F. Penninckx, "Laparoscopic versus open liver resection of hepatic neoplasms: comparative analysis of short-term results," *Surgical Endoscopy*, vol. 22, no. 10, pp. 2208–2213, 2008.

[7] A. J. Koffron, G. Auffenberg, R. Kung, and M. Abecassis, "Evaluation of 300 minimally invasive liver resections at a single institution: less is more," *Annals of Surgery*, vol. 246, no. 3, pp. 385–392, 2007.

[8] M. Abu Hilal, F. Di Fabio, M. Abu Salameh, and N. W. Pearce, "Oncological efficiency analysis of laparoscopic liver resection for primary and metastatic cancer: a single-center UK experience," *Archives of Surgery*, vol. 147, no. 1, pp. 42–48, 2012.

[9] F. M. Polignano, A. J. Quyn, R. S. M. De Figueiredo, N. A. Henderson, C. Kulli, and I. S. Tait, "Laparoscopic versus open liver segmentectomy: prospective, case-matched, intention-to-treat analysis of clinical outcomes and cost effectiveness," *Surgical Endoscopy*, vol. 22, no. 12, pp. 2564–2570, 2008.

[10] S. M. Strasberg, "Nomenclature of hepatic anatomy and resections: review of the Brisbane 2000 system," *Journal of Hepato-Biliary-Pancreatic Surgery*, vol. 12, no. 5, pp. 351–355, 2005.

[11] M. R. Lee, Y. H. Kim, Y. H. Roh et al., "Lessons learned from 100 initial cases of laparoscopic liver surgery," *Journal of the Korean Surgical Society*, vol. 80, no. 5, pp. 334–341, 2011.

[12] R. M. Cannon, C. R. Scoggins, G. G. Callender, K. M. McMasters, and R. C. G. Martin II, "Laparoscopic versus open liver resection of hepatic colorectal liver metastases," *Surgery*, vol. 152, no. 4, pp. 567–574, 2012.

[13] F. D. Bhojani, A. Fox, K. Pitzul et al., "Clinical and economic comparison of laparoscopic to open liver resections using a 2-to-1 matched pair analysis: an institutional experience," *Journal of the American College of Surgeons*, vol. 214, no. 2, pp. 184–195, 2012.

[14] M. Abu Hilal, F. Di Fabio, M. J. Teng, D. A. Godfrey, J. N. Primrose, and N. W. Pearce, "Surgical management of benign and indeterminate hepatic lesions in the era of laparoscopic liver surgery," *Digestive Surgery*, vol. 28, no. 3, pp. 232–236, 2011.

[15] A. Rao, G. Rao, and I. Ahmed, "Laparoscopic vs. open liver resection for malignant liver disease. A systematic review," *Surgeon*, vol. 10, pp. 194–201, 2012.

[16] D. Dindo, N. Demartines, and P.-A. Clavien, "Classification of surgical complications: a new proposal with evaluation in a cohort of 6336 patients and results of a survey," *Annals of Surgery*, vol. 240, no. 2, pp. 205–213, 2004.

[17] R. Saif, M. Jacob, S. Robinson, G. Sen, D. Manas, and S. White, "Laparoscopic Pringle's manoeuvre for liver resection how I do it," *Minimally Invasive Therapy and Allied Technologies*, vol. 20, no. 6, pp. 365–368, 2011.

[18] M. G. House, H. Ito, M. Gönen et al., "Survival after hepatic resection for metastatic colorectal cancer: trends in outcomes for 1,600 patients during two decades at a single institution," *Journal of the American College of Surgeons*, vol. 210, no. 5, pp. 744–752, 2010.

[19] M. A. Choti, J. V. Sitzmann, M. F. Tiburi et al., "Trends in long-term survival following liver resection for hepatic colorectal metastases," *Annals of Surgery*, vol. 235, no. 6, pp. 759–766, 2002.

[20] E. Vibert, T. Perniceni, H. Levard, C. Denet, N. K. Shahri, and B. Gayet, "Laparoscopic liver resection," *British Journal of Surgery*, vol. 93, no. 1, pp. 67–72, 2006.

[21] B. Launois and G. G. Jamieson, "The importance of Glisson's capsule and its sheaths in the intrahepatic approach to resection of the liver," *Surgery Gynecology and Obstetrics*, vol. 174, no. 1, pp. 7–10, 1992.

[22] M. Morino, I. Morra, E. Rosso, C. Miglietta, and C. Garrone, "Laparoscopic vs open hepatic resection: a comparative study," *Surgical Endoscopy*, vol. 17, no. 12, pp. 1914–1918, 2003.

[23] M. Shimada, M. Hashizume, S. Maehara et al., "Laparoscopic hepatectomy for hepatocellular carcinoma," *Surgical Endoscopy*, vol. 15, no. 6, pp. 541–544, 2001.

[24] I. Dagher, N. O'Rourke, D. A. Geller et al., "Laparoscopic major hepatectomy: an evolution in standard of care," *Annals of Surgery*, vol. 250, no. 5, pp. 856–860, 2009.

[25] J. Belghiti, A. Cortes, E. K. Abdalla et al., "Resection prior to liver transplantation for hepatocellular carcinoma," *Annals of Surgery*, vol. 238, no. 6, pp. 885–893, 2003.

[26] M. T. Seymour, S. P. Stenning, and J. Cassidy, "Attitudes and practice in the management of metastatic colorectal cancer in Britain. Colorectal Cancer Working Party of the UK Medical Research Council," *Clinical Oncology*, vol. 9, no. 4, pp. 248–251, 1997.

[27] R. Lochan, S. A. White, and D. M. Manas, "Liver resection for colorectal liver metastasis," *Surgical Oncology*, vol. 16, no. 1, pp. 33–45, 2007.

[28] N. O'Rourke, I. Shaw, L. Nathanson, I. Martin, and G. Fielding, "Laparoscopic resection of hepatic colorectal metastases," *HPB*, vol. 6, no. 4, pp. 230–235, 2004.

[29] Y. Fong, W. Jarnagin, K. C. Conlon, R. DeMatteo, E. Dougherty, and L. H. Blumgart, "Hand-assisted laparoscopic liver resection: lessons from an initial experience," *Archives of Surgery*, vol. 135, no. 7, pp. 854–859, 2000.

[30] H. Kaneko, S. Takagi, Y. Otsuka et al., "Laparoscopic liver resection of hepatocellular carcinoma," *American Journal of Surgery*, vol. 189, no. 2, pp. 190–194, 2005.

[31] S. M. Robinson, K. Y. Hui, A. Amer, D. M. Manas, and S. A. White, "Laparoscopic liver resection: is there a learning curve?" *Digestive Surgery*, vol. 29, no. 1, pp. 62–69, 2012.

18

Normothermic Ex Vivo Machine Perfusion for Liver Grafts Recovered from Donors after Circulatory Death: A Systematic Review and Meta-Analysis

Jordan J. Nostedt ⓘ,[1] Daniel T. Skubleny,[1] A. M. James Shapiro ⓘ,[1] Sandra Campbell,[2] Darren H. Freed,[3,4,5] and David L. Bigam ⓘ[1]

[1]Department of Surgery, Division of General Surgery, University of Alberta Hospital, 2D4.41 W.M.C, 8440-112 St., Edmonton, AB, Canada T6G 2B7
[2]John W. Scott Health Sciences Library, University of Alberta, 2K3.28 W.M.C, 8440-112 St., Edmonton, AB, Canada T6G 2B7
[3]Department of Physiology, University of Alberta, 7-55 Medical Sciences Building, Edmonton, AB, Canada T6G 2H7
[4]Department of Biomedical Engineering, University of Alberta, 1098 Research Transition Facility, 8308-114 St., Edmonton, AB, Canada T6G 2V2
[5]Department of Surgery, Division of Cardiac Surgery, University of Alberta and 4A7.056 Mazankowski Alberta Heart Institute, 11220-83 Ave, Edmonton, AB, Canada T6G 2B7

Correspondence should be addressed to David L. Bigam; dbigam@ualberta.ca

Academic Editor: Shusen Zheng

As a result of donation after circulatory death liver grafts' poor tolerance to cold storage, there has been increasing research interest in normothermic machine perfusion. This study aims to systematically review the current literature comparing normothermic perfusion to cold storage in donation after circulatory death liver grafts and complete a meta-analysis of published large animal and human studies. A total of nine porcine studies comparing cold storage to normothermic machine perfusion for donation after circulatory death grafts were included for analysis. There was a significant reduction in AST (mean difference −2291 U/L, CI (−3019, −1563); $P \leq 0.00001$) and ALT (mean difference −175 U/L, CI (−266, −85); $P = 0.0001$), for normothermic perfusion relative to static cold storage, with moderate ($I^2 = 61\%$) and high ($I^2 = 96\%$) heterogeneity, respectively. Total bile production was also significantly higher (mean difference = 174 ml, CI (155, 193); $P \leq 0.00001$). Further research focusing on standardization, performance of this technology following periods of cold storage, economic implications, and clinical trial data focused on donation after circulatory death grafts will be helpful to advance this technology toward routine clinical utilization for these grafts.

1. Introduction

Liver transplant remains the only definitive therapy for end stage liver disease. However the shortage of quality organs remains significant in the United States with 1673 patients dying while on the waitlist and a further 1227 removed, too sick to undergo transplant during 2015 [1]. Due to organ shortage, there has been a rise in the use of extended criteria donors (ECD). These donors include those with significant steatosis, advanced age, and donation after circulatory death (DCD) liver grafts [2].

DCD grafts represent an important source of organs to expand the donor pool. The number of DCD grafts used continues to increase; however there is also a rise in the percentage of DCD grafts recovered but not transplanted [1]. This is a result of these grafts' poor tolerance to static cold storage (SCS) [3], the current standard for organ preservation. DCD grafts are more prone to reperfusion injury and susceptible to ischemic biliary cholangiopathy. As a result, outcomes of DCD transplants have traditionally been marginal showing lower long-term patient and graft survival and increased biliary complications [4]. More recent results show improved graft and patient survival, though ischemic cholangiopathy is still a frequent complication of DCD grafts [5].

Ex vivo perfusion is now being studied as a method of increasing use of DCD grafts. Studies using hypothermic and subnormothermic perfusion have shown promising results in both large animal [6–9] and clinical studies [10]; however, in marginal grafts such as those from DCD, normothermic machine perfusion (NMP) showed superior graft function and preservation of biliary epithelium in animal models [11, 12]. In addition to organ preservation, NMP offers the advantage of being able to assess graft viability during perfusion under physiologic conditions where the graft is metabolically active. It also provides opportunity to deliver and monitor response to therapies in order to resuscitate marginal grafts prior to transplantation. These added benefits have led to growing research interest in NMP for DCD grafts in an effort to expand the organ donor pool. NMP for DCD grafts have been studied primarily in large animal studies where resource allocation only allows for small study subject numbers, and study design is critical to advance this complex technology. Although not used often in animal research, systematic reviews can have an important role for the development of future studies [13]. To our knowledge this is the first systematic review of NMP for DCD liver grafts with a meta-analysis of published data.

The aim of this paper is to systematically review the current literature comparing NMP to SCS in DCD liver grafts in large animal (pig) and human studies. The secondary aim is to complete a meta-analysis of NMP versus SCS livers in published DCD porcine liver perfusions.

2. Methods

2.1. Search Strategy. Searches were conducted in Ovid MEDLINE, OVID EMBASE, EBSCO CINAHL, WOS, SCOPUS, Proquest Dissertations and Theses, and PROSPERO by an expert librarian (SC) in June 2017 and updated in July 2017. Searches employed both controlled vocabularies (e.g., MeSH, EMTREE) and key words such as (DCD livers) and (ex vivo perfusion or normothermic perfusion). Search strategies were adapted for each database. Search strategies are available in the supporting information (S1). No limits were applied.

All full text, porcine, and human trials comparing NMP to SCS for the preservation of DCD livers were included for analysis. Studies that did not include DCD livers and those that focused only on hypothermic or subnormothermic machine perfusion were excluded.

2.2. Selection of Studies. Titles and abstracts from the primary search were reviewed independently by two authors (JN, DS) for studies that met inclusion criteria. When this was not clear from the titles and abstracts, full text articles were reviewed to determine inclusion.

2.3. Outcome Measures. Primary outcomes in ex vivo perfusion studies included assessment of alanine aminotransferase (ALT) and aspartate aminotransferase (AST) levels as markers of hepatocellular damage, as well as bile production and lactate clearance as markers of liver function. Secondary outcomes were histological preservation and hemodynamic stability indicated by hepatic arterial flow. Primary outcomes in orthotopic pig liver transplant studies included posttransplant peak AST, bile production, and graft survival. Secondary outcomes included histologic preservation. Where there was missing data for quantitative analysis, this information was requested via email from the publication corresponding authors. We received two responses but no further data for inclusion. Where possible, this data was estimated from published figures using Adobe Acrobat Reader DC software.

2.4. Assessment of Bias. Articles were assessed by two authors (JN, DS) using the Systematic Review Centre for Laboratory Animal Experimentation (SYRCLE) risk of bias assessment tool [14].

2.5. Statistical Analysis. A trained statistician performed statistical analysis. Outcomes assessed in the meta-analysis included AST, ALT, total bile production, and hepatic artery flow for perfusion studies, as well as peak AST for transplant studies. They are all continuous variables expressed as mean ± standard deviation (SD). The mean difference (MD) was used as a summary measure of efficacy between groups treated by NMP and SCS. When no SD was provided, a pooled SD was estimated as previously described [15]. Meta-analysis was performed using RevMan 5.3 software. Heterogeneity of studies was assessed and the following cut-offs were applied, low (>25%), moderate (>50%), and high (>75%) as described by Higgins et al. [16].

3. Results

3.1. Search Results. Three hundred and eighty-six titles were identified through our primary search, with 228 remaining for screening after the removal of duplicates. Of these, 201 titles were excluded for the following reasons: published abstract with no complete full text article, comparison of hypothermic or subnormothermic perfusion without NMP, and studies without DCD grafts. Nine articles that directly compared cold storage to NMP for DCD grafts were included for analysis (Figure 1). Six articles were perfusion studies [11, 17–21] and two pig transplant models [22, 23]. One article published results of both a perfusion model and pig transplant model [12]. There are no clinical trials directly comparing SCS to NMP specifically for DCD livers and as such the studies included for analysis were limited to porcine experimental studies. The results of included studies are summarized in Tables 1 and 2.

3.2. Pig Liver Ex Vivo Perfusion Studies. Pooled data showed a significant reduction in AST at the end of the simulated transplant phase in the NMP group relative to SCS (MD = −2291 U/L, CI (−3019, −1563); $P \leq 0.00001$). A similar trend was seen in ALT (MD= −175 U/L, CI (−266, −85); $P = 0.0001$). However the heterogeneity was moderate ($I^2 = 61\%$) and high ($I^2 = 90\%$), respectively, for these two variables (Figure 2).

TABLE 1: Summary of pig liver perfusion study results.

Perfusion studies	Perfusate	Preservation time (hr)	Simulated transplant phase (hr)	WIT (min)	N-NMP	N-SCS	AST (U/L) NMP	AST (U/L) SCS	ALT (U/L) NMP	ALT (U/L) SCS	NMP total bile (ml)	SCS total bile (ml)	NMP HA flow (ml/min)	SCS HA flow (ml/min)
Boehnert et al. 2013	Steen	4 SCS + 8 NMP vs. 12 SCS	12	60	6	6	--	--	*69 ± 21	*308 ± 45	--	--	340 ± 85	180 ± 35
Liu et al. 2014	Whole blood	10	24	60	5	5	*309	*3163 ± 1545	*25	*186 ± 98	219 ± 42.5	11.6 ± 16.3	23 ± 7 ml/min/100 g liver	13 ± 3 ml/min/100 g
Banan et al. 2015	Saline + whole blood	6	2	40	3	3	610 ± 121	1942 ± 641	63 ± 10	109 ± 10	--	--	*504	*480 ± 60
Nassar et al. 2015	Acellular solutions + whole blood	10	24	60	15	5	1029 ± 230	3150 ± 691	46 ± 8	184 ± 43	181 ± 18	12 ± 7	94 ± 7 ml/min/100 g	57 ± 14 ml/min/100 g
Liu et al. 2016	Steen + RBC	10	24	60	5	5	*931 ± 793	3151 ± 1547	*40	185 ± 97	174 ± 30	12 ± 16	--	--
Nassar et al. 2016	Whole blood	10	24	60	5	5	277 ± 69	3150 ± 1546	22 ± 2	185 ± 97	219 ± 43	12 ± 16	--	--
St Peter et al. 2002	Whole blood	24	24	60	4	4	259	3810	*66 ± 20	*398 ± 74	--	--	1400 ml/min	440 ml/min

* denotes values estimated from published figures where raw data are not available for analysis. -- denotes data not available for meta-analysis. AST/ALT values are taken at the end of the simulated transplant reperfusion phase. HA flows are ml/min unless units otherwise specified.

TABLE 2: Summary of pig orthotopic liver transplant studies.

Pig transplant studies	Preservation time (hr)	Duration of posttransplant monitoring	NMP n =	SCS n =	NMP peak AST (U/L)	SCS peak AST(U/L)
Schön et al. 2001	4	7 days	6	6	603 ± 141	1570 ± 171
Fondevila et al. 2011	4	5 days	6	6	692 ± 77	1500 ± 269
Boehnert et al. 2013	12	8 hours	6	6	524 ± 187	1809 ± 205

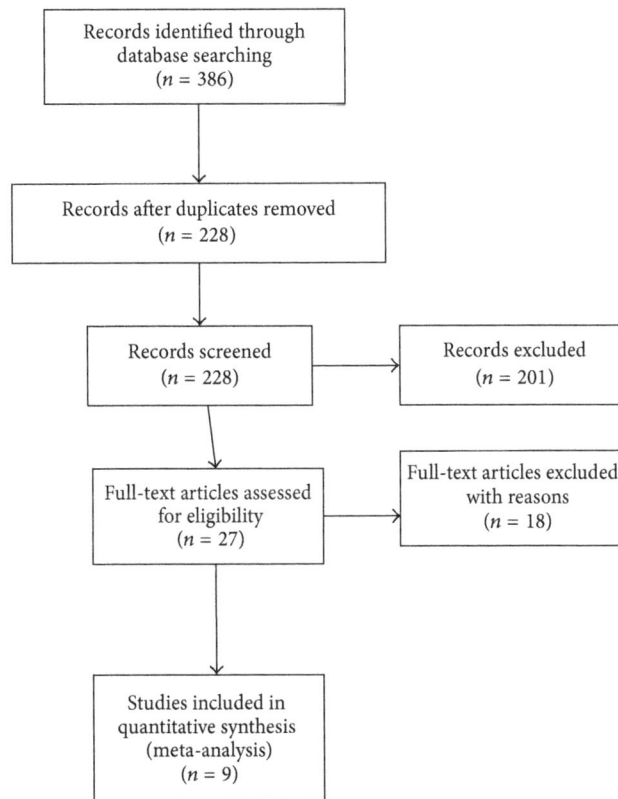

Records identified through database searching (n = 386)

Records after duplicates removed (n = 228)

Records screened (n = 228)

Records excluded (n = 201)

Full-text articles assessed for eligibility (n = 27)

Full-text articles excluded, with reasons (n = 18)

Studies included in quantitative synthesis (meta-analysis) (n = 9)

FIGURE 1: Study selection.

Total bile production following the simulated transplant phase was significantly higher in the NMP group (MD = 174 ml, CI (155, 193); P < 0.00001). There was low heterogeneity (I^2 = 45%) (Figure 2).

There was insufficient data available to perform meta-analysis for lactate clearance.

Limited data was available for hepatic arterial flow. The NMP group did demonstrate higher flows, although this did not reach statistical significance (P = 0.09) (Figure 2).

Different histological scoring systems were used by different centers and thus were not suitable for meta-analysis. All perfusion studies showed less necrosis and improved architectural preservation in the NMP group relative to SCS [11, 12, 17–21]. Similarly, NMP demonstrated improved preservation of the biliary epithelium and peribiliary plexus [11, 17, 20].

3.3. Pig Liver Orthotopic Transplant Studies. Posttransplant peak AST was lower in the NMP group (MD = −1019, CI (−1276, −762); P < 0.00001). There was a high level of heterogeneity (I^2 = 78%) (Figure 3). There was insufficient data available to compare bile production. Graft survival also was not assessed in the meta-analysis, as the recovery period in each of these studies was different (Table 2). Boehnert et al.

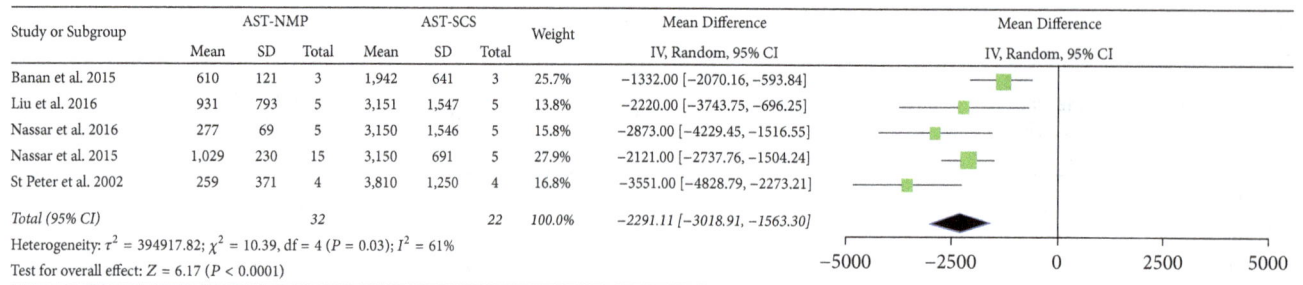

(a)

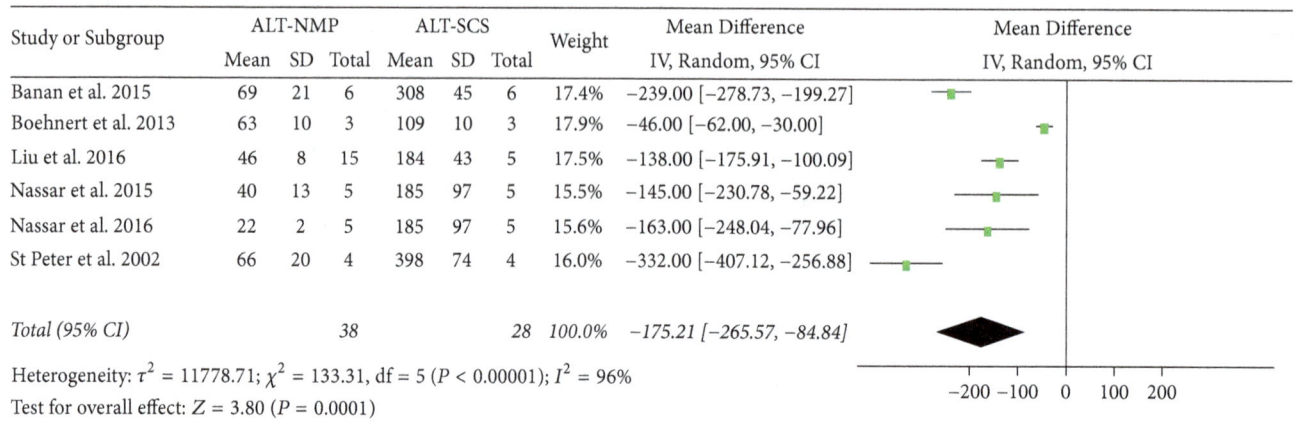

(b)

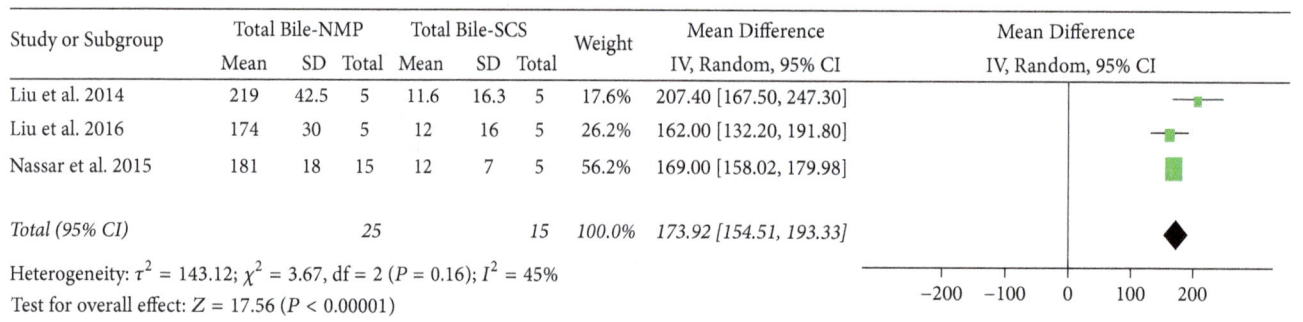

(c)

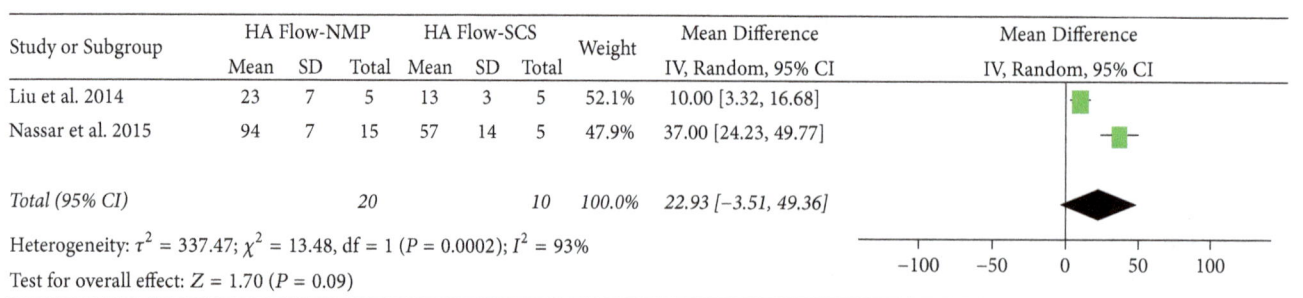

(d)

FIGURE 2: Forest plots showing pooled AST, ALT, and bile production data from porcine liver perfusion studies.

reported no difference in bile production in the eight hours following transplant after perfusing with acellular solution [12]. Schön et al. showed all grafts transplanted after 60 minutes of WIT and SCS suffered primary graft nonfunction [22].

In an uncontrolled DCD transplant model where normothermic extracorporeal membrane oxygenation was combined with either NMP or SCS, there was 100% five-day survival in the NMP group relative to 83% survival in the SCS group [23].

Study or Subgroup	Peak AST-NMP			Peak AST-SCS			Weight	Mean Difference	Mean Difference
	Mean	SD	Total	Mean	SD	Total		IV, Random, 95% CI	IV, Random, 95% CI
Boehnert et al. 2013	524	187	6	1,809	205	6	32.3%	−1285.00 [−1507.02, −1062.98]	
Fondevila et al. 2011	692	77	6	1,500	269	6	32.2%	−808.00 [−1031.89, −584.11]	
Schön et al. 2001	603	141	6	1,570	171	6	35.4%	−967.00 [−1144.34, −789.66]	
Total (95% CI)			18			18	100.0%	−1018.64 [−1275.65, −761.62]	

Heterogeneity: $\tau^2 = 40332.12$; $\chi^2 = 9.24$, df = 2 ($P = 0.010$); $I^2 = 78\%$
Test for overall effect: $Z = 7.77$ ($P < 0.00001$)

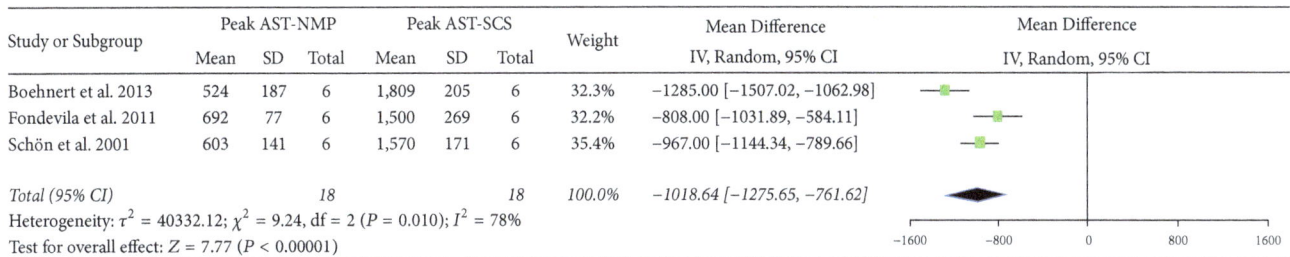

FIGURE 3: Forest plots showing pooled peak AST data from porcine orthotopic liver transplant studies.

NMP groups demonstrated less necrosis, sinusoidal swelling, and improved overall architectural preservation relative to SCS groups [22, 23]. One pig transplant model did not report histologic data [24].

3.4. Risk of Bias Assessment. The allocation process of animals was unclear in several studies [12, 21–23]; however no other significant sources of bias within the included studies were identified.

4. Discussion

The results of this review and meta-analysis must be interpreted with caution, as heterogeneity was high within the perfusion studies limiting the strength of conclusions that can be drawn. Experimental design for the included perfusion studies varied in several fundamental parameters. Major differences included surgical model, duration of preservation and reperfusion, and ex vivo circuit design.

Pigs used as liver donors were 30–40 kg and included landrace [18, 21] and Yorkshire [11, 12, 17, 19, 20], with male pigs used only by Boehnert et al. [25] and gender unspecified ones in one study [21]. The DCD model also varied between studies with the majority inducing cardiac arrest with potassium chloride injection [11, 17–21], while one study induced cardiac arrest via exsanguination [12].

Boehnert et al. work was the only perfusion study to compare SCS to NMP following a period of SCS [12]. The WIT in all included perfusion studies was 60 minutes except for Banan et al. [18] who compared SCS after 40 minutes of WIT to NMP following 20, 40, and 60 minutes of WIT. Following WIT livers were flushed with histidine-tryptophan-ketoglutarate [11, 17–20], University of Wisconsin [12], or Euro Collins [21] cold preservation solutions. Livers were flushed in situ [11, 12, 18, 19, 21] or ex situ [17, 20] with dual perfusion through the hepatic artery and portal vein [11, 17–20] or single arterial flush [21]. One study did not specify if dual vessel flush was used [12].

NMP was then carried out for either 6 [18], 8 [12], 10 [11, 17, 19, 20], or 24 [21] hours. Simulated transplant with whole blood reperfusion was for either 2 [18], 12 [12], or 24 [11, 17, 19–21] hours, which is of important note as transaminase levels were reported at the end of the reperfusion stage.

One study included a dialysis circuit as part of the perfusion setup [18]. Flow was driven by either dual centrifugal pumps [18], the combination of a centrifugal pump and roller pump[11, 17, 19, 20], or a centrifugal pump to perfuse the hepatic artery and the portal vein perfused by gravity [12, 21]. With regard to perfusate used, three studies used whole blood [11, 17, 21], two used dilute whole blood [18, 19], and one used acellular perfusate [12]. The study by Liu et al. is the only one to directly compare different perfusates [20], using Steen solution, Steen solution with washed red blood cells, and whole blood compared to SCS. Hepatocellular injury and liver function were significantly better in the Steen solution with red blood cells and whole blood groups relative to both SCS or Steen solution alone. There was no significant difference between the whole blood or Steen solution with washed red blood cells [20]. Within the included studies there was not enough available data to perform subgroup analysis based on type of perfusate used. However, the results with acellular perfusion [12] to our knowledge have not been replicated and more studies are still needed to determine the optimal NMP perfusate composition for DCD livers; however the results from Liu et al. [20] suggest the need for an oxygen carrier.

In porcine liver transplant models there was also significant study heterogeneity. The posttransplant observation period ranged from eight hours to seven days. Fondevila et al. [23] compared NMP to SCS following a period of normothermic extracorporeal machine oxygenation, which was significantly different from the other included transplant studies. Schön et al. compared SCS to NMP with no period of SCS and all grafts that were exposed to 4 hours of cold storage following 60 minutes of WIT suffered primary nonfunction [22]. This is in keeping with previous data suggesting that even brief periods of cold storage can impact positive effects of NMP [3]. The study by Boehnert et al., however, compared SCS alone to a period of SCS followed by NMP and reported less hepatocellular injury in the NMP group [12], but data from these grafts were only reported for eight hours after transplant and longer-term survival of the grafts was not assessed. In discarded human liver studies, NMP has shown the ability to recover function of damaged livers even after extensive periods of cold storage [26]. Further research to address NMP's ability to safely recover and transplant DCD grafts following periods of cold storage is needed. Devices available for NMP were reviewed by Ravikumar et al. [27] and portable perfusion devices are now available to try and eliminate cold storage time in the transplant sequence for these marginal organs. Whether NMP can successfully recover DCD grafts after periods of cold storage remains an important question that will impact the clinical implementation of ex vivo NMP. The economic impact of these systems has not yet been studied and will also remain a factor in clinical implementation of NMP for DCD grafts. The use of gradual rewarming has shown promise for this population of liver grafts [28–31] and may play an important role moving forward in utilizing machine perfusion after periods of SCS.

NMP has shown capacity to recover function in discarded DCD human liver studies [26, 32–35] and has been used to recover these grafts for clinical transplant [36, 37]. NMP has also been studied as a method to assess which marginal DCD grafts are safely transplantable. A set of viability criteria has been proposed by Mergental et al. [37]. Establishing a standardized set of criteria will be an important goal for clinical implementation of NMP for DCD grafts.

There are phase I clinical trials comparing NMP to SCS [38–40]; however these studies have only limited numbers of DCD and otherwise marginal grafts. To date no randomized control trials have been published comparing NMP to SCS specifically in DCD grafts. Results of a multicenter European randomized control trial (ISRCTN39731134) comparing NMP to SCS, once published, may be pivotal for this technology moving forward into clinical practice.

5. Limitations

There was a large amount of heterogeneity amongst the small number of studies as outlined above. These significant differences in experimental design limit the strength of conclusions that could be drawn from meta-analysis. Furthermore, multiple data points included for meta-analysis were estimated from published figures which may differ slightly from the measured values.

6. Conclusion

Meta-analysis of published porcine perfusion studies demonstrates that NMP is superior to SCS regarding the preservation of liver architecture and function in DCD grafts. Given significant differences between studies, these results are to be taken with caution. Further study is still required in order to optimize and standardize perfusate composition and to evaluate NMP's role in preservation following periods of cold storage. Clinical studies involving more DCD grafts will help bring this technology closer to clinical implementation. Economic factors need to be considered in subsequent studies to ensure feasibility within current healthcare systems.

Acknowledgments

The authors would like to thank Chunhong Tian for statistical assistance.

References

[1] W. R. Kim, J. R. Lake, and J. M. Smith, "OPTN/SRTR 2013 annual data report: liver," *American Journal of Transplantation*, vol. 15, 1, pp. 174–251, 2015.

[2] R. W. Busuttil and K. Tanaka, "The utility of marginal donors in liver transplantation," *Liver Transplantation*, vol. 9, no. 7, pp. 651–663, 2003.

[3] S. Reddy, J. Greenwood, N. Maniakin et al., "Non-heart-beating donor porcine livers: The adverse effect of cooling," *Liver Transplantation*, vol. 11, no. 1, pp. 35–38, 2005.

[4] D. P. Foley, L. A. Fernandez, G. Leverson et al., "Biliary complications after liver transplantation from donation after cardiac death donors: an analysis of risk factors and long-term outcomes from a single center," *Annals of Surgery*, vol. 253, no. 4, pp. 817–825, 2011.

[5] J. C. Coffey, K. N. Wanis, D. Monbaliu et al., "The influence of functional warm ischemia time on DCD liver transplant recipients' outcomes," *Clinical Transplantation*, vol. 31, no. 10, Article ID e13068, 2017.

[6] S. Op Den Dries, M. E. Sutton, N. Karimian et al., "Hypothermic oxygenated machine perfusion prevents arteriolonecrosis of the peribiliary plexus in pig livers donated after circulatory death," *PLoS ONE*, vol. 9, no. 2, Article ID e88521, 2014.

[7] K. Vekemans, Q. Liu, J. Brassil, M. Komuta, J. Pirenne, and D. Monbaliu, "Influence of Flow and Addition of Oxygen During Porcine Liver Hypothermic Machine Perfusion," *Transplantation Proceedings*, vol. 39, no. 8, pp. 2647–2651, 2007.

[8] E. Gringeri, P. Bonsignore, D. Bassi et al., "Subnormothermic machine perfusion for non-heart-beating donor liver grafts preservation in a swine model: A new strategy to increase the donor pool?" *Transplantation Proceedings*, vol. 44, no. 7, pp. 2026–2028, 2012.

[9] J. M. Knaak, V. N. Spetzler, N. Goldaracena et al., "Subnormothermic ex vivo liver perfusion reduces endothelial cell and bile duct injury after donation after cardiac death pig liver transplantation," *Liver Transplantation*, vol. 20, no. 11, pp. 1296–1305, 2014.

[10] J. V. Guarrera, S. D. Henry, B. Samstein et al., "Hypothermic machine preservation in human liver transplantation: The first clinical series," *American Journal of Transplantation*, vol. 10, no. 2, pp. 372–381, 2010.

[11] A. Nassar, Q. Liu, K. Farias et al., "Impact of Temperature on Porcine Liver Machine Perfusion From Donors After Cardiac Death," *Artificial Organs*, vol. 40, no. 10, pp. 999–1008, 2016.

[12] M. U. Boehnert, J. C. Yeung, F. Bazerbachi et al., "Normothermic acellular ex vivo liver perfusion reduces liver and bile duct injury of pig livers retrieved after cardiac death," *American Journal of Transplantation*, vol. 13, no. 6, pp. 1441–1449, 2013.

[13] R. B. M. de Vries, K. E. Wever, M. T. Avey, M. L. Stephens, E. S. Sena, and M. Leenaars, "The usefulness of systematic reviews of animal experiments for the design of preclinical and clinical studies," *ILAR Journal*, vol. 55, no. 3, pp. 427–437, 2014.

[14] C. R. Hooijmans, M. M. Rovers, R. B. M. De Vries, M. Leenaars, M. Ritskes-Hoitinga, and M. W. Langendam, "SYRCLE's risk of

bias tool for animal studies," *BMC Medical Research Methodology*, vol. 14, no. 1, article no. 43, 2014.

[15] T. A. Furukawa, C. Barbui, A. Cipriani, P. Brambilla, and N. Watanabe, "Imputing missing standard deviations in meta-analyses can provide accurate results," *Journal of Clinical Epidemiology*, vol. 59, no. 1, pp. 7–10, 2006.

[16] J. P. T. Higgins, S. G. Thompson, J. J. Deeks, and D. G. Altman, "Measuring inconsistency in meta-analyses," *British Medical Journal*, vol. 327, no. 7414, pp. 557–560, 2003.

[17] Q. Liu, A. Nassar, K. Farias et al., "Sanguineous normothermic machine perfusion improves hemodynamics and biliary epithelial regeneration in donation after cardiac death porcine livers," *Liver Transplantation*, vol. 20, no. 8, pp. 987–999, 2014.

[18] B. Banan, H. Chung, Z. Xiao et al., "Normothermic extracorporeal liver perfusion for donation after cardiac death (DCD) livers," *Surgery*, vol. 158, no. 6, pp. 1642–1650, 2015.

[19] A. Nassar, Q. Liu, K. Farias et al., "Ex vivo normothermic machine perfusion is safe, simple, and reliable: Results from a large animal model," *Surgical Innovation*, vol. 22, no. 1, pp. 61–69, 2015.

[20] Q. Liu, A. Nassar, K. Farias et al., "Comparing Normothermic Machine Perfusion Preservation with Different Perfusates on Porcine Livers from Donors after Circulatory Death," *American Journal of Transplantation*, vol. 16, no. 3, pp. 794–807, 2016.

[21] S. D. St Peter, C. J. Imber, I. Lopez, D. Hughes, and P. J. Friend, "Extended preservation of non-heart-beating donor livers with normothermic machine perfusion," *British Journal of Surgery*, vol. 89, no. 5, pp. 609–616, 2002.

[22] M. R. Schön, O. Kollmar, S. Wolf et al., "Liver transplantation after organ preservation with normothermic extracorporeal perfusion," *Annals of Surgery*, vol. 233, no. 1, pp. 114–123, 2001.

[23] C. Fondevila, A. J. Hessheimer, M.-H. J. Maathuis et al., "Superior preservation of DCD livers with continuous normothermic perfusion," *Annals of Surgery*, vol. 254, no. 6, pp. 1000–1007, 2011.

[24] M. U. Boehnert, J. Yeung, J.-M. Knaak et al., "Acellular Normothermic Ex Vivo Liver Perfusion (Nevlp) Decreases Hepatocyte and Bile Duct Injury in Livers Retrieved After Cardiac Death," *Hepatology*, vol. 54, 1, p. 386A, 2011.

[25] M. U. Boehnert, J. C. Yeung, J. M. Knaak, N. Selzner, and M. Selzner, "Normothermic acellular ex vivo liver perfusion (NEVLP) reduces liver and bile duct in DCD liver grafts," *American Journal of Transplantation*, vol. 13, no. 12, p. 3290, 2013.

[26] T. Vogel, J. G. Brockmann, A. Quaglia et al., "The 24-hour normothermic machine perfusion of discarded human liver grafts," *Liver Transplantation*, vol. 23, no. 2, pp. 207–220, 2017.

[27] R. Ravikumar, H. Leuvenink, and P. J. Friend, "Normothermic liver preservation: A new paradigm?" *Transplant International*, vol. 28, no. 6, pp. 690–699, 2015.

[28] T. Shigeta, N. Matsuno, H. Obara et al., "Impact of rewarming preservation by continuous machine perfusion: Improved post-transplant recovery in pigs," *Transplantation Proceedings*, vol. 45, no. 5, pp. 1684–1689, 2013.

[29] B. Banan, Z. Xiao, R. Watson et al., "Novel strategy to decrease reperfusion injuries and improve function of cold-preserved livers using normothermic ex vivo liver perfusion machine," *Liver Transplantation*, vol. 22, no. 3, pp. 333–343, 2016.

[30] H. Obara, N. Matsuno, T. Shigeta, T. Hirano, S. Enosawa, and H. Mizunuma, "Temperature controlled machine perfusion system for liver," *Transplantation Proceedings*, vol. 45, no. 5, pp. 1690–1692, 2013.

[31] T. Minor, P. Efferz, M. Fox, J. Wohlschlaeger, and B. Lüer, "Controlled oxygenated rewarming of cold stored liver grafts by thermally graduated machine perfusion prior to reperfusion," *American Journal of Transplantation*, vol. 13, no. 6, pp. 1450–1460, 2013.

[32] R. Bellomo, B. Marino, G. Starkey et al., "Extended normothermic extracorporeal perfusion of isolated human liver after warm ischaemia: a preliminary report," *Critical Care And Resuscitation: Journal of The Australasian Academy of Critical Care Medicine*, vol. 16, no. 3, pp. 197–201, 2014.

[33] B. Banan, R. Watson, M. Xu, Y. Lin, and W. Chapman, "Development of a normothermic extracorporeal liver perfusion system toward improving viability and function of human extended criteria donor livers," *Liver Transplantation*, vol. 22, no. 7, pp. 979–993, 2016.

[34] S. Op Den Dries, N. Karimian, M. E. Sutton et al., "Ex vivo normothermic machine perfusion and viability testing of discarded human donor livers," *American Journal of Transplantation*, vol. 13, no. 5, pp. 1327–1335, 2013.

[35] M. E. Sutton, S. Op Den Dries, N. Karimian et al., "Criteria for Viability Assessment of Discarded Human Donor Livers during Ex Vivo Normothermic Machine Perfusion," *PLoS ONE*, vol. 9, no. 11, Article ID e110642, 2014.

[36] C. J. E. Watson, V. Kosmoliaptsis, L. V. Randle et al., "Normothermic perfusion in the assessment and preservation of declined livers before transplantation: Hyperoxia and vasoplegia-important lessons from the first 12 cases," *Transplantation*, vol. 101, no. 5, pp. 1084–1098, 2017.

[37] H. Mergental, M. T. P. R. Perera, R. W. Laing et al., "Transplantation of Declined Liver Allografts Following Normothermic Ex-Situ Evaluation," *American Journal of Transplantation*, vol. 16, no. 11, pp. 3235–3245, 2016.

[38] R. Ravikumar, W. Jassem, H. Mergental et al., "Liver Transplantation After Ex Vivo Normothermic Machine Preservation: A Phase 1 (First-in-Man) Clinical Trial," *American Journal of Transplantation*, vol. 16, no. 6, pp. 1779–1787, 2016.

[39] M. Selzner, N. Goldaracena, J. Echeverri et al., "Normothermic ex vivo liver perfusion using steen solution as perfusate for human liver transplantation: First North American results," *Liver Transplantation*, vol. 22, no. 11, pp. 1501–1508, 2016.

[40] M. Bral, B. Gala-Lopez, D. Bigam et al., "Preliminary Single-Center Canadian Experience of Human Normothermic Ex Vivo Liver Perfusion: Results of a Clinical Trial," *American Journal of Transplantation*, vol. 17, no. 4, pp. 1071–1080, 2017.

19

Combined Liver and Multivisceral Resections

Martin de Santibañes,[1] **Agustin Dietrich,**[2] **and Eduardo de Santibañes**[1]

[1] *Department of Hepato-Biliary-Pancreatic Surgery & Liver Transplant Unit, Hospital Italiano de Buenos Aires, Perón 4190, 1181 Buenos Aires, Argentina*
[2] *Department of General Surgery, Hospital Italiano de Buenos Aires, Perón 4190, 1181 Buenos Aires, Argentina*

Correspondence should be addressed to Martin de Santibañes; martin.desantibanes@hospitalitaliano.org.ar

Academic Editor: Daniel Casanova

Background. Combined liver and multivisceral resections are infrequent procedures, which demand extensive experience and considerable surgical skills. *Methods.* An electronic search of literature related to this topic published before June 2013 was performed. *Results.* There is limited scientific evidence of the feasibility and clinical outcomes of these complex procedures. The majority of these cases are simultaneous resections of colorectal tumors with liver metastases. Combined liver and multivisceral resections can be performed with acceptable postoperative morbidity and mortality rates only in carefully selected patients. *Conclusion.* Lack of experience in these aggressive surgeries justifies a careful selection of patients, considering their comorbidities.

1. Introduction

Multivisceral resections associated with liver surgery are infrequent procedures that require considerable skills and extensive experience in general and liver surgery. Information regarding the feasibility and clinical outcomes of these combined procedures is very limited. The majority of cases come from colorectal carcinoma with synchronic liver metastases [1].

Over the last decade, there has been substantial progress in the understanding of liver anatomy and the technical aspects of major resections. Anaesthetic management and perioperative and intensive care have also significantly improved, making this kind of extensive surgeries feasible. However, it is important to carefully select the patients who will benefit from these major procedures. Properly defined selection criteria to do so are missing. The aim of this paper is to review the scientific evidence related to these complex procedures.

2. Surgical Indications for Combined Liver and Multivisceral Resections

Combined liver and multivisceral resections can arise in the case of an en bloc resection of tumors that have directly infiltrated other organs or in the circumstance of simultaneous resections of primary tumors along with distinct sites of metastatic extent. The last scenario has the advantage of offering a staged procedure, therefore avoiding a simultaneous multivisceral resection and its related risk. Table 1 shows the pathological etiologies that can be part of these clinical scenarios. The lack of experience in these aggressive approaches justifies a careful selection of patients, considering their comorbidity and procedure related complications rate.

3. Importance of Imaging in Patients' Selection

A radiological assessment enables a successful and effective stratification of patients that could result in better surgery outcomes. Multidetectors computed tomography (MDCT) and magnetic resonance imaging (MRI) have the advantage of allowing for preoperative staging and planning a surgical strategy. Both can evaluate the relationship between the primary tumor and the adjacent structures (stomach, colon, kidney, etc.), therefore anticipating multivisceral resections [2, 3] (Figures 1 and 2). They can also determine venous commitment (inferior vena cava, renal veins, superior mesenteric vein, and portal vein) or arterial invasion (celiac axis,

TABLE 1: Etiology for combined liver and multivisceral resections.

Primary tumors with liver infiltration

    Retroperitoneal sarcomas

    Renal tumor

    Adrenal tumor with liver and/or vena cava

    Tumors with splanchnic origin

Metastatic tumors

    Colorectal cancer

    Noncolorectal nonneuroendocrine metastases

    Neuroendocrine tumor

    Gist tumors

Liver tumor with splacnic infiltration

Hepatobiliary tumor that invade splacnic organs: hepatocarcinoma, cholangiocarcinoma, gallbladder carcinoma, hepatic sarcomas, and other mesenchymal tumors

hepatic artery, superior mesenteric artery, and aorta) to select candidates for neoadjuvant treatment [4].

They are valuable as well for the:

(i) assessment of liver tumor load (size, number of lesions, etc.) and evaluation of peritoneal and extra-hepatic disease [5, 6],

(ii) determination of liver volumes and estimation of hypertrophy degree of the future liver remnant (FLR) [2, 7, 8],

(iii) surgical planning of hepatic resection centered on the anatomical relationship of the tumor (vascular structures) [2] and radiological staging to increase the rate of resection with curative purpose [2, 9],

(iv) evaluation of biological tumour response to neoadju-vant/adjuvant chemotherapy [10],

(v) patients' followup after surgical resection.

Depending on the origin of the primary tumor (colorectal, neuroendocrine, etc.), it is important to exclude the presence of distant metastases (brain, lung, and bones) using other imaging methods such as positron emission tomography scan, Octreoscan, and bone scintigraphy.

4. Preoperative Stratification of Patient's Surgical Risk

4.1. Major Abdominal Surgery. Study of preoperative risk factors in major abdominal surgery can improve patient selection and postoperative outcomes. Borja-Cacho et al. [11] assessed the factors collected by the American College of Surgeons National Surgery Quality Improvement Program (ACS NSQIP) in major cancer surgeries to predict adverse operative events. This multicentric study highlights that older age (≥75 years) and ASA score (>3) can predict prolonged length of stay, major complications, and 30-day mortality. Cardiac and pulmonary diseases also present direct relationship with patients' postoperative outcomes in major abdominal surgeries [12]. This is caused by inadequate tissue

oxygenation during the perioperative course because of a cardiorespiratory malfunction [13]. Al-Refaie et al. [12] found similar results in the ACS NSQIP, reporting a higher incidence of higher operative mortality, greater frequency of major complications, and more prolonged hospital stays in older patients (>75 years).

In patients who underwent major abdominal surgeries, preoperative anesthetics evaluation becomes indispensable. The American Society of Anesthesiologists (ASA) physical status classification is the most prevalent and worldwide used score that stratifies patients according to their preoperative risk. Others describe ASA score as a strong predictor of hospital length stay [14]. There still remains the need to identify more preoperative risk assessment tools in order to predict with higher accuracy the incidence of postoperative complications [15].

4.2. Liver Resections. Schroeder et al. [16] analysed records of the National Surgical Quality Improvement in USA of postoperative morbidity and mortality in 587 patients who underwent liver resection, highlighting ASA score as a superior score than other indexes to predict postoperative morbidity. With respect to this, Belghiti et al. [17] among 747 hepatectomies (45% major liver resections) demonstrated that the ASA score not only was an independent risk factor for postoperative complications, but also significantly influenced patient mortality.

Obesity and diabetes are known related factors associated with hepatic steatosis and steatohepatitis [18], both associated with adverse outcomes after liver resection [19]. This popula-tion of patients also present a higher risk of anastomotic leaks, especially when undergoing rectal resections [20]. The use of body mass index (BMI) as a measure of patient obesity and as predictor of postoperative morbidity is clearly discussed. For ACS NSQIP, BMI has minimal association with short-term operative outcomes after major cancer surgery [21].

Specifically, even though neoadjuvant treatment appears to be well tolerated and often successful, some reports have informed that chemotherapeutic agents are associated with significant hepatotoxicity and resulting liver failure [22]. The histopathologic changes described in liver specimens include steatosis [23], sinusoidal injuries [24], and steatohepatitis [25]. These histologic changes may generate higher morbidity and even postoperative mortality.

4.3. Combined Resections. There is a critical difference in morbidity and mortality when simultaneous nonhepatic procedures were associated with major liver resections [26–28]. Although the lack of evidence in combined resections, prognosis risk factors like ASA score, associated pancreas and liver resections on elderly patients should be highlighted [11]. Additionally, the surgeons' experience and performance at high-volume hospitals are other complimentary factors. Birkmeyer et al. [29] analysed the relation between volume and outcomes in 2.5 millions major surgical procedures in USA, finding large differences in mortality between very-low-volume and very-high-volume hospitals. Perioperative outcomes of major pancreatic or hepatic resections present a

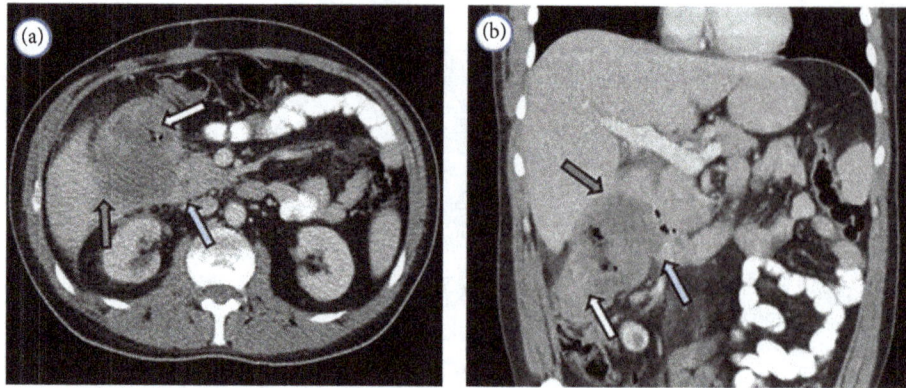

FIGURE 1: Abdominal and pelvic multidetector computed tomography (MDCT) in a patient with a large colonic tumor (white arrow), which compromises duodenum and pancreatic head (blue arrow) and the right liver (grey arrow).

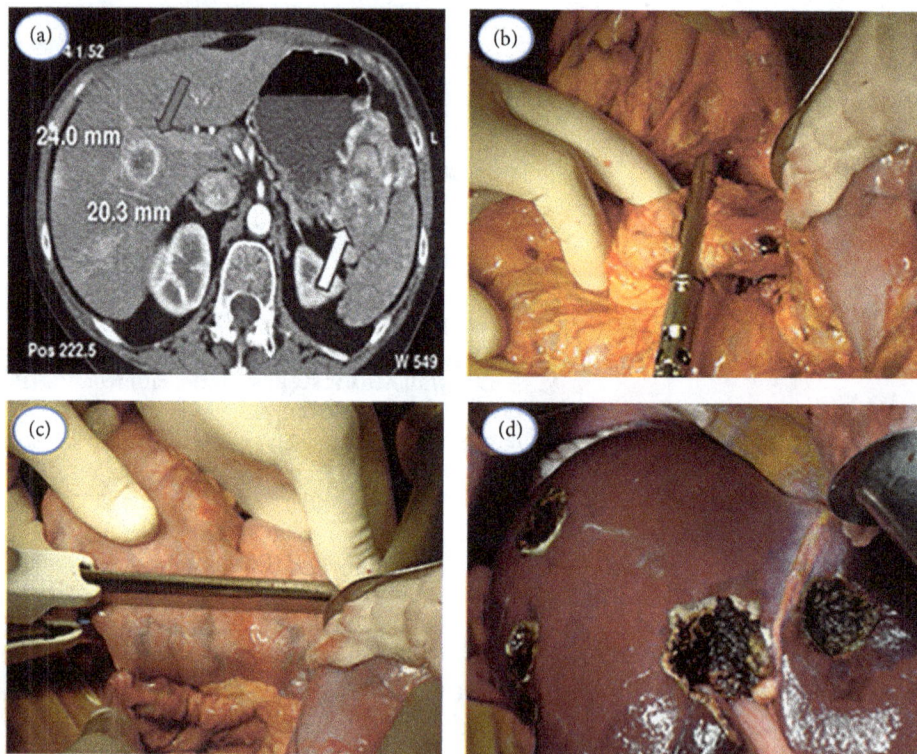

FIGURE 2: MCDT (a) and intraoperative images (b, c, and d) of a patient with an advanced pancreatic neuroendocrine tumour. (a) MCDT of a patient with diagnosis of a pancreatic neuroendocrine tumor, which involves the pancreas, splenic hilus, and the stomach (white arrow) with liver metastases (Grey arrow). (b) Distal pancreatectomy and splenectomy. (c) Atypical gastrectomy. (d) Multiple liver metastasectomies.

solid relationship with the number of performed procedures at a particular hospital [30–33]. Surgeon's volume seems to be an independent prognostic factor of patient's postoperative outcomes [34]. High-volume surgeons could improve postoperative outcomes after pancreatic or hepatic surgery [35, 36].

5. Intraoperative Risk Factors

Longer operation time, blood loss, and more frequent blood transfusions are commonly observed in multivisceral resections [37]. Operative time longer than 300 minutes due to

pancreatic malignancies was identified as an independent risk factor for the development of intra-abdominal complications [38] with a higher risk of septic events [39].

Blood loss remains a critical aspect during liver resection. Excessive bleeding and subsequent transfusions correlate with postoperative morbidity [40]. Jarnagin et al. [41] described blood loss as an independent predictor of perioperative morbidity and mortality in patients who underwent major liver resection associated with another surgical procedure. In the last years, intraoperative fluid management was reviewed [42, 43]. Adequate anaesthetic techniques to preserve a low central venous pressure, less than 5 mmhg, during extrahepatic dissection and parenchymal transection became necessary to minimize bleeding and the need of blood transfusion [44]. Monitoring lactate levels during the operative time represent an important parameter to control fluid administration [45].

6. Postoperative Patient Management

We already discussed the importance of high-volume centers in surgical outcomes. Dimick et al. [46] analyse the frequency of rounds by an intensivist in ICU of 35 hospitals, associating daily rounds with shorter lengths of stay and decreased frequency of postoperative complications. Another study evaluated the relationship between nurse-to-patient ratios in the ICU, showing that fewer nurses per patient increase number of postoperative respiratory related complications [47]. Linke et al. [48] highlighted the role of the surgeon as a leader of a multidisciplinary team in the ICU, not only for his unique knowledge of the patient's anatomy and physiology, but also to make a rapid diagnosis of surgical related complications.

Postoperative thrombosis is another critical issue in these patients. The routine use of venous thromboembolism chemoprophylaxis after hepatic surgery remains controversial, especially in complex resections, when the risk of postoperative bleeding complications influences bleeding more than the risk of postoperative thrombosis [49, 50]. However, due the short experience in liver resections associated with other abdominal procedures, indications of perioperative chemoprophylaxis should be evaluated individually.

7. Surgical Strategies

7.1. The Role of Staging Laparoscopy. Staging laparoscopy is a simple and minimally invasive method to recognize occult distant metastatic disease and prevent nontherapeutic laparotomies. However, during the last decade the ability of preoperative imaging to identify metastatic (<5 mm nodules) and locally advanced tumors (vascular invasion) has questioned the role of staging laparoscopy [51]. This method could be indicated in certain situations such as histological confirmation of peritoneal nodules, or high levels of tumor markers.

7.2. Abdominal Exploration and Oncological Surgical Principles. Extended midline incision or a bilateral subcostal incision with midline extension allows adequate access to the upper, lower, or both abdominal contents, depending on the location of the neoplasm. Vertical midline incisions can be combined with transverse laparotomies. Systematic exploration of the entire abdominal cavity is mandatory, in order to rule out unexpected tumor extension.

It is essential not to make irreversible manoeuvres without prior security of primary tumor resectability, especially if there is preoperative suspicion of vascular invasion. The "artery first approach" of the superior mesenteric artery may be helpful for this purpose, particularly in pancreatic malignancies [52].

Multivisceral resections follow the general principle of all oncological surgery attempting an en bloc tumor resection: to achieve clear margins a border of healthy tissue has to be included in the resection. If there are doubts with tumor-free margins, it is essential to make frozen biopsies. Other criteria include systematic lymphadenectomy. The extension of lymph node resections will depend on the origin of the primary tumor.

7.3. Liver Approach. Intraoperative liver ultrasound (IOLUS) represents an essential component of modern liver surgery. It has the potential to show preoperative undetected liver metastases in up to 10–20% of patients [53]. The IOLUS permits the evaluation of hepatic vascular anatomy and its relationship with tumor lesions, supervising the level of resection and the potential for resectability [54].

Associated vascular control techniques in liver surgery such as portal triad clamping and total hepatic vascular exclusion emerge as strategies to perform a safe liver resection minimizing blood loss, controlling hepatic inflow, outflow, or both [55, 56].

Commonly, major liver resections are mandatory to reach tumor-free surgical margins [57]. However, extended hepatectomy increases the risk of the development of postoperative liver failure (PLF) and has been shown to be a predominant cause of hepatectomy related mortality [58].

The assessed FLR volume to avoid PLF should be at least 20% of total liver volume in healthy livers and 30–40% in diseased livers [59, 60]. Portal vein occlusion represents the gold standard technique to induce liver hypertrophy of the FLR, allowing a safe preservation of hepatic reserve to decrease the incidence of PLF [61].

7.4. Simultaneous Resections. Due to lack of evidence of combined liver and multivisceral resections, surgical approaches in these scenarios remain controversial.

The largest experience comes from colorectal metastases. Many surgeons support a simultaneous approach as a safe treatment to liver metastases due to colorectal cancer [62–64]. Weber et al. [62] in his series of 97 patients with synchronous colorectal liver metastases divided patients treated with simultaneous approach and those who underwent a delayed resection, showing that morbidity and mortality rates were similar in both groups. In the same line, de Santibañes et al. [63] presented 185 consecutive patients who underwent simultaneous colorectal and hepatic resection for colorectal malignancy with low rates of postoperative morbidity and mortality (20.5% and 1.08%, resp.). Viganò et al. [64] showed similar results regarding morbidity and mortality. Maybe the most controversial factor and predictor of postoperative poor prognostic is the need to perform an extended hepatectomy. Reddy et al. [65] found an increased mortality and severe morbidity compared to minor hepatectomy in his series of 610 patients who underwent simultaneous or staged resections.

Locally advanced gastric carcinoma can be also associated with multivisceral resection, with acceptable perioperative morbidity, mortality (1.9–15%), and 5-year survival (0–40%)

[66]. A study showed that the most common combined resected organs were the spleen, pancreas, transverse colon, and liver and were not found to be predictors of poor survival on multivariate analysis [67].

Combined liver and multivisceral resections are infrequent procedures, which demand extensive experience and considerable surgical skills. The lack of experience in these aggressive surgeries justifies a careful selection of patients, considering their comorbidities and should be performed in high-volume centers.

References

[1] V. W. T. Lam, J. M. Laurence, T. Pang et al., "A systematic review of a liver-first approach in patients with colorectal cancer and synchronous colorectal liver metastases," *HPB*, 2013.

[2] W. Hartwig, T. Hackert, U. Hinz et al., "Multivisceral resection for pancreatic malignancies: risk-analysis and long-term outcome," *Annals of Surgery*, vol. 250, no. 1, pp. 81–87, 2009.

[3] C. M. Burdelski, M. Reeh, D. Bogoevski et al., "Multivisceral resections in pancreatic cancer: identification of risk factors," *World Journal of Surgery*, vol. 35, no. 12, pp. 2756–2763, 2011.

[4] E. F. Yekebas, D. Bogoevski, G. Cataldegirmen et al., "En bloc vascular resection for locally advanced pancreatic malignancies infiltrating major blood vessels: perioperative outcome and long-term survival in 136 patients," *Annals of Surgery*, vol. 247, no. 2, pp. 300–309, 2008.

[5] M. Kanematsu, H. Kondo, S. Goshima et al., "Imaging liver metastases: review and update," *European Journal of Radiology*, vol. 58, no. 2, pp. 217–228, 2006.

[6] C. Charnsangavej, B. Clary, Y. Fong, A. Grothey, T. M. Pawlik, and M. A. Choti, "Selection of patients for resection of hepatic colorectal metastases: expert consensus statement," *Annals of Surgical Oncology*, vol. 13, no. 10, pp. 1261–1268, 2006.

[7] Y. Kishi, E. K. Abdalla, Y. S. Chun et al., "Three hundred and one consecutive extended right hepatectomies: evaluation of outcome based on systematic liver volumetry," *Annals of Surgery*, vol. 250, no. 4, pp. 540–548, 2009.

[8] D. Ribero, E. K. Abdalla, D. C. Madoff, M. Donadon, E. M. Loyer, and J.-N. Vauthey, "Portal vein embolization before major hepatectomy and its effects on regeneration, resectability and outcome," *British Journal of Surgery*, vol. 94, no. 11, pp. 1386–1394, 2007.

[9] K. O. Ong and E. Leen, "Radiological staging of colorectal liver metastases," *Surgical Oncology*, vol. 16, no. 1, pp. 7–14, 2007.

[10] O. Strobel, V. Berens, U. Hinz et al., "Resection after neoadjuvant therapy for locally advanced, "unresectable" pancreatic cancer," *Surgery*, vol. 152, no. 3, supplement 1, pp. S33–S42, 2012.

[11] D. Borja-Cacho, H. M. Parsons, E. B. Habermann, D. A. Rothenberger, W. G. Henderson, and W. B. Al-Refaie, "Assessment of ACS NSQIP's predictive ability for adverse events after major cancer surgery," *Annals of Surgical Oncology*, vol. 17, no. 9, pp. 2274–2282, 2010.

[12] W. B. Al-Refaie, H. M. Parsons, W. G. Henderson et al., "Major cancer surgery in the elderly: results from the american college of surgeons national surgical quality improvement program," *Annals of Surgery*, vol. 251, no. 2, pp. 311–318, 2010.

[13] M. G. Mythen and A. R. Webb, "The role of gut mucosal hypoperfusion in the pathogenesis of post-operative organ dysfunction," *Intensive Care Medicine*, vol. 20, no. 3, pp. 203–209, 1994.

[14] C. S. F. Lorenzo, W. M. L. Limm, F. Lurie, and L. L. Wong, "Factors affecting outcome in liver resection," *HPB*, vol. 7, no. 3, pp. 226–230, 2005.

[15] F. J. García-Miguel, P. G. Serrano-Aguilar, and J. López-Bastida, "Preoperative assessment," *The Lancet*, vol. 362, no. 9397, pp. 1749–1757, 2003.

[16] R. A. Schroeder, C. E. Marroquin, B. P. Bute, S. Khuri, W. G. Henderson, and P. C. Kuo, "Predictive indices of morbidity and mortality after liver resection," *Annals of Surgery*, vol. 243, no. 3, pp. 373–379, 2006.

[17] J. Belghiti, K. Hiramatsu, S. Benoist, P. P. Massault, A. Sauvanet, and O. Farges, "Seven hundred forty-seven hepatectomies in the 1990s: an update to evaluate the actual risk of liver resection," *Journal of the American College of Surgeons*, vol. 191, no. 1, pp. 38–46, 2000.

[18] P. Angulo, "Medical progress: nonalcoholic fatty liver disease," *The New England Journal of Medicine*, vol. 346, no. 16, pp. 1221–1231, 2002.

[19] J.-N. Vauthey, T. M. Pawlik, D. Ribero et al., "Chemotherapy regimen predicts steatohepatitis and an increase in 90-day mortality after surgery for hepatic colorectal metastases," *Journal of Clinical Oncology*, vol. 24, no. 13, pp. 2065–2072, 2006.

[20] K. A. Gendall, S. Raniga, R. Kennedy, and F. A. Frizelle, "The impact of obesity on outcome after major colorectal surgery," *Diseases of the Colon and Rectum*, vol. 50, no. 12, pp. 2223–2237, 2007.

[21] W. B. Al-Refaie, H. M. Parsons, W. G. Henderson et al., "Body mass index and major cancer surgery outcomes: lack of association or need for alternative measurements of obesity?" *Annals of Surgical Oncology*, vol. 17, no. 9, pp. 2264–2273, 2010.

[22] M. Pocard, A. Vincent-Salomon, J. Girodet, and R.-J. Salmon, "Effects of preoperative chemotherapy on liver function tests after hepatectomy," *Hepato-Gastroenterology*, vol. 48, no. 41, pp. 1406–1408, 2001.

[23] L. McCormack, H. Petrowsky, W. Jochum, K. Furrer, and P.-A. Clavien, "Hepatic steatosis is a risk factor for postoperative complications after major hepatectomy: a matched case-control study," *Annals of Surgery*, vol. 245, no. 6, pp. 923–930, 2007.

[24] L. Rubbia-Brandt, V. Audard, P. Sartoretti et al., "Severe hepatic sinusoidal obstruction associated with oxaliplatin-based chemotherapy in patients with metastatic colorectal cancer," *Annals of Oncology*, vol. 15, no. 3, pp. 460–466, 2004.

[25] J.-N. Vauthey, T. M. Pawlik, D. Ribero et al., "Chemotherapy regimen predicts steatohepatitis and an increase in 90-day mortality after surgery for hepatic colorectal metastases," *Journal of Clinical Oncology*, vol. 24, no. 13, pp. 2065–2072, 2006.

[26] R. E. Schwarz, "Visceral organ resections combined with synchronous major hepatectomy: examples of safety and feasibility," *HPB*, vol. 5, no. 1, pp. 27–32, 2003.

[27] A. McKay, F. R. Sutherland, O. F. Bathe, and E. Dixon, "Morbidity and mortality following multivisceral resections in complex hepatic and pancreatic surgery," *Journal of Gastrointestinal Surgery*, vol. 12, no. 1, pp. 86–90, 2008.

[28] S. K. Reddy, A. S. Barbas, R. S. Turley et al., "Major liver resection in elderly patients: a multi-institutional analysis,"

Journal of the American College of Surgeons, vol. 212, no. 5, pp. 787–795, 2011.

[29] J. D. Birkmeyer, A. E. Siewers, E. V. A. Finlayson et al., "Hospital volume and surgical mortality in the United States," *The New England Journal of Medicine*, vol. 346, no. 15, pp. 1128–1137, 2002.

[30] C. B. Begg, L. D. Cramer, W. J. Hoskins, and M. F. Brennan, "Impact of hospital volume on operative mortality for major cancer surgery," *Journal of the American Medical Association*, vol. 280, no. 20, pp. 1747–1751, 1998.

[31] Y. Fong, M. Gonen, D. Rubin et al., "Long-term survival is superior after resection for cancer in high-volume centers," *Annals of Surgery*, vol. 242, no. 4, pp. 540–547, 2005.

[32] M. A. Choti, H. M. Bowman, H. A. Pitt et al., "Should hepatic resections be performed at high-volume referral centers?" *Journal of Gastrointestinal Surgery*, vol. 2, no. 1, pp. 11–20, 1998.

[33] J. B. Dimick, J. A. Cowan Jr., J. A. Knol, and G. R. Upchurch Jr., "Hepatic resection in the United States: indications, outcomes, and hospital procedural volumes from a nationally representative database," *Archives of Surgery*, vol. 138, no. 2, pp. 185–191, 2003.

[34] J. D. Birkmeyer, T. A. Stukel, A. E. Siewers, P. P. Goodney, D. E. Wennberg, and F. L. Lucas, "Surgeon volume and operative mortality in the United States," *The New England Journal of Medicine*, vol. 349, no. 22, pp. 2117–2127, 2003.

[35] R. W. Eppsteiner, N. G. Csikesz, J. P. Simons, J. F. Tseng, and S. A. Shah, "High volume and outcome after liver resection: surgeon or center?" *Journal of Gastrointestinal Surgery*, vol. 12, no. 10, pp. 1709–1716, 2008.

[36] R. W. Eppsteiner, N. G. Csikesz, J. T. McPhee, J. F. Tseng, and S. A. Shah, "Surgeon volume impacts hospital mortality for pancreatic resection," *Annals of Surgery*, vol. 249, no. 4, pp. 635–640, 2009.

[37] Y. Nakafusa, T. Tanaka, M. Tanaka, Y. Kitajima, S. Sato, and K. Miyazaki, "Comparison of multivisceral resection and standard operation for locally advanced colorectal cancer: analysis of prognostic factors for short-term and long-term outcome," *Diseases of the Colon and Rectum*, vol. 47, no. 12, pp. 2055–2063, 2004.

[38] W. Hartwig, T. Hackert, U. Hinz et al., "Multivisceral resection for pancreatic malignancies: risk-analysis and long-term outcome," *Annals of Surgery*, vol. 250, no. 1, pp. 81–87, 2009.

[39] T. Mynster, I. J. Christensen, F. Moesgaard, and H. J. Nielsen, "Effects of the combination of blood transfusion and postoperative infectious complications on prognosis after surgery for colorectal cancer," *British Journal of Surgery*, vol. 87, no. 11, pp. 1553–1562, 2000.

[40] L. Capussotti and R. Polastri, "Operative risks of major hepatic resections," *Hepato-Gastroenterology*, vol. 45, no. 19, pp. 184–190, 1998.

[41] W. R. Jarnagin, M. Gonen, Y. Fong et al., "Improvement in perioperative outcome after hepatic resection: analysis of 1,803 consecutive cases over the past decade," *Annals of Surgery*, vol. 236, no. 4, pp. 397–407, 2002.

[42] N. N. Rahbari, J. B. Zimmermann, T. Schmidt, M. Koch, M. A. Weigand, and J. Weitz, "Meta-analysis of standard, restrictive and supplemental fluid administration in colorectal surgery," *British Journal of Surgery*, vol. 96, no. 4, pp. 331–341, 2009.

[43] V. Nisanevich, I. Felsenstein, G. Almogy, C. Weissman, S. Einav, and I. Matot, "Effect of intraoperative fluid management on outcome after intraabdominal surgery," *Anesthesiology*, vol. 103, no. 1, pp. 25–32, 2005.

[44] J. A. Melendez, V. Arslan, M. E. Fischer et al., "Perioperative outcomes of major hepatic resections under low central venous pressure anesthesia: blood loss, blood transfusion, and the risk of postoperative renal dysfunction," *Journal of the American College of Surgeons*, vol. 187, no. 6, pp. 620–625, 1998.

[45] Y. WenKui, L. Ning, G. JianFeng et al., "Restricted perioperative fluid administration adjusted by serum lactate level improved outcome after major elective surgery for gastrointestinal malignancy," *Surgery*, vol. 147, no. 4, pp. 542–552, 2010.

[46] J. B. Dimick, P. J. Pronovost, R. F. Heitmiller, and P. A. Lipsett, "Intensive care unit physician staffing is associated with decreased length of stay, hospital cost, and complications after esophageal resection," *Critical Care Medicine*, vol. 29, no. 4, pp. 753–758, 2001.

[47] P. J. Pronovost, D. Dang, T. Dorman et al., "Intensive care unit nurse staffing and the risk for complications after abdominal aortic surgery," *Effective Clinical Practice*, vol. 4, no. 5, pp. 199–206, 2001.

[48] G. R. Linke, M. Mieth, S. Hofer et al., "Surgical intensive care unit: essential for good outcome in major abdominal surgery?" *Langenbeck's Archives of Surgery*, vol. 396, no. 4, pp. 417–428, 2011.

[49] R. S. Turley, S. K. Reddy, C. K. Shortell, B. M. Clary, and J. E. Scarborough, "Venous thromboembolism after hepatic resection: analysis of 5,706 patients," *Journal of Gastrointestinal Surgery*, vol. 16, no. 9, pp. 1705–1714, 2012.

[50] P. Mismetti, S. Laporte, J.-Y. Darmon, A. Buchmüller, and H. Decousus, "Meta-analysis of low molecular weight heparin in the prevention of venous thromboembolism in general surgery," *British Journal of Surgery*, vol. 88, no. 7, pp. 913–930, 2001.

[51] R. White, C. Winston, M. Gonen et al., "Current utility of staging laparoscopy for pancreatic and peripancreatic neoplasms," *Journal of the American College of Surgeons*, vol. 206, no. 3, pp. 445–450, 2008.

[52] J. Weitz, N. Rahbari, M. Koch, and M. W. Büchler, "The "Artery First" approach for resection of pancreatic head cancer," *Journal of the American College of Surgeons*, vol. 210, no. 2, pp. e1–e4, 2010.

[53] M. G. Van Vledder, T. M. Pawlik, S. Munireddy, U. Hamper, M. C. De Jong, and M. A. Choti, "Factors determining the sensitivity of intraoperative ultrasonography in detecting colorectal liver metastases in the modern era," *Annals of Surgical Oncology*, vol. 17, no. 10, pp. 2756–2763, 2010.

[54] G. Torzilli, T. Takayama, A.-M. Hui, K. Kubota, Y. Harihara, and M. Makuuchi, "A new technical aspect of ultrasound-guided liver surgery," *The American Journal of Surgery*, vol. 178, no. 4, pp. 341–343, 1999.

[55] H. Chen, N. B. Merchant, and M. S. Didolkar, "Hepatic resection using intermittent vascular inflow occlusion and low central venous pressure anesthesia improves morbidity and mortality," *Journal of Gastrointestinal Surgery*, vol. 4, no. 2, pp. 162–167, 2000.

[56] N. N. Rahbari, M. Koch, A. Mehrabi et al., "Portal triad clamping versus vascular exclusion for vascular control during hepatic resection: a systematic review and meta-analysis," *Journal of Gastrointestinal Surgery*, vol. 13, no. 3, pp. 558–568, 2009.

[57] S. K. Reddy, A. S. Barbas, R. S. Turley et al., "A standard definition of major hepatectomy: resection of four or more liver segments," *HPB*, vol. 13, no. 7, pp. 494–502, 2011.

[58] N. N. Rahbari, O. J. Garden, R. Padbury et al., "Posthepatectomy liver failure: a definition and grading by the International Study

Group of Liver Surgery (ISGLS)," *Surgery*, vol. 149, no. 5, pp. 713–724, 2011.

[59] B. Nordlinger, E. Van Cutsem, T. Gruenberger et al., "Combination of surgery and chemotherapy and the role of targeted agents in the treatment of patients with colorectal liver metastases: recommendations from an expert panel," *Annals of Oncology*, vol. 20, no. 6, pp. 985–992, 2009.

[60] P. S. Wolf, J. O. Park, F. Bao et al., "Preoperative chemotherapy and the risk of hepatotoxicity and morbidity after liver resection for metastatic colorectal cancer: a single institution experience," *Journal of the American College of Surgeon*, vol. 216, no. 1, pp. 41–49, 2013.

[61] A. Abulkhir, P. Limongelli, A. J. Healey et al., "Preoperative portal vein embolization for major liver resection: a meta-analysis," *Annals of Surgery*, vol. 247, no. 1, pp. 49–57, 2008.

[62] J. C. Weber, P. Bachellier, E. Oussoultzoglou, and D. Jaeck, "Simultaneous resection of colorectal primary tumour and synchronous liver metastases," *British Journal of Surgery*, vol. 90, no. 8, pp. 956–962, 2003.

[63] E. de Santibañes, D. Fernandez, C. Vaccaro et al., "Short-term and long-term outcomes after simultaneous resection of colorectal malignancies and synchronous liver metastases," *World journal of surgery*, vol. 34, no. 9, pp. 2133–2140, 2010.

[64] L. Viganò, M. Karoui, A. Ferrero, C. Tayar, D. Cherqui, and L. Capussotti, "Locally advanced mid/low rectal cancer with synchronous liver metastases," *World Journal of Surgery*, vol. 35, no. 12, pp. 2788–2795, 2011.

[65] S. K. Reddy, T. M. Pawlik, D. Zorzi et al., "Simultaneous resections of colorectal cancer and synchronous liver metastases: a multi-institutional analysis," *Annals of Surgical Oncology*, vol. 14, no. 12, pp. 3481–3491, 2007.

[66] S. S. Brar, R. Seevaratnam, R. Cardoso et al., "Multivisceral resection for gastric cancer: a systematic review," *Gastric Cancer*, vol. 15, no. 1, pp. S100–S107, 2012.

[67] F. Pacelli, G. Cusumano, F. Rosa et al., "Multivisceral resection for locally advanced gastric cancer: an Italian multicenter observational study," *JAMA Surgery*, vol. 148, no. 4, pp. 353–360, 2013.

20

The Falciform Ligament for Mesenteric and Portal Vein Reconstruction in Local Advanced Pancreatic Tumor: A Surgical Guide and Single-Center Experience

T. Malinka ⓘ,[1] **F. Klein** ⓘ,[1] **T. Denecke,**[2] **U. Pelzer** ⓘ,[3] **J. Pratschke,**[1] **and M. Bahra**[1]

[1]*Department of Surgery, Charité Campus Mitte and Charité Campus Virchow Klinikum,*
Charité-Universitätsmedizin Berlin, Berlin, Germany
[2]*Department of Radiology, Charité Campus Virchow Klinikum, Charité-Universitätsmedizin Berlin, Berlin, Germany*
[3]*Department of Hematology/Oncology/Tumor Immunology, Campus Virchow Klinikum,*
Charité-Universitätsmedizin Berlin, Berlin, Germany

Correspondence should be addressed to T. Malinka; thomas.malinka@charite.de

Academic Editor: Hobart W. Harris

Background. Since local tumor infiltration to the mesenteric-portal axis might represent a challenging assignment for curative intended resectability during pancreatic surgery, appropriate techniques for venous reconstruction are essential. In this study, we acknowledge the falciform ligament as a feasible and convenient substitute for mesenteric and portal vein reconstruction with high reliability and patency for local advanced pancreatic tumor. *Methods.* A retrospective single-center analysis. Between June 2017 and January 2018, a total of eleven consecutive patients underwent pancreatic resections with venous reconstruction using falciform ligament. Among them, venous resection was performed in nine cases by wedge and in two cases by full segment. Patency rates and perioperative details were reviewed. *Results.* Mean clamping time of the mesenteric-portal blood flow was 34 min, while perioperative mortality rate was 0%. By means of Duplex ultrasonography, nine patients were shown to be patent on the day of discharge, while two cases revealed an entire occlusion of the mesenteric-portal axis. Orthograde flow demonstrated a mean value of 34 cm/s. All patent grafts on discharge revealed persistent patency within various follow-up assessments. *Conclusion.* The falciform ligament appears to be a feasible and reliable autologous tissue for venous blood flow reconstruction with high postoperative patency. Especially the possibility of customizing graft dimensions to the individual needs based on local findings allows an optimal size matching of the conduit. The risk of stenosis and/or segmental occlusion may thus be further reduced.

1. Introduction

Pancreatic ductal adenocarcinoma is a common malignancy of the gastrointestinal tract and incidences are unfortunately evolving [1]. Despite continuous advancements in interdisciplinary treatment concepts, the majority of patients are still diagnosed at advanced tumor stages and overall long-term prognosis still remains limited [2]. As entire surgical tumor removal remains the best chance for disease-free and long-term survival, recent improvements in surgical expertise have thus been focused on increasing surgical radicality and margin-negative resections rates [3]. While hepatic metastasis, peritoneal carcinomatosis, and/or invasion of major vessels were traditionally considered as parameters for nonresectability, progress in surgical techniques has, however, lead to a debate to redefine modern resection criteria [4, 5]. Nowadays multivisceral resections (MVR) may be considered as feasible and reliable procedures with decreasing complication rates for selected patients [6]. According to this continuous progress, resections of the superior mesenteric vein (SMV), portal vein (PV), or coeliac axis are considered as a safe and reliable technique when performed at high-volume centers [7, 8]. Furthermore, recent studies have shown that survival rates for patients undergoing pancreatectomy with venous reconstruction were comparable to those undergoing pancreatectomy exclusively [9, 10]. However, in case of vascular resection, suitable reconstruction techniques are demanded in order to ensure unimpaired blood flow. When primary direct closure of the venous vessel is not feasible to restore continuity, complex segmental reconstruction, requiring autologous tissue or synthetic materials, is essential [8, 11, 12]. Previously we described bovine pericardium as an innovative and feasible option for venous reconstruction after pancreatic resection [13]. However, autologous materials appear most suitable to maintain venous blood flow continuity and therefore the retrieval of the most appropriate localization for withdrawal is still challenging [14, 15]. The falciform ligament is a broad and thin fold of the peritoneum, attaching the liver to the anterior parietal and diaphragmatic peritoneum, also separating the left and right lobe of the liver. Meaning "sickle-shaped", from Latin, it is a remnant of the embryonic ventral mesentery with its base being directed downward and backward and its apex upward and backward [16, 17]. Both sides are covered by layers of mesothelial cells and can become canalized in cases of portal hypertension [18, 19]. We herewith report on our initial experience with the falciform ligament as an autologous graft for portal and superior mesenteric vein reconstruction in extended pancreatic resections and provide a surgical guide based on our perioperative outcomes.

2. Methods

2.1. Patients' Inclusion Criteria and Data Collection. This was a retrospective single-center analysis conducted in a tertiary referral center for pancreatic surgery. Standard preoperative clinical diagnostics included a physical examination and routine laboratory testing. Computed tomography (CT) and/or magnet resonance imaging (MRI) were routinely used as radiological diagnostic tools to analyze tumor diagnosis as well as the stage of the disease. Indications for pancreatic resections were endorsed in an interdisciplinary consensus meeting. All included operations were performed by experienced pancreatic surgeons at the study site and all oncological procedures, as well as venous resections, were performed as open surgical procedures according to international standards [20]. There were no minimal-invasive pancreatectomies within the study group. Accordingly, between June 2017 and January 2018, we identified and reviewed an overall of eleven patients who had undergone en bloc tumor resection with simultaneous venous vascular resection and reconstruction of the venous blood continuity using a falciform ligament graft within our study period. Written informed consent was obtained from all patients.

The following data were collected for each patient: demographics (age, gender); underlying diagnosis; surgical procedure; neoadjuvant chemotherapy; results of the final histopathological examination, including TNM classification; operative details such as operation time, clamping time, and intraoperative transfusion; associated vein resection and reconstruction graft within surgical procedure; details of the perioperative course such as postoperative morbidity in terms of postoperative pancreatic fistula (POPF), postpancreatectomy haemorrhage (PPH), and abdominal collection

which were all classified according to International Study Group of Pancreatic Fistula (ISGPF) definitions [21, 22]; length of hospital stay (LOS) was calculated from the day of surgery until the day of discharge; patency of vein and results of orthograde flow measurement during Duplex ultrasonography.

2.2. Preconditioning, Technique, and Surgical Guide. When preoperative CT or MRI showed tumor involvement of the celiac axis and/or the common hepatic artery (CHA) but no affiliation to the superior mesenteric artery (SMA) or the gastroduodenal artery (GDA), patients were further evaluated for distal celiacopancreatectomy. If examinations revealed eligible conditions for resection, preoperative embolization of the celiac axis and the CHA was performed. Hereby the arterial blood supply to the liver and stomach was enhanced through collateral pathways from the SMA over the pancreaticoduodenal arcades to the GDA, the proper hepatic artery (PHA), the gastroepiploic artery, and the right gastric artery as previously described [23].

At the beginning of the operation, peritoneal metastases were initially excluded by complete exploration of the abdominal cavity. Access to the omental bursa was established by dissection of the gastrocolic ligament. After retraction of the stomach and inspection of the pancreas, local resectability of the lesion and the extent of the resection were determined based on local findings such as vascular and/or another organ infiltration. In cases of underlying malignant disease, a standard lymphadenectomy was performed. Dissection of the pancreas was done by electrocautery, or in cases of pancreatic left resections with a stapling device.

In the event of underlying venous infiltration, all veins draining into the impaired segment were clamped and en bloc resection including tumor and vein was conducted. In order to avoid edema in the bowel, cross-clamp time was kept to a minimum. Grafts of the falciform ligament were tailored to the individual needs based on local findings. Therefore, patches from the falciform ligament were retrieved by scissor and kept in saline. In order to shape cylindrical interposition grafts, patches were rolled over a tube and sutured. Preparation of the interposition graft, as well as patch insertion and anastomoses, were all completed by 6.0 Prolene® sutures (Ethicon, Norderstedt, Germany). Cases which required only partial resection of the venous circumference were provided by patch graft (Figure 1), whereas interposition grafts were used to replace segments affected with tumor infiltration of more than half the circumference of the vessel (Figure 2). A growth factor was applied in all anastomosis in order to allow expansion of the suture line as previously described [24]. In case of a pancreatoenteral anastomosis, either a pancreatojejunostomy or a pancreatogastrostomy was performed. Distal closure of the pancreas remnant by stapler was performed using linear stapling devices armed with a 60-mm cartridge (EndoGIA™, Auto-Suture, Covidien) reinforced by a bioabsorbable mesh (SEAMGUARD®, W.L. Gore, Flagstaff, AZ). Every patient received at least one intra-abdominal drain (Degania Silicone

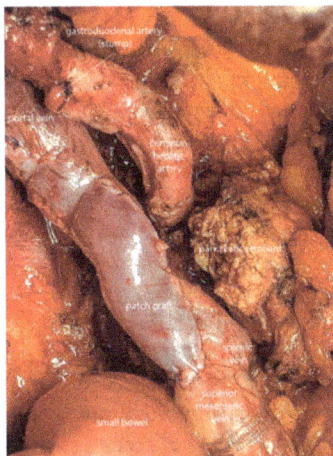

FIGURE 1: Intraoperative perspective after pylorus-preserving pancreaticoduodenectomy (PPPD) with partial resection of the portal vein and successful reconstruction by patch graft.

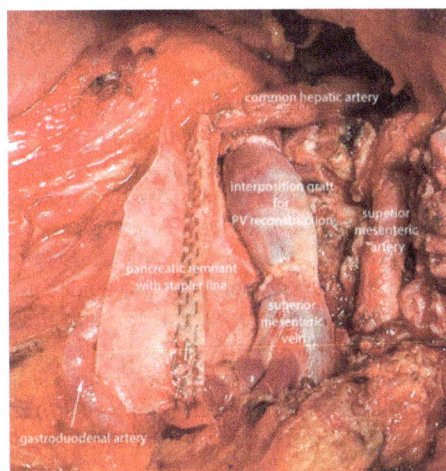

FIGURE 2: Intraoperative perspective after distal pancreatectomy with en bloc resection of the celiac trunk as well as portal vein segment and successful reconstruction by interposition graft.

Europe GmbH, Regensburg, Germany) to measure postoperative amylase levels and drain output in the postoperative course.

2.3. Standard Postoperative Care. Postoperative care was standardized. All patients were monitored for at least one day at a specialized surgical intensive care unit. Anticoagulant therapy after venous reconstruction was performed by continuous administration of unfractionated heparin (UFH) to achieve a PTT of 40-50 seconds for 5 days. Laboratory testing for coagulation variables was performed every 8 hours according to standard ICU care. Afterward, prevention of venous thromboembolism was achieved by subcutaneous application of low molecular weight heparin (LMWH) based on patient's requirement throughout the length of hospital stay. Specific procedure related anticoagulation therapy was discontinued after discharge and only continued if required

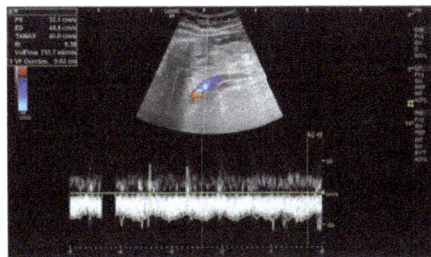

FIGURE 3: Duplex ultrasonography examination to verify unimpaired portal blood flow in the postoperative course.

by additional comorbidities or the underlying diagnose of the individual patient. Portal and superior mesenteric vein blood flow was evaluated by Duplex ultrasonography intraoperative, immediately postoperative as well as on the first and second postoperative day. Final Duplex ultrasonography was performed prior to discharge (Figure 3). If normal hilar portal blood flow along normal liver function was verified, graft patency was assumed sufficient. Contrast-enhanced abdominal computed tomography scanning was not performed regularly but rather on the clinical requirement. Amylase levels were monitored in the serum and in the intraoperatively placed abdominal drains on the second postoperative day. In the absence of signs of a pancreatic fistula, oral food intake was started depending on the clinical presentation and tolerance. The concept of enhanced recovery after surgery (ERAS) has not been applied within the study period. Adjuvant chemotherapy followed depending on the TNM category and clinical situation. All comprehensive procedures were reviewed in an interdisciplinary consensus meeting and patients were seen routinely for follow-up examinations in the outpatient clinic.

3. Results

3.1. Baseline Characteristics. Between June 2017 and January 2018, a total of eleven consecutive patients underwent pancreatic resections with venous reconstruction by the falciform ligament for extended pancreatic tumor disease at our institution; among them five patients underwent pylorus-preserving pancreaticoduodenectomy (PPPD), two patients received a pylorus preservation total pancreatectomy, two patients received a distal pancreatectomy with splenectomy, and two patients required an Appleby procedure in order to achieve radical tumor removal. There were six males and five females with a mean age of 63 years (43–82) in this group. Three patients received a neoadjuvant chemotherapy, exclusively by FOLFIRINOX, according to an endorsement by an interdisciplinary consensus meeting. Venous resection was performed in nine patients by wedge and in two patients by full segment resection. All venous reconstructions were performed utilizing portions of the falciform ligament. Histological examination showed ductal adenocarcinomas in ten patients, while one patient suffered from an invasive intraductal papillary mucinous carcinoma (IPMC) of the pancreas. In four cases complete resection of tumor tissue was achieved, while in seven cases residual tumor was present microscopically at retroperitoneal resection margins (Table 1).

3.2. Perioperative and Postoperative Data. The mean duration of the surgical procedure was 361 min, while mean clamping time of the mesenteric-portal blood flow was 34 min. In seven patients the portal vein was solely infiltrated by tumor, whereas in four cases tumor involvement of the confluence was determined. Nine cases were provided by patch graft, while two patients required an interposition graft due to a segmental tumor infiltration of more than half the circumference of the underlying venous vessel. In six patients a transfusion of red blood cells (RBC) and fresh frozen plasma (FFP) was necessary during the intraoperative course. Mean ICU length of stay and overall hospital stay was 4 (1-12) and 23 (12-59) days, respectively. The perioperative mortality rate was 0%. Two patients developed POPF grade B, while two patients sustained post pancreatectomy haemorrhage. In one case, a bleeding from the anastomosis of the interposition graft occurred and surgical revision was required. The other case demonstrated a bleeding from the gastroduodenal artery, although no pancreatic fistula was observed. Coiling of the stump of the GDA stopped PPH and no surgical intervention was necessary. Both cases of POPF grade B were managed by percutaneous drainage and fistula resolved in the course without further intervention. In one patient, a CT scan revealed an abdominal collection, which was approached by CT guided percutaneous drainage. By means of Duplex ultrasonography, nine patients were shown to be patent on the day of discharge, while two cases revealed an entire occlusion of the mesenteric-portal axis. Both patients presented ascites in the postoperative course and required diuretics. Reopening by interventional approach was unsuccessfully attempted in one patient. Both patients received anticoagulant therapy and could be discharged uneventfully. Orthograde flow demonstrated a mean value of 34 cm/s for patent grafts. All patent grafts on discharge revealed persistent patency within various assessments in our oncological outpatient clinic or direct communication with the general practitioner (Table 2). After discharge, eight patients were included in the study protocol of the Hyperthermia European Adjuvant Trial (HEAT; ClinicalTrials.gov Identifier: NCT01077427) for further treatment, based on the recommendations of the interdisciplinary consensus meeting. Two patients sustained FOLFIRINOX for their adjuvant treatment, while to one patient gemcitabine/nab-paclitaxel was administered (Table 2).

4. Discussion

Clinical outcome after pancreatic surgery has improved considerably over the last decades with a consistent reduction of postoperative morbidity and mortality [25]. While previous studies indicated no significant differences in terms of postoperative morbidity and long-term survival after pancreatectomy with mesenteric-portal vein resection, recent studies demonstrated beneficial outcomes and increased

resectability rates for patients with underlying pancreatic malignancies [5, 9, 26]. Since local tumor infiltration to the venous blood flow might represent a challenging assignment for curative intended resectability, appropriate techniques for venous reconstruction are essential [27, 28]. In this study, we acknowledge the falciform ligament as a feasible and convenient substitute for mesenteric and portal vein reconstruction with high patency and reliability in extended pancreatic tumor resections.

After venous resection has been performed, rearrangement of the mesenteric-portal axis is essential to ensure unimpaired blood flow continuity. Even though the primary direct closure of the venous vessel is frequently feasible, pancreatic surgeons partially encounter complex situations requiring additional tissue for reconstruction [14, 29, 30]. Various autologous grafts have been described in the literature, including the great saphenous vein, internal jugular vein, femoral vein, left renal vein, or gonadal veins [11, 12, 31–33]. Harvesting of these grafts may, however, be accompanied by relevant morbidity due to the impermanent into another anatomic region [12, 34, 35]. Postoperative edema, increased operative time, increased risk of bleeding or size mismatches resulting in deficient portal inflow with an increased risk of turbulence that might promote clotting of the graft are frequently reported [8]. In addition, synthetic grafts composed of polytetrafluoroethylene (PTFE) or polyethylene terephthalate (Dacron) contain a seriously substandard risk of thrombosis and infection and an elongated anticoagulation therapy postoperative is demanded [36]. Consequently, also synthetic grafts are not commonly recommended as grafts for mesenteric and portal vein reconstruction and therefore the most suitable tissue still remains to be identified [28, 37].

Previously we described bovine pericardium as a safe and feasible material for mesenteric and portal vein reconstruction during pancreatic surgery and indicated good patency and easy handling [13]. Although the introduced procedure is still frequently implemented in our tertiary referral center for pancreatic surgery, we targeted an even more autologous and cost-effective solution.

The falciform ligament, a remnant of the embryonic ventral mesentery, is a broad and thin fold of the peritoneum that is covered with epithelial layers on both sides featuring several advantages. Within our observation period, we discovered good graft patency, which is comparable with results of other studies using different autologous tissue or interposition grafts compounded by PTFE [32, 37]. However, retrieval, as well as implementation, is much easier and dimensions can be customized to the individual needs based on intraoperative findings. Furthermore, due to its autologous nature, the risk of infection and the necessity for long-term anticoagulation therapy postoperative is limited. In addition, cost-effective availability results in verifiable benefits in favor of the autologous falciform ligament. Surprisingly, our results are in contrast to a comparable study also targeting the falciform ligament as a graft for portal and mesenteric vein reconstruction. Zhiying et al. reported good graft patency until two weeks postoperatively, while an increased occlusion rate up two months postoperatively was observed [38]. Interpretations of differences to our

TABLE 1: Patient demographics, surgical procedure, and histopathologic results.

Patient	Age/Sex	Diagnosis	Surgical procedure	Neoadjuvant chemotherapy	Pathology (TNM)	Category
A	49/M	Ductal adenocarcinoma pancreatic body	Distal pancreatectomy, splenectomy, celiac trunk resection, portal vein wedge resection	No	pT2 pN1 (2/24) L1 V1 Pn1 G3	R1
B	66/M	Ductal adenocarcinoma pancreatic head	PPPD, portal vein wedge resection	No	pT2 pN1 (3/21) L1 V0 Pn1 G2	R1
C	82/M	IPMC	PPPD, portal vein wedge resection	No	pT1c pN0 (0/28) L0 V0 Pn0 G2	R0
D	63/M	Ductal adenocarcinoma pancreatic body	Distal pancreatectomy, splenectomy, celiac trunk resection, portal vein wedge resection	No	pT2 pN0 (0/11) L0 V1 Pn1 G2	R1
E	58/F	Ductal adenocarcinoma pancreatic tail	Distal pancreatectomy, splenectomy, Portal vein segment resection	Yes FOLFIRINOX (6#)	ypT2 ypN0 (0/11) L0 V1 Pn1 G2	R1
F	65/F	Ductal adenocarcinoma pancreatic body	Distal pancreatectomy, splenectomy, Portal vein wedge resection	No	pT2 pN2 (5/48) L0 V1 Pn1 G3	R1
G	70/M	Ductal adenocarcinoma pancreatic head	Pylorus preservation pancreatectomy, portal vein wedge resection	Yes FOLFIRINOX (10#)	ypT2 ypN2 (4/24) L0 V0 Pn0 G2	R0
H	63/F	Ductal adenocarcinoma pancreatic head	Pylorus preservation pancreatectomy, portal vein wedge resection	Yes FOLFIRINOX (6#)	ypT3 ypN1 (1/17) L0 V0 Pn1 G2	R1
I	72/F	Ductal adenocarcinoma pancreatic head	PPPD, portal vein wedge resection	No	pT3 pN1(1/12) L0 V1 Pn1 G2	R1
J	43/F	Ductal adenocarcinoma pancreatic head	PPPD, portal vein segment resection	No	pT2 pN0 (0/14) L0 V0 Pn1 G2	R0
K	63/M	Ductal adenocarcinoma pancreatic head	PPPD, portal vein wedge resection	No	pT3 N0 (0/28) R0 L0 V0 Pn1 G3	R0

TABLE 2: Perioperative and postoperative data after pancreatectomy with en bloc venous resection and reconstruction by falciform ligament.

Patient	Operative time (min)	Involved vein	Clamping (min)	Type of graft	RBC/FFP	Hospital/ICU length of stay (day)	Perioperative complications	Patency of Vein prior to discharge	Orthograde flow	Adjuvant chemotherapy	Diabetes mellitus	Outcome Patency
A	300	PV	35	Patch	3/6	37/5	Pancreatic fistula (Bassi B)	Occlusion	n.a.	HEAT	No	Occlusion
B	332	PV	30	Patch	0/0	10/2	None	Patent	Vmax = 27 cm/s	Gemcitabine/nab-paclitaxel	No	Patent (POD 147)
C	410	PV	25	Patch	2/4	20/9	PPH	Patent	Vmax = 32 cm/s	HEAT	Insulin-dependent	Patent (POD 118)
D	368	PV	30	Patch	4/8	28/2	Abdominal collection	Patent	Vmax = 28 cm/s	HEAT	No	Patent (POD 64)
E	336	PV	45	Interposition	0/0	12/1	None	Patent	Vmax = 21 cm/s	HEAT	No	Patent (POD 57)
F	314	Confluens	35	Patch	2/4	59/7	Pancreatic fistula (Bassi B)	Patent	Vmax = 57 cm/s	HEAT	No	Patent (POD 74)
G	368	Confluens	30	Patch	6/12	14/2	None	Patent	Vmax = 35 cm/s	FOLFIRINOX	Insulin-dependent	Patent (POD 88)
H	485	Confluens	30	Patch	4/8	15/2	None	Patent	Vmax = 44 cm/s	FOLFIRINOX	Insulin-dependent	Patent (POD 39)
I	348	PV	35	Patch	0/0	19/2	SSI	Patent	Vmax = 28 cm/s	HEAT	No	Patent (POD 30)
J	371	PV	50	Interposition	0/0	29/12	PPH	Occlusion	n.a.	HEAT	No	Occlusion
K	348	Confluens	30	Patch	0/0	18/2	None	Patent	Vmax = 32 cm/s	HEAT	No	Patent (POD 18)

findings are very difficult to distinguish and due to the small number of cases within both series, further studies need to trace long-term patency and overall outcome. Nevertheless, information regarding the chosen suture material, as well as placement of a growth factor, has not been depicted within their manuscript and could therefore possibly be accountable for the documented stenosis and occlusion in the follow-up. Although there is a significant heterogeneity regarding anticoagulation after venous reconstruction with pancreatic resection and currently no agreed approach available [36], continuous administration of unfractionated heparin (UFH) to achieve a PTT of 40-50 seconds for 5 days was conducted in our series by contrast. However, a significant impact on occlusion rates in the course remains debatable.

The most frequent complication in our series was the occurrence of a pancreatic fistula, which can be seen as being related to the pancreatic resection itself. However, two patients were consequently affected by PPH demanding further intervention. In one case bleeding occurred from the stump of the gastroduodenal artery, which was controlled by an angiographic procedure, while the other patient was impaired from a direct bleeding from the venous interposition graft due to an occult arrosion of the suture material. According to other series, PPH occurred frequently and appears to be independent of the chosen tissue for venous reconstruction [39].

Microscopic resection margin involvement (R1 resection) was present in 7 patients, of which all involved the retroperitoneal margins. However, superior mesenteric-portal vein resections including tangential resection with a patch or segmental resection with interposition graft revealed margin-free resections at this point in all eleven cases. Accordingly, the falciform ligament appears to be a safe and feasible substitute to achieve venous R0 resections when the tumor cannot be separated from the venous axis.

The present study is, of course, limited by common biases that are mainly due to the retrospective character of this analysis and the heterogonous time specification concerning long-term longevity. Therefore, further studies with increased numbers of cases need to determine observations.

In conclusion, pancreatectomy with resection of the mesenteric-portal axis due to tumor infiltration provides the chance for complete tumor resection. In our series, the falciform ligament appears to be a feasible and reliable autologous tissue for venous blood flow reconstruction with high postoperative patency and low risk of infection. Due to the possibility of customizing graft dimensions to the individual needs based on local findings, optimal size matching of the conduit is feasible and thus the formation of stenosis and segmental occlusion may be less likely. Although rates of patency in our patients are promising, conclusions on longevity still need to be evaluated in further enlarged observations.

Acknowledgments

The authors acknowledge support from the German Research Foundation (DFG) and the Open Access Publication Fund of Charité-Universitätsmedizin Berlin.

References

[1] L. Rahib, B. D. Smith, R. Aizenberg, A. B. Rosenzweig, J. M. Fleshman, and L. M. Matrisian, "Projecting cancer incidence and deaths to 2030: the unexpected burden of thyroid, liver, and pancreas cancers in the United States," Cancer Research, vol. 74, no. 11, pp. 2913–2921, 2014.

[2] D. Li, K. Xie, R. Wolff, and J. L. Abbruzzese, "Pancreatic cancer," The Lancet, vol. 363, no. 9414, pp. 1049–1057, 2004.

[3] C. W. Michalski, J. Weitz, and M. W. Büchler, "Surgery Insight: Surgical management of pancreatic cancer," Nature Clinical Practice Oncology, vol. 4, no. 9, pp. 526–535, 2007.

[4] S. Matsuno, S. Egawa, S. Fukuyama et al., "Pancreatic cancer registry in Japan: 20 years of experience," Pancreas, vol. 28, no. 3, pp. 219–230, 2004.

[5] G. Ramacciato, P. Mercantini, N. Petrucciani et al., "Does portal-superior mesenteric vein invasion still indicate irre-sectability for pancreatic carcinoma?" Annals of Surgical Oncology, vol. 16, no. 4, pp. 817–825, 2009.

[6] W. Hartwig, C. M. Vollmer, A. Fingerhut et al., "Extended pancreatectomy in pancreatic ductal adenocarcinoma: Definition and consensus of the International Study Group for Pancreatic Surgery (ISGPS)," Surgery, vol. 156, no. 1, pp. 1–14, 2014.

[7] Å. Andrén-Sandberg, "Tumors of the body and tail of the pancreas," North American Journal of Medical Sciences, vol. 3, no. 11, pp. 489–494, 2011.

[8] S. Hirono, M. Kawai, M. Tani et al., "Indication for the use of an interposed graft during portal vein and/or superior mesenteric vein reconstruction in pancreatic resection based on perioperative outcomes," Langenbeck's Archives of Surgery, vol. 399, no. 4, pp. 461–471, 2014.

[9] X. Z. Yu, J. Li, D. L. Fu et al., "Benefit from synchronous portal-superior mesenteric vein resection during pancreatico-duodenectomy for cancer: a meta-analysis," European Journal of Surgical Oncology, vol. 40, no. 4, pp. 371–378, 2014.

[10] Y. Zhou, Z. Zhang, Y. Liu, B. Li, and D. Xu, "Pancreatectomy combined with superior mesenteric vein-portal vein resection for pancreatic cancer: a meta-analysis," World Journal of Surgery, vol. 36, no. 4, pp. 884–891, 2012.

[11] J. B. Fleming, C. C. Barnett, and G. P. Clagett, "Superficial femoral vein as a conduit for portal vein reconstruction during pancreaticoduodenectomy," JAMA Surgery, vol. 140, no. 7, pp. 698–701, 2005.

[12] R. L. Smoot, J. D. Christein, and M. B. Farnell, "An innovative option for venous reconstruction after pancreaticoduodenec-tomy: The left renal vein," Journal of Gastrointestinal Surgery, vol. 11, no. 4, pp. 425–431, 2007.

[13] M. Jara, M. Malinowski, M. Bahra et al., "Bovine pericardium for portal vein reconstruction in abdominal surgery: A surgical guide and first experiences in a single center," Digestive Surgery, vol. 32, no. 2, pp. 135–141, 2015.

[14] G. M. Fuhrman, S. D. Leach, C. A. Staley et al., "Rationale for en bloc vein resection in the treatment of pancreatic adenocarcinoma adherent to the superior mesenteric-portal vein confluence," Annals of Surgery, vol. 223, no. 2, pp. 154–162, 1996.

[15] C. Pulitanò, M. Crawford, P. Ho et al., "The use of biological grafts for reconstruction of the inferior vena cava is a safe and

valid alternative: Results in 32 patients in a single institution," *HPB*, vol. 15, no. 8, pp. 628–632, 2013.

[16] B. F. Martin and R. G. Tudor, "The umbilical and paraumbilical veins of man," *Journal of Anatomy*, vol. 130, part 2, pp. 305–322, 1980.

[17] K. Ibukuro, H. Fukuda, K. Tobe, K. Akita, and T. Takeguchi, "The vascular anatomy of the ligaments of the liver: Gross anatomy, imaging and clinical applications," *British Journal of Radiology*, vol. 89, no. 1064, 2016.

[18] C. Morin, M. Lafortune, G. Pomier, M. Robin, and G. Breton, "Patent paraumbilical vein: Anatomic and hemodynamic variants and their clinical importance," *Radiology*, vol. 185, no. 1, pp. 253–256, 1992.

[19] K. Ibukuro, R. Tanaka, H. Fukuda, S. Abe, and K. Tobe, "The superior group of vessels in the falciform ligament: Anatomical and radiological correlation," *Surgical and Radiologic Anatomy*, vol. 30, no. 4, pp. 311–315, 2008.

[20] T. Malinka, F. Klein, A. Andreou, J. Pratschke, and M. Bahra, "Distal Pancreatectomy Combined with Multivisceral Resection Is Associated with Postoperative Complication Rates and Survival Comparable to Those After Standard Procedures," *Journal of Gastrointestinal Surgery*, vol. 22, no. 9, pp. 1549–1556, 2018.

[21] M. N. Wente, J. A. Veit, C. Bassi et al., "Postpancreatectomy hemorrhage (PPH): an International Study Group of Pancreatic Surgery (ISGPS) definition," *Surgery*, vol. 142, no. 1, pp. 20–25, 2007.

[22] C. Bassi, C. Dervenis, G. Butturini et al., "Postoperative pancreatic fistula: an international study group (ISGPF) definition," *Surgery*, vol. 138, no. 1, pp. 8–13, 2005.

[23] T. Denecke, A. Andreou, P. Podrabsky et al., "Distal pancreatectomy with en bloc resection of the celiac trunk for extended pancreatic tumor disease: An interdisciplinary approach," *CardioVascular and Interventional Radiology*, vol. 34, no. 5, pp. 1058–1064, 2011.

[24] T. E. Starzl, S. Iwatsuki, and B. W. Shaw, "A growth factor in fine vascular anastomoses," *Surgery, Gynecology, and Obstetrics*, vol. 159, pp. 164-165, 1984.

[25] W. Hartwig, T. Hackert, U. Hinz et al., "Multivisceral resection for pancreatic malignancies: risk-analysis and long-term outcome," *Annals of Surgery*, vol. 250, no. 1, pp. 81–87, 2009.

[26] M. Adham, D. F. Mirza, F. Chapuis et al., "Results of vascular resections during pancreatectomy from two European centres: An analysis of survival and disease-free survival explicative factorsThe first, second and third authors participated equally in the study report," *HPB*, vol. 8, no. 6, pp. 465–473, 2006.

[27] R. Ravikumar, C. Sabin, M. Abu Hilal et al., "Portal vein resection in borderline resectable pancreatic cancer: a United Kingdom multicenter study," *Journal of the American College of Surgeons*, vol. 218, no. 3, pp. 401–411, 2014.

[28] C. K. Chu, M. B. Farnell, J. H. Nguyen et al., "Prosthetic graft reconstruction after portal vein resection in pancreaticoduodenectomy: A multicenter analysis," *Journal of the American College of Surgeons*, vol. 211, no. 3, pp. 316–324, 2010.

[29] D. Kleive, A. E. Berstad, M. A. Sahakyan et al., "Portal vein reconstruction using primary anastomosis or venous interposition allograft in pancreatic surgery," *Journal of Vascular Surgery: Venous and Lymphatic Disorders*, vol. 6, no. 1, pp. 66–74, 2018.

[30] F. Wang, R. Arianayagam, A. Gill et al., "Grafts for Mesenterico-Portal vein resections can be avoided during pancreatoduodenectomy," *Journal of the American College of Surgeons*, vol. 215, no. 4, pp. 569–579, 2012.

[31] A. N. Krepline, K. K. Christians, K. Duelge et al., "Patency Rates of Portal Vein/Superior Mesenteric Vein Reconstruction After Pancreatectomy for Pancreatic Cancer," *Journal of Gastrointestinal Surgery*, vol. 18, no. 11, pp. 2016–2025, 2014.

[32] D. Y. Lee, E. L. Mitchell, M. A. Jones et al., "Techniques and results of portal vein/superior mesenteric vein reconstruction using femoral and saphenous vein during pancreaticoduodenectomy," *Journal of Vascular Surgery*, vol. 51, no. 3, pp. 662–666, 2010.

[33] Y. Yamamoto, Y. Sakamoto, S. Nara et al., "Reconstruction of the portal and hepatic veins using venous grafts customized from the bilateral gonadal veins," *Langenbeck's Archives of Surgery*, vol. 394, no. 6, pp. 1115–1121, 2009.

[34] W. Gao, X. Dai, C. Dai et al., "Comparison of patency rates and clinical impact of different reconstruction methods following portal/superior mesenteric vein resection during pancreatectomy," *Pancreatology*, vol. 16, no. 6, pp. 1113–1123, 2016.

[35] R. L. Smoot, J. D. Christein, and M. B. Farnell, "Durability of portal venous reconstruction following resection during pancreaticoduodenectomy," *Journal of Gastrointestinal Surgery*, vol. 10, no. 10, pp. 1371–1375, 2006.

[36] M. D. Chandrasegaram, G. D. Eslick, W. Lee et al., "Anticoagulation policy after venous resection with a pancreatectomy: A systematic review," *HPB*, vol. 16, no. 8, pp. 691–698, 2014.

[37] J. A. Stauffer, M. K. Dougherty, G. P. Kim, and J. H. Nguyen, "Interposition graft with polytetrafluoroethylene for mesenteric and portal vein reconstruction after pancreaticoduodenectomy," *British Journal of Surgery*, vol. 96, no. 3, pp. 247–252, 2009.

[38] Y. Zhiying, T. Haidong, L. Xiaolei et al., "The falciform ligament as a graft for portal–superior mesenteric vein reconstruction in pancreatectomy," *Journal of Surgical Research*, vol. 218, pp. 226–231, 2017.

[39] U. F. Wellner, B. Kulemann, H. Lapshyn et al., "Postpancreatectomy hemorrhage—incidence, treatment, and risk factors in over 1,000 pancreatic resections," *Journal of Gastrointestinal Surgery*, vol. 18, no. 3, pp. 464–475, 2014.

21

Quality of Life in Hepatocellular Carcinoma Patients Treated with Transarterial Chemoembolization

Saleem Ahmed,[1,2] **Nurun Nisa de Souza,**[3,4] **Wang Qiao,**[2] **Meidai Kasai,**[5] **Low Jee Keem,**[1] **and Vishal G. Shelat**[1]

[1]*Department of General Surgery, Tan Tock Seng Hospital, Singapore 308433*
[2]*Ministry of Health Holdings, 1 Maritime Square, Singapore 099253*
[3]*Duke-NUS Graduate Medical School, 8 College Road, Singapore 169857*
[4]*Singapore Clinical Research Institute, 31 Biopolis Way, Singapore 138669*
[5]*Department of Gastroenterological Surgery, Sendai Kousei Hospital, 8-15 Hirosemachi, Aoba-ku, Sendai-shi, Miyagi 9800873, Japan*

Correspondence should be addressed to Vishal G. Shelat; vgshelat@gmail.com

Academic Editor: Pablo Ramírez

Hepatocellular carcinoma (HCC) is one of the most commonly diagnosed cancers worldwide. Majority of patients with HCC are diagnosed in the advanced stages of disease and hence they are only suitable for palliative therapy. TACE (transarterial chemoembolization) is the most commonly used treatment for unresectable HCC. It is however unclear if TACE improves the quality of life (QoL) in patients with HCC. The aim of this review is to evaluate the impact of TACE on QoL of HCC patients.

1. Introduction

Hepatocellular carcinoma (HCC) is the 5th most common cancer worldwide and the 3rd most common cause of cancer-related death [1]. At diagnosis, fewer than 20% of patients are eligible for curative treatment [2]. The majority of patients receive palliation because of late-stage presentation, multiple comorbidities, associated hepatic dysfunction, and limited donor liver availability. The aim of palliative therapy is to provide symptomatic relief, extend survival, and improve QoL (quality of life).

Most advanced cancers are incurable and 95% of patients with advanced cancer report that QoL is at least as important as length of survival [3]. Palliative treatments may negatively influence QoL, especially if complications ensue. Poor QoL after treatment has a negative impact on the willingness of patients to continue and comply with future treatments. QoL is most influenced by health and healthcare interventions and hence QoL is an important clinical endpoint and it has become a component of clinical trials on chronic or incurable diseases [3].

TACE (transarterial chemoembolization) is the most widely used treatment for unresectable HCC [4] and is recommended as first-line treatment option for patients who meet the criteria for the intermediate stage of the Barcelona Clinic Liver Cancer (BCLC) staging system [5, 6]. Meta-analysis of six randomized controlled trials, including a total of 503 patients, showed survival benefit in patients who underwent TACE compared to the control group [7]. It is unclear if TACE helps in enhancing QoL of HCC patients by palliating several disturbing symptoms such as pruritis, fatigue, sleep disorders, sexual dysfunction, and abdominal discomfort [8]. Moreover, TACE can also cause postembolization syndrome, acute liver decompensation, or associated complications which can negatively affect the QoL. Hence it is important to study if HCC patients undergoing TACE enjoy a reasonably good QoL along with improved survival. The aim of this systematic review is to describe the current evidence and evaluate the impact of TACE on QoL of HCC patients.

2. Materials and Methods

2.1. Search Strategy. We searched medical databases including PubMed and SCOPUS for studies that discussed quality of life and/or survival rates of TACE. Search terms were (liver cancer OR hepatocellular carcinoma) AND (quality of life) AND (chemo* OR transarterial* OR infusional OR TACE) within the titles, abstracts, and keywords. In order to obtain a highly sensitive yield, we did not apply limits to our search. In addition, we hand searched the proceedings of conferences on liver diseases (International Hepato-Pancreato-Biliary Association) in 2011, 2012, and 2013.

All titles and abstracts of studies identified in the initial search were screened by lead author Vishal G. Shelat based on the following inclusion and exclusion criteria: (1) study population to consist of patients with hepatocellular carcinoma, (2) patients who were managed with transarterial chemoembolization, and (3) reported quality of life (QoL) outcomes using a discrete QoL tool. In studies reporting on outcomes for two or more groups including TACE as a control group, QoL outcomes of TACE group were included (2,9–12). Full-text papers of the selected studies were screened independently by Nurun Nisa de Souza and Vishal G. Shelat to assess eligibility. Any disagreements on eligibility were resolved by a third reviewer (Saleem Ahmed). Author Wang Qiao assisted in translation and analysis of the Chinese language study and Meidai Kasai assisted in translation and analysis of the Japanese language study.

We also included studies reporting on infusional chemotherapy without embolization [9, 10]. Exclusion criteria ruled out any study reporting on QoL in HCC patients treated by radiofrequency ablation, radioembolization, hepatic resection, or liver transplantation only. References of all the included studies were screened for potentially relevant studies not identified during initial search.

2.2. Data Extraction. The following variables were extracted from the studies where available: number of patients, age, sex, QoL questionnaire used, timing of the questionnaire administration, and dosage and type of chemotherapy agent used in TACE and QoL outcomes.

3. Results

We identified a total of 3469 studies (Figure 1) through electronic searches and from the reference lists of eligible articles. Of these, 3453 were excluded after reading titles and abstracts and further two studies were excluded for reporting QoL in patients who did not undergo TACE.

The description of the QoL tools used in the 14 publications studying the impact of TACE on QoL is detailed in Table 1. All studies except one (Shun et al.) used a single QoL instrument to assess impact of QoL in patients who underwent TACE [22]. Four authors used their own unique questionnaire [9, 10, 19, 20].

3.1. QoL Tools

3.1.1. Review of Studies Reporting on QoL in TACE Patients. Based upon the literature search, 14 studies were identified

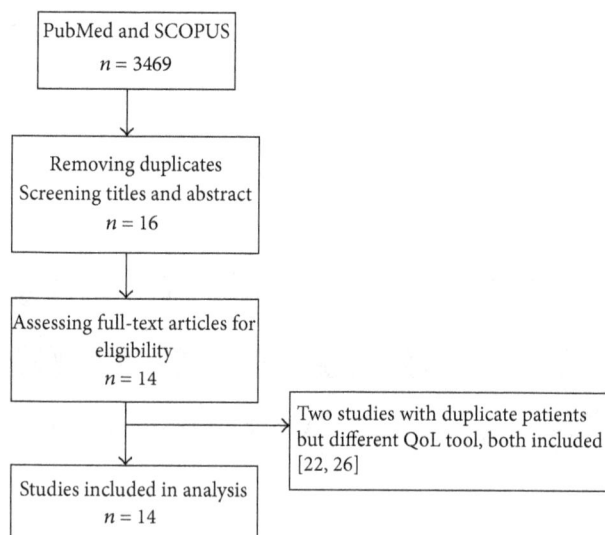

FIGURE 1: Study selection.

which reported on the use of QoL instruments to study the impact of TACE on QoL of HCC patients. Table 2 provides a summary of the studies, the sample size, comparative groups if any, disease profile, and the details of the TACE regime used in the study.

All studies that had one or more comparative groups compared the QoL of patients undergoing TACE alone versus other treatment strategies except the study by Wang et al. who compared TACE alone versus TACE and RFA in combination [23].

The study by Toyoda et al. studied the effect of repetitive continuous local intra-arterial injection chemotherapy with 5-FU and CDDP (5-FU 50 mg/day + CDDP 5–10 mg/day) via implantable reservoir on QoL. Owing to the small numbers for QoL analysis it did not produce statistically significant results. However, it found that among the 3 patients with partial remission 2 of them had an improvement in QoL scores. The overall at-home rate was 94% and the main reason for admission was to troubleshoot catheters.

Shun et al.'s study in 2012 shows that all 8 domains of QoL scores (short form 12 item health survey) improved over the three time periods studied (prior to discharge and at 4th and 8th weeks after discharge) except for vitality which improved only after 2 months after discharge. The study by Jianbo et al. showed that the QoL improved at 1 and 3 months in the physiology and symptom domains of the questionnaire compared with preintervention [20]. However, the psychology domains fell back to preintervention levels and the social domain was worse as compared to preintervention levels. Shun et al.'s study in 2005 supplements the data by Jianbo et al. on symptoms and fatigue by describing QoL scores in the more immediate period after intervention (up to day 6 after intervention) [20, 22]. It shows that the scores for fatigue, symptom distress, and depression peaked (worse) on day 2 and subsequently trended lower on day 6, although they were still higher than preintervention levels. Wible et al.'s study shows that at the 4th month after intervention there was

TABLE 1: Description of quality of life instruments used in HCC patients undergoing TACE.

Instruments	Domains (items)	Domain description
FACT-Hep QoL Questionnaire [11]	5 (45)	Emotional well-being, functional well-being, and physical well-being Social/family well-being Additional concerns
FACT-G QoL Questionnaire [12]	4 (28)	Emotional well-being, functional well-being, physical well-being, and social/family well-being
WHOQoL-BREF Questionnaire [13]	4 (26)	Physical health Psychological health Social relationships Environment
SF-36 [14]	8 (36)	Physical functioning Role physical Bodily pain General health Vitality Social functioning Role emotional Mental health
SF-12 [15]	8 (12)	Same as SF-36
Revised Piper Fatigue Scale (PFS) [16]	4 (27)	Behavioural/severity, affective meaning, sensory, and cognitive/mood
Modified Symptom Distress Scale (SDS-m) [17]	1 (13)	Symptoms: nausea (frequency, intensity), appetite, insomnia, pain (frequency, intensity), fatigue, bowel patterns, concentration, appearance, breathing, outlook, and cough
Hospital Anxiety and Depression Scale (HADS) [18]	2 (14)	Anxiety and depression
Kato et al. [19]	3 (10)	Physical health Social well-being Additional concerns regarding confidence in treatment
Tanabe et al. [10]	4 (4)	Physical function, psychological function, social function, and physical sensation
Toyoda et al. [9]	2 (10)	Symptoms Psychology Social function
Jianbo et al. [20]	4 (22)	Physiology Psychology Symptoms Social function

FACT: Functional Assessment of Cancer Therapy; WHO: World Health Organization; QoL: Quality of Life; SF: short form.

a significant improvement in mental health scores in contrast to the data by Jianbo et al., which show that the psychology domain scores fell back to preintervention levels at the third month [20, 24]. The study by Wible et al. also showed that there was no trend towards deterioration of patient's overall QoL over a 1-year period.

Eltawil et al.'s prospective observational study designed to assess both survival and QoL of primary HCC patients showed that there was a stable trend of QoL of patients undergoing repeat sessions of TACE over time [27]. The study did not see any statistically significant temporal trends for any of the four QoL domains, although there was tendency towards declining physical health after the 3rd session of TACE which is approximately 1 year after 1st session. This finding is supported by Wible et al. and Xing

et al., both showing that the patients are able to tolerate repeated TACE over a period of 1 year with no significant drop in QoL. However, Toro et al. compare QoL of patients who undergo different intervention and measure QoL over a 24-month period. Patients who underwent TACE show statistically significantly worse QoL in all domains at the 12th month and 24th month marks compared to the 3rd month in Toro et al.'s study [25]. Xie et al. have multiple time points for conducting the QoL questionnaire from the 1st month after procedure all the way to 24 months [28]. Generally, there is sharp decline in the physical and mental components in the 1st month; however, both recover in the 3rd month and 6th month and start to decline again in the 12th month mark with the worst scores being recorded at the 24th month mark.

TABLE 2: Impact of TACE on QoL in patients with HCC.

SN	Author	Study design and population	Intervention	Comparative groups or subset	Timing of questionnaire	Outcome
1	Kato et al. 1990 [19]	Prospective study Unresectable HCC $n = 16$	Patients with unresectable liver cancer: comparison of TAE, MMC microcapsule, and single shot intra-arterial doxorubicin	6: TAE; 6: MMC microcapsule; 4: single shot intra-arterial doxorubicin	Before TACE 1 week after 2 weeks after	Anorexia and depression worse in patients who underwent TACE with doxorubicin
2	Toyoda et al. 1993 [9]	Retrospective study Stage IVa HCC $n = 21$	Patients with stage IVa HCC who are unsuitable for surgery, PEIT, and TAE were selected for continuous intra-arterial chemotherapy	NA	Variable timing	Two patients in partial remission group had improvement in QoL
3	Tanabe et al. 2001 [10]	Retrospective study HCC recurrence after initial curative resection $n = 23$	Recurrence of HCC after HR: comparison of repeat HR versus HAI chemotherapy	13: HAI; 10: repeat HR	After TACE	Repeat HR provides good prognosis and favourable QoL compared to HAI in patients with resectable recurrence
4	Jianbo et al. 2002 [20]	Prospective study Primary HCC $n = 175$	TACE	NA	Before TACE 1 month after 3 months after	QoL is improved after TACE and can be maintained till 3 months after treatment in the physiology, psychology, and symptoms domain
5	Steel et al. 2004 [21]	Prospective nonrandomized cohort study Histology proven HCC $n = 28$	Patients with HCC: comparison of TACE and ^{90}Y radioembolization	14: TACE; 14: ^{90}Y radioembolization	Before TACE 3 months after 6 months after 12 months after	Treatment with Yttrium has a modest advantage with regard to QoL when compared to HAI with cisplatin
6	Shun et al. 2005 [22]	Prospective study Primary HCC $n = 40$	TACE 16 patients had 2–5 previous TACE procedures	NA	Before TACE 2 days after 4 days after 6 days after	Patient fatigue levels peaked at day 2. Factors responsible for increased fatigue levels include greater symptom distress, anxiety, and depression, higher Adriamycin dosage, longer duration of previous fatigue; and less education levels
7	Wang et al. 2007 [23]	Prospective randomized study Histology proven HCC $n = 83$	Patients with HCC: comparison of TACE and TACE + RFA	40: TACE; 43: TACE + RFA	Before TACE 3 months after 1st TACE	The overall QoL of HCC patients in TACE-RFA group was maintained at higher level than that of TACE group
8	Wible et al. 2010 [24]	Prospective study Primary HCC $n = 73$	TACE 23 patients underwent 3 or more TACE procedures	NA	Before TACE 4 months after 8 months after 12 months after	Patients with HCC are likely to perceive improved mental health during the first 4 months of primary TACE. If they undergo more than 2 procedures, they are likely to perceive improved mental health during the first 2 sessions. Patient-perceived vitality will likely worsen after initial procedure
9	Toro et al. 2012 [25]	Prospective study Primary HCC eligible for HR, RFA, TACE, or NT $n = 52$	Patients with HCC: comparison of HR, TACE, RFA, and NT	14: HR; 15: TACE; 9: RFA; 13: NT	Before TACE 3 months after 6 months after 12 months after 24 months after	RFA provides a worse QoL compared to HR but a higher QoL compared to TACE or NT

TABLE 2: Continued.

SN	Author	Study design and population	Intervention	Comparative groups or subset	Timing of questionnaire	Outcome
10	Shun et al. 2012 [26]	Prospective study Primary HCC patients receiving TACE $n = 89$	TACE	NA	3 days prior to discharge 4 weeks after discharge 8 weeks after discharge	Those at greatest risk for lower QoL include males and those who have higher levels of depression and anxiety after discharge
11	Eltawil et al. 2012 [27]	Prospective study Primary HCC not amenable to ablation or resection $n = 48$	TACE 6 patients underwent 3 or more TACE procedures	NA	Data collected every 3-4 months	QoL remained stable for almost a year and only started to decline after the 3rd TACE which coincided with progression of tumour; concluded that majority of patients were able to tolerate several TACE sessions without significant deterioration of QoL
12	Salem et al. 2013 [2]	Prospective study Primary HCC $n = 56$	Patients with HCC: comparison of TACE versus ^{90}Y radioembolization	29: ^{90}Y radioembolization; 27: TACE	Before TACE 2 weeks after 4 weeks after	QoL difference did not reach statistical significance; change in EES score was most pronounced; ^{90}Y radioembolization is better able to maintain health-related QoL.
13	Xie et al. 2015 [28]	Retrospective study Primary intermediate stage HCC $n = 102$	Patients with HCC: comparison of TACE versus HR	58: HR 44: TACE	Before TACE 1 month after 3 months after 6 months after 12 months after 24 months after	QoL was lower in the 1st month after procedure but recovered in the 3rd and 6th months but dropped again in the 12th month with lowest scores in the 24th month
14	Xing et al. 2015 [29]	Prospective study Unresectable HCC $n = 118$	TACE	NA	Before TACE 3 months after 6 months after 12 months after	QoL was preserved for up to 12 months after TACE

5-FU: 5-Fluorouracil; CDDP: cisplatin; HAI: hepatic artery infusion; HR: hepatic resection; MMC: mitomycin C; NA: not applicable; NS: not specified; NT: no treatment; QoL: quality of life; RFA: radiofrequency ablation; SD: standard deviation; TACE: transarterial chemoembolization; TAE: transarterial embolization.

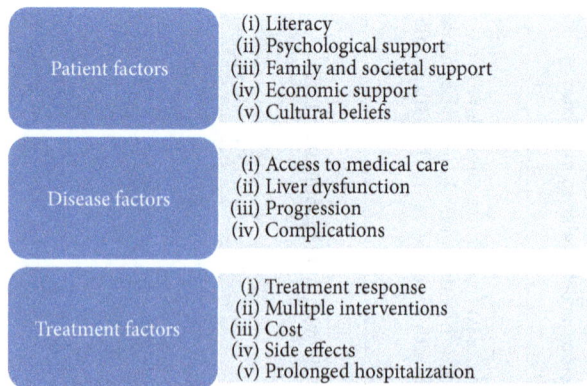

FIGURE 2: Factors influencing QoL in HCC patients treated with TACE.

The study by Kato et al. is the earliest study in our review to study effect of TACE on QoL. They use their own unique tool to study QoL. It is a 10-item questionnaire with a 5-point ordinal scale. There is no overall QoL score reported and each item in the questionnaire is compared individually. The study is one of 2 studies that study at-home rates as a surrogate measure of QoL. The results of the study by Kato et al. suggest that anorexia and depression symptoms were particularly worse in patients who underwent TACE with doxorubicin, while those who underwent TAE had much worse abdominal pain, fatigue, and uneasiness scores. Those patients who underwent MMC microcapsule therapy had the highest at-home rates of 86.6%, while those who underwent TACE with doxorubicin had the lowest at-home rates of 43.5%.

The studies included in this review tended to be with high risk of bias [30].

4. Discussion

QoL is both clinically and physiologically meaningful endpoint and is best defined from the patient's perspective [31]. Ferrel defines QoL in cancer as a personal sense of well-being encompassing a multidimensional perspective that generally includes physical, psychological, social, and spiritual dimensions or domains [32–35]. Changes in one domain can affect or influence other domains.

HCC is a common cancer and patients often present at late stages. TACE is the most common palliative treatment modality and recent meta-analysis has demonstrated survival benefit of TACE. There are limited data to show the effect of TACE on QoL [8]. It is important that current evidence on this topic is summarized and synthesised. Due to heterogeneity in existing reports, a meta-analysis is not possible. There is variation in selection of HCC patients, the TACE treatment protocols, and QoL measures employed in the 14 studies, which all contribute to heterogeneity and make direct comparison difficult. Figure 2 provides a summary of patient, disease, and treatment factors affecting QoL in HCC patients treated with TACE.

4.1. Study Populations. Eltawil et al.'s study included HCC patients with disease not amenable to ablation or resection, while the study by Toro et al. included patients with primary HCC who were eligible for resection, ablation, and TACE [25, 27]. Furthermore, the study by Toyoda et al. included only patients with stage IVa HCC, while the study by Tanabe et al. only looked at patients with HCC recurrence after initial curative resection [9, 10].

4.2. Treatment. The treatment protocols for TACE vary from institution to institution and also vary according to the time period studied. There is no strong evidence to favour one chemotherapy agent over another agent. This gives rise to variance in dose, concentration, rate of injection of drug, and even the choice of embolizing agent or its volume to be used if it is at all used [36]. There is even variance in the number of chemotherapy agents used: some authors such as Tanabe et al. use single agent chemotherapy, while others such as Jianbo et al. use combination of up to 3 chemotherapy agents [10, 20]. Intuitively, use of combination chemotherapy may produce synergistic effects with less toxicity due to lower dose of individual chemotherapeutic agents; however, there are few data to support this [37]. Toyoda et al.'s study was the only study to use continuous infusion of chemotherapy.

4.3. QoL Questionnaires. The choice of QoL questionnaires is also variable with 4 of the 14 studies using their own unique questionnaires and, even among those using standardized questionnaires, the number of items and content of the scales vary between instruments making direct comparison difficult [38]. Furthermore, the timing of administration of questionnaires and the chemotherapy agent used also may influence QoL. All this is compounded by the fact that some of the studies are statistically underpowered to provide conclusive results. Figure 2 demonstrates all the potential factors which can influence QoL of HCC patients treated with TACE. There is no study which is ideal and, therefore, we report a descriptive systematic review to evaluate impact of TACE on QoL of HCC patients.

4.4. QoL Assessment. QoL is subjective and multifaceted [8]. The ability to understand QoL is only as good as the tools available. QoL questionnaires are essential tools in quantifying the physical, social, psychological, and spiritual domains and can generally be categorised as generic, disease-specific, and symptom-specific. The generic instruments measure the complete range of diseases in different populations and are particularly useful in comparing QoL across different diseases [39]. The disease-specific instruments measure domains of QoL specific to a disease process. Carolinas Comfort Scale for hernias is an example of such a scale [40]. Symptom-specific instruments measure QoL changes specific to a symptom, for example, nausea [39].

A recent review of an online database of QoL tools (http://proqolid.org/) produced over 50 neoplasia-specific and 2 hepatobiliary-specific tools [41]. For a QoL instrument to be useful it must be able to satisfy the basic psychometric principles of validity, reliability, and responsiveness in the patient population studied [8, 42]. Clinical utility, ease of administration, and scoring are other important factors impacting the usefulness of the HRQoL instrument [42].

Despite the large number of neoplasia and hepatobiliary-specific QoL tools available, 4 out of 14 (29%) studies still used their own unique questionnaire [9, 10, 19, 20]. The high number of unique questionnaires could be due to 2 main reasons. Firstly, of the 4 studies that used their own unique questionnaires, 3 were non-English publications (2 Japanese and 1 Chinese). Lack of ready translated HRQoL questionnaires might have prompted the authors to use their own unique questionnaires. Moreover, since most HRQoL tools are developed in the West, they might have not undergone validation in the Asian setting, as QoL is subjective in nature and is influenced by the cultural and social norms of the population studied. Secondly, 2 of the papers (Kato et al. and Toyoda et al.) were published in the 1990s when the tools for HRQoL have not yet gained widespread prominence and most of the tools available then were generic in nature. Generic QoL instruments lack detail to assess the impact of symptoms specific to the disease state.

However, these issues are being addressed with the development of many HRQoL tools specifically aimed at patients with HCC. For example, QLQ-HCC18 of European Organisation for Research and Treatment of Cancer (EORTC) has been developed for use specifically in patients with HCC as a supplement module to EORTC QLQ-C30 [43]. It is the first questionnaire to include patients from both East and West during its development and included patients from Europe, Taiwan, and Hong Kong. To add further credibility, in addition to literature search, the questionnaire was developed using semistructured interviews with patients and healthcare professionals. In addition, it is currently available in Arabic, English, Chinese, and Taiwanese and is in the process of being validated. It is likely that more authors would be using internationally validated HRQoL tools with ready translations available in their own local languages. This would enable more meaningful comparison of study data across different languages and cultural settings.

Functional Assessment of Cancer Therapy (FACT) QoL tool is the most commonly used tool among the publications included in this review. FACT-G is a neoplasia-specific HRQoL tool developed in 1993 [12] and is one of the most widely used QoL instruments for cancer patients [8]. FACT-G was developed by answers generated from open-ended interviews with patients and oncology professionals. The 28-item questionnaire, in addition to a total score, also produces subscale scores for physical, social, and emotional well-being as well as satisfaction with treatment relationship. FACT-Hep is a hepatobiliary neoplasia-specific tool adapted from the Functional Assessment of Chronic Illness Therapy (FACIT) measurement system [3]. In addition to the questions contained in the original FACT-G scales, there are additional 18 questions to assess symptoms and QoL issues specific to patients with hepatobiliary cancers. The items are scored from 0 to 4, with higher overall and subscale scores pointing to better QoL. It is known to have good test-retest reliability. FACT-G and FACT-Hep together were used in 3 of the 12 studies.

Despite the difference in study variables, there are some general outcomes that are observed in the 14 studies. Firstly, as shown in the studies by Tanabe et al. and Toro et al., resection of tumour with a curative intent provides better overall QoL than TACE [10, 25]. While Toro et al. suggest that the overall QoL is worse in patients that underwent RFA compared to TACE, the combination of RFA and TACE was shown to be superior in terms of QoL outcomes compared to TACE alone in the study by Wang et al. [23, 25]. However, when compared with ^{90}Yttrium radioembolization, TACE offers inferior QoL outcomes [2, 21].

QoL is dynamic measurement encompassing many dimensions which change independently of each other over time. The timing of the administration of the QoL tool to the patients is important and can influence study outcomes. The time of administration of questionnaire after intervention can be divided into early (≤1 month after intervention), intermediate (1–3 months after intervention), and late (≥3 months after intervention). Administration of the questionnaire in the early stage may negatively influence scores for symptom and physical and psychological domains. This is because patients might experience pain from procedure and this coupled with complications can lead to physical, functional, and psychological distress. Shun et al. noted that scores for symptom distress, fatigue, anxiety, and depression peaked on 2nd day after intervention and subsequently trended lower on the 6th day after intervention [22]. Administration of questionnaire in the intermediate phase can have varying results depending on treatment response and patients' knowledge of treatment effectiveness. The studies that looked at the intermediate term such as the studies by Jianbo et al. and Wible et al. generally showed improved QoL [20, 24]. Administration of questionnaire in long term can be affected by many aspects including but not limited to disease progression and economic aspects. The studies that reported on long-term QoL showed differing results. The studies by Wible et al. and Xing et al. show no significant drop in QoL at 1 year, while the studies by Toro et al. and Xie et al. show statistically significantly worse QoL at the 1-year and 2-year time periods [24, 25, 29]. It is likely that psychological domain will be negatively influenced in patients who know that they have disease progression.

However, there is limited evidence to suggest that clinicians actually study the QoL in HCC patients undergoing palliative TACE. The existing studies are heterogeneous with regard to the type of QoL tool used and timing of administration of the questionnaire. This is further compounded with geopolitical, socioeconomic, and cultural values of global population.

5. Conclusion

QoL measurement has become an important outcome measurement in oncology, especially in the palliative setting. However, there is limited robust evidence to conclusively derive the impact of TACE on QoL in patients with HCC. It is important that hepatobiliary oncology community recognize measurement of QoL as an important aspect of multidisciplinary patient care and international collaboration is sought to standardize the measurement of QoL in HCC patients treated with palliative TACE.

Competing Interests

The authors declare that they have no competing interests.

References

[1] F. X. Bosch, J. Ribes, R. Cléries, and M. Díaz, "Epidemiology of hepatocellular carcinoma," *Clinics in Liver Disease*, vol. 9, no. 2, pp. 191–211, 2005.

[2] R. Salem, M. Gilbertsen, Z. Butt et al., "Increased quality of life among hepatocellular carcinoma patients treated with radioembolization, compared with chemoembolization," *Clinical Gastroenterology and Hepatology*, vol. 11, no. 10, pp. 1358.e1–1365.e1, 2013.

[3] N. Heffernan, D. Cella, K. Webster et al., "Measuring health-related quality of life in patients with hepatobiliary cancers: the functional assessment of cancer therapy-hepatobiliary questionnaire," *Journal of Clinical Oncology*, vol. 20, no. 9, pp. 2229–2239, 2002.

[4] K. Takayasu, S. Arii, I. Ikai et al., "Prospective cohort study of transarterial chemoembolization for unresectable hepatocellular carcinoma in 8510 patients," *Gastroenterology*, vol. 131, no. 2, pp. 461–469, 2006.

[5] European Association for the Study of the Liver and European Organisation for Research and Treatment of Cancer, "EASL-EORTC clinical practice guidelines: management of hepatocellular carcinoma," *Journal of Hepatology*, vol. 56, no. 4, pp. 908–943, 2012.

[6] J. Bruix and M. Sherman, "Management of hepatocellular carcinoma: an update," *Hepatology*, vol. 53, no. 3, pp. 1020–1022, 2011.

[7] J. M. Llovet and J. Bruix, "Systematic review of randomized trials for unresectable hepatocellular carcinoma: chemoembolization improves survival," *Hepatology*, vol. 37, no. 2, pp. 429–442, 2003.

[8] S. Gandhi, S. Khubchandani, and R. Iyer, "Quality of life and hepatocellular carcinoma," *Journal of Gastrointestinal Oncology*, vol. 5, no. 4, pp. 296–317, 2014.

[9] H. Toyoda, S. Nakano, I. Takeda et al., "The study of continuous local arterial-infusion chemotherapy with 5-FU + CDDP for patients with severely advanced HCC—for the elongation of the life-span and the improvement of QOL," *Gan To Kagaku Ryoho*, vol. 20, no. 11, pp. 1495–1498, 1993.

[10] G. Tanabe, S. Ueno, M. Maemura et al., "Favorable quality of life after repeat hepatic resection for recurrent hepatocellular carcinoma," *Hepato-Gastroenterology*, vol. 48, no. 38, pp. 506–510, 2001.

[11] N. Heffernan, D. Cella, K. Webster et al., "Measuring health-related quality of life in patients with hepatobiliary cancers: the functional assessment of Cancer Therapy-Hepatobiliary Questionnaire," *Journal of Clinical Oncology*, vol. 20, no. 9, pp. 2229–2239, 2002.

[12] D. F. Cella, D. S. Tulsky, G. Gray et al., "The functional assessment of cancer therapy scale: development and validation of the general measure," *Journal of Clinical Oncology*, vol. 11, no. 3, pp. 570–579, 1993.

[13] "Development of the World Health Organization WHOQOL-BREF quality of life assessment. The WHOQOL Group," *Psychological Medicine*, vol. 28, no. 3, pp. 551–558, 1998.

[14] J. E. Ware, K. K. Snow, M. Kosinski, and B. Gandek, *SF-36 Health Survey*, New England Medical Center Hospital, Health Institute, 1993.

[15] J. E. Ware Jr., M. Kosinski, and S. D. Keller, "A 12-item short-form health survey: construction of scales and preliminary tests of reliability and validity," *Medical Care*, vol. 34, no. 3, pp. 220–233, 1996.

[16] B. F. Piper, S. L. Dibble, M. J. Dodd, M. C. Weiss, R. E. Slaughter, and S. M. Paul, "The revised Piper Fatigue Scale: psychometric evaluation in women with breast cancer," *Oncology Nursing Forum*, vol. 25, no. 4, pp. 677–684, 1998.

[17] S. Holmes, "Use of a modified symptom distress scale in assessment of the cancer patient," *International Journal of Nursing Studies*, vol. 26, no. 1, pp. 69–79, 1989.

[18] A. S. Zigmond and R. P. Snaith, "The hospital anxiety and depression scale," *Acta Psychiatrica Scandinavica*, vol. 67, no. 6, pp. 361–370, 1983.

[19] T. Kato, M. Niwa, Y. Saito et al., "Evaluation of quality of life in arterial infusion chemotherapy of hepatocellular carcinoma," *Gan To Kagaku Ryoho*, vol. 17, no. 8, pp. 1623–1628, 1990.

[20] Z. Jianbo, L. Yanhao, C. Yong et al., "Evaluation of quality of life before and after interventional therapy in patients with primary hepatocellular carcinoma," *Chinese Journal of Radiology*, vol. 36, no. 10, pp. 873–876, 2002.

[21] J. Steel, A. Baum, and B. Carr, "Quality of life in patients diagnosed with primary hepatocellular carcinoma: hepatic arterial infusion of cisplatin versus 90-Yttrium microspheres (Therasphere®)," *Psycho-Oncology*, vol. 13, no. 2, pp. 73–79, 2004.

[22] S.-C. Shun, Y.-H. Lai, T.-T. Jing et al., "Fatigue patterns and correlates in male liver cancer patients receiving transcatheter hepatic arterial chemoembolization," *Supportive Care in Cancer*, vol. 13, no. 5, pp. 311–317, 2005.

[23] Y.-B. Wang, M.-H. Chen, K. Yan, W. Yang, Y. Dai, and S.-S. Yin, "Quality of life after radiofrequency ablation combined with transcatheter arterial chemoembolization for hepatocellular carcinoma: comparison with transcatheter arterial chemoembolization alone," *Quality of Life Research*, vol. 16, no. 3, pp. 389–397, 2007.

[24] B. C. Wible, W. S. Rilling, P. Drescher et al., "Longitudinal quality of life assessment of patients with hepatocellular carcinoma after primary transarterial chemoembolization," *Journal of Vascular and Interventional Radiology*, vol. 21, no. 7, pp. 1024–1030, 2010.

[25] A. Toro, E. Pulvirenti, F. Palermo, and I. Di Carlo, "Health-related quality of life in patients with hepatocellular carcinoma after hepatic resection, transcatheter arterial chemoembolization, radiofrequency ablation or no treatment," *Surgical Oncology*, vol. 21, no. 1, pp. e23–e30, 2012.

[26] S.-C. Shun, C.-H. Chen, J.-C. Sheu, J.-D. Liang, J.-C. Yang, and Y.-H. Lai, "Quality of life and its associated factors in patients with hepatocellular carcinoma receiving one course of transarterial chemoembolization treatment: a longitudinal study," *Oncologist*, vol. 17, no. 5, pp. 732–739, 2012.

[27] K. M. Eltawil, R. Berry, M. Abdolell, and M. Molinari, "Quality of life and survival analysis of patients undergoing transarterial chemoembolization for primary hepatic malignancies: a prospective cohort study," *HPB*, vol. 14, no. 5, pp. 341–350, 2012.

[28] Z. R. Xie, Y. L. Luo, F. M. Xiao, Q. Liu, and Y. Ma, "Health-related quality of life of patients with intermediate hepatocellular carcinoma after liver resection or transcatheter arterial chemoembolization," *Asian Pacific Journal of Cancer Prevention*, vol. 16, no. 10, pp. 4451–4456, 2015.

[29] M. Xing, G. Webber, H. J. Prajapati et al., "Preservation of quality of life with doxorubicin drug-eluting bead transarterial chemoembolization for unresectable hepatocellular carcinoma: longitudinal prospective study," *Journal of Gastroenterology and Hepatology*, vol. 30, no. 7, pp. 1167–1174, 2015.

[30] L. Hopp, "Risk of bias reporting in Cochrane systematic reviews," *International Journal of Nursing Practice*, vol. 5, pp. 683–686, 21.

[31] T. M. Gill and A. R. Feinstein, "A critical appraisal of the quality of quality-of-life measurements," *The Journal of the American Medical Association*, vol. 272, no. 8, pp. 619–626, 1994.

[32] B. Ferrell, M. Grant, G. Padilla, S. Vemuri, and M. Rhiner, "The experience of pain and perceptions of quality of life: validation of a conceptual model," *Hospice Journal*, vol. 7, no. 3, pp. 9–24, 1991.

[33] B. R. Ferrell, C. Wisdom, and C. Wenzl, "Quality of life as an outcome variable in the management of cancer pain," *Cancer*, vol. 63, no. 11, pp. 2321–2327, 1989.

[34] B. R. Ferrell, "The impact of pain on quality of life. A decade of research," *The Nursing Clinics of North America*, vol. 30, no. 4, pp. 609–624, 1995.

[35] B. R. Ferrell, K. H. Dow, and M. Grant, "Measurement of the quality of life in cancer survivors," *Quality of Life Research*, vol. 4, no. 6, pp. 523–531, 1995.

[36] Y.-S. Guan, Q. He, and M.-Q. Wang, "Transcatheter arterial chemoembolization: history for more than 30 years," *ISRN Gastroenterology*, vol. 2012, Article ID 480650, 8 pages, 2012.

[37] S. W. Shin, "The current practice of transarterial chemoembolization for the treatment of hepatocellular carcinoma," *Korean Journal of Radiology*, vol. 10, no. 5, pp. 425–434, 2009.

[38] S. Kaasa and J. H. Loge, "Quality-of-life assessment in palliative care," *The Lancet Oncology*, vol. 3, no. 3, pp. 175–182, 2002.

[39] L. D. MacKeigan and D. S. Pathak, "Overview of health-related quality-of-life measures," *American Journal of Hospital Pharmacy*, vol. 49, no. 9, pp. 2236–2245, 1992.

[40] A. E. T. Yeo and C. R. Berney, "Carolinas comfort scale for mesh repair of inguinal hernia," *ANZ Journal of Surgery*, vol. 82, no. 4, pp. 285–286, 2012.

[41] Mapi Research Trust, "PROQOLID, the Clinical Outcome Assessment (COA) Instruments Database," http://www.proqolid.org/.

[42] M. L. Slevin, "Quality of life: philosophical question or clinical reality?" *British Medical Journal*, vol. 305, no. 6851, pp. 466–469, 1992.

[43] J. M. Blazeby, E. Currie, B. C. Y. Zee, W.-C. Chie, R. T. Poon, and O. J. Garden, "Development of a questionnaire module to supplement the EORTC QLQ-C30 to assess quality of life in patients with hepatocellular carcinoma, the EORTC QLQ-HCC18," *European Journal of Cancer*, vol. 40, no. 16, pp. 2439–2444, 2004.

22

The Prognostic Significance of Lymphatics in Colorectal Liver Metastases

Vijayaragavan Muralidharan, Linh Nguyen, Jonathan Banting, and Christopher Christophi

Department of Surgery, The University of Melbourne and Austin Hospital, Lance Townsend Building Level 8, Studley Road, Heidelberg, Melbourne, VIC 3084, Australia

Correspondence should be addressed to Linh Nguyen; linh.nguyen@unimelb.edu.au

Academic Editor: Attila Olah

Background. Colorectal Cancer (CRC) is the most common form of cancer diagnosed in Australia across both genders. Approximately, 40%–60% of patients with CRC develop metastasis, the liver being the most common site. Almost 70% of CRC mortality can be attributed to the development of liver metastasis. This study examines the pattern and density of lymphatics in colorectal liver metastases (CLM) as predictors of survival following hepatic resection for CLM. *Methods.* Patient tissue samples were obtained from the Victorian Cancer Biobank. Immunohistochemistry was used to examine the spatial differences in blood and lymphatic vessel densities between different regions within the tumor (CLM) and surrounding host tissue. Lymphatic vessel density (LVD) was assessed as a potential prognostic marker. *Results.* Patients with low lymphatic vessel density in the tumor centre, tumor periphery, and adjacent normal liver demonstrated a significant disease-free survival advantage compared to patients with high lymphatic vessel density ($P = 0.01$, $P > 0.01$, and $P = 0.05$, resp.). Lymphatic vessel density in the tumor centre and periphery and adjacent normal liver was an accurate predictive marker of disease-free survival ($P = 0.05$). *Conclusion.* Lymphatic vessel density in CLM appears to be an accurate predictor of recurrence and disease-free survival.

1. Introduction

Almost 40%–60% of patients with colorectal cancer (CRC) develop metastasis, predominantly in the liver [1]. Tumor angiogenesis has been implicated as a major factor in the development and spread of these metastases. The recent discovery of vascular endothelial growth factor-C (VEGF-C) and VEGF receptor-3 (VEGFR-3) involvement in lymphatic vessel development [2] and specific lymphatic markers has provided new insights into the field of lymphangiogenesis [3]. Using these markers, studies have suggested that lymphangiogenesis plays an active role in the formation and spread of colorectal liver metastases (CLM) [4, 5]. The patterns of intratumoral lymphatics may have potential clinical significance as a predictive marker of disease recurrence and patient survival [5].

In this study, we investigated the patterns of tumor lymphangiogenesis using monoclonal D2-40 and LYVE-1 antibody, as a predictive marker for disease-free survival in patients with CLM. Blood vessels were examined using CD34 antibody to differentiate the blood vessels from the lymphatic vessels.

2. Patients and Methods

2.1. Case Selection. Tissue was obtained from the Victorian Cancer Biobank for 49 patients who underwent hepatic resection for CLM. Informed consent had been obtained from these patients at the time of surgery for long-term storage of specimen samples and subsequent research according to well-established protocols. Formal ethics approval was obtained from the Human Research Ethics Committee (HREC) of the Austin Hospital for the study (HREC submission number: H2012/04618). Patients' demographic information was obtained from data records.

2.2. Definition of Tumor Region. The tumor mass was divided into four regions for each parameter measured; tumor periphery, tumor centre, liver immediately adjacent to tumor, and host liver distal to tumor. Previously, we demonstrated that, following the treatment with a novel vascular destructive agent (VDA), OXi4503, the bulk of the tumor died leaving a viable rim of tumor cells at the periphery extending one hundred microns from the tumor-host interface towards the tumor centre [6]. Based on findings from our previous study, the tumor periphery is defined as the area covering the tumor-host interface and extending one hundred microns towards the tumor centre. The tumor centre is the remaining bulk of the tumor without considering the periphery. The liver immediately adjacent to the tumor is defined as the area at the tumor-host interface and extending one hundred microns away from the tumor. The host liver distal to the tumor is host liver which is farther than one hundred microns from the tumor.

2.3. Immunohistochemistry. Tissue samples from the specimen were fixed in 10% buffered formalin, embedded in paraffin, and cut into four μm thick sections. Sections were deparaffinized and rehydrated using standard techniques. Endogenous peroxidases were blocked using 3% peroxide for 30 minutes at room temperature.

D2-40 is a new selective monoclonal antibody for lymphatic endothelium which does not cross react with blood vessel endothelium [7]. For D2-40 and LYVE-1 staining, heat antigen retrieval was performed using TRIS buffer (50 mM) pH 9.5 for 15 minutes at 99°C. The sections were immunostained with mouse monoclonal antibody D2-40 used at 0.03475 mg/mL (D2-40, Dako, Victoria, Australia) and LYVE-1 used at 0.0067 mg/mL (Abcam, Cambridge, USA).

CD34 is an established endothelial vessel marker normally expressed on tumor vessels and host vessels undergoing neovasculature [8]. For CD34, no antigen retrieval was required. Normal goat serum (20%) was used to block non-specific binding. CD34 was used at 0.005 mg/mL (Abcam, Cambridge, USA).

A polymer-based detection kit containing goat anti-mouse immunoglobulins (IgG) coupled with horseradish peroxidase (HRP) (ENvision Plus, DakoCytomation Pty, Ltd, Botany, NSW, Australia) was used. The presence of vessels was visualized using diaminobenzidine (DAB) as a substrate. Appropriate negative controls were done simultaneously for each batch of slides.

2.4. Quantitation. Images of positively stained vessels were captured using a digital light microscope (Nikon Coolscope, Nikon Corporation, Japan) between 10x and 400x magnification. The images of tumor fields were captured to be representative of the entire tumor, using a raster pattern which allowed for captured fields to be random and avoid overlap. Between 20 and 30 fields per tumor were assessed. The images were analyzed using Image-Pro Plus (Version 5, Media Cybernetics, Perth Australia).

Vessels were assessed as the number of positively stained vessels per tumor area to provide a microvascular density index.

TABLE 1: Demographic and clinical characteristics.

Variable	Value*
Age (year)	61 (33–84)
Sex (male: female)	29: 20
Number of liver metastases	2 (1–10)
Total volume of tumour (mm^3)	12845 (502–867600)
Volume of largest tumour (mm^3)	8181 (381–904778)
Metachronous: synchronous	28: 21

*Data expressed as median (range) or n (%).

The lymphatic vessel density (LVD) assessments were performed by researchers blinded to the patient outcome data.

2.5. Statistical Analysis. All data are expressed as the mean ± SEM unless otherwise stated. Data were tested for normality. Pairwise comparisons of group means for parametric data were performed using analysis of variance (ANOVA) with post hoc analysis as appropriate. Nonparametric data were performed using Mann-Whitney U or Kruskal-Wallis tests, as appropriate.

Disease-free survival was calculated from the date of surgery to the date of progression or the date of last follow up. Overall survival was not used in this study as a result of a relatively small number of deaths (7/49) within the follow up period.

Receiver operating characteristic (ROC) analysis was conducted to assess the discriminative performance and the predictive capability of LVD in each region (tumor periphery, tumor centre, and adjacent liver) with tumor recurrence as the end point. Accuracy of a test is measured by the area under the ROC curve. An area under the curve (AUC) of 1 represents a perfect test; an area of 0.5 represents a worthless test. Cut-off points that maximized sensitivity and specificity were established by analyzing ROC curve coordinate points. Using optimal cut-off thresholds determined from ROC analysis, Kaplan-Meier survival curves were generated to compare survival between groups of high and low LVD in the three regions. A logistic regression model was performed using multivariate and univariate analysis.

P values of <0.05 were considered statistically significant. All statistical analyses were performed using SPSS (Statistics Package for Social Sciences, SPSS, Chicago, IL).

3. Results

3.1. Patient Characteristics. A total of 49 patients with histologically proven CLM were included in the study. Median follow-up time for all patients was 27 months (range 4–95 months). Five patients died during the follow-up period. Median time to death was 21 months (range 15–33 months). Patient demographics and clinical characteristics are summarized in Table 1.

All patients had been assessed by a multidisciplinary team consisting of radiologists, HPB surgeons, oncologists, and nuclear physicians prior to commencement of treatment.

(a)

(b)

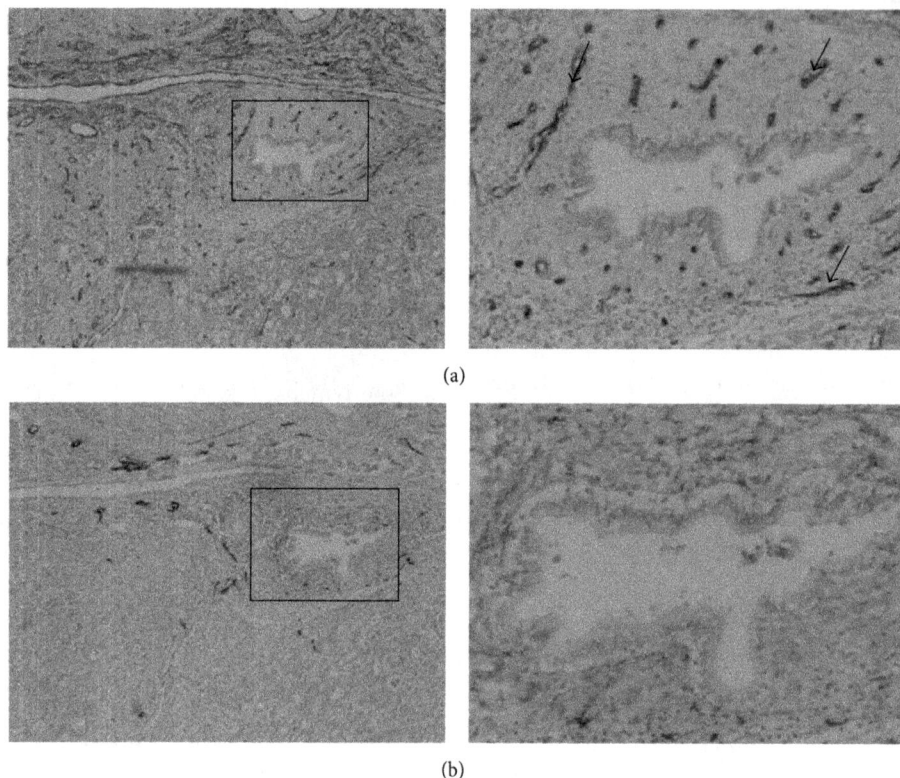

FIGURE 1: CD34 and D2-40 expression in colorectal liver metastases. (a) Strong staining of blood vessels using CD34, magnified insert. Arrows indicating CD34 positive blood vessels. (b) Lymphatic vessel staining using D2-40; magnified insert indicating the absence of lymphatic vessels in highly vascular region.

Standard indications for liver resection of CLM were followed after excluding extrahepatic metastases by multidetector computed tomography (MDCT) of chest and triple phase MDCT of abdomen and pelvis in addition to whole body positron emission tomography with fluorodeoxyglucose integrated with computed tomography (FDG PET/CT) scans. Patients received a combination chemotherapy regimen including oxaliplatin (FOLFOX or capecitabine/oxaliplatin) or irinotecan (FOLFIRI) based regimen.

3.2. Spatial Differences in Tumor Lymph Vessel Density. CD34 appears to only stain blood vessel endothelial cells, leaving lymphatic endothelial cells negative. Serial immunohistochemistry staining using CD34 and D2-40 antibodies demonstrates the specificity of the markers. No overlapping of vessels was observed between CD34 and D2-40 (Figure 1).

Quantification of D2-40 staining (Figure 2) revealed greater density at the tumor periphery compared to the tumor centre (49.22 ± 24.3 positive LVD/mm^2 versus 22.1 ± 11.5 positive LVD/mm^2, $P < 0.001$), adjacent liver (49.22 ± 24.3 positive LVD/mm^2 versus 4.3 ± 4.9 positive LVD/mm^2, $P < 0.001$), normal liver (distal to the tumor) (49.22 ± 24.3 positive LVD/mm^2 versus 6.7 ± 3.1 positive LVD/mm^2, $P < 0.001$), and benign liver (49.22 ± 24.3 positive LVD/mm^2 versus 8.7 ± 6.2 positive LVD/mm^2, $P < 0.001$). LYVE-1, a marker selective for lymphatic vessels, was also carried out.

LYVE-1 was found to be expressed in the liver sinusoids but absent from the tumor (Figure 3).

3.3. Low Lymphatic Vessel Density Is Associated with Disease-Free Survival Advantage. The ROC curve in Figures 4(a), 5(a) and 6(a) shows the ability of LVD in the tumor periphery, centre, and adjacent liver to be used as a prognostic marker to predict the likelihood of disease recurrence following hepatic resection. The ROC graph shows a statistically significant ability of peripheral ($P < 0.01$), central ($P < 0.05$), and adjacent liver ($P = 0.01$) LVD to predict disease recurrence. Peripheral LVD was the most discriminative, with an area under the curve (AUC) of 0.713, followed by LVD in the adjacent liver with an AUC equal to 0.708 and central LVD with an AUC equal to 0.692.

According to the optimal cut-off values provided by ROC analysis, patients were categorized into two groups: Low LVD and High LVD in different regions.

A further analysis was performed using Kaplan-Meier disease-free survival graphs. Low D2-40 stained LVD in the tumor periphery ($P < 0.01$), centre ($P = 0.01$), and liver adjacent to the tumor ($P = 0.018$) (Figures 4(b), 5(b) and 6(b), resp.) correlated significantly with disease-free survival.

Table 2 shows that patients, with high LVD in the periphery, centre, and liver adjacent to the tumor, appear to demonstrate close correlation to disease recurrence within the first and second year ($P < 0.05$) after resection. However, only

(a)

(b)

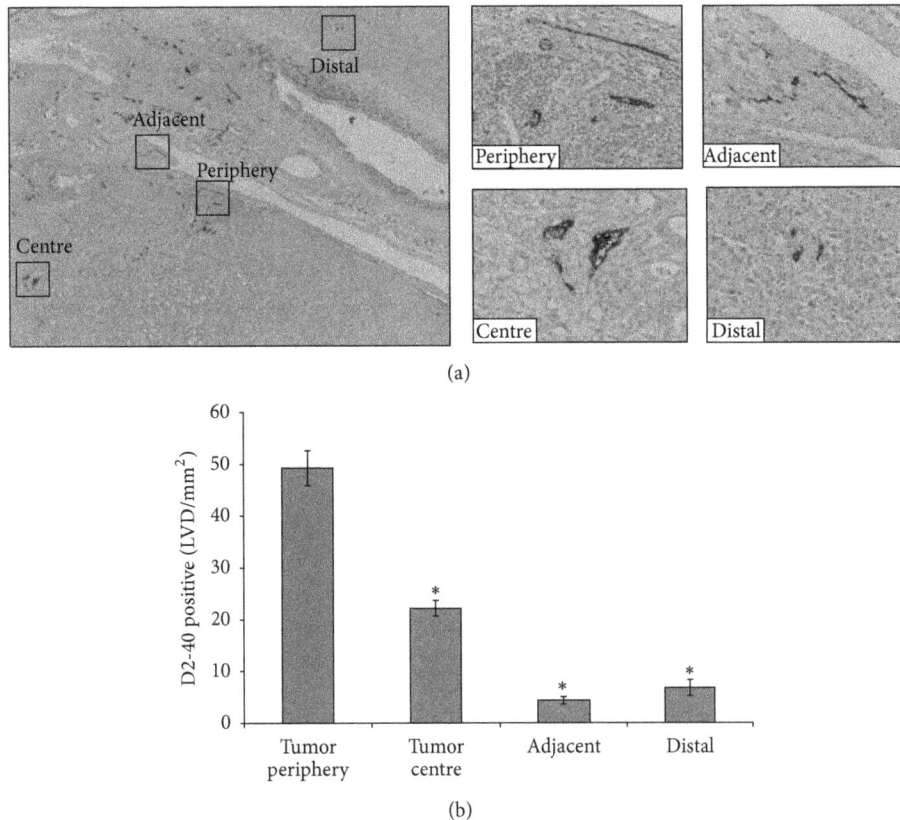

FIGURE 2: Higher lymphatic vessel density (LVD) in the tumor periphery compared to tumor centre, adjacent, and distal liver. (a) Paraffin embedded section showing lymphatic vessels stained with D2-40 at the tumor periphery and centre, adjacent, and distal liver; magnified inserts of area of interest shown (×400). (b) Enumeration of lymphatic vessel counts revealed higher LVD in the tumor periphery compared to tumor centre, adjacent and distal liver ($^*P < 0.001$).

TABLE 2: Lymphatic vessel density significantly correlates with disease recurrence.

	Tumour periphery	Tumour centre	Adjacent liver
1 year recurrence	0.014	0.007	0.007
2 year recurrence	0.050	0.028	0.034
3 year recurrence	0.009	0.080	0.097

The table summarizes the correlation of LVD in different regions to disease recurrence at 1, 2 and 3 years following resection.

patients with high LVD in the tumor periphery significantly correlated with disease-free survival within the third year ($P = 0.009$) after resection.

In Cox multivariate analysis, taking into consideration the other variables including sex, age, total tumor volume (TTV), largest tumor volume (LTV), and number of lesions, only high LVD in the normal liver adjacent to the tumor showed significant correlation ($P = 0.046$) to disease recurrence following resection (Table 3).

4. Discussion

The potential role of lymphangiogenesis in the process of tumor metastasis has been largely overshadowed by the role of angiogenesis [9]. For decades, angiogenesis, the formation of new blood vessels, has been the main focus of research in the pathogenesis of tumor metastases [10]. Over the decades, much knowledge has accumulated linking angiogenesis as an essential step in tumor growth and development [10]. It has been reported that, in the absence of active angiogenesis, the growing tumor may undergo necrosis and apoptosis beyond 1-$2 \, mm^2$ in diameter due to limitation imposed by diffusion [10]. Several studies have focused on the microvessel density (MVD) as a prognostic tool; Hasan et al. observed elevated levels of MVD in CRC to be associated with poor prognosis [11]. Our study is in concordance with those findings and demonstrates significant differences in MVD between different regions of the tumor and adjacent liver. This highlights the spatial differences within the tumor microenvironment and the heterogeneity of the tumor [12].

In contrast to the extensive characterization of molecular mechanisms involved in angiogenesis, research into the role and mechanisms of lymphangiogenesis in cancer has been hampered by singular lack of specific markers [13]. However, recent discovery of lymphangiogenic factor, vascular endothelial growth factor-C (VEGF-C), and specific lymphatic markers (LYVE-1 and D2-40) now allow researchers to identify and focus on the role of lymphangiogenesis in tumor

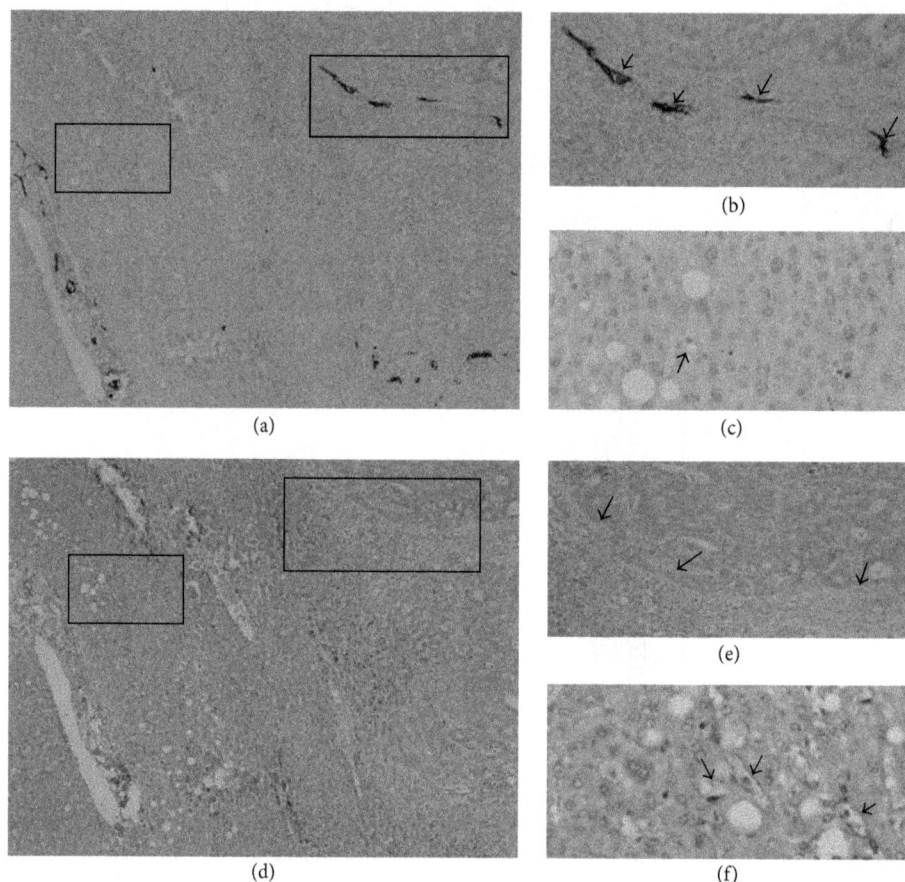

FIGURE 3: LYVE-1 not able to detect lymphangiogenesis in tumor. (a) Paraffin embedded section showing lymphatic vessels stained with D2-40 (×80). (b) Magnified insert highlighting the strong staining of D2-40 expressing lymphatics within the tumor (arrows) (×400). (c) D2-40 did not stain the liver sinusoids or hepatic blood vessels (arrow) (×400). (d) Serial sections stained using immunohistochemistry with LYVE-1; revealed LYVE-1 was not a specific marker for lymphangiogenesis in the liver (×80). (e) LYVE-1 was not able to detect lymphatic vessels in the tumor periphery where D2-40 was able to detect lymphatic vessels (arrows) (×400). (f) LYVE-1 was expressed in liver sinusoids and hepatic blood vessels (arrows) (×400).

TABLE 3: Cox multivariate regression analysis.

	B	SE	Wald	df	Sig.	Exp (B)	95.0% CI for Exp (B)	
Variables in the Equation								
							Lower	Upper
Age	0.001	0.021	0.002	1	0.964	1.001	0.960	1.044
Sex	−0.521	0.448	1.353	1	0.245	0.594	0.247	1.429
Lesions	0.158	0.252	0.394	1	0.530	1.171	0.715	1.919
Total tumor volume (TTV)	0.000	0.000	0.039	1	0.843	1.000	1.000	1.000
Largest tumor volume (LTV)	0.000	0.000	0.002	1	0.961	1.000	1.000	1.000
Synchronous/metachronous	0.374	0.477	0.616	1	0.433	1.454	0.571	3.700
Tumor periphery	−0.929	0.515	3.252	1	**0.071**	0.395	0.144	1.084
Tumor centre	−0.792	0.544	2.121	1	**0.145**	0.453	0.156	1.315
Adjacent liver	−0.883	0.443	3.982	1	**0.046**	0.413	0.174	0.984

Table demonstrates that when other variables are taken into account, only high LVD in adjacent liver was able to significantly predict disease recurrence.

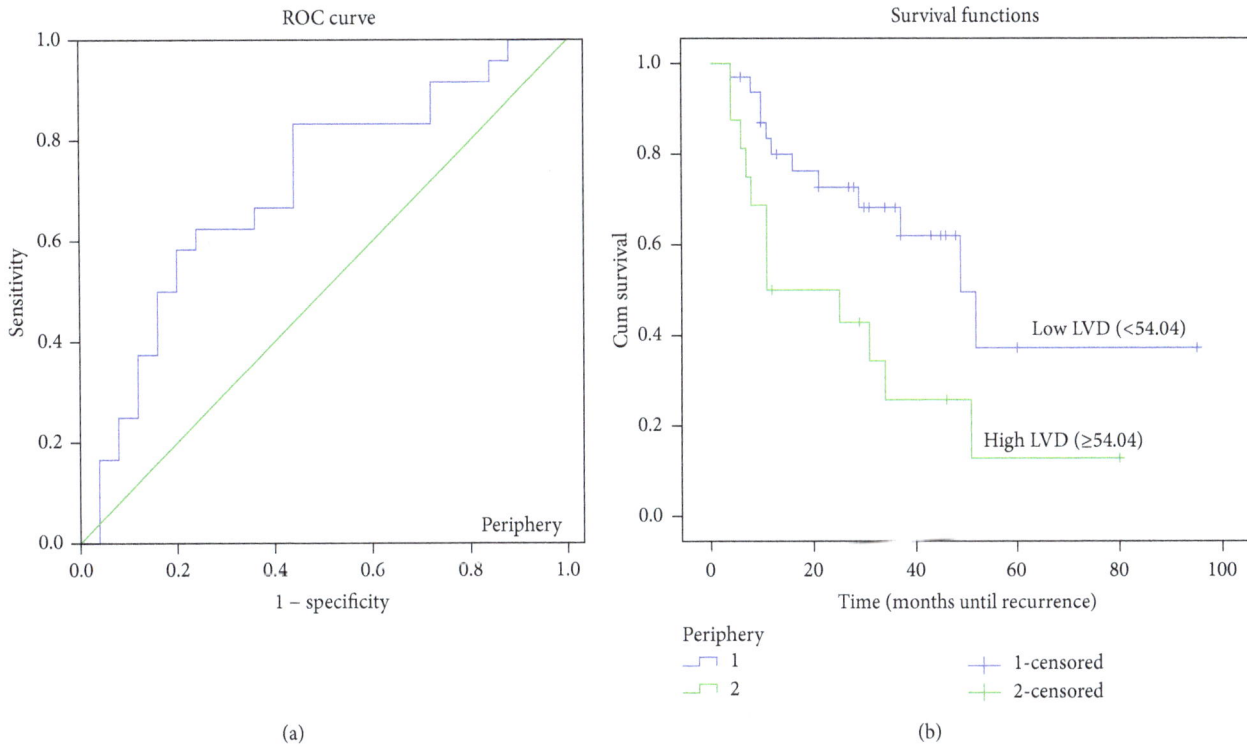

FIGURE 4: ROC curve and Kaplan-Meier survival curves of lymphatic vessel density (LVD) in the tumor periphery. (a) ROC curve showing the specificity and sensitivity of LVD in the periphery predicting recurrence (AUC = 0.713). (b) High LVD (>54.04) in the tumor periphery correlated with poorer prognosis ($P < 0.01$).

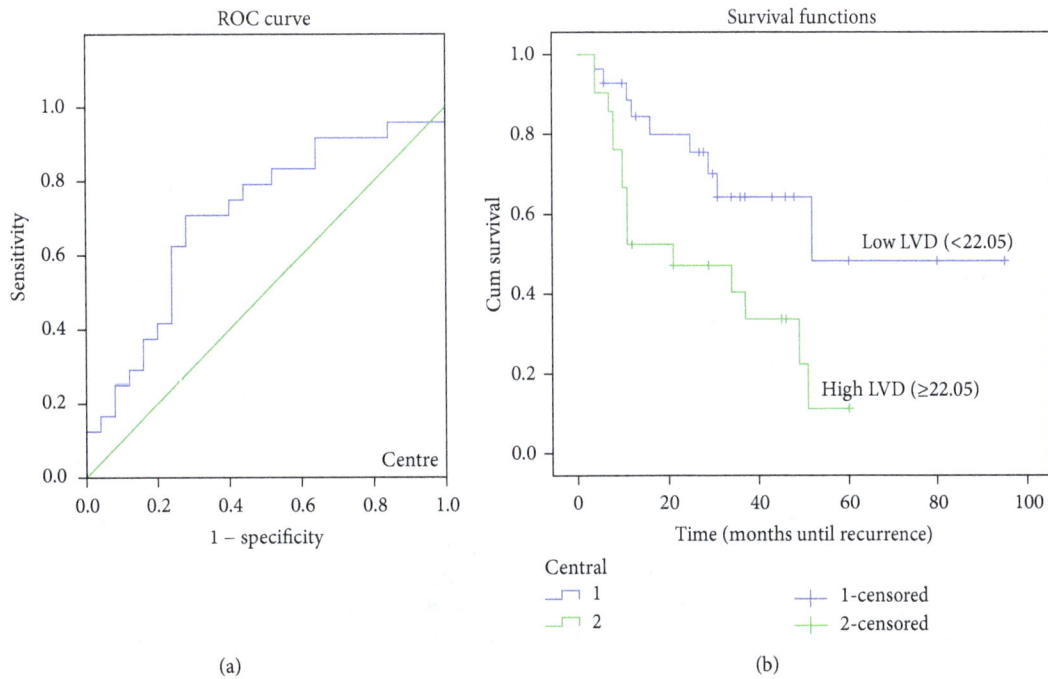

FIGURE 5: ROC curve and Kaplan-Meier survival curves of lymphatic vessel density (LVD) in the tumor centre. (a) ROC curve showing the specificity and sensitivity of LVD in the centre predicting recurrence (AUC = 0.692). (b) High LVD (>22.02) in the tumor periphery correlated with poorer prognosis ($P = 0.01$).

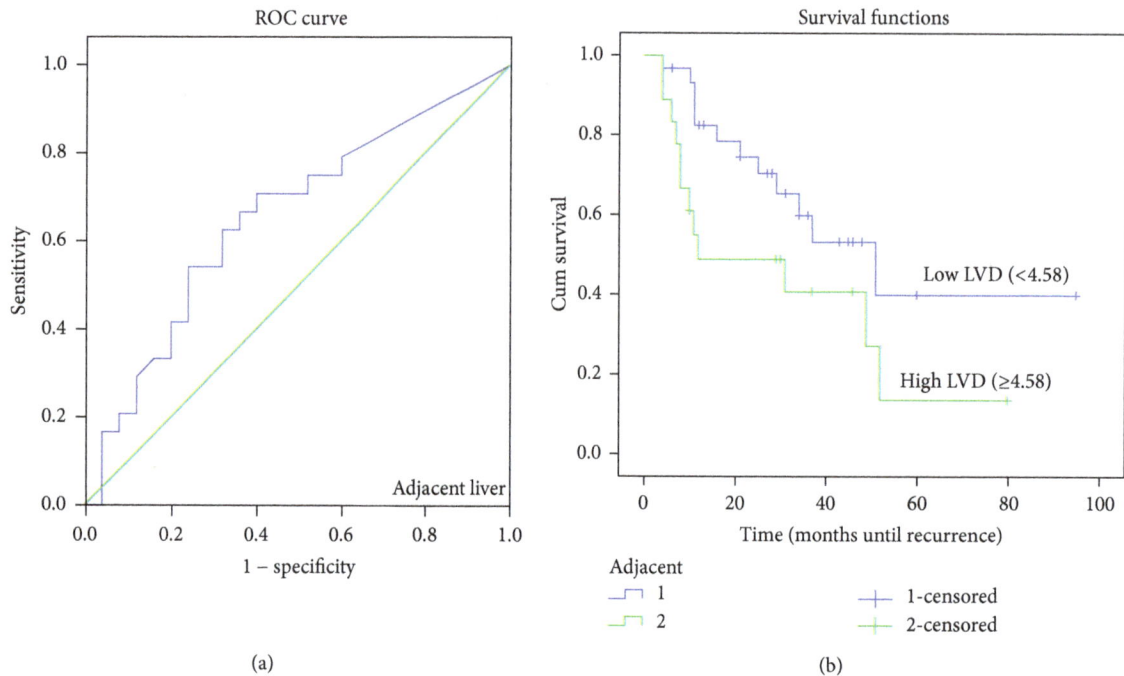

FIGURE 6: ROC curve and Kaplan-Meier survival curves of lymphatic vessel density (LVD) in the adjacent liver. (a) ROC curve showing the specificity and sensitivity of LVD in the centre predicting recurrence (AUC = 0.708). (b) High LVD (>22.02) in the tumor periphery correlated with poorer prognosis ($P = 0.01$).

metastases and to determine whether they have prognostic implications.

The recent introduction of LYVE-1 and D2-40 has paved the way for exciting research into the field of lymphangiogenesis: its mechanisms and the possible role these vessels play in the spread and dissemination of tumor cells [7, 13]. Despite the recent focus on lymphangiogenesis research, literature on the role of lymphatic vessels in tumor metastasis has been slow to accumulate with conflicting evidence.

Early studies reported the absence of lymphangiogenesis within the tumor, initially believed to be due to the high interstitial pressure created by rapidly proliferating tumor cells [9]. Due to the absence of intratumoral lymphatic vessels, it was suggested that lymphatic vessels at the periphery were responsible for the spread of tumors [14]. However, more recent studies have reported the presence of intratumoral lymphatics in several different cancers such as breast cancer [15] and colon cancer [16]. Dadras et al. investigated the possibility of using LVD as a marker for prognosis; the study reported high intratumoral LVD in metastatic lesions compared to primary lesions significantly correlated with poor disease-free survival in cutaneous melanoma [17]. In agreement, Saad et al. also reported the presence of intratumoral lymphatics in 46% of cases with stage 1 endocervical adenocarcinoma; however, they observed small and flattened vessels within the tumor, in contrast to the wide open lymphatic vessels found in the tumor periphery, casting a doubt of functionality of intratumoral lymphatic vessels [18]. In contrast to Dadras' findings, Saad et al. showed a significant correlation with peritumoral D2-40 LVD and depth of invasion. Intratumoral LVD was found to have no

significant correlation to clinicopathologic parameters [18]. Due to many conflicting results and the absence of a general consensus on the prognostic value of LVD, different types of cancers need to be investigated separately to identify the prognostic value of lymphangiogenesis.

Few studies have investigated LVD as a prognostic marker in CLM and the results have been contradictory [19–21]. Despite recent progress in this field, the potential use of LVD as a prognostic marker in CLM remains unclear. Investigating the expression of VEGF-C, a marker associated with lymphangiogenesis, Matsumoto et al. reported that VEGF-C overexpression significantly correlated with tumor invasion, lymphatic invasion, and lymph node metastases [19]. In contrast, using LYVE-1 as a marker for lymphatic vessels, Brundler et al. observed no significant correlation between LVD and clinical outcome and concluded that LVD had no prognostic value in esophageal adenocarcinoma [20]. One possible explanation for the results reported by Brundler et al. maybe due to the antibody used to identify lymphatic vessels. LYVE-1 does not appear to be a sensitive and reliable marker for lymphatic vessels in all solid tumors. In agreement with previous studies [22], we found that LYVE-1 did not specifically stain lymphatic vessels in the liver. LYVE-1 stained liver sinusoidal endothelial cells and was not able to identify lymphatic vessels in the tumor. LYVE-1 is a known hyaluronan (HA) receptor found on lymphatic endothelial cells; however, the liver sinusoidal endothelial cells play a major role in HA catabolism and as a result also display HA receptors [22]. In addition, Ichida et al. reported elevated HA levels associated with liver injury including cirrhosis and hepatocellular carcinoma (HCC) [23]. It is believed that reduced expression of the scavenging LYVE-1 HA receptors during liver injury and HCC leads to increased HA serum levels [22].

Indeed, in contrast to Brundler et al., Saad et al. reported a significant correlation between LVD and lymph node metastasis and lymphovascular invasion and tumor stage in esophageal adenocarcinoma using D2-40 as a marker for lymphatic vessels [24]. Due to these few and conflicting results, clear consensus on the potential use of LVD as a prognostic marker remains to be elucidated.

Using D2-40 as a specific marker for lymphatic vessels, our data demonstrated that LVD in the tumor periphery and centre and adjacent liver significantly correlated with disease-free survival. LVD in the tumor periphery and centre and adjacent liver correlated with recurrence within the first two years following resection, while LVD in the tumor periphery continued to correlate with disease recurrence three years after resection. However, in the multivariate analysis, only the LVD in the adjacent liver was significantly correlated with disease-free survival. The contradictory results regarding the prognostic significance of LVD in tumor metastases may be due to different patient cohorts, specific tumors included in the analysis, or the method/markers used to detect lymphatic vessels. One of the limitations of this study is that samples were obtained only from a single tumor from each patient. This, therefore, may not necessarily reflect the LVD in other tumors in the same patient and, hence, be a confounding factor.

5. Conclusion

This study has demonstrated that D2-40 is effective in identifying lymphatic vessels in human CLM. The monoclonal antibody strongly labeled lymphatic vessels without staining blood vessels as observed in the serial staining of D2-40 and CD34. D2-40 was, therefore, found to be an appropriate and selective marker for lymphatic vessels in CLM. Our results further demonstrate the potential predictive value of LVD detected by D2-40, as a prognostic marker CLM. Despite the limitations imposed by the retrospective nature of the study, relatively short follow-up period, and sampling of single lesions from each patient, the results have established a foundation for investigating what appears to be a potentially significant predictive factor in the long-term survival of patients with CLM. Determining the lymphatic development within tumors may further play a significant role in the selective use of biological agents [25] with the ability to target lymphatics being currently under development.

References

[1] R. S. Warren, H. Yuan, M. R. Matli, N. A. Gillett, and N. Ferrara, "Regulation by vascular endothelial growth factor of human colon cancer tumorigenesis in a mouse model of experimental liver metastasis," *Journal of Clinical Investigation*, vol. 95, no. 4, pp. 1789–1797, 1995.

[2] E. Kukk, A. Lymboussaki, S. Taira et al., "VEGF-C receptor binding and pattern of expression with VEGFR-3 suggests a role in lymphatic vascular development," *Development*, vol. 122, no. 12, pp. 3829–3837, 1996.

[3] S. S. Sundar and T. S. Ganesan, "Role of lymphangiogenesis in cancer," *Journal of Clinical Oncology*, vol. 25, no. 27, pp. 4298–4307, 2007.

[4] N. J. P. Beasley, R. Prevo, S. Banerji et al., "Intratumoral lymphangiogenesis and lymph node metastasis in head and neck cancer," *Cancer Research*, vol. 62, no. 5, pp. 1315–1320, 2002.

[5] S.-M. Maula, M. Luukkaa, R. Grénman, D. Jackson, S. Jalkanen, and R. Ristamäki, "Intratumoral lymphatics are essential for the metastatic spread and prognosis in squamous cell carcinomas of the head and neck region," *Cancer Research*, vol. 63, no. 8, pp. 1920–1926, 2003.

[6] T. Fifis, L. Nguyen, C. Malcontenti-Wilson et al., "Treatment with the vascular disruptive agent OXi4503 induces an immediate and widespread epithelial to mesenchymal transition in the surviving tumor," *Cancer Medicine*, vol. 2, no. 5, pp. 595–610, 2013.

[7] H. J. Kahn, D. Bailey, and A. Marks, "Monoclonal antibody D2-40, a new marker of lymphatic endothelium, reacts with Kaposi's sarcoma and a subset of angiosarcomas," *Modern Pathology*, vol. 15, no. 4, pp. 434–440, 2002.

[8] L. Fina, H. V. Molgaard, D. Robertson et al., "Expression of the CD34 gene in vascular endothelial cells," *Blood*, vol. 75, no. 12, pp. 2417–2426, 1990.

[9] M. S. Pepper, "Lymphangiogenesis and tumor metastasis: myth or reality?" *Clinical Cancer Research*, vol. 7, no. 3, pp. 462–468, 2001.

[10] J. Folkman, "Angiogenesis-dependent diseases," *Seminars in Oncology*, vol. 28, no. 6, pp. 536–542, 2001.

[11] J. Hasan, R. Byers, and G. C. Jayson, "Intra-tumoural microvessel density in human solid tumours," *British Journal of Cancer*, vol. 86, no. 10, pp. 1566–1577, 2002.

[12] L. Nguyen, T. Fifis, C. Malcontenti-Wilson et al., "Spatial morphological and molecular differences within solid tumors may contribute to the failure of vascular disruptive agent treatments," *BMC Cancer*, vol. 12, no. 1, p. 522, 2012.

[13] S. Banerji, J. Ni, S.-X. Wang et al., "LYVE-1, a new homologue of the CD44 glycoprotein, is a lymph-specific receptor for hyaluronan," *Journal of Cell Biology*, vol. 144, no. 4, pp. 789–801, 1999.

[14] T. P. Padera, A. Kadambi, E. di Tomaso et al., "Lymphatic metastasis in the absence of functional intratumor lymphatics," *Science*, vol. 296, no. 5574, pp. 1883–1886, 2002.

[15] P. Bono, V.-M. Wasenius, P. Heikkilä, J. Lundin, D. G. Jackson, and H. Joensuu, "High LYVE-1-positive lymphatic vessel numbers are associated with poor outcome in breast cancer," *Clinical Cancer Research*, vol. 10, no. 21, pp. 7144–7149, 2004.

[16] S. Kuroyama, N. Kobayashi, M. Ohbu, Y. Ohtani, I. Okayasu, and A. Kakita, "Enzyme histochemical analysis of lymphatic vessels in colon carcinoma: occurrence of lymphangiogenesis within the tumor," *Hepato-Gastroenterology*, vol. 52, no. 64, pp. 1057–1061, 2005.

[17] S. S. Dadras, T. Paul, J. Bertoncini et al., "Tumor lymphangiogenesis: a novel prognostic indicator for cutaneous melanoma metastasis and survival," *American Journal of Pathology*, vol. 162, no. 6, pp. 1951–1960, 2003.

[18] R. S. Saad, L. Kordunsky, Y. L. Liu, K. L. Denning, H. A. Kandil, and J. F. Silverman, "Lymphatic microvessel density as prognostic marker in colorectal cancer," *Modern Pathology*, vol. 19, no. 10, pp. 1317–1323, 2006.

[19] M. Matsumoto, S. Natsugoe, H. Okumura et al., "Overexpression of vascular endothelial growth factor-C correlates with lymph node micrometastasis in submucosal esophageal cancer," *Journal of Gastrointestinal Surgery*, vol. 10, no. 7, pp. 1016–1022, 2006.

[20] M.-A. Brundler, J. A. Harrison, B. de Saussure, M. de Perrot, and M. S. Pepper, "Lymphatic vessel density in the neoplastic progression of Barrett's oesophagus to adenocarcinoma," *Journal of Clinical Pathology*, vol. 59, no. 2, pp. 191–195, 2006.

[21] M. I. Auvinen, E. I. T. Sihvo, T. Ruohtula et al., "Incipient angiogenesis in Barrett's epithelium and lymphangiogenesis in Barrett's adenocarcinoma," *Journal of Clinical Oncology*, vol. 20, no. 13, pp. 2971–2979, 2002.

[22] C. M. Carreira, S. M. Nasser, E. di Tomaso et al., "LYVE-1 is not restricted to the lymph vessels: expression in normal liver blood sinusoids and down-regulation in human liver cancer and cirrhosis," *Cancer Research*, vol. 61, no. 22, pp. 8079–8084, 2001.

[23] T. Ichida, S. Sugitani, T. Satoh et al., "Localization of hyaluronan in human liver sinu-soids: a histochemical study using hyaluronan-binding protein.," *Liver*, vol. 16, pp. 365–371, 1996.

[24] R. S. Saad, J. L. Lindner, Y. Liu, and J. F. Silverman, "Lymphatic vessel density as prognostic marker in esophageal adenocarcinoma," *American Journal of Clinical Pathology*, vol. 131, no. 1, pp. 92–98, 2009.

[25] Y. Luo, L. Liu, D. Rogers et al., "Rapamycin inhibits lymphatic endothelial cell tube formation by down regulating vascular endothelial growth factor receptor 3 protein expression," *Neoplasia*, vol. 14, no. 3, pp. 228–237, 2012.

23

Hepatectomy Based on Future Liver Remnant Plasma Clearance Rate of Indocyanine Green

Yuichiro Uchida,[1] **Hiroaki Furuyama,**[1] **Daiki Yasukawa,**[1] **Hiroto Nishino,**[2] **Yasuhisa Ando,**[1] **Toshiyuki Hata,**[1] **Takafumi Machimoto,**[1] **and Tsunehiro Yoshimura**[1]

[1]*Department of Gastrointestinal and General Surgery, Tenri Yorozu Hospital, 200 Mishima-cho, Tenri, Nara 632-8552, Japan*
[2]*Division of Hepato-Biliary-Pancreatic and Transplant Surgery, Graduate School of Medicine, Kyoto University, 54 Shogoin-kawahara-cho, Kyoto 606-8507, Japan*

Correspondence should be addressed to Yuichiro Uchida; yuichiro.uchida3389@gmail.com

Academic Editor: Shuji Isaji

Background. Hepatectomy, an important treatment modality for liver malignancies, has high perioperative morbidity and mortality rates. Safe, comprehensive criteria for selecting patients for hepatectomy are needed. Since June 2011, we have used a cut-off value of ≥ 0.05 for future liver remnant plasma clearance rate of indocyanine green as a criterion for hepatectomy. The aim of this study was to verify the validity of this criterion. *Methods.* From June 2011 to December 2015, 212 hepatectomies were performed in Tenri Yorozu Hospital. Of these 212 patients, 107 who underwent preoperative computed tomography imaging volumetry, indocyanine green clearance test, and hepatectomy (excluding partial resection or enucleation) were retrospectively analyzed. *Results.* There was no postoperative mortality. Posthepatectomy liver failure occurred in 59 patients (55.1%) (International Study Group of Liver Surgery Grade A: 43 cases (40.2%), Grade B: 16 cases (15.0%), and Grade C: no cases). Operative morbidity greater than Clavien-Dindo Grade 3 occurred in 23 patients (21.5%). A low future liver remnant plasma clearance rate of indocyanine green was a good predictor for Grade B cases (area under curve = 0.804; 95% confidence interval, 0.712–0.895). *Conclusion.* Liver remnant plasma clearance rate of indocyanine green is a valid criterion for hepatectomy.

1. Introduction

Hepatectomy is an important treatment modality for liver malignancies. On the other hand, postoperative morbidity and mortality rates are still high. Posthepatectomy liver failure (PHLF), one of the most critical forms of morbidity, is closely correlated with postoperative mortality.

In 1993, Makuuchi's criteria [1] were proposed for hepatectomy in patients with underlying liver diseases. These criteria are based on presence or absence of ascites, preoperative total bilirubin concentration, and indocyanine green (ICG) retention rate at 15 minutes and have since been widely accepted in Japan. Makuuchi's criteria are probably appropriate for patients with basically healthy liver too and are used by many surgeons; however, patients who are ineligible for hepatectomy according to Makuuchi's criteria are frequently encountered. The safety of hepatectomy in such patients is still controversial. In 1980, Takasaki et al. reported that future liver remnant plasma clearance rate of ICG (rICGK) was useful for predicting posthepatectomy liver function [2]. It is easily calculated as follows: preoperative ICGK × % future remnant liver volume (RLV) and is also widely used in Japan. Nagino et al. and Yokoyama et al. reported that rICGK less than 0.05 is associated with a high incidence of perioperative mortality after hepatectomy for biliary cancer [3, 4], but the significance of rICGK on hepatectomy for other diseases has not been fully evaluated.

2. Methods

2.1. Patients. From June 2011 to December 2015, 212 patients underwent hepatectomy in Tenri Yorozu Hospital. Eighty-nine patients who had undergone limited resection (partial resection or enucleation) and 16 who had undergone different

TABLE 1: Patient characteristics.

Variables	($n = 107$)
Age, years	69 (38–86)
Sex, male, %	67.3
HBs antigen+, %	12.1
HCV antibody+, %	14.0
ICGK	0.151 (0.069–0.264)
ICGR15, %	11.9 (1.9–35.4)
TLV, mL	1181 (735–2169)
% RLV	59.3 (34.7–93.7)
rICGK	0.088 (0.050–0.199)
T-Bil, mg/dL	0.7 (0.2–2.5)
Alb, g/dL	3.9 (1.8–5.2)
Plt, $10^4/\mu$L	20.5 (8.3–72.0)
PT-INR	1.03 (0.93–1.93)
eGFR (mL/min)	76.0 (6.5–185.6)
Blood loss, mL	867 (50–7750)
Operation time, min	361 (151–748)
Indications for hepatectomy	($n = 107$)
Hepatocellular carcinoma	52
Metastatic liver tumor	29
Cholangiocarcinoma	14
Others	12

HBs antigen+: hepatitis B virus surface antigen positive, HCV antibody+: hepatitis C virus antibody positive, ICGR15: indocyanine green retention rate at 15 minutes, TLV: total liver volume, % RLV: remnant liver volume/total liver volume (%), T-Bil: total bilirubin, Alb: albumin, Plt: platelet count, PT-INR: international normalized ratio of prothrombin time, and eGFR: estimated glomerular filtration rate.

TABLE 2: Type of hepatectomy.

Type of hepatectomy	Total 107
Trisectionectomy	2
Hemihepatectomy	55
Right hemihepatectomy	34
Left hemihepatectomy	21
Sectionectomy	44
Right anterior + left medial	4
Right posterior	21
Left medial	10
Left lateral	9
Segmentectomy	6

Both trisectionectomies were right trisectionectomies. Segmentectomy included S3 (two patients), S2, S5, S6, and S5 + 6 (one patient each).

types of hepatectomy than had been planned preoperatively by computed tomography (CT) imaging were excluded because lack of data on future RLV prevented assessment of the validity of the rICGK ≥ 0.05 criterion in these patients. Thus, 107 patients who had undergone hepatectomy based on preoperative planning by computed tomography (CT) imaging volumetry were included in this study.

Patient characteristics, indications for hepatectomy, and types of hepatectomy are shown in Tables 1 and 2.

2.2. Resection Criteria. Only patients whose rICGK ≥ 0.05 were considered eligible for hepatectomy. Preoperative CT imaging volumetry was performed using SYNAPSE VINCENT version 2.0 (FUJIFILM, Tokyo, Japan). Preoperative portal embolism was performed in eight patients whose rICGK was less than 0.05. After this procedure, the rICGK became greater than 0.05 in all eight of these patients and all of them subsequently underwent hepatectomy. We have included these eight patients in this study.

2.3. Clinical Data Assessed. The clinical data we assessed included the following: age, sex, ICGK, ICG retention rate at 15 minutes (ICGR15), total liver volume, % RLV (future remnant liver volume/total liver volume − tumor volume × 100), rICGK, serum total bilirubin (T-Bil), serum albumin (Alb), platelet count (Plt), international normalized ratio of prothrombin time (PT-INR), estimated glomerular filtration rate (eGFR), intraoperative blood loss, and operation time.

2.4. Outcomes Evaluated. We assessed postoperative mortality and morbidity (greater than Clavien-Dindo Grade 3), PHLF, and postoperative hospital stay. PHLF was categorized according to the criteria of the International Study Group of Liver Surgery (ISGLF) [5]. Patients were also categorized as meeting or not meeting Makuuchi's criteria.

2.5. Statistical Analysis. Data are expressed as median and range. Differences between two groups were assessed by the Mann-Whitney U test and χ^2 test. Differences between three groups were assessed by one-way analysis of valiance and the Tukey multiple comparison procedure. Predictive value was assessed by calculating the area under the receiver operator characteristic (ROC) curve (AUC). Statistical analysis was performed using SPSS Statistics version 22.0 (IBM, NY, USA). A P value < 0.05 was considered statistically significant.

2.6. Study Design. The study design was approved by our institution's ethics review board (approval number 739) and the need for informed consent was waived in view of its retrospective nature.

3. Results

There was no postoperative mortality. There was one inhospital death that was not directly related to hepatectomy (it was due to pleural dissemination of renal cell carcinoma). PHLF was identified in 59 patients (55.1%), being Grade A in 43 (40.2%), B in 16 (15.0%), and C in none. Patient characteristics according to PHLF Grade A or Grade B and absence of PHLF (non-PHLF) are shown in Table 3. There were significant differences between these three groups in %RLV, rICGK, operative blood loss, and operation time. A significant difference was also observed between PHLF Grades A and B for rICGK (Figure 1). A low rICGK was a good predictor of development of PHLF Grade B (AUC, 0.804; 95% confidence interval, 0.712–0.895) The optimal cutoff value of rICGK was 0.073 for predicting both PHLF Grade B (sensitivity, 0.812 specificity, 0.736) and PHLF all grades

TABLE 3: Patient characteristics according to PHLF grade.

Variables	Non-PHLF ($n = 48$)	PHLF Grade A ($n = 43$)	PHLF Grade B ($n = 16$)	P value
Age, years	69 (38–82)	68 (40–86)	69 (56–93)	0.59
Sex, male, %	75.0	55.8	75	0.12
HBs antigen+, %	14.5	11.6	6.3	0.68
HCV antibody+, %	10.4	11.6	31.3	0.10
ICGK	0.154 (0.069–0.212)	0.156 (0.091–0.264)	0.137 (0.085–0.211)	0.21
ICGR15, %	9.9 (4.2–35.4)	10.2 (1.9–25.6)	12.9 (4.2–27.8)	0.39
TLV, mL	1214 (786–2025)	1133 (735–2086)	1320 (829–2169)	0.39
% RLV	68.9 (40.5–93.7)	55.9 (34.7–87.0)	44.0 (37.2–80.2)	<0.001
rICGK	0.095 (0.053–0.199)	0.079 (0.050–0.153)	0.067 (0.050–0.088)	<0.001
T-Bil, mg/dL	0.5 (0.2–2.5)	0.7 (0.3–1.9)	0.7 (0.4–2.2)	0.74
Alb, g/dL	4.1 (1.8–5.2)	4.1 (2.6–4.7)	3.9 (3.0–4.7)	0.31
Plt, $10^4/\mu$L	19.4 (8.3–72.0)	17.0 (9.7–41.5)	17.7 (8.6–45.5)	0.68
PT-INR	1.03 (0.93–1.93)	1.03 (0.94–1.35)	1.06 (0.94–1.31)	0.93
eGFR (mL/min)	75.8 (53.2–124.4)	74.1 (6.5–186.0)	69.3 (38.9–120.4)	0.54
Blood loss, mL	440 (50–2600)	500 (70–7750)	1385 (230–3400)	0.047
Operation time, min	328 (151–654)	348 (204–620)	401 (286–748)	0.02

P values between the three groups were assessed by one-way analysis of variance and the Tukey multiple comparison procedure.

TABLE 4: Postoperative outcomes according to PHLF grade.

	ALL ($n = 107$)	Non-PHLF ($n = 48$)	PHLF Grade A ($n = 43$)	PHLF Grade B ($n = 16$)
Postoperative hospital stay (days)	16 (9–186)	14.5 (9–70)	16 (10–123)	34.5 (16–186)
Postoperative morbidity (≥G3), %	21.5	8.3	27.9	43.7

Postoperative morbidity greater than Clavien-Dindo Grade 3 was evaluated.

(sensitivity, 0.525 specificity, 0.875) (Figure 2): patients whose rICGK was greater than 0.09 did not develop PHLF Grade B (Figure 3).

Patients who developed PHLF Grade B had significantly longer postoperative hospital stays (14.5 versus 43.7 days, $P < 0.001$) and significantly higher rates of morbidity greater than Clavien-Dindo Grade 3 (8.3 versus 43.7%, $P = 0.007$) than those who did not develop PHLF. There were no significant differences in postoperative hospital days and rates of morbidity greater than Clavien-Dindo Grade 3 between PHLF Grade A and non-PHLF groups (16.5 versus 14.5 days, $P = 0.429$; 27.9 versus 8.3%, $P = 0.062$) (Table 4).

The 29 patients who did not meet Makuuchi's criteria had significantly higher rates than those who did meet this criterion of developing PHLF ($P = 0.016$), but not of developing PHLF Grade B ($P = 0.054$) or morbidity greater than Clavien-Dindo Grade 3 ($P = 0.350$) (Figure 4).

4. Discussion

There was no postoperative mortality in this study. According to a Japanese national database, the perioperative mortality of hepatectomy performed for more than one segment (except for a lateral segment) is 4.0% [6]. Thus, the rICGK ≥ 0.05 criterion appears to be safe regarding zero mortality. However, there was a high incidence of PHLF. Previous studies have reported the incidence of PHLF as 9.0%–39.6% [7, 8]. Because patient characteristics have varied between studies, it is not valid to simply compare our findings with those of other studies; however, this is a noteworthy issue. Many of the cases

of PHLF in the present study were PHLF Grade A, which had relatively little influence on the patients' postoperative course. However, patients who developed PHLF Grade B had a high morbidity rate and longer postoperative hospital stay. Because major operative blood loss and long operating time are considered to contribute to development of PHLF, surgeons should try to minimize blood loss and improve their surgical techniques. A low rICGK had good predictive value for development of PHLF Grade B in this study. The optimal cut-off value was 0.073 for predicting PHLF Grade B and patients with rICGK ≥ 0.09 did not have any severe PHLF in our series. Because rICGK was used not to predict PHLF but to assess the eligibility for hepatectomy in our series, we think these values are not directly meaningful, but these findings are consistent with our clinical experience; Thus, patients with higher rICGK may not be at risk of severe PHLF and, in patients with rICGK < 0.07, more careful perioperative management should be performed to avoid PHLF. There was also a high incidence of postoperative morbidity greater than Clavien-Dindo Grade 3, which may at least in part be attributable to our perioperative management policy. We rarely place prophylactic drains after hepatectomy and perform CT scans routinely on postoperative Day 7. We frequently perform percutaneous drainage when we suspect a fluid collection. This policy results in a relatively high frequency of postoperative percutaneous drainage and these cases are counted as postoperative morbidity Grade 3 even when they do not actually have an infection or biliary leak.

We consider the rICGK ≥ 0.05 criterion to be more expansive than Makuuchi's criteria because 29 study patients

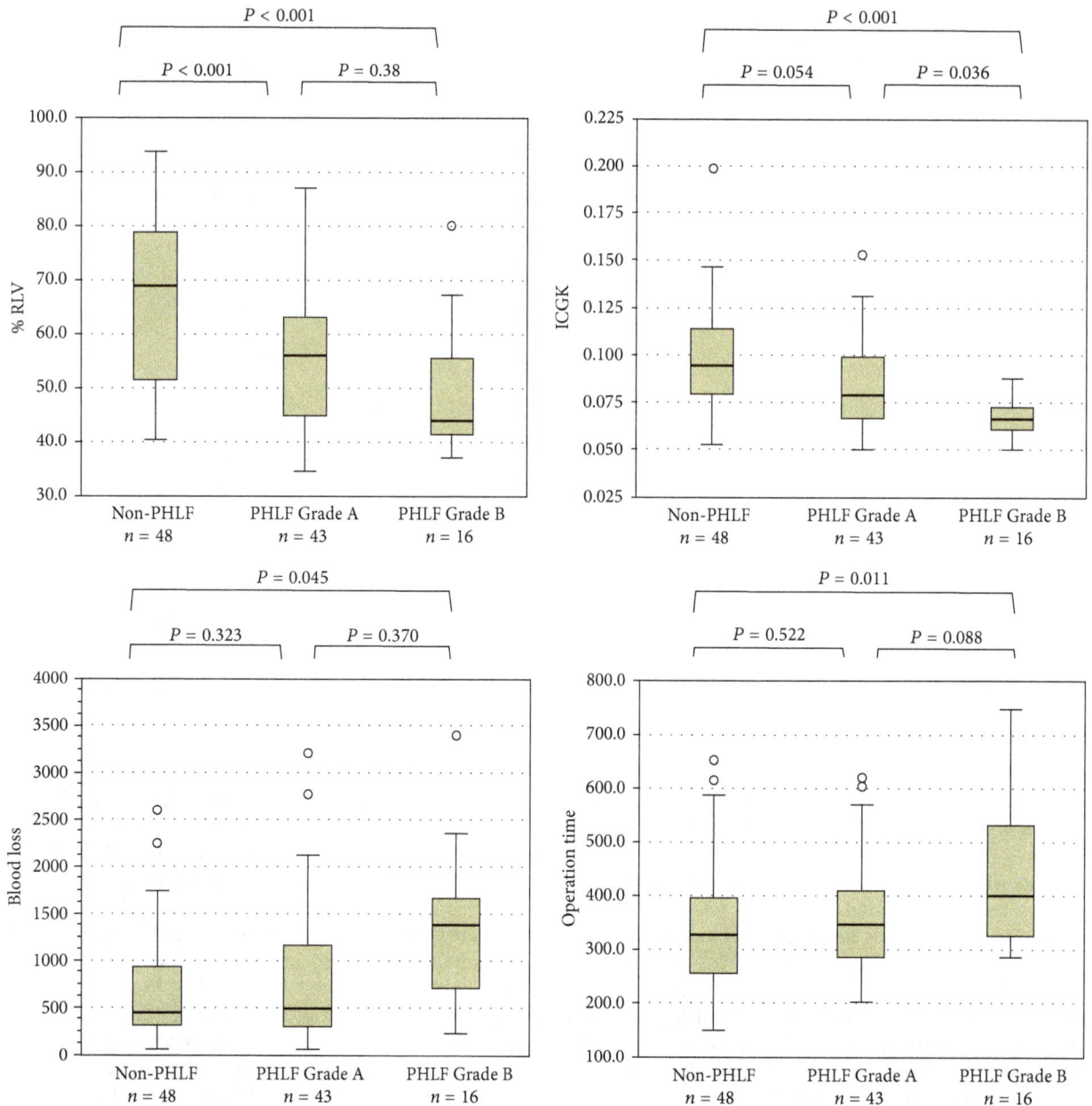

FIGURE 1: Distribution of factors significantly associated with development of PHLF. The rICGK of patients who developed PHLF Grade B was significantly lower than that of others. Blood loss volume is greater and operation time is longer in the PHLF Grade B than Grade A group, although not significant.

who did not meet Makuuchi's criteria did meet the rICGK $\geq$ 0.05 criterion. Although these patients tended to have poorer postoperative outcomes than patients who did meet Makuuchi's criteria, this difference was not significant. How far we can expand the indications for hepatectomy is controversial. Iguchi and colleagues reported results of hepatectomy for HCC based on the criterion of rICGK more than 0.03 [8]. In their study, patients whose rICGK was less than 0.05 had a significantly higher incidence and greater severity of PHLF than patients whose rICGK was more than 0.05. However, these two groups did not differ significantly in perioperative mortality or long-term oncological outcomes.

Patients with lower rICGK have a higher operative risk. However, because hepatectomy is the only potentially curative treatment modality for many liver malignancies, it is difficult to determine the optimal operative risk. The appropriate lower limit for rICGK may be different according to the underlying disease; we had too few patients in this study to assess this possibility.

In 2011, PHLF grading was proposed by the ISGLF. Since then, cross-sectional research on PHLF has become possible and such studies are increasingly being performed. Further accumulation of data and prospective studies investigating criteria for hepatectomy are expected.

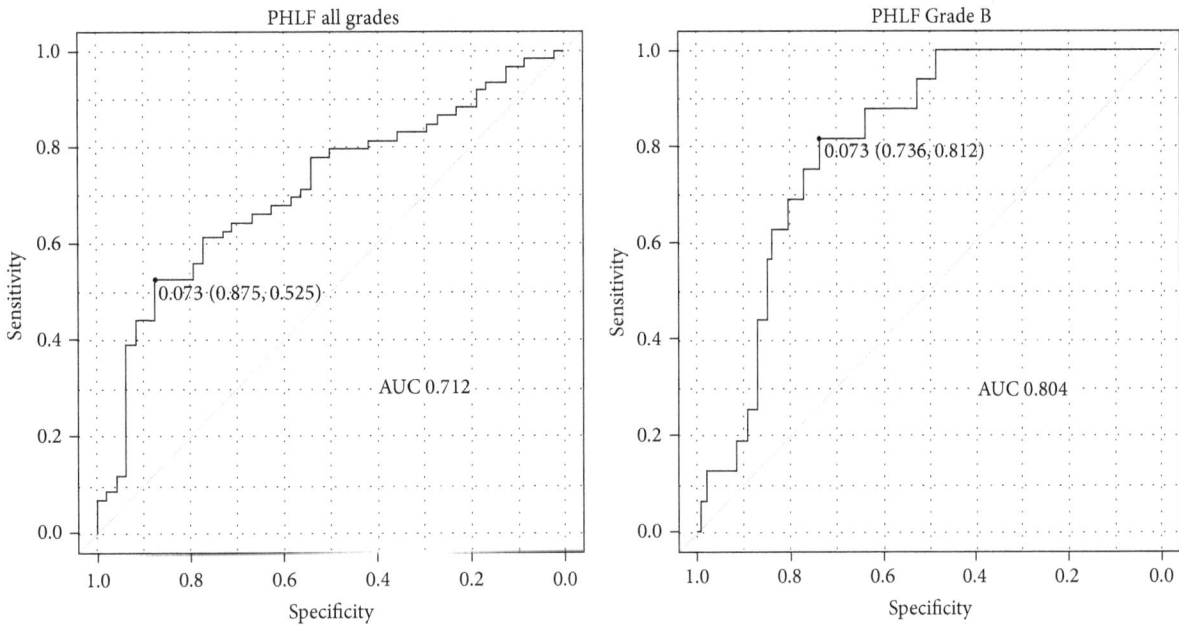

FIGURE 2: Receiver operating characteristic curve of rICGK for prediction of PHLF. Low rICGK has high predictive value for development of PHLF Grade B rather than PHLF of all grades (including PHLF Grade A).

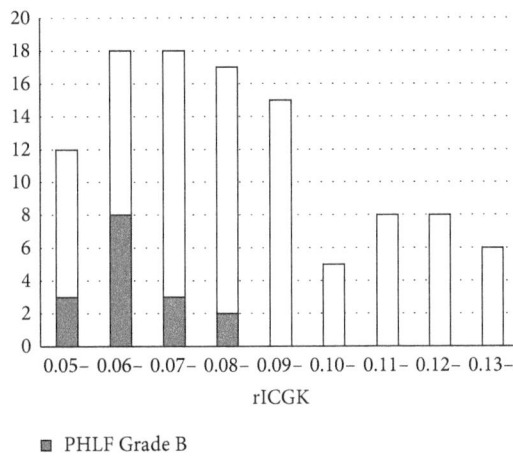

FIGURE 3: Histogram showing relationship between rICGK and PHLF Grade B. Patients whose rICGK was more than 0.09 did not develop severe PHLF (Grade B).

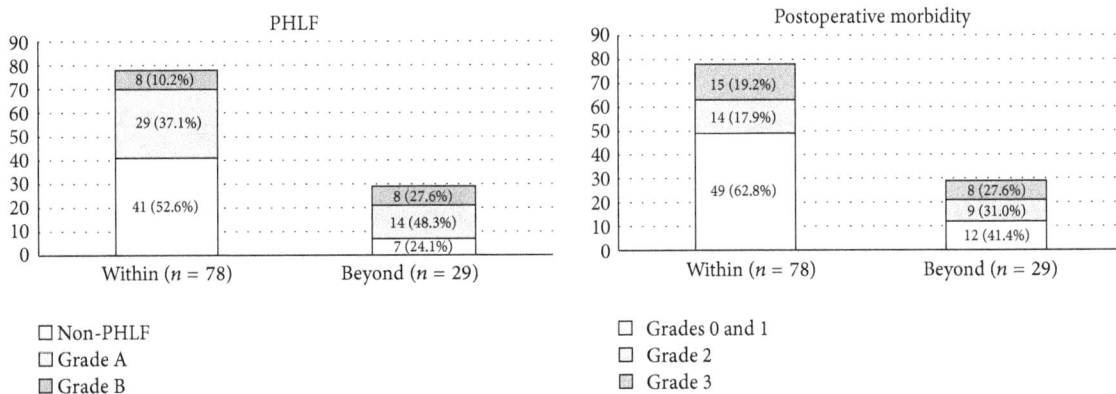

FIGURE 4: Postoperative morbidity according to Makuuchi's criterion. Patients who met Makuuchi's criterion had lower incidences of severe PHLF and postoperative morbidity than those who did not, although not significant.

This study has several limitations. It was a retrospective study and factors such as performance status and comorbidities were considered when assessing operative indications. Thus, some poor risk patients may have been excluded. The small sample size resulted in low statistical power for rare morbidities such as PHLF Grade C.

In conclusion, the rICGK ≥ 0.05 criterion is a sufficiently broad and safe criterion for selecting patients with various diseases for hepatectomy.

Competing Interests

None of the authors have any conflict of interests to declare.

References

[1] M. Makuuchi, T. Kosuge, T. Takayama et al., "Surgery for small liver cancers," *Seminars in Surgical Oncology*, vol. 9, no. 4, pp. 298–304, 1993.

[2] T. Takasaki, S. Kobayashi, S. Suzuki et al., "Predetermining postoperative hepatic function for hepatectomies," *International Surgery*, vol. 65, no. 4, pp. 309–313, 1980.

[3] M. Nagino, J. Kamiya, H. Nishio, T. Ebata, T. Arai, and Y. Nimura, "Two hundred forty consecutive portal vein emboliza-tions before extended hepatectomy for biliary cancer: surgical outcome and long-term follow-up," *Annals of Surgery*, vol. 243, no. 3, pp. 364–372, 2006.

[4] Y. Yokoyama, H. Nishio, T. Ebata, T. Igami, G. Sugawara, and M. Nagino, "Value of indocyanine green clearance of the future liver remnant in predicting outcome after resection for biliary cancer," *British Journal of Surgery*, vol. 97, no. 8, pp. 1260–1268, 2010.

[5] N. N. Rahbari, O. J. Garden, R. Padbury et al., "Posthepatectomy liver failure: a definition and grading by the International Study Group of Liver Surgery (ISGLS)," *Surgery*, vol. 149, no. 5, pp. 713–724, 2011.

[6] M. Gotoh, H. Miyata, H. Hashimoto et al., "National Clinical Database feedback implementation for quality improvement of cancer treatment in Japan: from good to great through transparency," *Surgery Today*, vol. 46, no. 1, pp. 38–47, 2016.

[7] Y. Tomimaru, H. Eguchi, K. Gotoh et al., "Platelet count is more useful for predicting posthepatectomy liver failure at surgery for hepatocellular carcinoma than indocyanine green clearance test," *Journal of Surgical Oncology*, vol. 113, no. 5, pp. 565–569, 2016.

[8] K. Iguchi, E. Hatano, K. Yamanaka, S. Tanaka, K. Taura, and S. Uemoto, "Validation of the conventional resection criteria in patients with hepatocellular carcinoma in terms of the incidence of posthepatectomy liver failure and long-term prognosis," *Digestive Surgery*, vol. 32, no. 5, pp. 344–351, 2015.

24

Prevalence of Steatosis Hepatis in the *Eurotransplant* Region: Impact on Graft Acceptance Rates

Simon Moosburner ⑩,[1] **Joseph M. G. V. Gassner,**[1] **Maximilian Nösser,**[1]
Julian Pohl,[1] **David Wyrwal,**[1] **Felix Claussen,**[1] **Paul V. Ritschl,**[1,2] **Duska Dragun,**[3]
Johann Pratschke,[1] **Igor M. Sauer** ⑩,[1] **and Nathanael Raschzok** ⑩[1,2]

[1]*Department of Surgery, Campus Charité Mitte | Campus Virchow-Klinikum, Experimental Surgery and Regenerative Medicine, Charité – Universitätsmedizin Berlin 13353, Germany*
[2]*BIH Charité Clinician Scientist Program, Berlin Institute of Health (BIH), Berlin 10178, Germany*
[3]*Berlin Institute of Health and Department of Nephrology and Critical Care Medicine, Charité Universitätsmedizin, Berlin 13353, Germany*

Correspondence should be addressed to Igor M. Sauer; igor.sauer@charite.de

Academic Editor: Shu-Sen Zheng

Due to the shortage of liver allografts and the rising prevalence of fatty liver disease in the general population, steatotic liver grafts are considered for transplantation. This condition is an important risk factor for the outcome after transplantation. We here analyze the characteristics of the donor pool offered to the *Charité – Universitätsmedizin Berlin* from 2010 to 2016 with respect to liver allograft nonacceptance and steatosis hepatis. Of the 2653 organs offered to our center, 19.9% (n=527) were accepted for transplantation, 58.8% (n=1561) were allocated to other centers, and 21.3% (n = 565) were eventually discarded from transplantation. In parallel to an increase of the incidence of steatosis hepatis in the donor pool from 20% in 2010 to 30% in 2016, the acceptance rates for steatotic organs increased in our center from 22.3% to 51.5% in 2016 (p < 0.001), with the majority (86.9%; p > 0.001) having less than 30% macrovesicular steatosis hepatis. However, by 2016, the number of canceled transplantations due to higher grades of steatosis hepatis had significantly increased from 14.7% (n = 15) to 63.6% (42; p < 0.001). The rising prevalence of steatosis hepatis in the donor pool has led to higher acceptance rates of steatotic allografts. Nonetheless, steatosis hepatis remains a predominant phenomenon in discarded organs necessitating future concepts such as organ reconditioning to increase graft utilization.

1. Introduction

Orthotopic liver transplantation (OLT), which is the only curative therapy option in patients with end-stage liver disease, is increasingly limited by the discrepancy between organ demand and availability [1, 2]. Donation after cardiac death, split-liver transplantation, living donor liver transplantation, and transplantation of grafts from extended criteria donors have been developed to expand the donor pool [3, 4]. In spite of these developments, and due to the increase in donor age and stagnation of donations, the number of patients on the waiting list constantly exceeds the organ supply [5]. While the number of liver transplantations decreased, more restrictive listing policies have led to sicker patients on the waiting list,

with high rates of mortality and impaired outcome after liver transplantation [6–8].

Steatosis hepatis, also known as fatty liver disease, is considered an important risk factor for graft dysfunction after liver transplantation, and more than 50% of grafts with histologically confirmed moderate or severe macrosteatosis are usually not used for transplantation [9]. Nonalcoholic fatty liver disease, which is the hepatic manifestation of the metabolic syndrome, is already the second most common cause for liver transplantation in the USA and currently the only increasing etiology with increasing incidence [10–13]. With the rising prevalence of steatosis hepatis in potential donors, graft utilization is expected to fall from 78% to 44% by 2030 [10]. However, data on the current nonacceptance rate of liver grafts due to steatosis hepatis in the *Eurotransplant* region are not well documented in the literature. Based on large retrospective database analyses, transplantation of liver grafts with macrovesicular steatosis > 30% is only recommended from donors with less overall risk factors [14, 15]. Even though macrovesicular steatosis is a recognized risk factor for primary nonfunction and early allograft dysfunction (EAD) [14–21], the extent of the postoperative impairment remains disputed. It is generally accepted that severe macrovesicular steatosis ≥ 60% leads to higher rates of primary nonfunction and EAD, and to reduced 1- and 3-year recipient and graft survival [16, 22, 23], while mild steatotic organs seem to be safe to transplant [14, 15, 24].

Germany in particular has seen a drastic 30% decline in organ donation, from 1200 donors in 2011 to only 857 donors in 2016. This aggravates the need to offer grafts from extended criteria donors to meet the demand for liver allografts. The question arises if expanding the donor pool with such donors has actually yielded higher rates of transplantations or just higher rates of notaccepted livers. To address this question and to update the knowledge concerning liver graft utilization and reasons for nonacceptance in the *Eurotransplant* region [25], we here analyzed all grafts offered to our high-volume center from 2010 to 2016 with regard to allocation, i.e., acceptance, nonacceptance, or discarded organs, with a special focus on grafts with steatosis hepatis.

2. Materials and Methods

2.1. Study Site and Ethical Board Approval. This single center retrospective data analysis was performed in the Department of Surgery, Campus Charité Mitte | Campus Virchow-Klinikum of the Charité – Universitätsmedizin Berlin (Berlin, Germany). The study protocol was approved by the local ethics committee (Ethics committee of the Charité, EA2/010/17).

2.2. Organ Offers. Data for all livers from 2010 to 2016 offered by *Eurotransplant* to the Charité – Universitätsmedizin Berlin was requested from *Eurotransplant* and analyzed. All donors included in the analysis were from brain death donors (DBD). Donor data included in analysis were donor age, body mass index (BMI), hepatitis B (HBV) status, hepatitis C (HCV) status, aspartate-aminotransferase (AST), alanine-aminotransferase (ALT), gamma-glutamyl transferase (GGT), international normalized ratio (INR), c-reactive protein (CRP), creatinine, sodium, history of diabetes mellitus, or smoking, cardiopulmonary resuscitation, cause of death, duration of intensive care unit (ICU) stay, signs for steatosis hepatis in ultrasonography, steatosis hepatis in histopathology report, and the allocation phase, i.e., whether the offered donor liver was procured or transplanted at all.

2.3. Organ Acceptance. All liver offers made to the Charité – Universitätsmedizin Berlin are recorded and in case of nonacceptance the reason is remarked. Clinic records were screened from 2010 to 2016. Reason of nonacceptance was

categorized into "donor medical," "weight/size," "recipient medical," "logistics," or "other reasons." "Donor medical" was further subclassified into "age," "biochemical parameters," "cardiopulmonary resuscitation," "steatosis hepatis," "infection," "malignancy," "substance abuse," "ICU stay," or "other reasons." Liver allografts were accepted on a case-by-case basis for each individual patient, considering donor age, weight, and size relative to recipient age, as well as the virologic status of the donor (especially HCV and human immunodeficiency virus). Additionally, the expected cold ischemia time (CIT) and the presence of steatosis hepatis influenced the acceptance decision.

2.4. Classification of Steatosis Hepatis. Steatosis hepatis is classified into two groups: (I) any description of steatosis hepatis, i.e., ultrasound or histopathological report; (II) cases with histopathological confirmation. The histopathological confirmed cases were further graded by the degree of macrovesicular steatosis hepatis as previously reported by Chu et al. and Briceño et al. [24, 26]. Macrovesicular steatosis < 5% was classified as "no steatosis," followed by < 30% as "mild steatosis," ≥ 30% as "moderate steatosis," and ≥ 60% as "severe steatosis." In addition, 1-year graft and recipient survival rates were calculated. Graft survival was defined as the absence of recipient death or retransplantation. Early allograft dysfunction was calculated for all recipients and defined as bilirubin ≥ 10mg/dl or INR ≥ 1.6 on POD 7 or AST/ALT >2000 IU/l during the first 7 days [17].

2.5. Statistical Analysis. Data is presented as mean ± standard deviation (SD) for normal distribution of data. Not normally distributed data is reported in median and interquartile range. Categorical variables were measured in proportions and counts. After testing for normality, continuous parametric variables were analyzed with the Student's t-test and nonparametric variables using the Wilcoxon rank-sum test. Grouped variables were analyzed with the one-way ANOVA or the Kruskal-Wallis test according to normality. Categorical variables were analyzed using the Pearson χ^2 test.

A binary logistic regression analysis for liver acceptance was carried out. Age was classified into groups of <50 years and above 50 into decades: 50-59, 60-69, 70-79, and >80. BMI was classified in a similar way: < 18.5, 18.5-24.9, 25-29.9, 30-34.9, 35-39.9, and >40. All reported *P* values are two-sided; overall a *P* value < 0.05 was considered significant. Graphs were plotted using GraphPad Prism Version 6.04 for Macintosh (GraphPad Software, La Jolla, CA, USA) and calculations were carried out using IBM SPSS Statistics for Macintosh Version 24.0 (IBM Corp., Armonk, NY, USA).

3. Results

3.1. Increasing Number of Cancelled Transplantations. From 2010 to 2016 liver grafts from 2653 donors were offered to the Charité – Universitätsmedizin Berlin. Organs from 527 donors (19.9%) were accepted and successfully transplanted (Figure 1(a)). From the remaining 2126 (80.1%) of offered donor organs, 1561 (73.4%) were allocated and transplanted at

All Organ
Offers 2010 - 2016

Not Accepted Organ
Offers 2010 - 2016

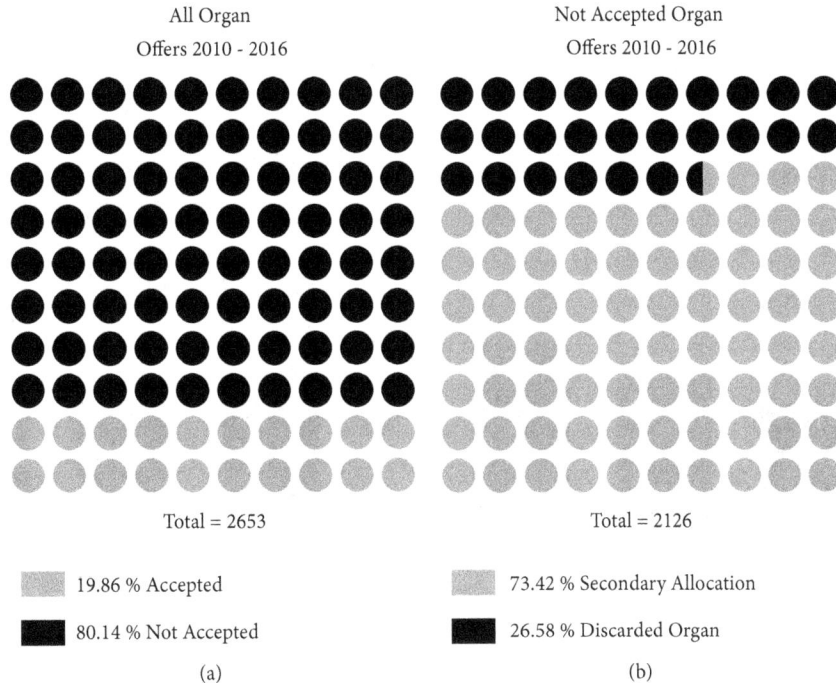

Total = 2653

Total = 2126

19.86 % Accepted

73.42 % Secondary Allocation

80.14 % Not Accepted

26.58 % Discarded Organ

(a)

(b)

FIGURE 1: Organs offered and accepted 2010-2016. (a) All liver allografts offered to our center, accepted and not accepted. (b) All nonaccepted liver allografts, secondary allocation to another center or discarded from allocation.

other centers and 565 (26.6%) donors could not be allocated and were not used for transplantation (Figure 1(b)). Of all organs not used for transplantation, 304 (53.8%) were not procured at all.

At our center the number of livers accepted and transplanted significantly decreased (p < 0.001) from 2010 (102, i.e., 32.9%) to 2016 (66, i.e., 10.9%), while the number of nonaccepted organ offers more than doubled (208 and 536, respectively) in the same time period. Although the number of patients awaiting OLT at our center decreased from 157 in 2010 to 98 in 2016, respectively, there were more overall offers.

3.2. Reasons for Liver Allograft Nonacceptance.
Medical issues of the donors, such as age, biochemical parameters, or steatosis hepatis, were the primary reason for graft nonacceptance. Steatosis hepatis, as reported by the explant surgeon based on macroscopic or histopathological assessment of the graft, did not differ significantly from 2010 (15.0%) to 2016 (11.8%), but the number of cancelled liver transplantations due to macrovesicular steatosis hepatis of the graft significantly increased from 2010 to 2016 (p < 0.001) from 15 to 42.

3.3. Donors of Discarded Organs Are Older and Present with Higher Rates of Steatosis Hepatis.
In analysis of allocation groups, i.e., transplanted in our center, allocated elsewhere, or discarded, age differed significantly across groups with discarded organs having the highest age (56.0 ± 21.3, p < 0.001). In regard to steatosis hepatis, 49.7% of discarded organs had reports of steatosis hepatis compared to 28.3% transplanted at our center and 27% transplanted elsewhere after secondary allocation (Figure 2(b)). Age and steatosis

hepatis were significantly associated (p < 0.001); almost half of donors (45.2%) above the age of 65 had reports of steatosis hepatis, compared to 26.5% in donors under the age of 65 (Figure 2(a)).

Cause of death due to trauma was the least likely cause for organs to be discarded 12.6% vs. 15.9%, 19.8, respectively, p < 0.001. Furthermore, the laboratory parameters AST, GGT, bilirubin, INR, and creatinine were all significantly higher (p < 0.001) in the group of discarded organs (Table 1).

3.4. Increasing Prevalence of Steatosis Hepatis in Accepted Organs.
From 2010 to 2016 the proportion of accepted and transplanted steatotic livers increased significantly (p < 0.001, Figures 3(a) and 3(b)). While 22.3% (n = 22) of livers transplanted in 2010 had evidence of steatosis hepatis, this number rose to 51.5 % (n = 66) by 2016. During the same time the proportion of discarded organs which were steatotic significantly decreased (p = 0.04) from 61.2% (n = 30) in 2010 to 46.8% (n=66) in 2016. In the overall offered donor pool, steatosis hepatis differed in between years (p = 0.007), with an increase of the prevalence from 24.0% in 2013 to 34.7% in 2016 (Figure 3(c)).

3.5. Histopathological Reports of Steatosis Hepatis Influence Acceptance Rates.
Histopathological reports of donors were available in 28.9% (n = 766) of cases. In discarded liver grafts 42.5% of organs had a pathology report present compared to only in 24.7% in transplanted liver grafts. Moderate or severe steatosis hepatis was present in discarded organs in 43.8% (n = 105) of cases with 17.5% (n = 42) of those being severely steatotic, i.e., ≥ 60% macrovesicular steatosis (Table 2).

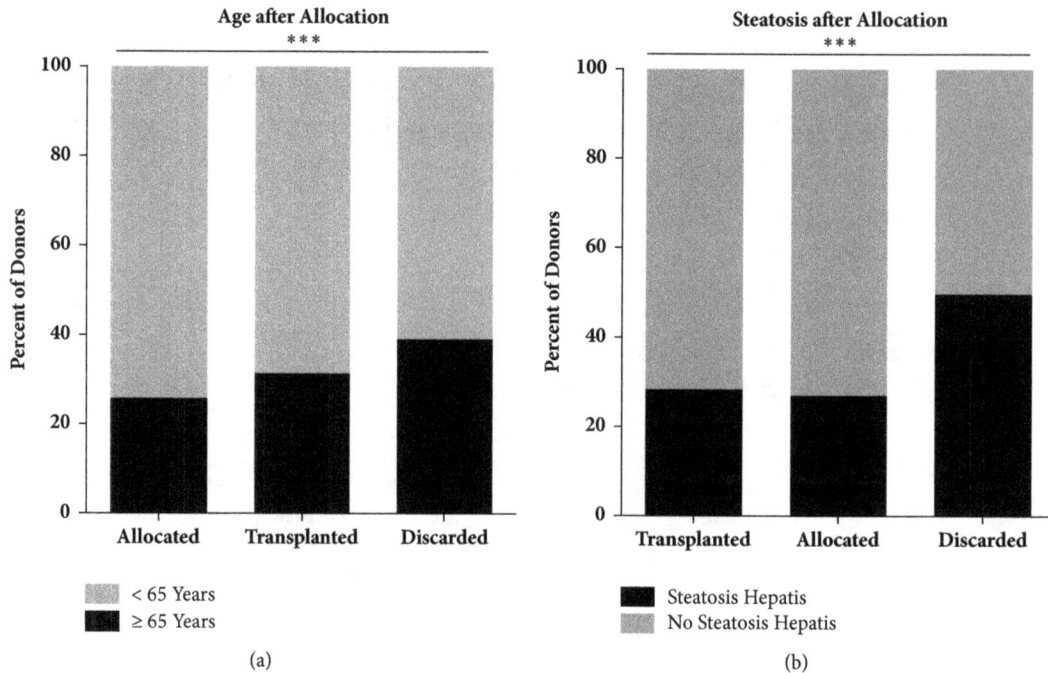

FIGURE 2: Age and steatosis as influencing factors of acceptance rates. (a) Significantly higher proportion of discarded liver allografts from senior donors (39.1% ∗ ∗ ∗ p < 0.001). (b) Steatosis hepatis is significantly more frequently present in discarded organs (49.7%, ∗ ∗ ∗ p < 0.001).

TABLE 1: Donor data overview.

	Total	Allocated	Transplanted	Discarded	P value
N	2653	1561	527	565	
Gender (m) (n, %)	1418 (53.5)	816 (52.3)	268 (51.0)	334 (59.3)	0.007
Age[1]	51.3 ± 20.6	49.0 ± 20.8	53.25 ± 18.2	56.0 ± 21.3	< 0.001
Cause of Death					< 0.001
Trauma (n, %)	464 (17.5)	309 (19.8)	84 (15.9)	71 (12.6)	
Cerebrovascular (n, %)	1308 (49.3)	716 (45.9)	288 (54.6)	304 (53.8)	
Anoxia (n, %)	379 (14.3)	219 (14.0)	74 (14.0)	86 (15.2)	
Other (n, %)	502 (18.9)	317 (20.3)	81 (15.4)	104 (18.4)	
BMI (kg/m2)[1]	25.5 ± 4.9	25.0 ± 4.3	25.6 ± 4.6	26.8 ± 6.3	< 0.001
ICU stay (days)[2]	3.0 (5)	3 (5)	3 (6)	3 (4)	0.25
AST (U/l)[2]	52.0 (76)	49.0 (71)	47.0 (78)	64.5 (102)	< 0.001
ALT (U/l)[2]	34.0 (60)	34.0 (57)	34.0 (59)	36 (70)	0.08
GGT (U/l)[2]	44.0 (93)	39.0 (78)	47.0 (100)	70.0 (161)	< 0.001
Bilirubin (μmol/l)[2]	8.7 (10)	8.2 (10)	9.2 (10)	12.0 (14)	< 0.001
INR[2]	1.18 (02.4)	1.16 (0.25)	1.19 (0.27)	1.2 (0.29)	< 0.001
Creatinine (μmol/l)[2]	70.7 (57.3)	68.0 (55.75)	73.2 (51.85)	79.8 (68.58)	< 0.001
CRP (mg/l)[2]	139.9 (162.65)	136.8 (164.75)	142.5 (152.4)	143.6 (175.23)	0.29
Na+[+] (mmol/l)[2]	148.0 (76.0)	148.0 (11)	147.0 (10)	148.0 (12)	0.15
CPR (n, %)	177 (11)	128 (8.2)	14 (2.7)	35 (6.2)	< 0.001
Steatosis Hepatis in sonography or pathology (n, %)	828 (32.1)	409 (27.0)	146 (28.3)	273 (49.7)	< 0.001
Steatosis Hepatis confirmed only in pathology (n, %)	665 (26.6)	334 (22.4)	114 (22.9)	217 (42.4)	< 0.001

[1]Data is presented as mean ± standard deviation. [2]Data is presented as median (interquartile range). Abbreviations: ALT: alanine-aminotransferase; AST: aspartate-aminotransferase; BMI: body mass index; CPR: cardiopulmonary resuscitation; CRP: C-reactive protein; GGT: gamma-glutamyl transferase; ICU: intensive care unit; INR: international normalized ratio; Na+: serum sodium.

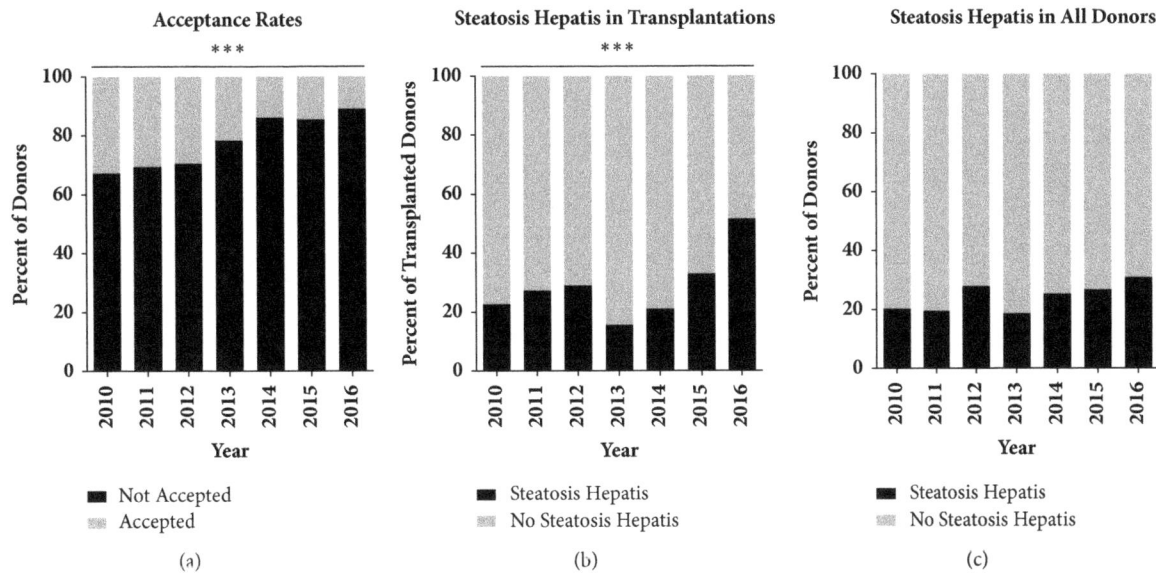

FIGURE 3: Steatosis hepatis prelavence and influence on acceptance rates. (a) Declining acceptance rate for all liver allografts during study period ($* * *$ p < 0.001). (b) Significant increase in steatosis hepatis in transplantations in our center ($* * *$ p < 0.001). (c) Trend in rising steatosis hepatis prevalence in donor population after 2012.

TABLE 2: Steatosis hepatis in donors with available histopathological report.

	Organs Discarded	Transplanted	P value
n	240	526	
No Steatosis Hepatis (n, %)	42 (17.5%)	183 (34.8%)	
Mild Steatosis (n, %)	93 (38.8%)	274 (52.1%)	< 0.001
Moderate Steatosis (n, %)	63 (26.3%)	50 (9.5%)	
Severe Steatosis (n, %)	42 (17.5%)	19 (3.6%)	

Data is presented as counts (proportions).

3.6. Steatosis Hepatis Is a Significant Predictor of Liver Nonuse in Multivariate Model.
A logistic regression was performed to determine the effects of age, BMI, cause of death, history of smoking and/or diabetes, blood levels of AST, GGT, bilirubin, INR, creatinine, HCV, HBV, and steatosis hepatis on the probability of liver grafts being accepted for transplantation. The created model was statistically significant χ^2 = 226.25 p < 0.001 and explained 28.0% (Nagelkerke R^2) of the variance in organ acceptance while correctly classifying 79.7% of cases (Table 3). Donor age below 50 was a significant predictor of organ acceptance (p = 0.004, OR = 2.77, 95% CI = 1.29-5.53); ages above 50 were not significantly associated with organ acceptance. In cases of normal or overweight donor BMI this was equally the case (normal weight: p = 0.001, OR = 7.32, 95% CI = 2.26-3.3; overweight: p = 0.003, OR = 5.6, 95% CI = 1.77-7.73). Compared to donors with positive HCV antibodies, the odds for acceptance were highest in cases of donors being negative for HCV antibodies (p < 0.001, OR = 11.79, 95% CI = 4.49-30.93)

Additionally, lack of steatosis hepatis increased odds for acceptance significantly (p < 0.001, OR = 1.88, 95% CI = 1.33-2.65). Relevant biochemical parameters were levels of AST,

GGT, bilirubin, and INR which all presented increased odds for organ acceptance with lower values.

A similar logistic regression was performed with all cases with available histopathological reports. This model was statistically significant χ^2(4) = 119.19, p < 0.001 and explained 40.2% (Nagelkerke R^2) of the variance in organ acceptance while correctly classifying 78.8% of cases. Macrovesicular steatosis of the graft below 5% was associated with higher organ acceptance (p < 0.001; OR 16.68, 95% CI = 5.01–55.43). In this model only blood levels of creatinine, AST, bilirubin, HCV status, and age were significantly associated with organ acceptance.

3.7. Macrovesicular Steatosis Is Predictive for EAD after Transplantation.
The incidence of EAD significantly increased (p = 0.013) with regard to the degree of macrovesicular steatosis of the graft. EAD occurred in 13 recipients (21.3%) of grafts with no steatosis, 23 patients (39.0%) that received grafts with mild macrovesicular steatosis, and 9 recipients (56.3%) of grafts with moderate and severe macrovesicular steatosis (Figure 4(a)). Cold ischemia time greater than 8 hours combined with moderate macrovesicular steatosis led

TABLE 3: Multivariate logistic regression of organ acceptance.

	Organ Acceptance	
	P value	OR (95% CI)
Age (years)		
< 50	0.004	2.77 (1.29; 5.53)
50 – 59	0.372	1.34 (0.68; 2.80)
60 – 69	0.172	1.63 (0.81; 3.30)
70 – 79	0.567	1.22 (0.62; 2.37)
>80	Reference	
BMI		
< 18.5	0.50	1.62 (0.40; 6.52)
18.5 – 24.9	0.001	7.32 (2.26; 23.77)
25.0 – 29.9	0.003	5.60 (1.77; 17.73)
30 – 34.9	0.12	2.56 (0.78; 8.41)
35 – 39.9	0.51	1.61 (0.40; 6.55)
≥ 40.0	Reference	
Cause of Death		
Trauma	0.76	1.72 (0.94; 3.14)
Cerebrovascular Accident	0.72	1.09 (0.68; 1.73)
Anoxia	0.12	1.61 (0.88; 2.94)
Other	Reference	
Smoking (yes)	0.4	1.12 (0.82; 1.67)
Diabetes mellitus (yes)	0.88	0.96 (0.59; 1.57)
No Steatosis hepatis	< 0.001	1.88 (1.33; 2.65)
HCV antibody negative	< 0.001	11.79 (4.49; 30.93)
HBV core antibody negative	0.09	1.62 (0.94; 2.81)
AST	0.01	1.0 (1.0; 1.0)
GGT	< 0.001	1.0 (1.0; 1.0)
Bilirubin	< 0.001	0.97 (0.96; 0.98)
INR	0.04	0.79 (0.62; 0.99)
Creatinine	0.47	1.0 (1.0; 1.0)
Na+	0.07	0.98 (0.96; 1.0)
CRP	0.76	1.0 (1.0; 1.0)

Data is presented as odds ratios (OR) and 95% confidence intervals (CI). Abbreviations: AST: aspartate-aminotransferase; BMI: body mass index; CRP: C-reactive protein; GGT: gamma-glutamyl transferase; HBV: hepatitis B virus; HCV: hepatitis C virus; INR: international normalized ratio; Na+: serum sodium.

to EAD in 9 (69.2%) cases compared to 28 (30.4%) cases with cold ischemia time less than 8 hours (p = 0.006). EAD led to significantly decreased 1-year recipient (p < 0.001) and graft survival (p < 0.001) (Figure 4(b)). In univariate analysis, severe macrovesicular steatosis compared to any other grades of steatosis or no steatosis had a significant effect on 1-year graft survival (p = 0.03; 33.3% vs. 75%) and recipient survival (p = 0.04; 33.3% vs 72.0%), while lower degrees of macrovesicular steatosis had no effect on graft survival (p = 0.13, Figure 4(c)).

4. Discussion

The increasing shortage of suitable organs for transplantation necessitates constant reevaluation and expansion of organ acceptance criteria. The results of our study show a steady increase in the overall number of liver graft offers but a decline in the acceptance rate from 2010 to 2016. The increase

in the number of organs offered to our center is in huge discrepancy with the factual number of organ donations in the Eurotransplant region and the decreasing number of realized liver transplantations. This trend can be explained by multiple or repeating offers of marginal organs from extended criteria donors to different transplant centers and may be attributed to a more restrictive policy for acceptance of organs from extended criteria donors for high-MELD patients, which are prioritized in the Eurotransplant allocation system.

Steatosis hepatis is a critical factor for declining an organ offer. The rising prevalence of steatosis hepatis in the general population is well documented [27, 28]: The overall prevalence today is between 20% and 30% in Europe and 46% in the United States [10, 29]. De Graaf et al. reported a rate of 62% microvesicular and 38% macrovesicular steatosis in liver allografts from deceased donors from 2001 to 2007 in Australia [16]. Among potential living donors, the prevalence of biopsy-proven nonalcoholic fatty liver disease ranged from

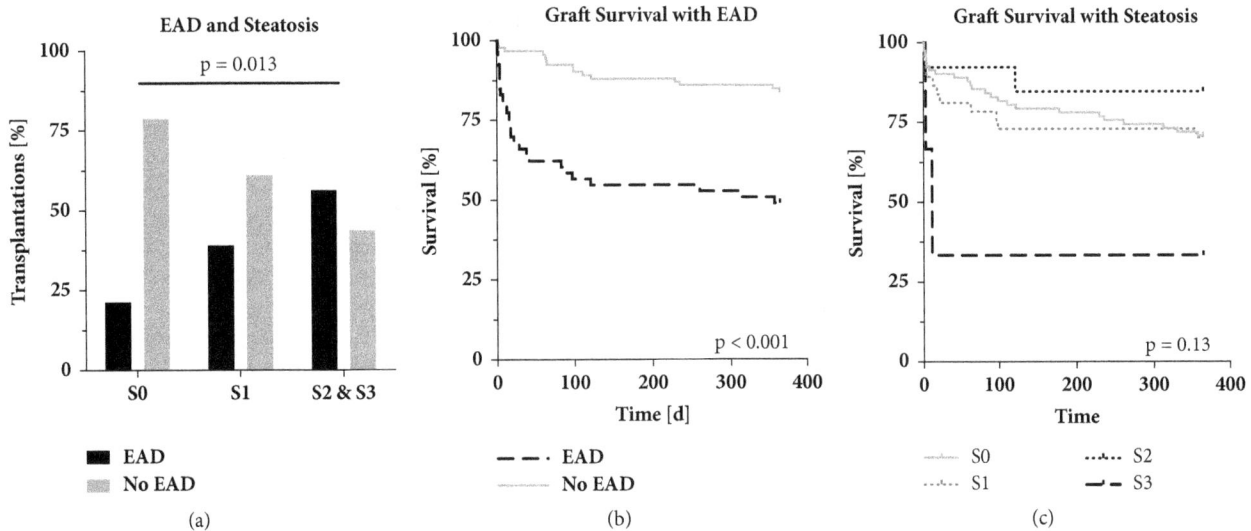

FIGURE 4: Steatosis hepatis prelavence and influence on graft survival. (a) Increased rates of EAD in steatotic liver grafts (p = 0.013). (b) Kaplan-Meier analysis of graft survival of patients with and without early allograft dysfunction (EAD) (p < 0.001). (c) Kaplan-Meier analysis of graft survival in steatotic liver grafts (p = 0.13). S0, no steatosis; S1, mild steatosis; S2, moderate steatosis; S3, severe steatosis. EAD, early allograft dysfunction.

15% to 53% in different studies and disqualified 3% to 21% of potential liver grafts [10]. In contrast, the extent of steatosis on the nonacceptance rate of donated livers is not well documented in the literature. Of note, such an evaluation is limited by the fact that there is no standardized protocol for evaluation of steatosis hepatis of potential liver grafts. The assessment of liver steatosis in potential deceased donors is usually limited to the sonographic inspection or analysis in computed tomography scans. Histopathological verification cannot be performed on a routine basis in hospitals conducting organ retrieval due to logistic reasons. Even though, in our cohort, if steatosis hepatis was reported from ultrasound or macroscopic examination, it was confirmed in 92.5% of cases with a histopathological analysis, nevertheless, liver grafts are rejected by the transplant center based on a nonstandardized assessment of steatosis hepatis. We here show that even though the proportion of steatotic donor organs transplanted in our recipients increased significantly from 2013 to 2016, 12 liver grafts were still rejected due to steatosis hepatis in 2016, which accounted for a potential increase of 63.6% liver transplantations not transplanted due to steatosis of the graft. Compared to 2010, this rate of not-realized transplantations increased by 49%. Efforts to counteract steatosis hepatis are therefore of immediate clinical relevance and should be therapeutically targeted, e.g., by conditioning of steatotic liver grafts by machine perfusion during the preservation period [30].

Our evaluation of reason for nonacceptance confirms previous reports from Orman et al. concerning age and BMI [9]. However, the history of diabetes mellitus was not significantly associated with organ acceptance in our study cohort. The effect of DCD donors on acceptance could not be investigated, as transplantation in Germany is strictly DBD donors only. Additionally, we could show that a significantly

larger proportion of steatotic organs were discarded and that prevalence of steatosis hepatis increased over time. In multivariate analysis, we found a significant trend to declining organs with moderate or severe macrovesicular steatosis and a positive trend for acceptance of organs with macrovesicular steatosis hepatis levels below 30%.

Interestingly enough steatosis hepatis coincided with major limitations in organ quality such as increased liver injury parameters and decreased renal function parameters. Donors with steatosis hepatis also had increased ICU stay duration and were older. This combination is challenging, as each factor for itself is known to negatively impact survival after liver transplantation [15, 31, 32]. Unlike in the United States, recipient survival after liver transplantation has been worse since the introduction of the MELD score [33–35]. Irregularities uncovered in the German liver allocation program since 2012 have changed the donor pool and led to fewer suitable donors and reduced overall organ quality [33]. Our data on graft acceptance rate reflects this trend and shows a 21.8% drop of acceptance from 2010 to 2016, while organ offer numbers doubled in the same time.

Our evaluation of the outcome of macrovesicular liver grafts confirms previous reports, showing significantly higher rates of EAD compared to grafts with no steatosis. Unlike previously reported [16, 23, 36], we observed this effect not only for severe but also for mild and moderate steatotic grafts. However, the definition of EAD is not standardized. As previously reported from Westerkamp et al., the combination of long CIT and moderate or severe macrovesicular steatosis had detrimental effects on the outcome after transplantation [37]. These effects, which we already observe in grafts with mild steatosis, could demand adapted allocation and preservation procedures to reduce CIT and subsequently reduce expected ischemia-reperfusion injury [18, 19].

5. Conclusion

In conclusion, our analysis shows a significant decline in liver allograft acceptance rate at our center. In parallel to the increase of steatosis hepatis in the donor pool there was a significant increase of steatosis hepatis acceptance at our center especially in cases with histopathological confirmation of less than 30% macrovesicular steatosis. Moreover, we show a strong association of macrovesicular graft steatosis and the development of EAD, especially in cases with prolonged CIT. Although our results are limited by the retrospective and single center analysis, we propose the present data to be at least relevant for Germany and the *Eurotransplant* region, where high MELD patients and organs from extended criteria donors affect the outcome of liver transplantation. Therapeutic concepts are necessary to address the rising prevalence of steatotic grafts and the inferior outcome associated with transplantation of such grafts. These concepts should range from limiting the effects of cold ischemia to the graft by *ex vivo* machine perfusion to the metabolic reconditioning of steatotic organs prior to transplantation [38].

Abbreviations

ALT: Alanine-aminotransferase
AST: Aspartate-aminotransferase
BMI: Body mass index
CPR: Cardiopulmonary resuscitation
CRP: C-reactive protein
DBD: Donation after brain death
DCD: Donation after cardiac death
EAD: Early allograft dysfunction
GGT: Gamma-glutamyl transferase
HCV: Hepatitis C virus
HBV: Hepatitis B virus
ICU: Intensive care unit
INR: International normalized ratio
IQR: Interquartile range
OLT: Orthotopic liver transplantation
SD: Standard deviation
UNOS: United Network for Organ Sharing.

Acknowledgments

The authors want to thank Jacob de Boer from Eurotransplant, Thomas Mehlitz, Birgit Kulawick, and Michael Hippler-Benscheidt for their assistance in this study. Nathanael Raschzok and Paul Ritschl are participants of the BIH Charité Clinician Scientist Program funded by the Charité – Universitätsmedizin Berlin and the Berlin Institute of Health. This work was supported by institutional funding of the Charité – Universitätsmedizin Berlin. We acknowledge support from the German Research Foundation (DFG) and the Open Access Publication Fund of Charité – Universitätsmedizin Berlin.

References

[1] D. Habka, D. Mann, R. Landes, A. Soto-Gutierrez, and S. Gruttadauria, "Future Economics of Liver Transplantation: A 20-Year Cost Modeling Forecast and the Prospect of Bioengineering Autologous Liver Grafts," *PLoS ONE*, vol. 10, no. 7, p. e0131764, 2015.

[2] E. S. Orman, M. E. Mayorga, S. B. Wheeler et al., "Declining liver graft quality threatens the future of liver transplantation in the United States," *Liver Transplantation*, vol. 21, no. 8, pp. 1040–1050, 2015.

[3] D. A. Sass and D. J. Reich, "Liver Transplantation in the 21st Century: Expanding the Donor Options," *Gastroenterology Clinics of North America*, vol. 40, no. 3, pp. 641–658, 2011.

[4] D. Pezzati, D. Ghinolfi, P. De Simone, E. Balzano, and F. Filipponi, "Strategies to optimize the use of marginal donors in liver transplantation," *World Journal of Hepatology*, vol. 7, no. 26, pp. 2636–2647, 2015.

[5] Eurotransplant, "Deceased liver donors used, by year, by donor country," Eurotransplant Statistics Report Library, Leiden, 2017.

[6] Eurotransplant, *Active liver waiting list (at year-end) in All ET, by year, by country*, 2016.

[7] K. B. Klein, T. D. Stafinski, and D. Menon, "Predicting survival after liver transplantation based on pre-transplant MELD score: A systematic review of the literature," *PLoS ONE*, vol. 8, no. 12, 2013.

[8] P. Sharma, D. E. Schaubel, Q. Gong, M. Guidinger, and R. M. Merion, "End-stage liver disease candidates at the highest model for end-stage liver disease scores have higher wait-list mortality than status-1A candidates," *Hepatology*, vol. 55, no. 1, pp. 192–198, 2012.

[9] E. S. Orman, A. S. Barritt, S. B. Wheeler, and P. H. Hayashi, "Declining liver utilization for transplantation in the United States and the impact of donation after cardiac death," *Liver Transplantation*, vol. 19, no. 1, pp. 59–68, 2013.

[10] R. Pais, A. S. Barritt, Y. Calmus et al., "NAFLD and liver transplantation: Current burden and expected challenges," *Journal of Hepatology*, vol. 65, no. 6, pp. 1245–1257, 2016.

[11] C. D. Williams, J. Stengel, M. I. Asike et al., "Prevalence of nonalcoholic fatty liver disease and nonalcoholic steatohepatitis among a largely middle-aged population utilizing ultrasound and liver biopsy: a prospective study," *Gastroenterology*, vol. 140, no. 1, pp. 124–131, 2011.

[12] M. H. Le, P. Devaki, N. B. Ha et al., "Prevalence of non-alcoholic fatty liver disease and risk factors for advanced fibrosis and mortality in the United States," *PLoS ONE*, vol. 12, no. 3, p. e0173499, 2017.

[13] N. Chalasani, Z. Younossi, and J. E. Lavine, "The diagnosis and management of non-alcoholic fatty liver disease: practice guideline by the American Association for the Study of Liver Diseases, American College of Gastroenterology, and the American Gastroenterological Association," *Hepatology*, vol. 55, no. 6, pp. 2005–2023, 2012.

[14] A. L. Spitzer, O. B. Lao, A. A. S. Dick et al., "The biopsied donor liver: incorporating macrosteatosis into high-risk donor assessment," *Liver Transplantation*, vol. 16, no. 7, pp. 874–884, 2010.

[15] P. Dutkowski, A. Schlegel, K. Slankamenac et al., "The use of fatty liver grafts in modern allocation systems: risk assessment by the balance of risk (BAR) score," *Annals of Surgery*, vol. 256, no. 5, pp. 861–869, 2012.

[16] E. L. de Graaf, J. Kench, P. Dilworth et al., "Grade of deceased donor liver macrovesicular steatosis impacts graft and recipient outcomes more than the Donor Risk Index," *Journal of Gastroenterology and Hepatology*, vol. 27, no. 3, pp. 540–546, 2012.

[17] K. M. Olthoff, L. Kulik, B. Samstein et al., "Validation of a current definition of early allograft dysfunction in liver transplant recipients and analysis of risk factors," *Liver Transplantation*, vol. 16, no. 8, pp. 943–949, 2010.

[18] R. C. Gehrau, V. R. Mas, C. I. Dumur et al., "Donor hepatic steatosis induce exacerbated ischemia-reperfusion injury through activation of innate immune response molecular pathways," *Transplantation*, vol. 99, no. 12, pp. 2523–2533, 2015.

[19] M. J. J. Chu, A. J. R. Hickey, A. R. J. Phillips, and A. S. J. R. Bartlett, "The Impact of Hepatic Steatosis on Hepatic Ischemia-Reperfusion Injury in Experimental Studies: A Systematic Review," *BioMed Research International*, vol. 2013, Article ID 192029, 12 pages, 2013.

[20] M. K. Angele, M. Rentsch, W. H. Hartl et al., "Effect of graft steatosis on liver function and organ survival after liver transplantation," *The American Journal of Surgery*, vol. 195, no. 2, pp. 214–220, 2008.

[21] U. Kulik, F. Lehner, J. Klempnauer, and J. Borlak, "Primary nonfunction is frequently associated with fatty liver allografts and high mortality after re-transplantation," *Liver International*, vol. 37, no. 8, pp. 1219–1228, 2017.

[22] M. Gabrielli, F. Moisan, M. Vidal et al., "Steatotic livers. can we use them in OLTX? Outcome data from a prospective baseline liver biopsy study," *Annals of Hepatology*, vol. 11, no. 6, pp. 891–898, 2012.

[23] J. P. Deroose, G. Kazemier, P. Zondervan, J. N. M. IJzermans, H. J. Metselaar, and I. P. J. Alwayn, "Hepatic steatosis is not always a contraindication for cadaveric liver transplantation," *HPB*, vol. 13, no. 6, pp. 417–425, 2011.

[24] M. J. Chu, A. J. Dare, A. R. Phillips, and A. S. Bartlett, "Donor hepatic steatosis and outcome after liver transplantation: a systematic review," *Journal of Gastrointestinal Surgery*, vol. 19, pp. 1713–1724, 2015.

[25] P. Waage and S. Novak, Organspende und Transplantation in Deutschland [Organ donation and transplantation in Germany]. Frankfurt/Main: Deutsche Stiftung Organtransplantation. https://www.dso.de/uploads/tx_dsodl/DSO_JB_2015_Web_2.pdf.

[26] J. Briceno, J. Padillo, S. Rufián, G. Solórzano, and C. Pera, "Assignment of steatotic livers by the mayo model for end-stage liver disease," *Transplant International*, vol. 18, no. 5, pp. 577–583, 2005.

[27] P. Paschos and K. Paletas, "Non alcoholic fatty liver disease and metabolic syndrome," *Hippokratia*, vol. 13, no. 1, pp. 9–19, 2009.

[28] T. Williams, "Metabolic Syndrome: Nonalcoholic Fatty Liver Disease," *FP Essent*, vol. 435, pp. 24–29, 2015.

[29] The GBD 2015 Obesity Collaborators, "Health Effects of Overweight and Obesity in 195 Countries over 25 Years," *The New England Journal of Medicine*, vol. 377, no. 1, pp. 13–27, 2017.

[30] N. I. Nativ, T. J. Maguire, G. Yarmush et al., "Liver defatting: An alternative approach to enable steatotic liver transplantation," *American Journal of Transplantation*, vol. 12, no. 12, pp. 3176–3183, 2012.

[31] A. M. Cameron, R. M. Ghobrial, H. Yersiz et al., "Optimal utilization of donor grafts with extended criteria: A single-center experience in over 1000 liver transplants," *Annals of Surgery*, vol. 243, no. 6, pp. 748–753, 2006.

[32] K. J. Halazun, A. A. Rana, B. Fortune et al., "No country for old livers? Examining and optimizing the utilization of elderly liver grafts," *American Journal of Transplantation*, vol. 18, no. 3, pp. 669–678, 2018.

[33] F. Tacke, D. C. Kroy, A. P. Barreiros, and U. P. Neumann, "Liver transplantation in Germany," *Liver Transplantation*, vol. 22, no. 8, pp. 1136–1142, 2016.

[34] M. Taniguchi, "Liver transplantation in the MELD era–analysis of the OPTN/UNOS registry," *Clinical transplants*, pp. 41–65, 2012.

[35] W. Schoening, M. Helbig, N. Buescher et al., "Eurotransplant donor-risk-index and recipient factors: Influence on long-term outcome after liver transplantation - A large single-center experience," *Clinical Transplantation*, 2016.

[36] F. E. Sharkey, I. Lytvak, T. J. Prihoda, K. V. Speeg, W. K. Washburn, and G. A. Halff, "High-grade microsteatosis and delay in hepatic function after orthotopic liver transplantation," *Human Pathology*, vol. 42, no. 9, pp. 1337–1342, 2011.

[37] A. C. Westerkamp, M. T. De Boer, A. P. Van Den Berg, A. S. H. Gouw, and R. J. Porte, "Similar outcome after transplantation of moderate macrovesicular steatotic and nonsteatotic livers when the cold ischemia time is kept very short," *Transplant International*, vol. 28, no. 3, pp. 319–329, 2015.

[38] N. Gilbo, G. Catalano, M. Salizzoni, and R. Romagnoli, "Liver graft preconditioning, preservation and reconditioning," *Digestive and Liver Disease*, vol. 48, no. 11, pp. 1265–1274, 2016.

25

Diagnostic Laparoscopy with Ultrasound Still Has a Role in the Staging of Pancreatic Cancer: A Systematic Review of the Literature

Jordan Levy,[1] Mehdi Tahiri,[1,2] Tsafrir Vanounou,[1,2] Geva Maimon,[2] and Simon Bergman[1,2]

[1]Division of General Surgery, Jewish General Hospital, McGill University, Montreal, QC, Canada H3T 1E2
[2]Lady Davis Institute for Medical Research, Montreal, QC, Canada H3T 1E2

Correspondence should be addressed to Simon Bergman; simon.bergman@mcgill.ca

Academic Editor: Attila Olah

Background. The reported incidence of noncurative laparotomies for pancreatic cancer using standard imaging (SI) techniques for staging remains high. The objectives of this study are to determine the diagnostic accuracy of diagnostic laparoscopy with ultrasound (DLUS) in assessing resectability of pancreatic tumors. *Study Design.* We systematically searched the literature for prospective studies investigating the accuracy of DLUS in determining resectability of pancreatic tumors. *Results.* 104 studies were initially identified and 19 prospective studies (1,573 patients) were included. DLUS correctly predicted resectability in 79% compared to 55% for SI. DLUS prevented noncurative laparotomies in 33%. Of those, the most frequent DLUS findings precluding resection were liver metastases, vascular involvement, and peritoneal metastases. DLUS had a morbidity rate of 0.8% with no mortalities. DLUS remained superior to SI when analyzing studies published only in the last five years (100% versus 81%), enrolling patients after the year 2000 (74% versus 58%), or comparing DLUS to modern multidimensional CT (100% versus 78%). *Conclusion.* DLUS seems to still have a role in the preoperative staging of pancreatic cancer. With its ability to detect liver metastases, vascular involvement, and peritoneal metastases, the use of DLUS leads to less noncurative laparotomies.

1. Introduction

Pancreatic cancer represents an aggressive disease that is resectable in only 10–20% of patients at the time of diagnosis [1, 2]. While resection can be curative in some, it may also be abandoned intraoperatively due to the presence of occult advanced disease [3]. Careful selection of patients for surgery is important in order to avoid unnecessary procedures and their associated morbidities. In addition, with the advent of minimally invasive procedures for symptomatic relief and palliation, such as endoscopic and percutaneous biliary stenting and laparoscopic duodenal and biliary bypass, the need to correctly identify unresectable patients prior to laparotomy has been further emphasized [4].

Diagnostic laparoscopy (DL) was introduced in many preoperative staging algorithms for pancreatic carcinoma over 20 years ago [5]. Its value seemed to have been considerably enhanced with the adjunct of laparoscopic ultrasound (LUS) [4, 6]. Despite the growing body of research in the use of diagnostic laparoscopy with ultrasound (DLUS) for preoperative staging of pancreatic cancers, its application remains controversial [7]. Several studies support its use, as it is a sensitive tool in detecting small hepatic lesions, vascular invasion, and malignant lymphadenopathy [8]. However, many have argued, especially with the advent of multidimensional computed tomography (CT), that standard imaging (SI) modalities may be sufficient and just as reliable in staging of pancreatic cancer, obviating the need of an additional operative procedure [9].

We performed a systematic review of prospective studies investigating the use of DLUS in staging pancreatic cancer. The objectives of this study are (1) to determine the diagnostic accuracy of DLUS in assessing resectability of pancreatic tumors, (2) to compare the reported resection rates of DLUS to standard preoperative imaging, and (3) to determine how the accuracy of these modalities has evolved over time.

2. Methods

2.1. Data Sources and Searches. A focused literature search using Medline and EMBASE databases, through June 2014, was conducted. Prospective studies evaluating the accuracy of diagnostic laparoscopy followed by laparoscopic ultrasound in determining resectability of pancreatic cancer were included. The search strategy combined the terms "laparoscopic ultraso*" and "pancrea*" and "cancer" or "tumor*" or "malignancy" and "stage" or "staging" in the English language. This strategy was complemented by manually searching the references of the studies identified in the primary search. Study eligibility criteria were (1) that it was prospective; (2) that its objective was to investigate the accuracy of DLUS in determining resectability of pancreatic tumors; (3) that it reported intraoperative DLUS findings; and (4) that surgery was considered the gold standard for resectability.

2.2. Data Extraction. Data from each study was independently extracted by two reviewers. Disagreements were resolved by consensus or, when necessary, by a third reviewer. The reviewers systematically extracted information on author, date of publication, institution, study design, enrolment years, patient demographics, type of preoperative imaging, laparoscopic ultrasound probe and monitor specifications, morbidity associated with DLUS, and failure rates in performing DLUS. The reviewers also extracted statistical data, including sensitivity, specificity, and predictive values of DLUS and SI. We respected the following rigorous criteria for our analysis: (1) all patients declining or unfit (determined by the surgical team at that time) for DLUS or laparotomy were excluded. (2) All patients in whom laparoscopic ultrasound was not achieved were excluded, unless diagnostic laparoscopy had already proven unresectability before LUS was required. (3) In certain studies, patients were classified as "doubtfully resectable"; those patients were treated similarly to the resectable group and were thus included in our study as such. (4) Benign lesions discovered at DLUS or laparotomy were considered as "resected" for the purpose of the analysis.

2.3. Statistical Analysis. Both imaging techniques, DLUS and SI, are being used to determine the resectability of a pancreatic cancer. Hence, for our purposes, the term "true positive" refers to a cancer that was deemed resectable by a staging technique and was actually resected. Similarly, a "true negative" refers to a cancer deemed unresectable by SI or DLUS and confirmed as unresectable according to operative findings, cytopathology, frozen section, or grossly suspicious findings during either staging technique. Sensitivity is defined as the number of true positives over the number of resectable cancers. Specificity is defined as the number of true negatives over the total number of unresectable cancers. The positive predictive value is the number of true positives over the total number of cancers deemed resectable by imaging. Negative predictive value is the number of true negatives over the total number of cancers deemed unresectable by imaging. Our measure of resection rate is equivalent to the positive predictive value, as defined above. To calculate the overall resection rate across all applicable studies, the data were weighted according to each study's sample size.

3. Results

3.1. Study Selection and Baseline Characteristics. Study selection occurred according to the Preferred Reporting Items for Systematic Review and Meta-Analyses (PRISMA) diagram (Figure 1). The search initially identified a total of 99 abstracts, with additional five abstracts found after a manual search through the references. These abstracts were reviewed and screened for relevance. 43 full-text and potentially relevant articles were retrieved and evaluated for eligibility following exclusion of review articles ($n = 29$), nonrelevant articles ($n = 24$), conference outlines or abstracts ($n = 4$), letters to the editor ($n = 2$), critical appraisal ($n = 1$), and duplicate abstract ($n = 1$). Of the 43 full-text studies retrieved, 18 studies met the inclusion criteria and were included in the analysis. Studies were excluded because they did not provide relevant analytical data necessary for the calculation of the sensitivity and specificity of DLUS as a diagnostic tool ($n = 20$) or were not prospective studies ($n = 5$). One of the 18 prospective studies included in the systematic review reported a two-part study occurring at different times on different study populations [10]. It was thus considered as two separate studies, bringing the total to 19 prospective studies and 1,573 patients.

Eleven of 19 studies were published after January 1, 2000. The average patient age ranged from 55 to 66 years old. The percentage of male patients ranged from 25 to 64%. The location of the pancreatic tumor was found most commonly in the pancreatic head, followed by the ampullary region, body, and tail, and rarely in the uncinate process (Table 1).

3.2. Execution of Preoperative Staging. CT scan was the investigation of choice in the assessment of resectability in all but one study (18/19), which was completed in a center where mesenteric angiography was frequently performed [25]. 79% (15/19) of studies reported using at least one additional staging procedure following CT [4, 6, 11, 13–20, 22–25]: abdominal ultrasound (15/19) [4, 6, 11, 13–20, 22–25], endoscopic retrograde pancreatography (10/19) [4, 6, 14, 16–20, 22, 24], endoscopic ultrasound (5/19) [13, 14, 18, 19, 23], visceral angiography (7/19) [4, 6, 14, 16, 23–25], and magnetic resonance imaging (MRI) (5/19) [14–17, 20], although the additional procedures were not performed in all patients.

Diagnostic laparoscopy was first carried out to explore the peritoneal cavity in search of malignant ascites, peritoneal metastases, visceral implants, or suspicious lymph nodes. The LUS probe was then inserted. Most often, the probe used linear array with a frequency of 5–7.5 MHz and frequently had Doppler capabilities. The liver was scanned in search of undiagnosed micrometastases and the biliary tree explored for any abnormalities. The pancreas was scanned to better characterize the primary lesion and determine local extensions into peripancreatic tissues including duodenum, mesocolon, stomach, and spleen. In less than one-third of the studies did the authors explicitly report exploring

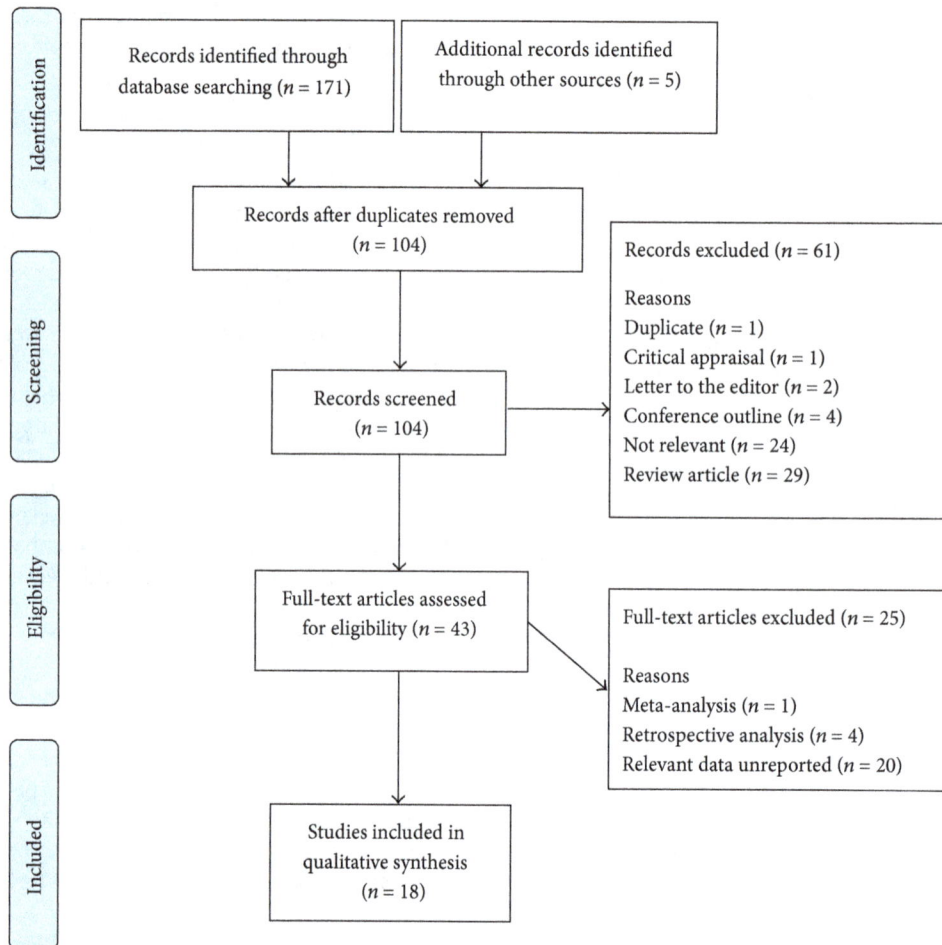

FIGURE 1: Search diagram.

the lesser sac by retroduodenal or infragastric approaches. Blood vessels, including the celiac axis, superior mesenteric artery, and the portal venous system, were characterized according to their relation to the tumor and whether they were encased, thrombosed, stenosed, infiltrated, or frankly invaded. Associated lymph node basins were also investigated.

Nine studies described DLUS timing [6, 11–13, 16, 18, 19, 21, 24]. In five studies it occurred as a separate procedure prior to laparotomy [6, 12, 18, 19, 24]; in two studies it occurred in the same setting immediately prior to laparotomy [11, 16]. In two studies it occurred both immediately before and as a separate procedure [13, 21]. Procedure time varied between 15 and 90 minutes depending on surgeon experience and whether biopsies and lesser sac dissection were performed.

3.3. Morbidity and Mortality. Complication rates were minimal at 0.8% (9/1076), including 2 port-site hemorrhages, 2 episodes of pancreatitis, 2 wound infections, 1 enterotomy, 1 aspiration pneumonia, and 1 bile leak following biopsy [4, 6, 16, 17, 24]. There were no procedure-related mortalities.

3.4. Resectability Criteria. Nonresectability criteria differed between studies. All studies considered liver and peritoneal

and other distant metastases unresectable. Seven studies only considered distant lymphadenopathy as unresectable [11, 13, 14, 16, 17, 21, 22] while two studies included regional involvement [4, 19]; the rest of the studies did not specify. Size was only considered in three studies [4, 12, 25]. Most studies considered any vascular involvement as unresectable, except four studies in which some degree of portal vein or superior mesenteric vein was considered resectable [14, 16, 22, 24]. All but one study [11] discussed confirmation of nonresectability due to liver, peritoneal, or lymph node metastases by biopsy proven histopathology.

3.5. Rates of Resection. Studies including data on SI are summarized in Table 2. CT was used in 99.7% (1569/1573) of patients to determine resectability; 4 patients underwent angiography without CT. Of these, the data for 1442 patients from 15 studies were available for analysis [4, 6, 10–14, 16, 18, 19, 21, 22, 24, 25]. Eight of 15 studies only included "SI resectable" patients in their analysis without presenting the initial study population screened by SI, precluding a sensitivity and specificity analysis [4, 10, 11, 18, 21, 24, 25]. Following imaging, 911 patients were considered resectable and of these, only 505 were resected at laparotomy, corresponding to a

TABLE 1: Study characteristics.

Author	Year of publication	Years of enrolment	Study design	Country	Sample size	Mean age	% male	Location/tumor type
Barabino et al. [10]	2011	1995–1999	Prospective	Italy	40	NR	NR	Periampullary 40
Barabino et al. [10]	2011	2002–2007	Prospective	Italy	64	NR	NR	Periampullary 64
Piccolboni et al. [11]	2010	2005–2008	Prospective	Italy	48	NR	NR	NR
Doucas et al. [12]	2007	2001–2004	Prospective	UK	100	63	52%	Head 90, body, or tail 10
Fristrup et al. [13]	2006	2002–2004	Prospective	Denmark	148	66*	54%	NR
Doran et al. [14]	2004	1997–2002	Prospective	UK	239	64*	60%	NR
Zhao et al. [15]	2003	NR	Prospective	China	22	55	64%	Head 22
Kwon et al. [16]	2002	1996–2000	Prospective	Japan	118	59	64%	Head 39, body 13
Lavonius et al. [17]	2001	1997–1999	Prospective	Finland	27	63	48%	Head 21, body 2, chronic pancreatitis 4
Taylor et al. [18]	2001	1996–2000	Prospective	UK	51	66	57%	Head 42, ampullary 9
Schachter et al. [19]	2000	1996–1999	Prospective	Israel	94	63	46%	Head 40, body, or tail 19 UP 5, ampullary 3
Velasco et al. [20]	2000	NR	Prospective	USA	33	NR	NR	NR
Norton et al. [21]	1999	NR	Prospective	USA	50	NR	NR	NR
Minnard et al. [22]	1998	1993–1995	Prospective	USA	90	65*	47%	Head 64, body 19, ampullary 4, tail 3
Champault et al. [23]	1997	1994–1996	Prospective	France	26	61	46%	Head 26
Pietrabissa et al. [24]	1996	1994-1995	Prospective	Italy	21	65	62%	Head 14, body, or tail 7
Bemelman et al. [6]	1995	1993-1994	Prospective	Netherlands	350	NR	NR	Head 60, ampullary 13
John et al. [4]	1995	1991–1993	Prospective	UK	40	59*	45%	NR
Murugiah et al. [25]	1993	1991-1992	Prospective	UK	12	58	25%	Head 12

*Median age.
AdenoCA = adenocarcinoma, NOS = not otherwise specified, CCA = cholangiocarcinoma, NET = neuroendocrine tumor, UP = uncinate process, NR = not reported.

resection rate of 55% (29%–85%) [4, 6, 10–14, 16, 18, 19, 21, 22, 24, 25].

Table 3 summarizes DLUS data. 1076 patients were initially considered for DLUS. However, five patients declined further investigations and were excluded from the study; failures due to dense adhesions occurred in nine patients, while 12 patients were deemed unfit for surgery and were also excluded from formal analysis. Ultimately, 1050 patients were investigated using DLUS. 646 patients were deemed resectable and 513 were finally resected, corresponding to a resection rate of 79% (41%–100%). Of note, even those studies employing additional diagnostic procedures following CT did not show superior accuracy than DLUS. Such

complementary studies, such as EUS, once represented an important role in pancreatic cancer staging and have now fallen out of favor with certain institutions recommending against its routine use in staging [26].

3.6. DLUS versus SI. 14 studies presented data on SI and DLUS findings in a sequential manner such that the study population could be followed up from SI to DLUS [4, 6, 10–14, 16, 18, 19, 21, 24, 25]. In 781 patients deemed resectable by SI, DLUS correctly prevented noncurative laparotomies in 254 (33%). In this group, the most common findings precluding resection were liver metastases, vascular involvement, and peritoneal metastases.

TABLE 2: Analysis of SI.

Author	Year	# receiving SI	Analysis sample	Resectability			
				Sensitivity	Specificity	PPV	NPV
Barabino et al. [10]	2011	40*	40	NA	NA	33% (13/40)	NA
Barabino et al. [10]	2011	64*	64	NA	NA	78% (50/64)	NA
Piccolboni et al. [11]	2010	48*	48	NA	NA	85% (41/48)	NA
Doucas et al. [12]	2007	100	94	71% (20/28)	26% (17/66)	29% (20/69)	68% (17/25)
Fristrup et al. [13]	2006	148	148	100% (38/38)	64% (70/110)	49% (38/78)	100% (70/70)
Doran et al. [14]	2004	239	227	96% (127/132)	46% (44/95)	71% (127/178)	90% (44/49)
Zhao et al. [15]	2003	22	NR	NA	NA	NA	NA
Kwon et al. [16]	2002	118	118	100% (39/39)	84% (66/79)	75% (39/52)	100% (66/66)
Lavonius et al. [17]	2001	27	NR	NA	NA	NA	NA
Taylor et al. [18]	2001	51*	49	NA	NA	53% (26/49)	NA
Schachter et al. [19]	2000	94	94	100% (33/33)	44% (27/61)	49% (33/67)	100% (27/27)
Velasco et al. [20]	2000	33	NR	NA	NA	NA	NA
Norton et al. [21]	1999	50*	50	NA	NA	52% (26/50)	NA
Minnard et al. [22]	1998	90	90	100% (40/40)	34% (17/50)	55% (40/73)	100% (17/17)
Champault et al. [23]	1997	26	NR	NA	NA	NA	NA
Pietrabissa et al. [24]	1996	21*	21	NA	NA	62% (13/21)	NA
Bemelman et al. [6]	1995	350	347	100% (22/22)	85% (277/325)	31% (22/70)	100% (277/277)
John et al. [4]	1995	40*	40	NA	NA	30% (12/40)	NA
Murugiah et al. [25]	1993	12*	12	NA	NA	42% (5/12)	NA

*Size of initial population screened not available. Only patients deemed resectable as per SI were included.
NA = Not applicable, NR = Not Reported.

TABLE 3: Analysis of DLUS.

Author	Year	Analysis sample	Resectability			
			Sensitivity	Specificity	PPV (resection rate)	NPV
Barabino et al. [10]	2011	40	100% (13/13)	93% (25/27)	87% (13/15)	100% (25/25)
Barabino et al. [10]	2011	9	100% (1/1)	100% (8/8)	100% (1/1)	100% (8/8)
Piccolboni et al. [11]	2010	48	100% (41/41)	100% (7/7)	100% (41/41)	100% (7/7)
Doucas et al. [12]	2007	94	100% (28/28)	64% (42/66)	54% (28/52)	100% (42/42)
Fristrup et al. [13]	2006	78	100% (38/38)	65% (26/40)	73% (38/52)	100% (26/26)
Doran et al. [14]	2004	227	98% (130/132)	57% (54/95)	76% (130/171)	96% (54/56)
Zhao et al. [15]	2003	22	100% (9/9)	92% (12/13)	90% (9/10)	100% (12/12)
Kwon et al. [16]	2002	52	100% (39/39)	100% (13/13)	100% (39/39)	100% (13/13)
Lavonius et al. [17]	2001	24	100% (11/11)	69% (9/13)	73% (11/15)	100% (9/9)
Taylor et al. [18]	2001	49	100% (26/26)	91% (21/23)	93% (26/28)	100% (21/21)
Schachter et al. [19]	2000	67	100% (33/33)	88% (30/34)	89% (33/37)	100% (30/30)
Velasco et al. [20]	2000	33	100% (22/22)	82% (9/11)	92% (22/24)	100% (9/9)
Norton et al. [21]	1999	50	100% (26/26)	92% (22/24)	93% (26/28)	100% (22/22)
Minnard et al. [22]	1998	90	100% (40/40)	98% (49/50)	98% (40/41)	100% (49/49)
Champault et al. [23]	1997	26	100% (5/5)	100% (21/21)	100% (5/5)	100% (21/21)
Pietrabissa et al. [24]	1996	21	100% (13/13)	100% (8/8)	100% (13/13)	100% (8/8)
Bemelman et al. [6]	1995	70	100% (22/22)	33% (16/48)	41% (22/54)	100% (16/16)
John et al. [4]	1995	38	92% (11/12)	88% (23/26)	79% (11/14)	96% (23/24)
Murugiah et al. [25]	1993	12	100% (5/5)	86% (6/7)	83% (5/6)	100% (6/6)

3.7. DLUS versus DL. The added benefit of laparoscopic ultrasound (LUS) to diagnostic laparoscopy (DL) was investigated and clearly reported in three studies. In these studies, diagnostic laparoscopy with ultrasound (DLUS) identified 64 unresectable patients, of which 37 were discovered using ultrasound after being overlooked by diagnostic laparoscopy (DL) alone. Signifying that 58% of these accurate staging procedures were directly attributable to the addition of ultrasound to diagnostic laparoscopy. The findings precluding resection in these 37 patients were 17 vascular involvements,

14 liver metastases, 5 malignant lymphadenopathies, and 1 transverse mesocolon invasion [6, 13, 21].

3.8. Controlling for Advances in Diagnostic Imaging. As imaging studies have improved substantially in recent years, subgroup analyses of studies published in the last five years, enrolling patients after 2000 and those using multidimensional CT (MDCT), were carried out. In studies published between 2009 and 2014 (two studies), the resection rates using DLUS and SI were 100% and 81% (78%–85%), respectively [10, 11]. In those studies enrolling patients only after the year 2000 (four studies), the resection rates were 74% (54%–100%) and 58% (29%–85%) for DLUS and SI, respectively [10–13]. In the only prospective study specifically comparing DLUS to multidimensional CT (and no previous model of CT), the resection rates were 100% and 78%, respectively [10].

4. Discussion

Currently, DLUS is not routinely used in preoperative staging of pancreatic tumors. Some institutions selectively incorporate it into staging protocols, while others do not use it at all. Our study was designed to determine the accuracy of DLUS in determining resectability of pancreatic tumors. We included only the most rigorous prospective studies, in which DLUS, SI, and laparotomy findings were clearly reported.

Overall, by weighted analysis, DLUS improved the resection rate of pancreatic malignancies from 55% to 79% with no increase in mortality and a 0.8% complication rate. DLUS remained more accurate when restricting our analysis to more recent studies, in which SI had presumably improved.

A meta-analysis published in 2010 evaluating the role of DL and LUS in the preoperative staging of pancreaticobiliary cancer demonstrated that it improved resection rates of pancreatic malignancies from 61% to 80% [27]. These results are largely consistent with our systematic review. Our study differs in that we included only prospective studies and focused on comparing operative findings and resection rates following DLUS to SI. In addition, we have updated the literature search with all eligible studies published after the meta-analysis.

4.1. Modernized Standard Imagine. It is possible that the studies included in this systematic review are not representative of modern staging techniques, as they did not all employ MDCT. It is important to acknowledge that modern techniques for CT imaging offer higher-resolution images with more detail of vascular involvement and metastatic disease. Advances in CT imaging, namely, multiphase imaging technique including noncontrast, arterial, pancreatic parenchymal, and portal venous phases with cuts less than 3 mm through the abdomen, have improved its ability to predict resectability of pancreatic tumors [28, 29]. A prospective study comparing MDCT Angiography with MDCT 3D Reconstruction reported resection rates of 94% and 100%, respectively. However, MDCT Angiography also overestimated unresectability in 32% of patients, which may be in part due to overestimating vascular invasions [30]. The authors

suggest that older grading schemes like those presented by Lu et al. [31] and Loyer et al. [32], which assess circumferential contiguity, tissue planes, mass effects, and occlusions, may be improved by visualizing tumor infiltration and vascular smoothness. An assessment readily made by LUS.

A study investigating MDCT for pancreatic head tumors found that only 40% of their "CT resectable" group was resected and that this was due to MDCT underestimating vascular involvement and local invasion. A subgroup analysis of patients that were unequivocally resectable improved the resection rate to 56% [33].

The use of MRI has increased dramatically in recent years and is considered by some to be standard of care along with MDCT cross-sectional imaging [34]. Using MRI with a pancreas protocol, at a high volume center, leads to a resection rate of 73%. The most common causes of intraoperative unresectability were vascular involvement and distant metastases, two findings aptly diagnosed by DLUS [29].

4.2. Timing and Cost Analysis. We believe that the optimal approach to include DLUS in the staging protocol is immediately prior to planned resection, which would minimize risks related to a second surgical procedure and general anesthesia. It may prove to be cost-effective as the patient would ultimately spend fewer days in hospital and most importantly decrease theoretical risk of progression in between procedures and delay in chemoradiation [35, 36]. In a recent cost-efficacy analysis of diagnostic laparoscopy prior to laparotomy for pancreatic cancer, the authors found that the total cost for introducing diagnostic laparoscopy was 1,480$ less per patient and provided better quality of life [37].

5. Limitations

This study has several limitations. The studies were heterogeneous, in their resectability criteria, use of multimodal imaging protocols, and the quality of their CT technology. In recent years there has been a paucity of literature on the subject and thus direct comparison of DLUS with more modern SI techniques is not possible. An important issue with DLUS is that the excellent results reported here may not be easily transferable to other centers where experience with this technique may be limited. The true benefit of DLUS may be difficult to achieve in all cases given the required expertise to perform and interpret this test correctly. In one study spanning three years, the average time to perform DLUS with lesser sac dissection in 67 patients was 30 minutes. The time to perform improved to 21 from 39 minutes in the last six months of the study [19].

6. Conclusion

Based on the highest quality studies available at this time, DLUS seems to still have a role in the preoperative staging of pancreatic cancer alongside SI techniques. With its ability to detect occult liver metastases, vascular involvement, and peritoneal metastases, the use of DLUS may lead to less noncurative laparotomies. Further research is warranted to compare DLUS to Pancreas Protocol MDCT and MRI.

Abbreviations

CT: Computed tomography
DL: Diagnostic laparoscopy
DLUS: Diagnostic laparoscopy with ultrasound
LUS: Laparoscopic ultrasound
MDCT: Multidimensional computed tomography
SI: Standard imaging.

Disclosure

This study was presented at SAGES 2015 and CSF 2015.

Competing Interests

The authors declare that they have no competing interests.

References

[1] A. Jemal, R. Siegel, J. Xu, and E. Ward, "Cancer statistics, 2010," *CA: Cancer Journal for Clinicians*, vol. 60, no. 5, pp. 277–300, 2010.

[2] J. P. Neoptolemos, D. D. Stocken, H. Friess et al., "A randomized trial of chemoradiotherapy and chemotherapy after resection of pancreatic cancer," *The New England Journal of Medicine*, vol. 350, no. 12, pp. 1200–1210, 2004.

[3] M. Sugiyama, H. Hagi, and Y. Atomi, "Reappraisal of intra-operative ultrasonography for pancreatobiliary carcinomas: assessment of malignant portal venous invasion," *Surgery*, vol. 125, no. 2, pp. 160–165, 1999.

[4] T. G. John, J. D. Greig, D. C. Carter, and O. J. Garden, "Carcinoma of the pancreatic head and periampullary region: tumor staging with laparoscopy and laparoscopic ultrasonography," *Annals of Surgery*, vol. 221, no. 2, pp. 156–164, 1995.

[5] A. Cuschieri, "Laparoscopy for pancreatic cancer: does it benefit the patient," *European Journal of Surgical Oncology*, vol. 14, no. 1, pp. 41–44, 1988.

[6] W. A. Bemelman, L. T. de Wit, O. M. van Delden et al., "Diagnostic laparoscopy combined with laparoscopic ultrasonography in staging of cancer of the pancreatic head region," *British Journal of Surgery*, vol. 82, no. 6, pp. 820–824, 1995.

[7] W. Richardson, D. Stefanidis, S. Mittal, and R. D. Fanelli, "SAGES guidelines for the use of laparoscopic ultrasound," *Surgical Endoscopy*, vol. 24, no. 4, pp. 745–756, 2010.

[8] A. Foroutani, A. M. Garland, E. Berber et al., "Laparoscopic ultrasound vs triphasic computed tomography for detecting liver tumors," *Archives of Surgery*, vol. 135, no. 8, pp. 933–938, 2000.

[9] S. C. Mayo, D. F. Austin, B. C. Sheppard, M. Mori, D. K. Shipley, and K. G. Billingsley, "Evolving preoperative evaluation of patients with pancreatic cancer: does laparoscopy have a role in the current era?" *Journal of the American College of Surgeons*, vol. 208, no. 1, pp. 87–95, 2009.

[10] M. Barabino, R. Santambrogio, A. Pisani Ceretti, R. Scalzone, M. Montorsi, and E. Opocher, "Is there still a role for laparoscopy combined with laparoscopic ultrasonography in the staging of pancreatic cancer?" *Surgical Endoscopy*, vol. 25, no. 1, pp. 160–165, 2011.

[11] D. Piccolboni, F. Ciccone, A. Settembre, and F. Corcione, "Laparoscopic intra-operative ultrasound in liver and pancreas resection: analysis of 93 cases," *Journal of Ultrasound*, vol. 13, no. 1, pp. 3–8, 2010.

[12] H. Doucas, C. D. Sutton, A. Zimmerman, A. R. Dennison, and D. P. Berry, "Assessment of pancreatic malignancy with laparoscopy and intraoperative ultrasound," *Surgical Endoscopy and Other Interventional Techniques*, vol. 21, no. 7, pp. 1147–1152, 2007.

[13] C. W. Fristrup, M. B. Mortensen, T. Pless et al., "Combined endoscopic and laparoscopic ultrasound as preoperative assessment of patients with pancreatic cancer," *HPB*, vol. 8, no. 1, pp. 57–60, 2006.

[14] H. E. Doran, L. Bosonnet, S. Connor et al., "Laparoscopy and laparoscopic ultrasound in the evaluation of pancreatic and periampullary tumours," *Digestive Surgery*, vol. 21, no. 4, pp. 305–313, 2004.

[15] Z.-W. Zhao, J.-Y. He, G. Tan, H.-J. Wang, and K.-J. Li, "Laparoscopy and laparoscopic ultrasonography in judging the resectability of pancreatic head cancer," *Hepatobiliary and Pancreatic Diseases International*, vol. 2, no. 4, pp. 609–611, 2003.

[16] A. H. Kwon, H. Inui, and Y. Kamiyama, "Preoperative laparoscopic examination using surgical manipulation and ultrasonography for pancreatic lesions," *Endoscopy*, vol. 34, no. 6, pp. 464–468, 2002.

[17] M. I. Lavonius, S. Laine, S. Salo, P. Sonninen, and J. Ovaska, "Role of laparoscopy and laparoscopic ultrasound in staging of pancreatic tumours," *Annales Chirurgiae et Gynaecologiae*, vol. 90, no. 4, pp. 252–255, 2001.

[18] A. M. Taylor, S. A. Roberts, and J. McK Manson, "Experience with laparoscopic ultrasonography for defining tumour resectability in carcinoma of the pancreatic head and periampullary region," *British Journal of Surgery*, vol. 88, no. 8, pp. 1077–1083, 2001.

[19] P. P. Schachter, Y. Avni, M. Shimonov, G. Gvirtz, A. Rosen, and A. Czerniak, "The impact of laparoscopy and laparoscopic ultrasonography on the management of pancreatic cancer," *Archives of Surgery*, vol. 135, no. 11, pp. 1303–1307, 2000.

[20] J. M. Velasco, H. Rossi, T. J. Hieken, and M. Fernandez, "Laparoscopic ultrasound enhances diagnostic laparoscopy in the staging of intra-abdominal neoplasms," *American Surgeon*, vol. 66, no. 4, pp. 407–411, 2000.

[21] J. A. Norton, "Intraoperative methods to stage and localize pancreatic and duodenal tumors," *Annals of Oncology*, vol. 10, supplement 4, pp. S182–S184, 1999.

[22] E. A. Minnard, K. C. Conlon, A. Hoos, E. C. Dougherty, L. E. Hann, and M. F. Brennan, "Laparoscopic ultrasound enhances standard laparoscopy in the staging of pancreatic cancer," *Annals of Surgery*, vol. 228, no. 2, pp. 182–187, 1998.

[23] G. Champault, "The use of laparoscopic ultrasound in the assessment of pancreatic cancer," *Wiadomości Lekarskie*, vol. 50, supplement 1, part 1, pp. 195–203, 1997.

[24] A. Pietrabissa, G. Di Candio, P. C. Giulianotti, A. Carobbi, U. Boggi, and F. Mosca, "Operative technique for the laparoscopic staging of pancreatic malignancy," *Minimally Invasive Therapy and Allied Technologies*, vol. 5, no. 3, pp. 274–280, 1996.

[25] M. Murugiah, S. Paterson-Brown, J. A. Windsor, W. F. Anthony Miles, and O. J. Garden, "Early experience of laparoscopic ultrasonography in the management of pancreatic carcinoma," *Surgical Endoscopy*, vol. 7, no. 3, pp. 177–181, 1993.

[26] NCCN, *Pancreatic Adenocarcinoma*, Version 1, 2016, http://www.nccn.org/professionals/physician_gls/pdf/pancreatic.pdf.

[27] D. Hariharan, V. A. Constantinides, F. E. M. Froeling, P. P. Tekkis, and H. M. Kocher, "The role of laparoscopy and laparoscopic ultrasound in the preoperative staging of pancreaticobiliary cancers—a meta-analysis," *European Journal of Surgical Oncology*, vol. 36, no. 10, pp. 941–948, 2010.

[28] N. J. McNulty, I. R. Francis, J. F. Platt, R. H. Cohan, M. Korobkin, and A. Gebremariam, "Multi-detector row helical CT of the pancreas: effect of contrast-enhanced multiphasic imaging on enhancement of the pancreas, peripancreatic vasculature, and pancreatic adenocarcinoma," *Radiology*, vol. 220, no. 1, pp. 97–102, 2001.

[29] D. M. Walters, D. J. Lapar, E. E. De Lange et al., "Pancreas-protocol imaging at a high-volume center leads to improved preoperative staging of pancreatic ductal adenocarcinoma," *Annals of Surgical Oncology*, vol. 18, no. 10, pp. 2764–2771, 2011.

[30] C.-H. Fang, W. Zhu, H. Wang et al., "A new approach for evaluating the resectability of pancreatic and periampullary neoplasms," *Pancreatology*, vol. 12, no. 4, pp. 364–371, 2012.

[31] D. S. K. Lu, H. A. Reber, R. M. Krasny, B. M. Kadell, and J. Sayre, "Local staging of pancreatic cancer: criteria for unresectability of major vessels as revealed by pancreatic-phase, thin-section helical CT," *American Journal of Roentgenology*, vol. 168, no. 6, pp. 1439–1443, 1997.

[32] E. M. Loyer, C. L. David, R. A. Dubrow, D. B. Evans, and C. Charnsangavej, "Vascular involvement in pancreatic adenocarcinoma: reassessment by thin-section CT," *Abdominal Imaging*, vol. 21, no. 3, pp. 202–206, 1996.

[33] S. L. Smith, A. Basu, D. M. Rae, and M. Sinclair, "Preoperative staging accuracy of multidetector computed tomography in pancreatic head adenocarcinoma," *Pancreas*, vol. 34, no. 2, pp. 180–184, 2007.

[34] S. V. Shrikhande, S. G. Barreto, M. Goel, and S. Arya, "Multimodality imaging of pancreatic ductal adenocarcinoma: a review of the literature," *HPB*, vol. 14, no. 10, pp. 658–668, 2012.

[35] A. A. Gumbs, A. M. Rodriguez Rivera, L. Milone, and J. P. Hoffman, "Laparoscopic pancreatoduodenectomy: a review of 285 published cases," *Annals of Surgical Oncology*, vol. 18, no. 5, pp. 1335–1341, 2011.

[36] R. Venkat, B. H. Edil, R. D. Schulick, A. O. Lidor, M. A. Makary, and C. L. Wolfgang, "Laparoscopic distal pancreatectomy is associated with significantly less overall morbidity compared to the open technique: a systematic review and meta-analysis," *Annals of Surgery*, vol. 255, no. 6, pp. 1048–1059, 2012.

[37] T. T. Jayakrishnan, H. Nadeem, R. T. Groeschl et al., "Diagnostic laparoscopy should be performed before definitive resection for pancreatic cancer: a financial argument," *HPB*, vol. 17, no. 2, pp. 131–139, 2015.

26

Surgical Strategy for Isolated Caudate Lobectomy: Experience with 16 Cases

Gendong Tian,[1] Qiong Chen,[2] Yuan Guo,[1] Mujian Teng,[1] and Jie Li[1]

[1] *Hepatobiliary and Liver Transplantation Department, The Affiliated Qianfoshan Hospital, Shandong University,*
No. 16766 Jingshi Road, Jinan, Shandong 250014, China
[2] *General Surgery Department, The First People's Hospital of Jinan City, No. 132 Minghu Road, Jinan, Shandong 250014, China*

Correspondence should be addressed to Gendong Tian; tiangendong@163.com

Academic Editor: Harald Schrem

Introduction. Surgical resection is the most effective treatment for neoplasm in the caudate lobe. Isolated caudate lobectomy is still a challenge for hepatobiliary surgeons. No widely accepted surgical strategy for the procedure has been developed yet. *Objective.* To get a better understanding of isolated caudate lobectomy and to optimize the procedure. *Materials and Methods.* 16 cases of isolated caudate lobectomy were reviewed to summarize the surgical experience. *Results.* All the 16 cases of isolated caudate lobectomy were carried out successfully, among which left side approach was adopted in two cases (12.5%), right side approach in three cases (18.75%), and both sides approach in 11 cases (68.75%). No severe complications occurred. *Conclusion.* The majority of neoplasms confined to the caudate lobe can be resected safely by left and right side approach with proper anatomic surgical procedure, usually in the sequence of mobilization, outflow control, inflow control, and division of the hepatic parenchyma. Fully mobilizing the caudate lobe from the inferior vena cava (IVC) is of great importance. Division of the retrohepatic ligament and the venous ligament facilitated the procedure.

1. Introduction

The caudate lobe lies deep in the liver, between the hepatic hila and the retrohepatic inferior vena cava (IVC), and is adjacent to the major hepatic veins in its upper part. Although the caudate lobe constitutes only a small part of the whole liver, it has the same histologic structure and the same incidence of developing benign and malignant neoplasms as other hepatic segments in proportion to their volume. Percutaneous ethanol injection and radiofrequency ablation (RFA) for tumors in the caudate lobe are difficult to be carried out because of their spatial peculiarity [1]. Multiple bilateral blood supplies from hepatic artery and portal vein make transcatheter arterial chemoembolization (TACE) less effective for malignant tumors in the lobe than those in the main lobes. Surgical resection is left the only radical solution for symptomatic benign tumors and malignant tumors confined to the lobe. Isolated caudate lobectomy, a parenchyma-sparing procedure, is still a challenge for hepatobiliary surgeons, especially in cirrhotic patients. Relatively safe and reliable

surgical techniques for the procedure have not been developed thoroughly. 16 cases of isolated caudate lobectomy in our departments from January 2010 to December 2013 were reviewed to optimize the operation.

According to Kumon's nomenclature [2], the caudate lobe consists of 3 portions: the Spiegel lobe (i.e., Couinaud's segment I), the paracaval portion (i.e., Couinaud's segment IX [3]), and the caudate process. The Spiegel lobe locates behind the lesser omentum, to the left of the retrohepatic IVC. The paracaval portion, which is attached to the anterior surface of the retrohepatic IVC by the retrohepatic ligament and the short hepatic veins, lies to the right of the Spiegel lobe. The upper tip of the caudate lobe extends behind the major hepatic veins. The caudate process, the smallest part of the three, is a thin tongue-like projection between the IVC and the portal vein. Kumon's definition is adopted here for better understanding. Isolated caudate lobectomy is to remove either part or total of the lobe surgically (i.e., isolated partial or complete caudate lobectomy).

TABLE 1: Diagnosis, size, location, and surgical approach of 16 cases of isolated caudate lobectomy.

Case number	Diagnosis	Size (cm)#	Location*	Approach
1	Hepatocellular carcinoma	3	Type 4	R
2	Hepatocellular carcinoma	3.5	Type 3	L and R
3	Hepatocellular carcinoma	6	Type 2	L and R
4	Hepatocellular carcinoma	4	Type 2	L and R
5	Hepatocellular carcinoma	2	Type 1	L
6	Hepatocellular carcinoma	5	Type 5	L and R
7	Hepatocellular carcinoma	4.5	Type 4	L and R
8	Hepatic cavernous hemangioma	5	Type 3	L and R
9	Hepatic cavernous hemangioma	8.5	Type 5	L and R
10	Hepatic cavernous hemangioma	7	Type 5	L and R
11	Hepatic cavernous hemangioma	5.5	Type 4	L and R
12	Hepatocellular adenoma	3	Type 2	L
13	Inflammatory pseudotumor	2	Type 4	R
14	Hepatic hamartoma	12	Type 4	L and R
15	Mixed hepatocellular carcinoma and cholangiocellular carcinoma	4.5	Type 3	L and R
16	Metastatic colonic cancer	3	Type 4	R

L: left side approach; R: right side approach; L and R: left and right side approach.
#Indicated in the maximum diameter.
*According to Hasegawa et al.'s classification [4].

Hasegawa et al. classified hepatocellular carcinomas spread from the caudate lobe into five types [4], which were frequently adopted to describe all neoplasms that originated in the caudate lobe. They were as follows:

(1) type 1 lesions: lesions in the upper part of the Spiegel lobe;

(2) type 2 lesions: lesions in the lower part of the Spiegel lobe;

(3) type 3 lesions: lesions in the paracaval portion;

(4) type 4 lesions: lesions in the caudate process;

(5) type 5 lesions: lesions spread from the whole caudate lobe.

2. Patients and Methods

2.1. Patients. 16 cases of isolated caudate lobectomy were performed for neoplasms confined to the caudate lobe, including seven cases of hepatocellular carcinoma (7/16, 43.75%), four cases of hepatic cavernous hemangioma (4/16, 25%), one case of hepatocellular adenoma (1/16, 6.25%), one case of inflammatory pseudotumor (1/16, 6.25%), one case of hepatic hamartoma (1/16, 6.25%), one case of mixed hepatocellular carcinoma and cholangiocellular carcinoma (1/16, 6.25%), and one case of metastatic colonic cancer (1/16, 6.25%). Hepatitis B virus surface antigen was positive in all the seven cases of hepatocellular carcinoma and in the case of mixed hepatocellular carcinoma and cholangiocellular carcinoma, respectively, and hepatitis B virus surface antibody was positive in the case of hepatocellular adenoma. The tumors were measured in the maximum diameter from 2 cm to

12 cm (4.91 cm in average). According to Hasegawa et al.'s classification [4], there were one case of type 1 lesions, three cases of type 2 lesions, three cases of type 3 lesions, six cases of type 4 lesions, and three cases of type 5 lesions (Table 1).

2.2. Surgical Procedure for Isolated Caudate Lobectomy. Isolated resection of the caudate lobe consisted of four major steps: mobilization of the lobe, outflow control by dividing the short hepatic veins behind the lobe, inflow control by dividing the portal triads to the lobe, and division of the hepatic parenchyma between the caudate lobe and the main liver. Left side approach, or right side approach, or both left and right sides approach were adopted in the operation. The sequence of the four steps and the surgical approach alternated according to the tumor's location, size, texture, and nature.

2.2.1. Approaches to the Caudate Lobe

Left Side Approach. Left side approach was adopted for resection of small masses that originated in the Spiegel lobe, especially type 2 lesions. After entering the abdominal cavity through a reversed L-shaped incision on the right upper quadrant of the belly, the round, falciform, left triangular, left coronary and hepatogastric ligaments were separated. The hepatoduodenal ligament was retracted to the right to expose the Spiegel lobe. The retroperitoneum covering the left wall of the retrohepatic IVC was incised to free the left margin of the Spiegel lobe. The retrohepatic ligament was divided when necessary (Figure 1). The venous ligament was divided to free the upper tip of the caudate lobe [5]. Then, the Spiegel

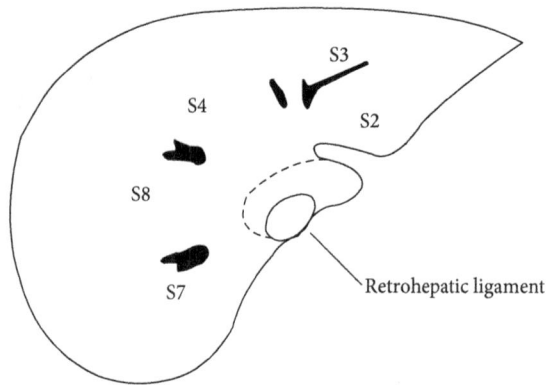

FIGURE 1: Schematic cross-sectional diagram of the caudate lobe, showing the retrohepatic ligament and the relationship between the caudate lobe and the main liver.

lobe was easily elevated from the retrohepatic IVC to expose the short hepatic veins to direct view as they were divided and ligated caudal cranially. The left portal hilum was lifted ventrally to expose the portal triads to the Spiegel lobe, which were divided and ligated subsequently. The liver parenchymal bridge was transected by CUSA.

Right Side Approach. Right side approach was adopted for resection of small masses that originated in the caudate process. After entering the abdominal cavity through a reversed L-shaped incision, the round, falciform, right triangular, right coronary and hepatorenal ligaments were divided in turn. The right adrenal gland was detached from the liver with care. The retroperitoneum covering the infrahepatic IVC was incised. The liver was elevated from the retrohepatic IVC and rotated to the left to show the short hepatic veins, which were divided and ligated in a cranial direction. The possible inferior right hepatic vein (IRHV), which often enters the IVC near the right adrenal gland vein, was divided also. The retrohepatic ligament was divided when necessary from the left lateral surface of the IVC through an incision on the lesser omentum. The hepatoduodenal ligament was retracted to the left to expose the caudate process. If the portal triads to the caudate process could be dissected easily, they would be divided in advance; in reverse, they were controlled during dividing the liver parenchyma by CUSA.

Left and Right Side Approach. Left and right side approach was adopted for resection of the majority of caudate masses. A reversed L-shaped incision on the right upper quadrant was adequate in most both sides approach cases. The transverse arm of the incision might be extended to the left subcostal region if necessary. The falciform ligament was dissected to the ventral surface of the suprahepatic IVC to show the loose space between the right hepatic vein and the confluence of the left and middle hepatic veins. The liver was fully mobilized by separation of all the peritoneal attachments. The right adrenal gland was detached from the liver. The retroperitoneum covering the infrahepatic IVC and the left wall of the retrohepatic IVC (referred to as Makuuchi's fascia in Japanese literature [6]) was incised caudal cranially to the superior recess of

the lesser sac to expose the entire retrohepatic IVC. At this time, the suprahepatic and infrahepatic IVC were taped if needed. The venous ligament was divided near the root of the left hepatic vein. The confluence of the left and middle hepatic veins, which enters the anterior left lateral wall of the suprahepatic IVC, was encircled by passing a vascular tape through the latent space surrounded by the dorsal surface of the two hepatic veins, the ventral surface of the IVC, and the tip of the caudate lobe. The retrohepatic ligament was divided. The liver was lifted and all the short hepatic veins (including the IRHV) were taken down and suture-ligated. The hepatoduodenal ligament was loosened, and the duodenum and the pancreatic head were partly mobilized by Kocher maneuver for better exposure of large caudate masses. The portal triads to the caudate lobe were dissected and ligated. After the liver parenchyma between the caudate lobe and the main liver was transected, the tumors were removed en bloc.

2.2.2. Dividing the Retrohepatic Ligament. The retrohepatic ligament attaches the Spiegel lobe to segment VI behind the retrohepatic IVC. Division of the ligament enabled the elevation of the caudate lobe from the caval vein. Usually the retrohepatic ligament is divided from the left side of the IVC. But when an enlarged Spiegel lobe embraced the IVC dorsally, it should be divided from the right side more conveniently [7].

2.2.3. Dividing the Venous Ligament. The venous ligament (i.e., the Arantius' ligament) lies in the sulcus of the ligamentum venosum and connects the left portal vein to the root of the left hepatic vein. The venous ligament was divided near the left hepatic vein to partly release the tip of the caudate lobe and to facilitate the isolation of the confluence of the left and middle hepatic veins [5].

2.2.4. Pringle Maneuver. The hepatic pedicle was encircled with a vascular tape for possible temporary inflow control of the liver.

2.2.5. Controlling the IVC. After complete mobilization of the liver and incision of the retroperitoneum that covers the infrahepatic IVC and the left wall of the retrohepatic IVC, the suprahepatic and infrahepatic IVC were isolated and encircled with vascular tapes easily in case of possible temporary total hepatic blood occlusion.

2.2.6. Dividing the Short Hepatic Veins, the Portal Triads to the Caudate Lobe, and the Liver Parenchyma. The short hepatic veins were dissected, divided, and ligated caudal cranially. These veins were best approached from the right side when there was a huge tumor [7]. Suture with transfixing stitch was obligatory for a large short hepatic vein. The whole liver was detached from the IVC besides the three main hepatic veins. The portal hila were lifted to expose the portal triads to the caudate lobe, which originate mainly from the left hilum and secondarily from the bifurcation (Figure 2) [8]. Then, the portal triads were divided and ligated serially. The parenchymal bridge between the caudate lobe and segments

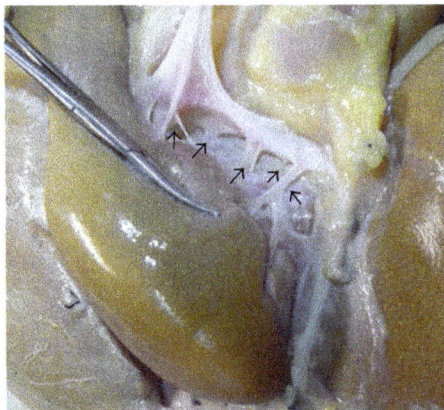

FIGURE 2: The portal branches to the caudate lobe (arrows), indicating that the portal branches to the caudate lobe originate mainly from the left hilum. Picture from unrelated specimen.

IV, VIII, and VII was transected by CUSA. Some small inflow vasculatures and draining vessels to the main hepatic veins, which were difficult to be dissected and ligated beforehand, were divided during transecting the liver parenchyma.

3. Results

All 16 cases of isolated caudate lobectomy were accomplished successfully without death and severe complications. Left side approach was adopted in two cases (2/16, 12.5%) and right side approach in three cases (3/16, 18.75%), while both sides approach in 11 cases (11/16, 68.75%). Estimated intraoperative blood loss ranged from 100 mL to 850 mL (356.25 mL in average) and transfusion varied from 0 to 800 mL (137.5 mL in average). Pringle maneuver was adopted in six cases for temporary inflow control of the liver (occlusion time ranged from 6 min to 13 min). The confluence of the left and middle hepatic veins (and the right hepatic vein in two cases) was taped in five cases for regional outflow control. The suprahepatic and infrahepatic IVC were encircled with vascular tapes in two cases, but neither needed total hepatic blood occlusion of the hepatic hila and the IVC at the same time. Small leakage in the retrohepatic IVC or the major hepatic veins was encountered in five cases, which was repaired with Prolene suture. Total operative time ranged from 150 min to 270 min (211.25 min in average). Ascites and/or right pleural effusion developed after operation in four cases. No bile leakage was encountered, which was reported as the major complication after isolated caudate lobectomy [6]. The seven cases of hepatocellular carcinoma and the case of mixed hepatocellular carcinoma and cholangiocellular carcinoma were followed up from 6 to 28 months, with one death case due to liver failure and upper gastrointestinal hemorrhage in the 26th month after operation and two cases of recurred hepatocellular carcinoma in the main liver, who thereafter received TACE, percutaneous RFA, and systemic chemotherapy. Patients with benign caudate diseases all survived in good condition.

4. Discussion

Isolated caudate lobectomy demands elaborate anatomy of the liver and exquisite skill of operation. The regular hepatectomy techniques are seldom employed in the operation [8]. The surgical strategy chosen for each patient must be based on the patient's idiographic situation. In the 16 cases of isolated caudate lobectomy, left side approach was adopted in two cases, right side approach in three cases, and combined left and right sides approach in 11 cases. Left side approach is adopted for small lesions in the lower part of the Spiegel lobe and right side approach for small lesions in the caudate process. Combined left and right sides approach is recommended for the majority of neoplasms in the caudate lobe [5, 9], especially for those that are bigger than 4 cm in diameter, those originating in the paracaval portion or in the whole caudate lobe, or those that are thought to be malignant tumors, which require total caudate lobectomy for clearance of the tumors. Symptomatic and continuously enlarging hepatic cavernous hemangioma also requires total caudate lobectomy before it reaches a nonresectable size. In fact, complete caudate lobectomy is technically easier and controllable than partial resection of the lobe [8]. Loosening the hepatoduodenal ligament and performing the Kocher maneuver help to expose the caudate lobe better and provide more space for the operation. When a bulky caudate tumor protrudes into the space between the right and middle hepatic veins or compresses the major hepatic veins severely, the anterior transhepatic approach should be employed in addition [10, 11] or combined lobectomy should be adopted.

Thorough medical imaging study of CT or/and MRI scan and type-B ultrasonography before operation is mandatory to illuminate the anatomic relationship between the masses and the hepatic hila, the major hepatic veins, and the retrohepatic IVC and to rule out metastases of malignant tumors. MRI scan provides more helpful information concerning the main vessels and the bile ducts. Although thrombosis in the portal vein is not thought to be a contraindication for isolated caudate lobectomy [12], ruling out thrombus in the portal vein and the IVC is important for the choice of strategy of treatment. Usually it is easy to dissect and divide the short hepatic veins along a tumor-free plane on the ventral surface of the retrohepatic IVC unless the tumor has involved the caval wall substantially [8]. Unlike the high incidence of thrombosis in the portal vein or the retrohepatic IVC in advanced hepatocellular carcinoma in the main liver or hilar cholangiocarcinoma which have involved the caudate lobe, the incidence of thrombosis is much lower than that expected for caudate tumors.

Dissection and division of the short hepatic veins are the major difficulty in isolated caudate lobectomy [9]. Complete mobilization of the liver is essential. Exposure of the entire course of the retrohepatic IVC by incising the covered retroperitoneum is of utmost importance. The superior recess of the lesser sac extends rightwards behind the Spiegel lobe and the retrohepatic IVC. The suprahepatic IVC is readily taped after the incision of this part of retroperitoneum. The short hepatic veins are first divided before the portal triads to separate the caudate lobe from the IVC, in case of removing the lobe quickly after temporary hemostasis of a possible huge bleeding from a parenchymal laceration or a tear in the major hepatic veins by Pringle maneuver. The length of the short hepatic veins is in proportion to their diameter reversely. Small short hepatic veins are easily isolated and divided. Large short hepatic veins should be tied and sutured on the hepatic side. On the caval side, the large dissected end should be repaired with Prolene suture after applying a side-wall vascular clamp. The largest short hepatic vein drains the bulkiest part of the caudate lobe, which locates predominantly in the middle of the Spiegel lobe and secondarily around the central part of the paracaval portion. The IRHV usually has a relatively large diameter also. A medium-sized short hepatic vein that drains the tip of the caudate lobe to the left hepatic vein or the nearby IVC is sometimes found, which should be ligated with care so as not to be torn. Small crevasse in the IVC is repaired with ease after hemostasis by finger press. A broken hepatic vein is repaired more conveniently after the caudate lobe is moved out as it is facilitated by Pringle maneuver. If combined with occlusion of the confluence of the left and middle hepatic veins (and sometimes the right hepatic vein), a more clear operative field is presented with less possibility of air embolism. In contrast, inflow control by dividing the portal triads to the caudate lobe is somewhat easy.

The caudate lobe attaches to the IVC circumferently by retrohepatic ligament and adheres to the caudal side of left liver by the venous ligament. When the caudate lobe is small or when the tumor locates mainly in the caudate process, the retrohepatic ligament is divided from the left side easily. But when the caudate lobe is enlarged, especially when it embraces the retrohepatic IVC dorsally with a bulky Spiegel lobe, the retrohepatic ligament should be divided from the right side [7]. Division of the retrohepatic ligament makes it much easier to elevate the caudate lobe from the ventral surface of the retrohepatic IVC, facilitates the exposure and division of the short hepatic veins, and contributes to the isolation of the main hepatic veins likewise [13]. The IRHV should be divided beforehand, which will facilitate the management of the other short hepatic veins from the right side. The division of the venous ligament loosens the cranial polar of the caudate lobe, facilitates mobilizing the caudate lobe from the left side, provides more space for encircling the left and middle hepatic veins, and minimizes the possibility of injuring the veins [5].

Hepatocellular carcinoma usually occurs after hepatitis B in China, no matter where the first tumor appears. After the original hepatic cancer in the caudate lobe is resected, the tumor may easily recur in the main liver lobes. Close follow-up of these patients at an interval of one to two months is necessary. Chemotherapy, transarterial embolization or chemoembolization, percutaneous RFA, and alcohol injection are adopted to reduce the possibility of recurrence or to treat a recurred tumor. Many authors have reported comparable (or even better) survival rate after isolated resection of caudate hepatocellular carcinoma with those in the main liver [1, 14, 15], which suggests that isolated caudate lobectomy for hepatocellular carcinoma in the caudate lobe is practical.

In summary, left and right side approach is adopted for isolated resection of most neoplasms in the caudate lobe. Mobilizing the whole caudate lobe is more important than enucleating the tumor itself in the operation. Considering the patients' safety as well as eradication of the diseases, the best surgical strategy is the one that is uncomplicated and easy to be mastered by most hepatobiliary surgeons, with fewer traumas and complications. And under the principle of mobilizing the caudate lobe firstly, controlling the outflow and then inflow vessels secondly, and dividing the liver parenchyma thirdly, it is advised that the relatively easier and safer step should be carried out first. Likewise, two steps can be carried out alternately. For example, some short hepatic veins can be divided while dividing the retrohepatic ligament; and some portal triads to the caudate lobe can be divided while dividing the liver parenchyma. Patients with malignant tumors should be followed up regularly after operation for recurrence and for adjuvant therapy.

References

[1] T. Yamamoto, S. Kubo, T. Shuto et al., "Surgical strategy for hepatocellular carcinoma originating in the caudate lobe," *Surgery*, vol. 135, no. 6, pp. 595–603, 2004.

[2] M. Kumon, "Anatomy of the caudate lobe with special reference to portal vein and bile duct," *Acta Hepatologica Japonica*, vol. 26, no. 9, pp. 1193–1199, 1985.

[3] C. Couinaud, "The paracaval segments of the liver," *Journal of Hepato-Biliary-Pancreatic Surgery*, vol. 1, no. 2, pp. 145–151, 1994.

[4] H. Hasegawa, T.-D. Cervens, S. Yamasaki, T. Kosuge, T. Takayama, and K. Shimada, "Surgical strategy for hepatocellular carcinoma of the caudate lobe," *Journal de Chirurgie*, vol. 128, no. 12, pp. 533–540, 1991.

[5] L.-N. Xu and Z.-Q. Huang, "Resection of hepatic caudate lobe hemangioma: experience with 11 patients," *Hepatobiliary and Pancreatic Diseases International*, vol. 9, no. 5, pp. 487–491, 2010.

[6] T. van Gulik and H. Lang, "Isolated resection of segment 1 of the liver," *Digestive Surgery*, vol. 22, no. 3, pp. 143–146, 2005.

[7] J. Lerut, J. A. Gruwez, and L. H. Blumgart, "Resection of the caudate lobe of the liver," *Surgery Gynecology and Obstetrics*, vol. 171, no. 2, pp. 160–162, 1990.

[8] E. Chaib, M. A. F. Ribeiro Jr., F. de S Collet e Silva, W. A. Saad, and I. Cecconello, "Surgical approach for hepatic caudate lobectomy: review of 401 cases," *Journal of the American College of Surgeons*, vol. 204, no. 1, pp. 118–127, 2007.

[9] E. Chaib, M. A. F. Ribeiro Jr., F. D. S. C. Silva, W. A. Saad, and I. Cecconello, "Caudate lobectomy: tumor location, topographic classification, and technique using right- and left-sided approaches to the liver," *American Journal of Surgery*, vol. 196, no. 2, pp. 245–251, 2008.

[10] J. Hu, X. Miao, D. Zhong, W. Dai, and W. Liu, "Anterior approach for complete isolated caudate lobectomy," *Hepato-Gastroenterology*, vol. 52, no. 66, pp. 1641–1644, 2005.

[11] E. Chaib, M. A. F. Ribeiro Jr., Y. E. D. M. de Souza, and L. A. C. D'Albuquerque, "Anterior hepatic transection for caudate lobectomy," *Clinics*, vol. 64, no. 11, pp. 1121–1125, 2009.

[12] P. Liu, J. Yang, W. Niu, F. Xie, Y. Wang, and Y. Zhou, "Surgical treatment of huge hepatocellular carcinoma in the caudate lobe," *Surgery Today*, vol. 41, no. 4, pp. 520–525, 2011.

[13] M. Makuuchi, J. Yamamoto, T. Takayama et al., "Extrahepatic division of the right hepatic vein in hepatectomy," *Hepato-Gastroenterology*, vol. 38, no. 2, pp. 176–179, 1991.

[14] M. Sakoda, S. Ueno, F. Kubo et al., "Surgery for hepatocellular carcinoma located in the caudate lobe," *World Journal of Surgery*, vol. 33, no. 9, pp. 1922–1926, 2009.

[15] T. Ikegami, T. Ezaki, T. Ishida, S. Aimitsu, M. Fujihara, and M. Mori, "Limited hepatic resection for hepatocellular carcinoma in the caudate lobe," *World Journal of Surgery*, vol. 28, no. 7, pp. 697–701, 2004.

27

Pancreatic Resections in Renal Failure Patients: Is It Worth the Risk?

K. S. Norman,[1] S. R. Domingo,[1,2] and L. L. Wong[1,3]

[1] *Department of Surgery, University of Hawaii John A. Burns School of Medicine, Honolulu, HI 96813, USA*
[2] *Queens Medical Center, Honolulu, HI 96813, USA*
[3] *University of Hawaii Cancer Center, Honolulu, HI 96813, USA*

Correspondence should be addressed to L. L. Wong; hepatoma@aol.com

Academic Editor: Christos G. Dervenis

Background. Chronic kidney disease affects 20 million US patients, with nearly 600,000 on dialysis. Long-term survival is limited and the risk of complex pancreatic surgery in this group is questionable. Previous studies are limited to case reports and small case series and a large database may help determine the true risk of pancreatic surgery in this population. *Methods.* The American College of Surgeons National Surgical Quality Improvement Program database was queried (2005–2011) for patients who underwent pancreatic resection. Renal failure was defined as the clinical condition associated with rapid, steadily increasing azotemia (rise in BUN) and increasing creatinine above 3 mg/dL. Operative trends and short-term outcomes were reviewed for those with and without renal failure (RF). *Results.* In 18,533 patients, 28 had RF. There was no difference in wound infections, neurologic or cardiovascular complications. Compared to non-RF patients, those with RF had more unplanned intubation (OR 4.89, 95% CI 1.85–12.89), bleeding requiring transfusion (OR 3.12, 95% CI 1.37–14.21), septic shock (OR 8.86, 95% CI 3.75–20.91), higher 30-day mortality (21.4% versus 2.3%, $P < 0.001$) and longer hospital stay (23 versus 12 days, $P < 0.001$). *Conclusions.* RF patients have much higher morbidity and mortality after pancreatic resections and surgeons should consider this before proceeding.

1. Introduction

Although the incidence of end stage renal disease (ESRD) has remained relatively stable in the United States, the prevalence has increased, such that 593,000 people are currently living on hemodialysis, on peritoneal dialysis, or with a functioning kidney transplant. Improvements in renal-replacement therapy, overall treatment, and access to care have increased patient survival in ESRD. In the prevalent population, mortality rates have declined by nearly 25 percent over the last two decades. Patients are living longer on renal replacement therapy and the population currently on dialysis is increasing in age. The overall incidence of dialysis patients is 340 per million persons but since 2000, the adjusted incidence rate of ESRD has increased by 12.2% for those patients 75 years or older (1773 per million persons) [1, 2].

Because of the rising number of aging dialysis patients, there will likely be an increased need for use of hospital resources and cancer care in this population. Multiple studies have consistently showed increased complications and mortality in renal patients undergoing general, vascular, and cardiac surgical procedures [3–8]. Patient selection and vigilant management are recommended in this population.

The question of whether patients with renal failure should undergo major cancer surgery has not been specifically addressed in the medical literature. The complexity of the surgery and overall prognosis of the type of cancer involved will need to be considered in choosing options for these patients. Few studies address outcomes of pancreatic surgery in patients with renal dysfunction and all were single center studies consisting of small series of patients [9–11]. The purpose of this study is to utilize a large, nationwide database

TABLE 1: Patient characteristics.

	Total (n = 18533)	Group RF (n = 28)	Group non-RF (n = 18505)	P value
Mean age (SD)	61.8 (13.9)	67.9 (13.5)	61.8 (13.9)	P = 0.02
Age 65 or older (%)	8659 (46.7%)	16 (57.1%)	8627 (46.6%)	NS (P = 0.34)
Males (%)	8922 (48.1%)	17 (60.7%)	8905 (48.1%)	NS (P = 0.41)
Diabetes	4197 (22.6%)	11 (39.3%)	4186 (22.6%)	P = 0.040
History of smoking	4065 (21.9%)	6 (21.4%)	4059 (21.9%)	NS (P = 0.95)
History of alcohol use	478 (2.6%)	0	478 (2.6%)	NS (P = 0.45)
History of COPD	815 (4.4%)	3 (10.7%)	812 (4.4%)	NS (P = 0.12)
Myocardial infarction within 6 mo.	56 (0.3%)	3 (10.7%)	53 (0.3%)	P < 0.0001
Hypertension requiring medications	9620 (51.9%)	24 (85.7%)	9596 (51.9%)	P < 0.0001
Congestive heart failure	51 (0.3%)	0	51 (0.3%)	NS (P = 0.86)
Transient ischemic attack	338 (1/8%)	1 (3.6%)	337 (1.8%)	NS (P = 0.55)
Cerebrovascular disease	255 (1.4%)	1 (3.6%)	254 (1.4%)	NS (P = 0.43)
Currently on steroids	383 (2.1%)	3 (10.7%)	380 (2.1%)	P = 0.02
Bleeding disorder	507 (2.7%)	6 (21.4%)	501 (2/7%)	P < 0.0001
Disseminated cancer	617 (3.3%)	6 (21.4%)	611 (3.3%)	P < 0.0001
Prior radiation therapy	376 (2.0%)	0	376 (2.0%)	NS (P = 0.48)
Prior chemotherapy	350 (1.9%)	2 (7.1%)	348 (1.9%)	NS (P = 0.09)
Transfusion before surgery	149 (0.8%)	3 (10.7%)	146 (0.8%)	P = 0.001

to determine outcomes of pancreatic resection in patients with renal failure to assist surgeons and oncologists in selecting the optimal patients for these procedures.

2. Materials and Methods

Data for this study was obtained from the American College of Surgeons National Surgical Quality Improvement Program (ACS NSQIP). ACS NSQIP is a prospective, multi-institutional, and clinical registry created by the Veterans Health Administration in 1994 for quality improvement purposes. Over 130 preoperative variables through 30-day postoperative variables are collected on randomly assigned patients, including patient demographics, surgical profile, preoperative risk assessment, laboratory values, operative information, and 30-day morbidity and mortality rates. A highly trained Surgical Clinical Reviewer (SCR) collects the data. All reviewers receive extensive initial training prior to starting data collection and ongoing training via continuing education. ACS NSQIP monitors accrual rates and data sampling methodologies and conducts audits on a random basis, ensuring highly reliable data [12].

ACS NSQIP participant files for the years 2005–2011 were reviewed and Current Procedure Terminology (CPT) codes were used to identify all patients who underwent pancreatic procedures (48100-48999). We excluded pancreatic biopsy and pancreatic debridement as these were presumably done for unresectable pancreatic malignancies or necrotizing pancreatitis. From the remaining pancreatic cases, two groups were created: patients who had pancreatic resection with renal failure (group RF) and those who underwent pancreatic resection with normal renal function (group non-RF).

Renal failure was defined as an increased creatinine above 3 mg/dL on laboratory studies within 24 hours prior to

surgery and patients on dialysis. Dialysis dependent patients were those with acute or chronic renal failure requiring peritoneal dialysis, hemodialysis, hemofiltration, hemodiafiltration, or ultrafiltration within two weeks prior to surgery.

Patient demographics included sex, age, smoking, and alcohol use. The comorbidities considered were diabetes, chronic obstructive pulmonary disease (COPD), congestive heart failure (CHF), hypertension requiring medications, disseminated cancer, and transfusions within 3 days prior to surgery. Postoperative complications of interest were superficial surgical site infection, deep incisional surgical site infection, organ space surgical site infection, wound disruption, pneumonia, urinary tract infections, unplanned intubation, pulmonary embolism, deep vein thrombosis, cardiac arrest requiring cardiopulmonary resuscitation, myocardial infarction, intraoperative or postoperative transfusions, sepsis, and septic shock.

Finally other outcome measures reviewed included operative time, return to the operating room, hospital length of stay, 30-day mortality, and time from operation to death in those patients who expired.

2.1. Statistical Analysis. RF versus non-RF groups were compared for baseline characteristics. Numerical values were compared using Student t-test. Categorical and dichotomous variables were compared using chi-square testing. Associated risks were expressed as odds ratios (OR) with a 95% confidence interval (CI). All reported P values are two-tailed, and for all tests, $P < 0.05$ was considered statistically significant.

With nominal regression, we used preoperative variables of sex, age > 65 years, history of diabetes, smoking, congestive heart failure, use of steroids, albumin < 3.0 gm/dL, bilirubin > 2.0 mg/dL, AST > 90 U/L, hematocrit < 30%, platelet count < 200 × 10³/cc, and prothrombin time > 14

TABLE 2: Preoperative laboratory studies. All values with standard deviation.

	Group RF ($n = 28$)	Group non-RF ($n = 18505$)	P value
Sodium (mmol/L)	138.1 (3.8)	138.9 (3.2)	NS ($P = 0.187$)
BUN (mg/dL)	45.2 (22.0)	14.8 (7.3)	$P < 0.0001$
Creatinine (mg/dL)	4.0 (2.03)	0.94 (0.5)	$P < 0.0001$
Albumin (gm/dL)	3.0 (0.9)	3.8 (0.7)	$P < 0.0001$
Total bilirubin (mg/dL)	2.0 (3.19)	1.57 (2.51)	NS ($P = 0.42$)
Alanine aminotransferase (U/L)	92.4 (145.0)	49.7 (67.7)	$P = 0.002$
Alkaline phosphatase (U/L)	234.3 (266.3)	162.4 (161.0)	$P = 0.026$
WBC ($\times 108$/L)	10.3 (7.23)	7.4 (2.9)	$P < 0.0001$
Hematocrit (%)	30.8 (5.6)	38.0 (5.1)	$P < 0.0001$
Platelet count ($\times 10^3$/mL)	218.5 (107.9)	265.4 (97.0)	$P = 0.012$
Partial thromboplastin time (seconds)	33.2 (9.6)	29.6 (5.8)	$P = 0.004$
Prothrombin time (seconds)	14.8 (3.9)	12.6 (2.4)	$P < 0.0001$

TABLE 3: Postoperative complications.

	Total ($n = 18533$)	Group RF ($n = 28$)	Group non-RF ($n = 18505$)	P value
Superficial/skin infection	1524 (8.2%)	1 (3.6%)	1523 (8.2%)	NS ($P = 0.37$)
Deep surgical site infection	361 (1.9%)	1 (3.6%)	360 (1.0%)	NS ($P = 0.53$)
Intra-abdominal infection	1887(10.2%)	2 (7.1%)	1885 (10.2%)	NS ($P = 0.60$)
Wound dehiscence	271 (1.5%)	0	271 (1.5%)	NS ($P = 0.52$)
Postoperative pneumonia	888 (4.8%)	1 (3.6%)	887 (4.8%)	NS ($P = 0.76$)
Need for reintubation	793 (4.3%)	5 (17.9%)	788 (4.3%)	$P < 0.0001$
Pulmonary embolism	210 (1/1%)	0	210 (1.1%)	NS ($P = 0.57$)
Urinary tract infection	934 (5.0%)	1 (3.6%)	933 (5.0%)	NS ($P = 0.72$)
Myocardial infarction	115 (0.6%)	0	115 (0.6%)	NS ($P = 0.68$)
Cardiac arrest	204 (1.1%)	3 (10.7%)	201 (1.1%)	$P < 0.0001$
Cerebrovascular accident	50 (0.3%)	0	50 (0.3%)	NS ($P = 0.78$)
Deep venous thrombosis	416 (2.2%)	2 (7.1%)	414 (2.2%)	NS ($P = 0.08$)
Bleeding requiring transfusion	2108 (11.4%)	8 (28.6%)	2100 (11.3%)	$P = 0.004$
Sepsis	1854 (10.0%)	1 (3.6%)	1853 (10.0%)	NS ($P = 0.26$)
Septic shock	678 (3.7%)	7 (25.0%)	671 (3.7%)	$P < 0.0001$
Return to OR	1141 (6.2%)	4 (14.3%)	1137 (6.2%)	NS ($P = 0.08$)

seconds and the presence of renal failure to determine if any of these factors were associated with 30-day mortality.

3. Results

During the 7-year period, 2005–2011, there were 18,533 patients who underwent pancreatic resection. Males to females were 8922 to 9585 and mean age was 61.8 years. Of this entire cohort, 28 patients were identified as having renal failure. Specific procedures included partial removal of pancreas (13), pancreatectomy (6), pancreatectomy with pancreatojejunotomy (3), distal pancreatectomy (3), and proximal pancreatectomy (3).

Patient demographics and comorbidities are as listed in Table 1. RF patients were older and were more likely to have diabetes, myocardial infarction within the previous 6 months, hypertension requiring medications, use of steroids, bleeding

disorder, disseminated cancer, and a blood transfusion prior to surgery.

Preoperative laboratory studies are as shown in Table 2. RF patients had significantly worse initial bleeding parameters with higher protime and partial thromboplastin time, as well as a lower platelet count. Initial WBC and hematocrit were also lower in RF patients. RF patients had similar bilirubin but higher AST, alkaline phosphatase, and lower albumin prior to pancreas surgery.

Postoperative complications and outcome are detailed in Tables 3 and 4. Most notably, RF patients were more likely to need reintubation, have a cardiac arrest, and have bleeding that required blood transfusion. Although RF patients were not any more likely to have surgical site infections, wound infections, or sepsis, they were more likely to have septic shock. RF patients were more likely to require a return to the operating room. Hospital length of stay and 30-day mortality were significantly higher in RF patients. Of all patients who

TABLE 4: Outcome measures.

	Group RF (n = 28)	Group non-RF (n = 18505)	P value
Operative time in minutes (SD)	316 (139.7)	324 (142.7)	NS (P = 0.913)
Hospital length of stay in days (SD)	23 (25.7)	12.0 (11.0)	P < 0.001
Days from operation to death (SD)	7.83 (7.36)	13.3 (8.54)	NS (P = 0.36)
30-day mortality	6/28 (21.4%)	425/18505 (2.3%)	P < 0.001

TABLE 5: Predictors of 30-day mortality.

	Odds ratio (95% CI)	P value
Renal failure	6.13 (2.32–16.18)	P < 0.001
History of congestive heart failure	4.72 (2.13–10.50)	P < 0.001
Age 65 or higher	2.44 (1.98–3.01)	P < 0.001
Albumin < 3.0 gm/dL	1.94 (1.47–2.56)	P < 0.001
History of steroid use	1.93 (1.18–3.16)	P = 0.009
Hematocrit < 30%	1.69 (1.24–2.28)	P = 0.001
Protime > 14 seconds	1.59 (1.25–2.02)	P < 0.001
Diabetes	1.33 (1.08–1.64)	P = 0.008
Bilirubin > 2.0 mmol/L	1.02 (0.79–1.32)	NS (P = 0.87)

died in this study, those with RF expired in a mean of 7.8 days compared to 13.3 days in non-RF patients.

Using nominal regression, the factors predictive of 30 day mortality included age 65 or higher, presence of diabetes, history of CHF, steroid use, albumin < 3.0 gm/dL, bilirubin > 2.0 mg/L, Hct < 30%, protime > 14 seconds, and renal failure (see Table 5). The presence of RF had the highest odds ratio at 6.13.

4. Discussion

Advances in renal replacement therapy and better management of diabetes and cardiovascular problems have allowed patients with RF to live longer with their chronic illnesses, but they now may be living long enough to develop neoplasms that require surgical intervention. While previous large studies have addressed surgical procedures in dialysis patients, less is known about how these RF patients fare in pancreatic resections.

Previous studies have demonstrated increased surgical morbidity and mortality in patients with renal failure who are dialysis dependent. In the largest study, Gajdos et al. used NSQIP to investigate the effect of long-term dialysis on general surgical procedures. The 1506 dialysis patients had 12.7% mortality (30-day) compared to 1.5% in the 164,094 patients with normal renal function. Dialysis patients also had a higher pulmonary complications, reoperations, cardiovascular complications, surgical site infections, and hospital length of stay. While this study had a large number of dialysis patients, it included a variety of general surgical procedures with varying levels of complexity and is done for both benign and malignant reasons [7].

Pancreatic surgeries are among the most complex of the abdominal procedures. Many factors contribute to this risk but the effect of renal dysfunction has been variably reported. Age has been the most commonly cited risk factor for outcome in pancreatic surgery [13–16]. Diabetes, the reason for pancreatic resection (benign versus malignant), hospital volume, preoperative biliary drainage, and resection of other organs have all been mentioned as contributing to prognosis [9, 11, 17–19]. Renal failure and dysfunction have been shown to contribute to poor outcome in pancreatic head resections in 3 single center studies, but these studies had 300 cases or fewer in each series [9–11].

Two studies attempted to combine multiple risk factors in developing tools to assess patients' risk for pancreatic surgery. Are et al. using the Nationwide Inpatient Sample (NIS) database developed a nomogram to predict outcome for patients undergoing pancreatic resection for malignancy. Renal failure was the factor with the highest number points assigned in the nomogram [20]. On the other hand, Parikh et al. using NSQIP developed a risk calculator to predict outcome after pancreatic resection. Renal failure was not mentioned as a risk factor, but American Society of Anesthesiologists (ASA) classification, functional health status, sepsis, surgical extent, age, dyspnea, body mass index, coronary heart disease, gender, and bleeding disorder were the most important [21].

Two additional studies reviewed outcomes after pancreatic surgery utilizing the NIS and discussed the effect of renal failure. McPhee analyzed in-hospital mortality in patients who underwent pancreatectomy for neoplasm between 1998 and 2003. Of 39,463 patients, 395 (1%) had renal failure and mortality rate of RF patients was 36.1% compared to the overall mortality rate of 5.9% [22]. Teh et al. evaluated the NIS database for major pancreatic resections done for benign and malignant disease between the years of 1988 and 2003. Among the cohort of 103,222 patients, 1% had renal insufficiency and this patient subset had increased in-hospital mortality (OR 6.3), perioperative complications (OR 2.3), and increased mortality following a major complication (OR 3.5) [23]. While these studies are helpful in stratifying renal failure as a risk, the clinical variables and specific outcomes in these RF patients are not described in detail.

Our study clearly demonstrates that renal failure increased morbidity and mortality for patients undergoing pancreatic resection. Although only a cohort of 28 patients, 21% of these patients died in a mean of 7.8 days after surgery. Renal failure increased the 30-day mortality by 6-fold. Patients with renal failure also had a significantly higher rate of postoperative complications with an increased risk of unplanned reintubation, cardiac arrest, septic shock, and need for transfusion. Those patients who did survive remained hospitalized for almost twice as long as patients without RF.

This study did have limitations, as it utilized an administrative database and can only be as precise as the trained staff who enter the data. Although the number of pancreatic resections was large, the number of cases with RF was relative small and the data may have diminished accuracy especially in subcategories and with some of the laboratory values. In addition, NSQIP is able to define a preoperative creatinine but cannot tell us if creatinine is due to a chronic kidney disease or if this is an acute or relatively recent renal dysfunction. One might assume that a patient with acute progressive renal failure would not be subjected to a major pancreatic resection, but unfortunately this study cannot provide us with the exact information. The grouping of the procedures by NSQIP based on procedural codes was quite nonspecific and there was likely variability in coding by the staff. It is likely that "partial removal of pancreas" may have included both distal pancreatic resections and pancreaticoduodenectomies with varying extents of each procedure. A major limitation of the study is that NSQIP database did not report the exact pathology of the resected specimen or the details of the operative procedure. It is unclear if some of these cases represented benign or premalignant lesions such as cystic tumors or neuroendocrine tumors which may have significantly less risk and better short, and long-term outcome. Finally, although NSQIP can identify general complications, it is not a database that can delineate procedure-specific complications so important complications such as pancreatic leaks and fistulas could not be assessed.

5. Conclusions

In conclusion, this study establishes a significant negative effect of renal failure on outcome in pancreatic resections. It will be difficult to acquire larger cohorts of patients with this particular problem and NSQIP is really not able to assess risk based on specific diagnoses requiring pancreatic resection. Each RF patient should be assessed for overall risk and especially in the context of expected long-term survival based on the specific pancreatic diagnosis. Those patients who opt for pancreatic resection should be optimized in terms of bleeding parameters and should be monitored carefully for respiratory, bleeding, and septic complications. Strong consideration should be made for nonoperative therapies or no treatment in those patients who have prohibitive risk or limited long-term survival.

Disclosures

Dr. L. L. Wong is supported by Bayer Healthcare (Speakers Bureau). Drs. S. R. Domingo and K. S. Norman have no financial disclosures. This paper was not presented at any meeting or previous communication.

Acknowledgment

The authors wish to thank Wanda Muranaka and Dr. Whitney Limm for assistance with this project.

References

[1] United States Renal Data System, *USRDS 2012 Annual Data Report: Atlas of Chronic Kidney Disease and End-Stage Renal Disease in the United States*, National Institutes of Health, National Institute of Diabetes and Digestive and Kidney Diseases, Bethesda, Md, USA, 2012.

[2] *Kidney Diseases Statistics for the United States*, NIH Publication No. 12-3895, National Kidney and Urologic Diseases Information Clearinghouse, Bethesda, Md, USA, 2012.

[3] C. Gajdos, M. T. Hawn, D. Kile et al., "The risk of major elective vascular surgical procedures in patients with end-stage renal disease," *Annals of Surgery*, vol. 257, no. 4, pp. 766–773, 2013.

[4] L. Labrousse, C. de Vincentiis, F. Madonna, C. Deville, X. Roques, and E. Baudet, "Early and long term results of coronary artery bypass grafts in patients with dialysis dependant renal failure," *European Journal of Cardio-Thoracic Surgery*, vol. 15, no. 5, pp. 691–696, 1999.

[5] J. F. M. Bechtel, C. Detter, T. Fischlein et al., "Cardiac surgery in patients on dialysis: decreased 30-day mortality, unchanged overall survival," *Annals of Thoracic Surgery*, vol. 85, no. 1, pp. 147–153, 2008.

[6] S. Drolet, A. R. MacLean, R. P. Myers, A. A. M. Shaheen, E. Dixon, and W. D. Buie, "Morbidity and mortality following colorectal surgery in patients with end-stage renal failure: a population-based study," *Diseases of the Colon and Rectum*, vol. 53, no. 11, pp. 1508–1516, 2010.

[7] C. Gajdos, M. T. Hawn, D. Kile, T. N. Robinson, and W. G. Henderson, "Risk of major nonemergent inpatient general surgical procedures in patients on long-term dialysis," *Archives of Surgery*, vol. 15, pp. 1–7, 2012.

[8] C. R. Schneider, W. Cobb, S. Patel, D. Cull, C. Anna, and R. Roettger, "Elective surgery in patients with end stage renal disease: what's the risk?" *The American Surgeon*, vol. 75, no. 9, pp. 790–793, 2009.

[9] U. Adam, F. Makowiec, H. Riediger, W. D. Schareck, S. Benz, and U. T. Hopt, "Risk factors for complications after pancreatic head resection," *The American Journal of Surgery*, vol. 187, no. 2, pp. 201–208, 2004.

[10] J. P. Lerut, P. R. Gianello, J. B. Otte, and P. J. Kestens, "Pancreaticoduodenal resection. Surgical experience and evaluation of risk factors in 103 patients," *Annals of Surgery*, vol. 199, no. 4, pp. 432–437, 1984.

[11] D. J. Gouma, R. C. I. van Geenen, T. M. van Gulik et al., "Rates of complications and death after pancreaticoduodenectomy: risk factors and the impact of hospital volume," *Annals of Surgery*, vol. 232, no. 6, pp. 786–795, 2000.

[12] ACS NSQIP, Data Collection, Analysis and Reporting, ACS NSQIP, Chicago, Ill, USA, http://site.acsnsqip.org.

[13] T. S. Riall, "What is the effect of age on pancreatic resection?" *Advances in Surgery*, vol. 43, no. 1, pp. 233–249, 2009.

[14] M. P. Spencer, M. G. Sarr, and D. M. Nagorney, "Radical pancreatectomy for pancreatic cancer in the elderly. Is it safe and
justified," *Annals of Surgery*, vol. 212, no. 2, pp. 140–143, 1990.

[15] M. Oliverius, Z. Kala, M. Varga, R. Gürlich, V. Lanska, and H.
Kubesova, "Radical surgery for pancreatic malignancy in the
elderly," *Pancreatology*, vol. 10, no. 4, pp. 499–502, 2010.

[16] T. S. Riall, D. M. Reddy, W. H. Nealon, and J. S. Goodwin, "The
effect of age on short-term outcomes after pancreatic resection:
a population-based study," *Annals of Surgery*, vol. 248, no. 3, pp.
459–467, 2008.

[17] R. M. Cannon, R. LeGrand, R. B. Chagpar et al., "Multi-institutional analysis of pancreatic adenocarcinoma demonstrating
the effect of diabetes status on survival after resection," *HPB*, vol.
14, no. 4, pp. 228–235, 2012.

[18] F. Maire, P. Hammel, B. Terris et al., "Prognosis of malignant
intraductal papillary mucinous tumours of the pancreas after
surgical resection. Comparison with pancreatic ductal adenocarcinoma," *Gut*, vol. 51, no. 5, pp. 717–722, 2002.

[19] F. P. Herter, A. M. Cooperman, T. N. Ahlborn, and C. Antinori,
"Surgical experience with pancreatic and periampullary cancer,"
Annals of Surgery, vol. 195, no. 3, pp. 274–281, 1982.

[20] C. Are, C. Afuh, L. Ravipati, A. Sasson, F. Ullrich, and L. Smith,
"Preoperative nomogram to predict risk of perioperative mor-
tality following pancreatic resections for malignancy," *Journal of
Gastrointestinal Surgery*, vol. 13, no. 12, pp. 2152–2162, 2009.

[21] P. Parikh, M. Shiloach, M. E. Cohen et al., "Pancreatectomy risk
calculator: an ACS-NSQIP resource," *HPB*, vol. 12, no. 7, pp.
488–497, 2010.

[22] J. T. McPhee, J. S. Hill, G. F. Whalen et al., "Perioperative
mortality for pancreatectomy: a national perspective," *Annals of
Surgery*, vol. 246, no. 2, pp. 246–253, 2007.

[23] S. H. Teh, B. S. Diggs, C. W. Deveney, and B. C. Sheppard,
"Patient and hospital characteristics on the variance of perioperative outcomes for pancreatic resection in the United
States: a plea for outcome-based and not volume-based referral
guidelines," *Archives of Surgery*, vol. 144, no. 8, pp. 713–721, 2009.

28

Bovine Serum Albumin-Glutaraldehyde Sealed Fish-Mouth Closure of the Pancreatic Remnant during Distal Pancreatectomy

Fritz Klein, Igor Maximilian Sauer, Johann Pratschke, and Marcus Bahra

Department of Surgery, Charité-Universitätsmedizin Berlin, Augustenburger Platz 1, 13353 Berlin, Germany

Correspondence should be addressed to Fritz Klein; fritz.klein@charite.de

Academic Editor: Pablo Ramírez

Introduction. Postoperative pancreatic fistula formation remains the major complication after distal pancreatectomy. At our institution, we have recently developed a novel bovine serum albumin-glutaraldehyde sealed hand sutured fish-mouth closure technique of the pancreatic remnant during distal pancreatectomy. The aim of this study was to analyze the impact of this approach with regard to technical feasibility and overall postoperative outcome. *Patients and Methods.* 32 patients who underwent a bovine serum albumin-glutaraldehyde sealed hand sutured fish-mouth closure of the pancreatic remnant during distal pancreatectomy between 2012 and 2014 at our institution were analyzed for clinically relevant postoperative pancreatic fistula formation (Grades B and C according to ISGPF definition) and overall postoperative morbidity. *Results.* Three out of 32 patients (9.4%) developed Grade B pancreatic fistula, which could be treated conservatively. No Grade C pancreatic fistulas were observed. Postpancreatectomy hemorrhage occurred in 1 patient (3.1%). Overall postoperative complications > Clavien II were observed in 5 patients (15.6%). There was no postoperative mortality. *Conclusion.* The performance of a bovine serum albumin-glutaraldehyde sealed hand sutured fish-mouth closure of the pancreatic remnant was shown to be technically feasible and may lead to a significant decrease of postoperative pancreatic fistula formation after distal pancreatectomy.

1. Introduction

Distal Pancreatectomy (DP) is performed as the standard procedure in patients with malignant, cystic, or neuroendocrine tumors and/or chronic pancreatitis in the body and tail of the pancreas [1]. Continuous progress in peri- and postoperative management as well as in surgical expertise has led to a decline in operation associated mortality to 0–7% even in patients with an advanced stage of disease in which DP was combined with additional vascular or visceral resections [2–4]. Postoperative morbidity after DP however remains high and is reported to range from 35% to 60% [5, 6]. Clinically relevant postoperative pancreatic fistula formation (POPF) Grades B and C which occur in up to 21% of all patients especially have a major impact on postoperative outcome and may lead to additional complications such as delayed gastric emptying, intra-abdominal abscess formation, sepsis, or hemorrhage from major visceral vessels and may therefore contribute not just to a prolonged hospital stay but eventually to a fatal postoperative outcome [5, 7–10]. The surgical technique as well as the status of the pancreatic remnant (soft versus hard parenchyma), patient age and body-mass index, patient care at a high-volume center, chronic pancreatitis, and the extent of lymphadenectomy, and visceral resection have been identified as predicting factors for POPF [7, 11, 12]. Numerous surgical techniques and variants for pancreatic remnant closure have been described for possible POPF reduction including hand-sewn suturing, various stapler methods, or a combination of both. Furthermore, pancreatoenteric anastomosis or the application of fibrin sealants or meshes, falciform ligament or gastric serosa patches, or the use of saline-coupled bipolar electrocautery and ultrasonic dissection had been evaluated [13–20]. However, no gold-standard technique with regard to POPF reduction has been established yet. Inspired by the well-established use of bovine serum albumin-glutaraldehyde (BioGlue®) sealing in

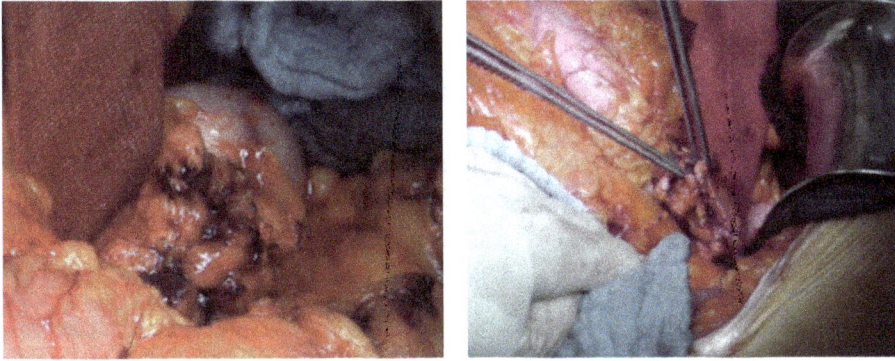

FIGURE 1: Fish-mouth shaped cutting surface of the pancreatic remnant.

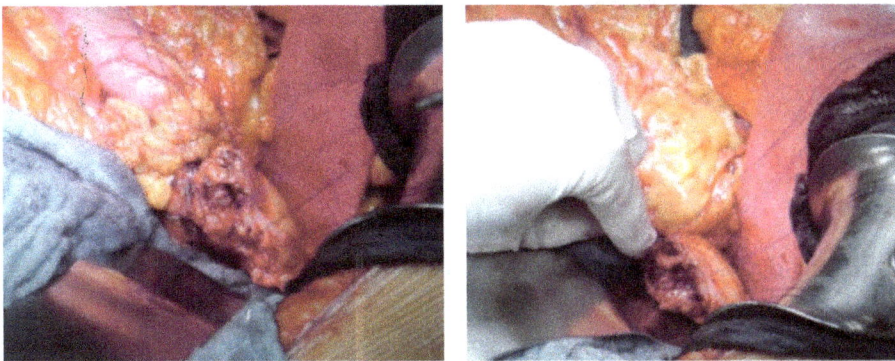

FIGURE 2: Single U-shaped 4-0 Prolene sutures placed along the cutting surface.

cardiovascular surgery we have recently developed a novel technique of a bovine serum albumin-glutaraldehyde sealed fish-mouth closure of the pancreatic remnant during distal pancreatectomy in attempt to further reduce POPF. BioGlue (25% bovine serum albumin and 10% glutaraldehyde; Cryolife Inc., Kennesaw, GA, USA) was approved by the FDA in 1998 for surgical application and is utilized in cardiovascular and pulmonary surgery, that is, for application during aortic root reconstruction and valve placement as well as for control of alveolar air leaks [21, 22]. Clinical and histopathological studies have demonstrated that this semisynthetic surgical adhesive upon application polymerises with native tissues including pancreatic tissue and thereby creates a flexible mechanical seal which strengthens and holds tissues together with an additive haemostatic property [23, 24]. The aim of this study was to analyze the technical feasibility of this novel surgical approach as well as to investigate a possible benefit with regard to POPF and overall postoperative outcome.

2. Patients and Methods

We retrospectively analyzed 33 consecutive patients who underwent a bovine serum albumin-glutaraldehyde (BioGlue) sealed fish-mouth closure of the pancreatic remnant during distal pancreatectomy for primary malignant or cystic tumors of the pancreas as well as for chronic pancreatitis

at the Department of General, Visceral and Transplantation Surgery, Charité-Universitätsmedizin Berlin, Campus Virchow, between January 1, 2012, and January 1, 2015. All operations were performed by five experienced visceral surgeons who were all educated about the technical steps of this novel procedure as part of the inclusion criteria of this study. This study was performed in accordance with the Declaration of Helsinki and its amendments and approved by the institutional ethic committee.

2.1. Surgical Technique. DP was performed as open surgery in each patient. The extent of the pancreatic resection, as well as the need for additional lymphadenectomy and splenectomy, was determined based on the underlying disease and/or cancer stages. The pancreatic resection was performed in all cases using electrocautery in an incision line, which creates a fish-mouth shaped cutting surface of the pancreatic remnant (Figure 1). After achievement of local hemostasis, subsequent closure of the main pancreatic duct (MDP) was performed by a stitch ligation using 4-0 polypropylene sutures (Prolene, Johnson & Johnson Medical GmbH, Norderstedt, Germany). As a next step single U-shaped 4-0 polypropylene sutures were placed along the cutting surface (Figure 2). The bovine serum albumin-glutaraldehyde (BioGlue, Cryolife Inc., Kennesaw, GA, USA) was then administered into the fish-mouth cavity of the pancreatic remnant in a step-by-step approach

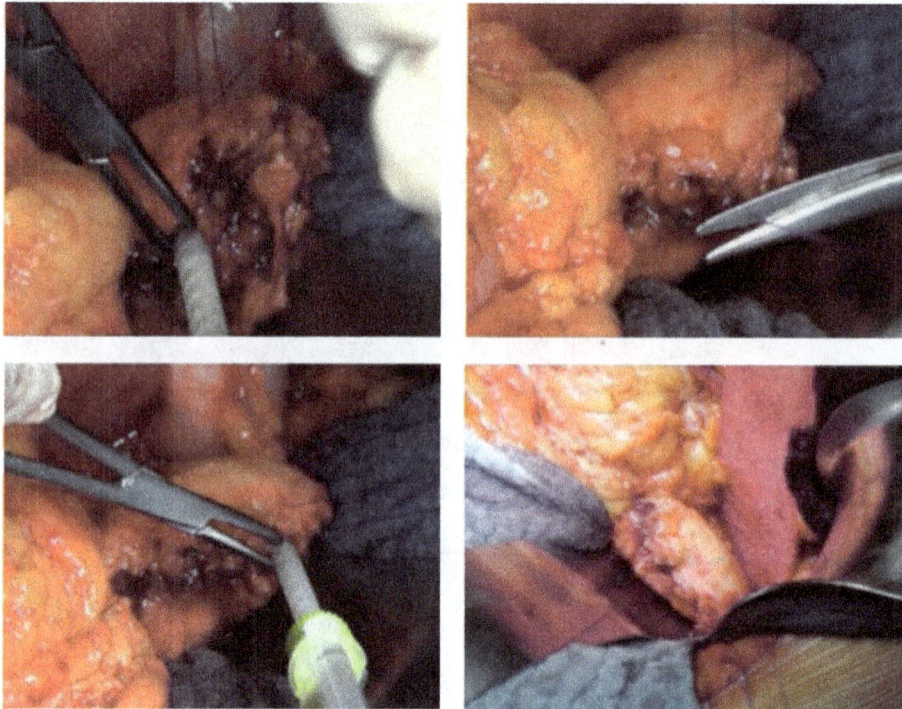

FIGURE 3: Bovine serum albumin-glutaraldehyde (BioGlue) administration into the fish-mouth cavity of the pancreatic remnant before the tying of each suture.

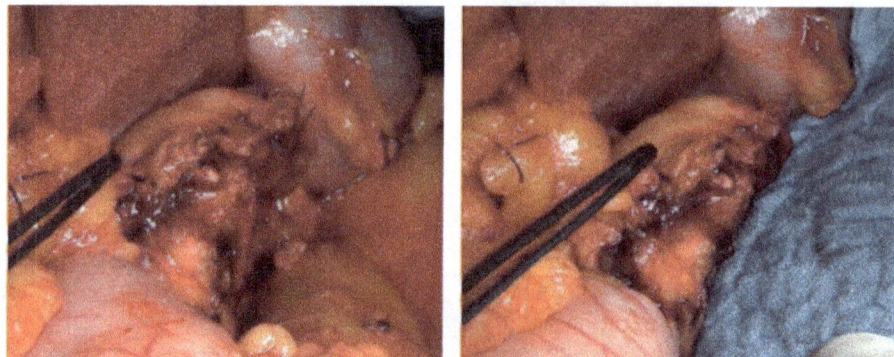

FIGURE 4: Pancreatic remnant after bovine serum albumin-glutaraldehyde sealed fish-mouth closure.

before the tying of each suture (Figure 3). No additional covering of the pancreatic remnant was performed (Figure 4). An intra-abdominal drain was placed at the pancreatic stump and if additional splenectomy was performed another intra-abdominal drain was positioned against the left subdiaphragmatic region.

2.2. Standard Postoperative Care. The levels of amylase and/or lipase in the blood and in the intra-abdominal drains were routinely measured on the 2nd and 5th postoperative day or immediately in the presence of laboratory or clinical signs of infection. Oral food intake was usually begun on the second postoperative day depending on the patient condition and bowel function. The drains were usually removed within

6 postoperative days if the output was clear and if there were no signs or symptoms of infection. We did not perform a standardized Somatostatin analogue (e.g., octreotide) prophylaxis for POPF prevention and pancreatic enzyme were only supplemented in the event of clinical signs of exocrine pancreatic insufficiency.

We also did not use a standardized protocol for POPF treatment. The drains were left in situ or replaced interventionally and continuous rinsing of the drain was initiated until the drain secretion was clear and the amylase/lipase had declined back to normal values. A cessation of oral food intake and/or eventually octreotide administration during POPF treatment was decided on individual basis in each patient.

The patients who had undergone an additional splenectomy received haemophilus, pneumococcal, and meningococcal vaccination according to current guidelines [25].

All patients were observed in our outpatient department for a postoperative period of at least 30 days.

2.3. Data Collection and Study Endpoints. Data collection in all patients included relevant information on their medical history, the pathological examination with regard to the underlying disease and resection margin status and the overall postoperative clinical outcome with documentation of any significant procedure related morbidity, the need for reintervention or reoperation, and the length of hospital stay. Postoperative morbidity was classified according to the Clavien-Dindo classification [26]. POPF and postpancreatectomy hemorrhage (PPH) were defined based on the ISGPF definitions [27, 28].

Besides a general analysis of the technical feasibility of this novel approach the primary outcome of our study was to investigate the rate of clinically relevant POPF equivalent to POPF Grades B and C. All other complications within 30 days of the operation were also recorded.

2.4. Statistical Analysis. Statistical analysis was performed using PASW statistics 19 (SPSS Software, IBM Company, Chicago, IL, USA). Continuous variables were reported using mean or median values where appropriate with range, whereas categorical variables were described using frequencies and percent.

3. Results

3.1. Patient Baseline and Preoperative Data. Between January 1, 2012, and January 1, 2015, 32 consecutive patients underwent a bovine serum albumin-glutaraldehyde sealed fish-mouth closure of the pancreatic remnant during distal pancreatectomy.

There were 15 males (47%) and 17 females (53%) with a median age of 62 years (32–77). The indication for distal pancreatectomy was pancreatic adenocarcinoma in 11 patients (34%), intraductal papillary mucinous neoplasm (IPMN) of the pancreas in 7 patients (22%), chronic pancreatitis in 3 patients (9%), neuroendocrine tumors (NET) of the pancreas in 2 patients (6%), mucinous cystic neoplasms (MCN) of the pancreas in 3 patients (9%), cyst adenoma in 4 patients (13%), cyst adenocarcinoma in 1 patient (3%), and leiomyosarcoma in 1 patient (3%). Two of the 32 patients (6%) underwent endoscopic retrograde cholangiopancreatography (ERCP) with endoscopic papillotomy (EPT) and endoscopic pancreas stent placement prior to the operation (Table 1).

3.2. Peri- and Postoperative Course. A splenectomy was performed in 27 of the 32 patients (84%). Seven patients (22%) underwent an additional multivisceral resection with partial or total gastrectomy in 4 patients (13%), colon resection in 5 patients (16%), and/or partial adrenalectomy in 3 patients (9%). The mean operation time was 199 minutes (116–282 minutes). No patient required intraoperative administration of packed red blood cells. The pancreas tissue texture was

TABLE 1: Demographics and preoperative characteristics.

	BioGlue sealed hand sutured fish-mouth closure technique during distal pancreatectomy
Number of patients	32
Median age (years; range)	62 (32–77)
Gender (male : female)	15 (47%) : 17 (53%)
Indication	
Pancreatic adenocarcinoma	11 (34%)
IPMN	7 (22%)
Chronic pancreatitis	3 (9%)
NET	2 (6%)
MCN	3 (9%)
Cyst adenoma	4 (13%)
Others	2 (6%)
Preoperative ERCP with EPT and pancreatic stent placement	2 (6%)

found to be soft in 13 patients (41%) and hard in 19 patients (59%) according to the intraoperative assessment of the operating surgeon. Major postoperative morbidity > Clavien II occurred in 5 of the 32 patients (16%). Three patients (9%) developed a clinically relevant POPF Grade B. Each of the three patients could be treated conservatively with a however prolonged hospital stay of 40, 71, and 93 days. No Grade C pancreatic fistulas were observed. Postpancreatectomy hemorrhage Grade A occurred in one patient (3%) as an intraluminal bleeding, which did not require therapeutic consequences. Two patients underwent reoperations, due to an insufficiency of a colon anastomosis in one patient and an abdominal fascial dehiscence in another patient. There was no postoperative mortality. The median length of hospital stay was 12 days (7–93) (Table 2).

4. Discussion

Postoperative pancreatic fistula formation remains the most relevant complication after distal pancreatectomy with a major impact on postoperative quality of life as well as on health care costs. In patients with an underlying malignant disease POPF may in addition lead to a delayed onset of further essential adjuvant treatment which has been identified as an independent risk factor for early peritoneal recurrence and decreased overall survival [29].

Numerous surgical techniques have therefore been described in an attempt to possibly decrease the incidence and impact of POPF. However, even two recent prospective randomized trials failed to identify an ideal technique for the procedure with the pancreatic remnant. The DISPACT trial compared a stapler versus hand-sewn closure of the pancreatic remnant and the incidence of clinically relevant POPF Grades B and C was reported with 20% and 21% in each group [5]. Analogously Carter et al. analyzed the effect of the use of an autologous falciform ligament patch with fibrin glue for both stapler and hand-sewn closure of the

TABLE 2: Operative data and clinical outcome.

	BioGlue sealed hand sutured fish-mouth closure technique during distal pancreatectomy ($n = 32$)
Mean operation time (minutes; range)	199 (116–282)
Splenectomy	27 (84%)
Additional visceral resection	7 (22%)
Partial/total gastrectomy	4 (13%)
Colon resection	5 (16%)
Partial adrenalectomy	3 (9%)
Pancreas tissue texture	
Soft	13 (41%)
Hard	19 (59%)
Postoperative morbidity > Clavien II	5 (16%)
Clinically relevant POPF	3 (9%)
POPF Grade B	3 (9%)
POPF Grade C	0
PPH	1 (3%)
Reoperation	2 (6%)
Median hospital stay (days; range)	12 (7–73)
Mortality	0

pancreatic remnant and reported a rate of clinically relevant POPF Grades B and C in 18% of their patients which did not differ significantly from the control group [30]. The question of an optimal surgical technique for distal pancreatectomy therefore remains to be debated controversially. At our institution we have recently developed a novel technique of a bovine serum albumin-glutaraldehyde (BioGlue) sealed fish-mouth closure of the pancreatic remnant during distal pancreatectomy, which was analyzed in this study. We could demonstrate that our technique was feasible with a distinct positive impact on clinically relevant POPF. Only three of our 32 patients (9%) developed a POPF Grade B, which could be treated conservatively, and no POPF Grade C was observed. With a clinically relevant POPF rate below 10% our results are thus to be seen promising especially in comparison to the results of the present prospective as well as retrospective studies [5, 13–15, 17–20, 30]. The concept of bovine serum albumin-glutaraldehyde application in pancreatic surgery is not new. Fisher et al. have previously investigated the use of BioGlue in an attempt to possibly reduce POPF and demonstrated general safety but no relevant clinical benefit [31]. Most patients in this study however underwent pancreaticoduodenectomy (PD) instead of DP and the bovine serum albumin-glutaraldehyde was only applied on the completed anastomosis. We modified this technique by creating a fish-mouth shaped pancreatic remnant with a ligated main pancreatic duct (MPD). The bovine serum albumin-glutaraldehyde (BioGlue) was then applied into

the fish-mouth cavity before the tying of previously placed single U-shaped sutures. Analogously to Ohwada et al. we believe that our technique enables the bovine serum albumin-glutaraldehyde adhesive to stay within the anastomosis region as opposed to the external application described by Fisher et al. in which the BioGlue may rather likely dissolve [32].

The creation of a fish-mouth shaped cutting margin of the pancreatic remnant may of course be challenging especially in a rather thin gland and may also be associated with an increased bleeding tendency [33]. Also the identification and routinely performed ligation of the main pancreatic duct which is considered an individual factor for POPF reduction may not always be possible [34]. We did however not experience any intraoperative problems of this kind.

The use of bovine serum albumin-glutaraldehyde (BioGlue) as a sealant is of course rather expensive especially in comparison to widely used fibrin glue. However, several studies showed that the use of fibrin for sealing the cutting surface after PD or DP as well as for occlusion of the main pancreatic duct was not associated with a reduction of POPF [18, 35]. In addition to the limited clinical evidence fibrin may be considered a poor adhesive for pancreatic surgery because it takes a long time to set up and may therefore be swiped or washed away easily. Bovine serum albumin-glutaraldehyde in contrast reaches maximal strength within 2 minutes after application with an additional benefit of local hemostatic properties [31]. We believe that a quick transformation of the liquid glue to a flexible hydrogel is especially important in this setting to prevent a loss of attachment to the applied surface.

Complications of bovine serum albumin-glutaraldehyde (BioGlue) application reported in cardiovascular and pulmonary surgery include nerve damage, local or embolic vascular obstruction, and foreign body reactions [36, 37]. Lämsä et al. have previously analyzed the histological effects of tissue adhesives on the pancreas and reported acinar cell vacuolization and necrosis together with moderate edema and leukocyte infiltration in each adhesive tested with however no relevant differences between fibrin and bovine serum albumin-glutaraldehyde (BioGlue) [24]. In our study we did not observe any of such complications reaching a clinical manifestation especially no clinical or laboratory signs of a postoperative pancreatitis.

It should of course be noted that any kind of additional physical barrier may lead to a delayed onset or at least clinical presentation of POPF [30]. As part of our internal treatment standard patients were however only discharged if all parameters indicating infection were low and the patient was feeling well which is reflected by a prolonged median hospital stay of 12 days in our study. In addition patients were observed in our outpatient department for a postoperative period of at least 30 days. A potentially undetected delayed onset of POPF may thus be excluded in our patient population.

A reduction in the incidence of POPF may of course not just be achieved by restricting on surgical technical factors alone. Several studies have reported an improved postoperative outcome if EPT or pancreatic stent placement were performed prior to DP [38]. This potential benefit is however outweighed by an increased risk for directly intervention related morbidity which is reported to occur in up to 57% of all patients [39]. In our study ERCP with EPT and/or stent placement was thus only performed in 2 of our 32 patients (6%) and only considered in patients with suspected benign diseases in an attempt to avoid any additional risk for a potential delayed onset of treatment in patients with an underlying malignant disease. The statistical power of our study is of course limited by the small sample size of patients. Also the retrospective study design may have led to an unintended selection bias. However, as a conclusion of our study we could demonstrate that our technique of a bovine serum albumin-glutaraldehyde sealed fish-mouth closure of the pancreatic remnant was technically feasible and safe with a high potential to decrease the incidence as well as the impact of clinically relevant POPF after DP.

Competing Interests

Dr. Klein has received honorarium for an oral presentation by Cryolife Inc. No other authors report competing interests or funding to disclose. No benefits in any form have been received or will be received from a commercial party related directly or indirectly to the subject of this article.

Authors' Contributions

Fritz Klein collected the data and wrote the manuscript. Igor Maximilian Sauer collected the data. Johann Pratschke and Marcus Bahra designed and performed the research.

References

[1] K. D. Lillemoe, S. Kaushal, J. L. Cameron, T. A. Sohn, H. A. Pitt, and C. J. Yeo, "Distal pancreatectomy: indications and outcomes in 235 patients," *Annals of Surgery*, vol. 229, no. 5, pp. 693–700, 1999.

[2] J. H. Balcom IV, D. W. Rattner, A. L. Warshaw, Y. Chang, and C. Fernandez-Del Castillo, "Ten-year experience with 733 pancreatic resections: changing indications, older patients, and decreasing length of hospitalization," *Archives of Surgery*, vol. 136, no. 4, pp. 391–398, 2001.

[3] W. Hartwig, T. Hackert, U. Hinz et al., "Multivisceral resection for pancreatic malignancies: risk-analysis and long-term outcome," *Annals of Surgery*, vol. 250, no. 1, pp. 81–87, 2009.

[4] F. Klein, M. Glanemann, W. Faber, S. Gül, P. Neuhaus, and M. Bahra, "Pancreatoenteral anastomosis or direct closure of the pancreatic remnant after a distal pancreatectomy: a single-centre experience," *HPB*, vol. 14, no. 12, pp. 798–804, 2012.

[5] M. K. Diener, C. M. Seiler, I. Rossion et al., "Efficacy of stapler versus hand-sewn closure after distal pancreatectomy (DISPACT): a randomised, controlled multicentre trial," *The Lancet*, vol. 377, no. 9776, pp. 1514–1522, 2011.

[6] U. F. Wellner, F. Makowiec, O. Sick, U. T. Hopt, and T. Keck, "Arguments for an individualized closure of the pancreatic remnant after distal pancreatic resection," *World Journal of Gastrointestinal Surgery*, vol. 4, no. 5, pp. 114–120, 2012.

[7] M. Distler, S. Kersting, F. Rückert et al., "Chronic pancreatitis of the pancreatic remnant is an independent risk factor for pancreatic fistula after distal pancreatectomy," *BMC Surgery*, vol. 14, no. 1, article 54, 2014.

[8] C. R. Ferrone, A. L. Warshaw, D. W. Rattner et al., "Pancreatic fistula rates after 462 distal pancreatectomies: staplers do not decrease fistula rates," *Journal of Gastrointestinal Surgery*, vol. 12, no. 10, pp. 1691–1698, 2008.

[9] H. Nathan, J. L. Cameron, C. R. Goodwin et al., "Risk factors for pancreatic leak after distal pancreatectomy," *Annals of Surgery*, vol. 250, no. 2, pp. 277–281, 2009.

[10] J. Kleeff, M. K. Diener, K. Z'graggen et al., "Distal pancreatectomy: risk factors for surgical failure in 302 consecutive cases," *Annals of Surgery*, vol. 245, no. 4, pp. 573–582, 2007.

[11] H. P. Knaebel, M. K. Diener, M. N. Wente, M. W. Büchler, and C. M. Seiler, "Systematic review and meta-analysis of technique for closure of the pancreatic remnant after distal pancreatectomy," *British Journal of Surgery*, vol. 92, no. 5, pp. 539–546, 2005.

[12] R. Yoshioka, A. Saiura, R. Koga et al., "Risk factors for clinical pancreatic fistula after distal pancreatectomy: analysis of consecutive 100 patients," *World Journal of Surgery*, vol. 34, no. 1, pp. 121–125, 2010.

[13] B. N. Fahy, C. F. Frey, H. S. Ho, L. Beckett, and R. J. Bold, "Morbidity, mortality, and technical factors of distal pancreatectomy," *American Journal of Surgery*, vol. 183, no. 3, pp. 237–241, 2002.

[14] L. J. Harris, H. Abdollahi, T. Newhook et al., "Optimal technical management of stump closure following distal pancreatectomy: a retrospective review of 215 cases," *Journal of Gastrointestinal Surgery*, vol. 14, no. 6, pp. 998–1005, 2010.

[15] D. A. Iannitti, N. G. Coburn, J. Somberg, B. A. Ryder, J. Monchik, and W. G. Cioffi, "Use of the round ligament of the liver to decrease pancreatic fistulas: a novel technique," *Journal of the American College of Surgeons*, vol. 203, no. 6, pp. 857–864, 2006.

[16] A. Sa Cunha, N. Carrere, B. Meunier et al., "Stump closure reinforcement with absorbable fibrin collagen sealant sponge (TachoSil) does not prevent pancreatic fistula after distal pancreatectomy: the FIABLE multicenter controlled randomized study," *The American Journal of Surgery*, vol. 210, no. 4, pp. 739–748, 2015.

[17] Y. Kluger, R. Alfici, B. Abbley, D. Soffer, and D. Aladgem, "Gastric serosal patch in distal pancreatectomy for injury: a neglected technique," *Injury*, vol. 28, no. 2, pp. 127–129, 1997.

[18] Y. Suzuki, Y. Kuroda, A. Morita et al., "Fibrin glue sealing for the prevention of pancreatic fistulas following distal pancreatectomy," *Archives of Surgery*, vol. 130, no. 9, pp. 952–955, 1995.

[19] I. Makino, H. Kitagawa, H. Nakagawara et al., "The management of a remnant pancreatic stump for preventing the development of postoperative pancreatic fistulas after distal pancreatectomy: current evidence and our strategy," *Surgery Today*, vol. 43, no. 6, pp. 595–602, 2013.

[20] Y. Suzuki, Y. Fujino, Y. Tanioka et al., "Randomized clinical trial of ultrasonic dissector or conventional division in distal pancreatectomy for non-fibrotic pancreas," *British Journal of Surgery*, vol. 86, no. 5, pp. 608–611, 1999.

[21] K. J. Zehr, "Use of bovine albumin-glutaraldehyde glue in cardiovascular surgery," *Annals of Thoracic Surgery*, vol. 84, no. 3, pp. 1048–1052, 2007.

[22] P. Tansley, F. Al-Mulhim, E. Lim, G. Ladas, and P. Goldstraw, "A prospective, randomized, controlled trial of the effectiveness of BioGlue in treating alveolar air leaks," *Journal of Thoracic and Cardiovascular Surgery*, vol. 132, no. 1, pp. 105–112, 2006.

[23] S. A. LeMaire, S. A. Carter, T. Won, X. Wang, L. D. Conklin, and J. S. Coselli, "The threat of adhesive embolization: BioGlue leaks through needle holes in aortic tissue and prosthetic grafts," *Annals of Thoracic Surgery*, vol. 80, no. 1, pp. 106–111, 2005.

[24] T. Lämsä, H.-T. Jin, J. Sand, and I. Nordback, "Tissue adhesives and the pancreas: biocompatibility and adhesive properties of 6 preparations," *Pancreas*, vol. 36, no. 3, pp. 261–266, 2008.

[25] E. G. Mourtzoukou, G. Pappas, G. Peppas, and M. E. Falagas, "Vaccination of asplenic or hyposplenic adults," *British Journal of Surgery*, vol. 95, no. 3, pp. 273–280, 2008.

[26] P. A. Clavien, J. Barkun, M. L. de Oliveira et al., "The clavien-dindo classification of surgical complications: five-year experience," *Annals of Surgery*, vol. 250, no. 2, pp. 187–196, 2009.

[27] C. Bassi, C. Dervenis, G. Butturini et al., "Postoperative pancreatic fistula: an international study group (ISGPF) definition," *Surgery*, vol. 138, no. 1, pp. 8–13, 2005.

[28] M. N. Wente, J. A. Veit, C. Bassi et al., "Postpancreatectomy hemorrhage (PPH)—an International Study Group of Pancreatic Surgery (ISGPS) definition," *Surgery*, vol. 142, no. 1, pp. 20–25, 2007.

[29] S. Nagai, T. Fujii, Y. Kodera et al., "Recurrence pattern and prognosis of pancreatic cancer after pancreatic fistula," *Annals of Surgical Oncology*, vol. 18, no. 8, pp. 2329–2337, 2011.

[30] T. I. Carter, Z. V. Fong, T. Hyslop et al., "A dual-institution randomized controlled trial of remnant closure after distal pancreatectomy: does the addition of a falciform patch and fibrin glue improve outcomes?" *Journal of Gastrointestinal Surgery*, vol. 17, no. 1, pp. 102–109, 2013.

[31] W. E. Fisher, C. Chai, S. E. Hodges, M.-F. Wu, S. G. Hilsenbeck, and F. C. Brunicardi, "Effect of BioGlue on the incidence of pancreatic fistula following pancreas resection," *Journal of Gastrointestinal Surgery*, vol. 12, no. 5, pp. 882–890, 2008.

[32] S. Ohwada, T. Ogawa, Y. Tanahashi et al., "Fibrin glue sandwich prevents pancreatic fistula following distal pancreatectomy," *World Journal of Surgery*, vol. 22, no. 5, pp. 494–498, 1998.

[33] T. Hackert and M. W. Buchler, "Remnant closure after distal pancreatectomy: current state and future perspectives," *Surgeon*, vol. 10, no. 2, pp. 95–101, 2012.

[34] M. M. Bilimoria, J. N. Cormier, Y. Mun, J. E. Lee, D. B. Evans, and P. W. T. Pisters, "Pancreatic leak after left pancreatectomy is reduced following main pancreatic duct ligation," *British Journal of Surgery*, vol. 90, no. 2, pp. 190–196, 2003.

[35] B. Suc, S. Msika, A. Fingerhut et al., "Temporary fibrin glue occlusion of the main pancreatic duct in the prevention of intra-abdominal complications after pancreatic resection: prospective randomized trial," *Annals of Surgery*, vol. 237, no. 1, pp. 57–65, 2003.

[36] W. Fürst and A. Banerjee, "Release of glutaraldehyde from an albumin-glutaraldehyde tissue adhesive causes significant in vitro and in vivo toxicity," *Annals of Thoracic Surgery*, vol. 79, no. 5, pp. 1522–1528, 2005.

[37] A. DeAnda, J. A. Elefteriades, N. W. Hasaniya, O. M. Lattouf, and R. R. Lazzara, "Improving outcomes through the use of surgical sealants for anastomotic sealing during cardiovascular surgery," *Journal of Cardiac Surgery*, vol. 24, no. 3, pp. 325–333, 2009.

[38] N. Abe, M. Sugiyama, Y. Suzuki et al., "Preoperative endoscopic pancreatic stenting for prophylaxis of pancreatic fistula development after distal pancreatectomy," *American Journal of Surgery*, vol. 191, no. 2, pp. 198–200, 2006.

[39] T. Okamoto, T. Gocho, Y. Futagawa et al., "Does preoperative pancreatic duct stenting prevent pancreatic fistula after surgery? A cohort study," *International Journal of Surgery*, vol. 6, no. 3, pp. 210–213, 2008.

29

Living-Donor Liver Transplantation and Hepatitis C

Nobuhisa Akamatsu[1,2] and Yasuhiko Sugawara[2]

[1] *Department of Hepato-Biliary-Pancreatic Surgery, Saitama Medical Center, Saitama Medical University, 1981 Tsujido-cho, Kamoda, Kawagoe, Saitama 350-8550, Japan*
[2] *Artificial Organ and Transplantation Division, Department of Surgery, Graduate School of Medicine, University of Tokyo, 7-3-1 Hongo, Bunkyo-ku, Tokyo 113-8655, Japan*

Correspondence should be addressed to Yasuhiko Sugawara; yasusugatky@yahoo.co.jp

Academic Editor: Andrea Lauterio

Hepatitis-C-virus- (HCV-) related end-stage cirrhosis is the primary indication for liver transplantation in many countries. Unfortunately, however, HCV is not eliminated by transplantation and graft reinfection is universal, resulting in fibrosis, cirrhosis, and finally graft decompression. In areas with low deceased-donor organ availability like Japan, living-donor liver transplantation (LDLT) is similarly indicated for HCV cirrhosis as deceased-donor liver transplantation (DDLT) in Western countries and accepted as an established treatment for HCV-cirrhosis, and the results are equivalent to those of DDLT. To prevent graft failure due to recurrent hepatitis C, antiviral treatment with pegylated-interferon and ribavirin is currently considered the most promising regimen with a sustained viral response rate of around 30% to 35%, although the survival benefit of this regimen remains to be investigated. In contrast to DDLT, many Japanese LDLT centers have reported modified treatment regimens as best efforts to secure first graft, such as aggressive preemptive antiviral treatment, escalation of dosages, and elongation of treatment duration.

1. Introduction

Since the first successful application of living donor liver transplantation (LDLT) in 1990 [1] and subsequent successful LDLT for adult recipient in 1994 [2], the use of live donors for liver transplantation has been widely applied to adult recipients where the availability of deceased-donors is severely restricted, like in Japan [3], and also accepted as a solution to the cadaveric donor shortage in Western countries [4].

End-stage liver disease caused by chronic hepatitis C virus (HCV) infection is the leading cause of liver transplantation in developed countries [5, 6], including Japan [7]. Unfortunately, liver transplantation does not cure HCV-infected recipients, but re-infection of HCV universally occurs and disease progression is accelerated compared with that in the nontransplant population, resulting in poor outcomes for HCV-infected recipients [8].

The aim of this paper was to overview the current trends and controversies in LDLT for patients with HCV in relation to the perspectives from deceased-donor liver transplantation (DDLT).

2. Natural History of Hepatitis C after Orthotopic Liver Transplantation

Accumulating perspectives of disease recurrence in HCV-infected recipients have been obtained in DDLT within the last two decades. HCV reinfection occurs just after reperfusion followed by a rapid increase in HCV ribonucleic acid (RNA) levels within 4 postoperative months [9]. The histologic features of liver injury usually resemble those of nontransplant HCV hepatitis typically developing after 3 months, but the clinical presentation, severity, and outcome are extremely heterogeneous and more profound compared to those in immune competent patients [10]. Progression to cirrhosis usually takes 9 to 12 years after liver transplantation with a linear progression of histologic fibrosis [10, 11]. A less common, but well-documented, form of recurrence is called fibrosing cholestatic hepatitis (<10%), possibly mediated by a direct cytopathic mechanism under an extremely high viral load and immune-compromised condition. Graft failure occurs in 50% of recipients within a few months after fibrosing cholestatic hepatitis develops [12]. Some HCV-reinfected recipients, however, show no apparent disease progression for at least the first decade and their graft injury remains mild or even absent despite a high vira burden.

Overall, cirrhosis develops in approximately 25% of liver transplant recipients (range 8%–44%) after 5 to 10 years and this percentage is likely to increase with an increase in the follow-up period [10, 11]. Once cirrhosis is complete, survival time is severely decreased and decompression is encountered with cumulative rates at 1 and 3 years of 40% and 60%, respectively, which finally results in graft failure [11, 13].

The development of decompensated cirrhosis due to recurrent hepatitis C is now the most frequent cause of graft failure, patient death, and the need for retransplantation in HCV-infected recipients [11, 13–17]. As a result, survival is significantly decreased compared with other indications, an overall 10% difference at 3 years [18]. In the most recent United Network for Organ Sharing/Organ Procurement and Transplantation Network (UNOS/OPTN) study from the United States, 3-year survival is 78% among 7459 HCV-positive recipients compared with 82% among 20734 HCV-negative recipients ($P < 0.0001$; http://www.unos.org) [19].

The poor outcome of HCV-positive recipients has resulted in the divergence in transplant outcomes between HCV-positive recipients and HCV-negative recipients. Improvements in organ preservation, surgical techniques, and postoperative care have dramatically improved the survival of HCV-negative recipients over the last two decades, whereas this has not been the case in HCV-positive recipients for whom outcome has remained unchanged or even worsened over time [19–22].

3. Current Status of LDLT

In areas with low deceased-donor organ availability like Japan, the indication of LDLT for HCV cirrhosis is similar to that of DDLT [7], whereas in Western countries, LDLT is conducted in an attempt to alleviate the shortage of donor organs and decrease the mortality among patients awaiting transplants, accounting for only 3% to 4% of all liver transplants [23].

According to the Japan Liver Transplantation Society [24], a total of 6097 LDLTs, comprising 98% of all liver transplants, have been performed till the end of 2010 in Japan. Among those, 3796 were adult cases including 1200 (32%) cases of HCV-related disease as a leading indication for adult LDLT. The 1, 3, 5, and 10 year survival rates of all adult LDLT and those of HCV-positive adults were 81%, 75%, 72%, and 66%, and 78%, 72%, 68%, and 59%, respectively, without difference.

In the United States, nearly 3000 LDLTs have been performed by the end of 2009, with decreased number of

cases annually, comprising only 4.5% of all liver transplants [23, 25, 26].

4. LDLT as a Risk Factor for Recurrent Hepatitis C Studies Comparing Outcomes of LDLT and DDLT

Based on the significant negative impact of recurrent hepatitis C on recipients' outcome, it is critical to identify the factors related to severe recurrent hepatitis C [8, 13]. In the transplant setting, many factors contribute to disease progression compared with nontransplant patients [13], including, viral-related factors [10, 27–36], donor age [17, 37–43], recipient-related factors [32, 44–49], graft and surgical factors [40, 50–57], and immunosuppressive agents [58–75] (Table 1) however, many aspects remain unclear and require further investigation [8]. Among those, the possibility of increased severity of recurrent HCV in LDLT patients had been one of the hottest debates. The benefit of LDLT might be offset if the outcome of LDLT for HCV-positive recipients is worse than that of DDLT.

Early studies raised some negative concerns regarding the outcomes of LDLT in HCV patients, such as a poorer graft outcome and earlier and more aggressive HCV recurrence after LDLT compared with DDLT [144–146]. Several theories have been proposed to explain the differences in HCV recurrence between LDLT and DDLT recipients. One possible explanation is that the intense hepatocyte proliferation that occurs in partial liver grafts may lead to increased viral translation and replication [145, 147–149]. Genetic donor-recipient similarity is another proposed mechanism for more severe HCV recurrence [150, 151]. Recent studies, however, comparing outcomes of LDLT and DDLT in HCV-infected patients have not only failed to identify LDLT as a risk factor for more intense viral recurrence with impaired outcome, but also revealed improved results in LDLT recipients [39, 84–95], which do not support the aforementioned speculations. Alternatively, recent studies favored the theory that outcomes of LDLT for HCV cirrhosis could be better than those of DDLT due to the younger donor age and shorter ischemic time of LDLT grafts. The studies comparing outcomes between LDLT and DDLT in HCV-infected recipients are summarized in Table 2.

While several earlier studies demonstrated impaired patient/graft survival and severe histologic findings in LDLT [144–146], the majority of studies reported equal or even improved outcomes both in patient/graft survival and in fibrosis progression in LDLT [39, 84–95]. Since the large UNOS database study [87] demonstrated comparable short-term (24 months) survival between LDLT and DDLT, subsequent studies with considerable follow-up period have been published demonstrating comparable or even superior outcome in LDLT. Five-year patient survival ranged 71% to 84% in HCV-positive LDLT recipients among studies with sufficient follow-up period [39, 86, 94, 95]. Additionally, as Terrault et al. [92] reported, the learning curve for the LDLT procedure may have a considerable impact on the outcome of LDLT for HCV cirrhosis, which has been repeatedly pointed

TABLE 1: Factors associated with the severity of recurrent hepatitis C after liver transplantation.

Variables	Effect on recurrent hepatitis C
Donor and graft factors	
Age [17, 37–43]	More severe disease (>40, >50, >65)
Steatosis [56, 57, 76–79]	Few studies
Prolonged ischemic time [54, 55, 80–83]	More severe disease
HCV+ graft [6, 22, 40, 50–53, 76]	No influence
Reduced size versus whole liver (LDLT versus DDLT) [39, 84–95]	No difference
Pretransplant recipient factors	
Genotype 1b [8, 32, 33, 35, 40]	Controversial
Pre-LT higher viral load [21, 28, 96, 97]	Unclear
Age [32, 44, 98]	Few studies
Race [45, 46, 99]	Few studies
Sex [20, 47, 48]	Few studies
HIV coinfection [100–107]	No influence
IL-28B gene polymorphism [49, 108–111]	More severe disease in CT and TT genotype
Posttransplant recipient factors	
Post-LT higher viral load [10, 27–31]	More severe disease
CMV infection [22, 29, 32, 112–116]	Unclear
Diabetes mellitus (Metabolic syndrome) [29, 117–121]	More severe disease
Immunosuppression	
Steroid bolus/OKT3 [6, 21, 22, 58, 59, 122–124]	More severe disease
Maintenance steroid [34, 60–62, 122]	Severe disease when rapidly tapered
Steroid free regimen [63–68, 125–127]	No influence
Tacrolimus versus cyclosporine [69–75]	No difference
Anti-IL-2 receptor antibodies [63, 126, 128–131]	Controversial
Azathioprine/mycophenolate mofetil [132–140]	Controversial
mTOR inhibitors [141–143]	Few studies

CMV: cytomegalovirus; DDLT: deceased-donor liver transplantation; HCV: hepatitis C virus; HIV: human immunodeficiency virus; LDLT: living-donor liver transplantation; LT: liver transplantation; mTOR: mammalian target of rapamycin.

out by recent authors. Actually, none of reports after 2005 has found impaired outcome in LDLT.

These data should be interpreted with caution, however, because of the important clinical distinction between LDLT and DDLT. At the time of transplantation, DDLT recipients are far sicker than LDLT recipients as represented by a significantly higher MELD score, donor age is higher, and graft ischemic time is longer. Indeed, significantly poorer preoperative condition and older donor age in DDLT recipients were indicated in 7 and 6 studies, respectively, among 16 studies listed in Table 2. Additionally, cold ischemia time is significantly longer in DDLT than that in LDLT in all studies. All these factors, as presented in Table 1, are considered independent prognostic factors for severe HCV recurrence and impaired patient/graft outcome. Actually, Jain et al. [95], who recently reported that both patient/graft survival and histologic findings are better in LDLT, found in a subanalysis of the study that adjusting for MELD score (<25) and donor age (<50) resulted in similar outcomes.

Based on accumulating reports demonstrating comparable outcome of LDLT and DDLT for HCV cirrhosis, and refinement of surgical techniques and management in LDLT, hepatitis C recurrence by itself does not seem to explain the differences in patient/graft survival between LDLT and DDLT, and even improved outcomes could be achieved in LDLT due to the better quality of the graft, younger donors, and less sick recipient condition at the time of transplantation. Furthermore, based on these benefits of LDLT, donor selection to improve outcome of LDLT for HCV positive recipients could be assumed. Selecting younger donors [17] or donors with favorable IL-28B genotype [108, 109] could be possible future issues; however, with the severe lack of live donors, it seems impractical in clinical setting at present. Anyway, LDLT could be strongly recommended for HCV-positive patients whenever it is available.

5. Antiviral Treatment

Antiviral treatments for recurrent hepatitis C after liver transplantation include eradication of the HCV virus before transplantation with the use of pretransplant antiviral treatment, eradication of HCV virus early after transplantation preemptively to prevent graft damage, and treatment for established recurrent hepatitis C in the acute, or more commonly, chronic phase. Regardless of the antiviral treatment timing, interferon (INF), especially pegylated-INF (PEG-INF), in conjunction with ribavirin (RBV), is currently accepted as a standard key drug in achieving high sustained

TABLE 2: Studies comparing living-donor liver transplantation and deceased-donor liver transplantation in patients with hepatitis C cirrhosis.

Author	Year	n (LDLT/DDLT)	MELD score (LDLT/DDLT)	Donor age (LDLT/DDLT)	Cold ischemia time (h) (LDL/DDLT)	Follow-up (mo)	Histologic progression	Patient survival LDLT/DDLT (%)	Graft survival LDLT/DDLT (%)	Comments
Gaglio et al. [144]	2003	68 (23/45)	12.6/28*	NA	NA	24	NA	87/89	87/85	No difference in outcomes, increased risk of cholestatic hepatitis in LDLT
García-Retortillo et al. [145]	2004	117 (22/95)	11 (5–24)/11 (2–28)	31 (19–58)/47 (13–86)#	NA	22	Significantly severe in LDLT	NA	NA	Severe hepatitis C recurrence in LDLT
Thuluvath and Yoo [146]	2004	619 (207/412)	NA	$35.8 \pm 0.4/38.9 \pm 18.1$†	$3.9 \pm 7.3/8.4 \pm 4.5$†	24	NA	79/81	74/73	Lower graft survival in LDLT
Humar et al. [85]	2005	51 (12/39)	17 (14–27)/24 (17–40)*	$37.7 \pm 9.2/42.8 \pm 16.2$#	$10.2 \pm 4.2/<1$†	28.3	Significantly severe in DDLT	92/90	NA	LDLT may be at a low risk for HCV recurrence
Shiffman et al. [84]	2004	76 (23/53)	$13.5 \pm 1.1/16.2 \pm 1.0$	$47.6 \pm 2/47.8 \pm 0.8$	NA	36	No difference	79/82	76/82	No difference in outcomes
Maluf et al. [86]	2005	126 (29/97)	$13.2 \pm 1.1/21 \pm 0.8$*	NA	$0.6 \pm 0.2/7.5 \pm 2.8$†	72	NA	67/70	64/69	No difference in survival, more rejection in DDLT and biliary complications in LDLT
Russo et al. [87]	2004	4234 (279/3955)	NA (TB, PT and Cre were significantly worse in DDLT)	37/40#	8.1/2.6†	24	NA	83/81	72/75	No difference in outcomes
Bozorgzadeh et al. [88]	2004	100 (35/65)	$14.9 \pm 4/15.9 \pm 5.3$	$34.6 \pm 9.7/49.2 \pm 20.4$	NA	39	No difference	89/75	83/64	No difference in outcomes
Van Vlierberghe et al. [89]	2004	43 (17/26)	$15 \pm 9/15 \pm 8$	$31 \pm 8/48 \pm 17$	$3.1 \pm 1.3/11.1 \pm 2.6$†	12	No difference	No difference (Presented with only figure)	No difference (Presented with only figure)	No difference in outcomes in short-term
Schiano et al. [90]	2005	26 (11/15)	14 (9–19)/18 (10–31) $P = 0.05$	33 (20–54)/47 (13–73)	0.6 (0.3–1.0)/10 (4.4–20)†	24	NA	73/80	73/80	No difference in survival, accelerated viral load increase in LDLT
Guo et al. [91]	2006	67 (15/52)	$16.9 \pm 6.9/19.0 \pm 8.3$	NA	NA	24	No difference	93/96	87/94	No difference in outcomes
Terrault et al. [92]	2007	275 (181/94)	14 (6–40)/18 (7–40)*	38 (19–57)/41 (9–72)	0.8 (0.1–8)/6.7 (0.2–10)†	36	No difference	74/82	68/80	No significant difference in patient/graft survival in experienced LDLT centers
Schmeding et al. [93]	2007	289 (20/269)	NA	$38.6 \pm 15.2/44.2 \pm 12$	NA	60	No difference	Better in DDLT ($P = 0.011$)	Better in DDLT ($P = 0.006$)	LDLT does not increase the risk and severity of HCV recurrence. No difference in patient/graft survival when HCC beyond Milan excluded.
Selzner et al. [94]	2008	201 (46/155)	14 (7–39)/17 (6–40)	38 (19–59)/46 (11–79)#	1.5 (0.5–4.9)/7.5 (1.1–16)†	60	Significantly severe in DDLT	84/78	76/74	Donor age, rather than transplant approach, affects the progression of HCV
Gallegos-Orozco et al. [39]	2009	200 (32/168)	$14.6 \pm 4.7/25.5 \pm 5.9$*	$35 \pm 12/40 \pm 16$ $P = 0.05$	NA	60	No difference	81/81	NA	LDLT is a good option for HCV cirrhosis
Jain et al. [95]	2011	100 (35/65)	$14.5 \pm 3.9/16.8 \pm 7.3$*	$34.3 \pm 9.3/47.2 \pm 19.8$#	11 ± 3.1 in DDLT	84	Significantly severe in DDLT at all time points	77/65	71/46	Both patient/graft survival and histologic findings were better in LDLT

* MELD score is significantly higher in DDLT.

Donor age is significantly higher in DDLT.

† Cold ischemia time is significantly longer in DDLT.

Cre: creatinine; DDLT: deceased-donor liver transplantation; LDLT: living-donor liver transplantation; MELD: model for end-stage liver disease; NA: not available; PT: prothombin-time; TB: total bilirubin.

viral response (SVR) rate according to the perspectives obtained in nontransplant populations.

Former two strategies, however, have almost been abandoned in Western countries. Pretransplant treatment is severely limited by poor liver function, a high prevalence of nonresponders, severe cytopenia, and complications, including life-threatening infections [152], and to date, only six studies [153–158] have been published in this phase with differences in the treatment duration (6–14 months versus 2-3 months) and in regimens used (INF only, INF/RBV, or PEG-INF/RBV). Regardless of the approach used, the results are similar, resulting in the prevention of HCV re-infection in about 20% of treated patients with high discontinuation rate and high dose reduction rate [152]. Considering the less severe disease of LDLT recipients as discussed earlier, pretransplant antiviral treatment seems more preferable for LDLT recipients to improve outcome; however, no such trial has been published so far in LDLT setting. This issue also seems remain to be investigated in future studies as with the case in live donor selection issues.

Prophylactic or preemptive antiviral treatment generally means antiviral treatment with INF/PEG-INF and RBV started early posttransplant, without requiring evidence of recurrent hepatitis C. In published studies [159–164] of preemptive antiviral therapy, SVR rates are reported to range from 8% to 34% (5% to 43% for genotype 1 and 14% to 100% for genotypes 2 or 3), with the rates of dose reduction and drug discontinuation are approximately 70% and 30%, respectively, due to the existence of cytopenia, renal dysfunction, rejection, or extrahepatic complications, and high levels of immunosuppression in this time window. The most recently published prospective, multicenter, randomized study (PHOENIX study) by Bzowej et al. [165] was designed to compare the efficacy, tolerability, and safety of an escalating dose regimen of PEG-INF alpha 2a/RBV for 48 weeks for preemptive antiviral treatment versus no treatment, which showed only 22% SVR in the prophylaxis patients with the rate of marked HCV recurrence at 120 weeks (62% in prophylaxis patients versus 65% in observation patients), and comparable fibrosis progression 120 weeks as well as similar patient/graft survival in both study arms. Dose reduction and discontinuation were required in 70% and 28%, respectively. Based on these results, European and United States transplant societies do not support the routine use of preemptive antiviral therapy.

Consequently, initiating antiviral therapy with PEG-INF/RBV after the confirmation of recurrent hepatitis C in the graft by liver biopsies is the mainstay for the treatment of recurrent disease in Western countries [35, 166–190]. Most of the data come from uncontrolled studies with different designs regarding time to start treatment, regimen used, and follow-up, but treatment duration is generally 48 to 52 weeks. Therefore, the results were also very different, with SVR rates ranging 0% to 56% (median: 33%), discontinuation rates ranging 4% to 58%, and dose reduction rate ranging 28% to 100%. In addition, the survival benefit of the treatment has not been confirmed in most studies so far, and it is compelling to conclude that there is currently no evidence to support the antiviral treatment for recurrent graft hepatitis C due to the lack of clinical benefit and frequent adverse effects, as concluded by the recent Cochrane meta-analysis [191]. On the other hand, recent retrospective cohort studies with a considerable follow-up duration found improved patient/graft survival in patients who obtained an SVR after antiviral treatment [35, 192–194]. Further randomized clinical trials with appropriate trial methodology and adequate follow-up duration are necessary to confirm an actual survival benefit of antiviral treatment.

6. Reports from Japanese LDLT Centers

Although retransplantation is the only potentially curative option for those with decompressed cirrhosis due to recurrent hepatitis C, in contrast to Western countries where re-DDLT is spared as a last resort [195, 196], it is extremely unlikely in Japan to perform retransplantation for patients with recurrent end-stage hepatitis C, if not absolutely impossible. These backgrounds might have led to various modified strategies for the treatment of recurrent disease as best efforts to secure first graft, such as aggressive preemptive antiviral treatment, escalation of dosages, and elongation of treatment duration.

We have reported preemptive INF/RBV treatment for HCV-positive LDLT recipients [161, 197–199]. Preemptive treatment was started just after recipient's condition had become stable (approximately one month after LDLT) with low-dose INF alpha 2b and RBV (400 mg/day) followed by escalation to PEG-INF (1.5 μg/kg per week) and RBV (800 mg/day) depending on patient's tolerance. The treatment duration was not settled, and was continued for additional 12 months after the serum HCV-RNA became negative. The response was considered to be SVR provided negative serologic results for another 6 months after discontinuation of therapy. That is, nonstopping peg-INF/RBV approach was applied for non-responders. Among 122 HCV-positive LDLT recipients, 42 (34%) achieved SVR and those with SVR showed significantly improved survival when compared to those without SVR (cumulative 5-year survival rate; 97% versus 66%) [199].

Kyoto group also reported modified PEG-INF/RBV treatment with individualized extension, while they started antiviral treatment for cases with biopsy-proven recurrent disease [200–202]. They started with PEG-INF (1.5 μg/kg per week) and RBV (400–800 mg/day) for 12 months for all patients with recurrent hepatitis. Then, full dose treatment was continued for additional 8–22 months for those whose serum HCV-RNA became negative within 12 months, while patients who did not become negative for serum HCV RNA within 12 months continued to receive a low-dose PEG-INF (0.5–0.75 μg/kg per week) with or without reduced RBV (200 mg/day) as maintenance treatment. Among 80 patients with recurrent hepatitis C after LDLT, SVR was achieved in 31 (39%), while remaining 49 (61%) received maintenance therapy among those 26 (53%) discontinued. In comparison to fibrosis progression, no difference was observed between SVR group and maintenance treatment group with improved or stable fibrosis in both groups, while those who withdrew from maintenance showed significantly deteriorated fibrosis [202].

Kyushu group performed antiviral treatment for 80 patients among 106 consecutive HCV-positive recipients, excluding 26 cases of early death, negative HCV RNA, and refusal for treatment [203]. Basically, they started with PEG-INF (0.5 µg/kg per week) and RBV (200 mg/day), then escalated to PEG-INF (1.5 µg/kg per week) and RBV (800 mg/day), with the treatment duration of 48 weeks and over 72 weeks for those with early viral response and for those without it, respectively. They reported overall SVR rate of 35%. They found both significantly severe fibrosis and impaired graft survival in those who did not show viral nor biochemical response.

Other Japanese centers [204–207] have also reported similar modified antiviral treatment with PEG-INF and RBV including dose escalation, treatment for all HCV-positive cases, and extension of treatment. Additionally, simultaneous splenectomy during LDLT operation in an attempt to improve tolerance to antiviral treatment, SVR rate and further graft survival should be noticed [198, 208, 209].

7. Conclusion

Hepatitis C is here to stay and will remain the most common indication for liver transplantation. In the areas where cadaveric organs are extremely limited like in Japan, indication of LDLT is same as that of DDLT, and recent studies have proved that LDLT can be performed as safely and effectively as DDLT for HCV-infected patients in experienced centers. Further investigation for more effective and tolerable antiviral treatment is warranted to secure the first live donor graft to the possible extent.

Abbreviations

DDLT:	Deceased-donor liver transplantation
HCV:	Hepatitis C virus
HIV:	Human immunodeficiency virus
INF:	Interferon
LDLT:	Living-donor liver transplantation
MELD:	Model for end-stage liver disease
MMF:	Mycophenolate mofetil
mTOR:	Mammalian target of rapamycin
PEG-INF:	Pegylated-interferon
RBV:	Ribavirin
RNA:	Ribonucleic acid
SVR:	Sustained viral response
UNOS/OPTN:	The United Network for Organ Sharing/Organ Procurement and Transplantation Network.

References

[1] R. W. Strong, S. V. Lynch, T. H. Ong, H. Matsunami, Y. Koido, and G. A. Balderson, "Successful liver transplantation from a living donor to her son," *New England Journal of Medicine*, vol. 322, no. 21, pp. 1505–1507, 1990.

[2] Y. Hashikura, M. Makuuchi, S. Kawasaki et al., "Successful living-related partial liver transplantation to an adult patient," *Lancet*, vol. 343, no. 8907, pp. 1233–1234, 1994.

[3] Y. Sugawara and M. Makuuchi, "Advances in adult living donor liver transplantation: a review based on reports from the 10th anniversary of the adult-to-adult living donor liver transplantation meeting in Tokyo," *Liver Transplantation*, vol. 10, no. 6, pp. 715–720, 2004.

[4] R. M. Merion, "Current status and future of liver transplantation," *Seminars in Liver Disease*, vol. 30, no. 4, pp. 411–421, 2010.

[5] R. Adam, P. McMaster, J. G. O'Grady et al., "Evolution of liver transplantation in Europe: report of the European liver transplant registry," *Liver Transplantation*, vol. 9, no. 12, pp. 1231–1243, 2003.

[6] R. H. Wiesner, M. Sorrell, F. Villamil et al., "Report of the first international liver transplantation society expert panel consensus conference on liver transplantation and hepatitis C," *Liver Transplantation*, vol. 9, no. 11, pp. S1–S9, 2003.

[7] Y. Sugawara and M. Makuuchi, "Living donor liver transplantation to patients with hepatitis C virus cirrhosis," *World Journal of Gastroenterology*, vol. 12, no. 28, pp. 4461–4465, 2006.

[8] M. Berenguer, R. Charco, J. M. Pascasio et al., "Spanish society of liver transplantation (SETH) consensus recommendations on hepatitis C virus and liver transplantation," *Liver International*, vol. 32, no. 5, pp. 712–713, 2012.

[9] M. Garcia-Retortillo, X. Forns, A. Feliu et al., "Hepatitis C virus kinetics during and immediately after liver transplantation," *Hepatology*, vol. 35, no. 3, pp. 680–687, 2002.

[10] E. J. Gane, B. G. Portmann, N. V. Naoumov et al., "Long-term outcome of hepatitis C infection after liver transplantation," *New England Journal of Medicine*, vol. 334, no. 13, pp. 815–820, 1996.

[11] M. Berenguer, M. Prieto, J. M. Rayón et al., "Natural history of clinically compensated hepatitis C virus-related graft cirrhosis after liver transplantation," *Hepatology*, vol. 32, no. 4, part 1, pp. 852–858, 2000.

[12] T. K. Narang, W. Ahrens, and M. W. Russo, "Post-liver transplant cholestatic hepatitis C: a systematic review of clinical and pathological findings and application of consensus criteria," *Liver Transplantation*, vol. 16, no. 11, pp. 1228–1235, 2010.

[13] B. Roche and D. Samuel, "Risk factors for hepatitis C recurrence after liver transplantation," *Journal of Viral Hepatitis*, vol. 14, no. 1, pp. 89–96, 2007.

[14] L. M. Forman, J. D. Lewis, J. A. Berlin, H. I. Feldman, and M. R. Lucey, "The association between hepatitis C infection and survival after orthotopic liver transplantation," *Gastroenterology*, vol. 122, no. 4, pp. 889–896, 2002.

[15] M. Ghabril, R. Dickson, and R. Wiesner, "Improving outcomes of liver retransplantation: an analysis of trends and the impact of hepatitis C infection," *American Journal of Transplantation*, vol. 8, no. 2, pp. 404–411, 2008.

[16] M. Berenguer, "Natural history of recurrent hepatitis C," *Liver Transplantation*, vol. 8, no. 10, supplement 1, pp. S14–S18, 2002.

[17] M. Berenguer, M. Prieto, F. S. Juan et al., "Contribution of donor age to the recent decrease in patient survival among HCV-infected liver transplant recipients," *Hepatology*, vol. 36, no. 1, pp. 202–210, 2002.

[18] A. Rubin, V. Aguilera, and M. Berenguer, "Liver transplantation and hepatitis C," *Clinics and Research in Hepatology and Gastroenterology*, vol. 35, no. 12, pp. 805–812, 2011.

[19] P. J. Thuluvath, K. L. Krok, D. L. Segev, and H. Y. Yoo, "Trends in post-liver transplant survival in patients with hepatitis C between 1991 and 2001 in the United States," *Liver Transplantation*, vol. 13, no. 5, pp. 719–724, 2007.

[20] L. S. Belli, A. K. Burroughs, P. Burra et al., "Liver transplantation for HCV cirrhosis: improved survival in recent years and increased severity of recurrent disease in female recipients: results of a long term retrospective study," *Liver Transplantation*, vol. 13, no. 5, pp. 733–740, 2007.

[21] M. Berenguer, L. Ferrell, J. Watson et al., "HCV-related fibrosis progression following liver transplantation: increase in recent years," *Journal of Hepatology*, vol. 32, no. 4, pp. 673–684, 2000.

[22] D. Samuel, X. Forns, M. Berenguer et al., "Report of the monothematic EASL conference on liver transplantation for viral hepatitis," *Journal of Hepatology*, vol. 45, no. 1, pp. 127–143, 2006.

[23] K. M. Olthoff, M. M. Abecassis, J. C. Emond et al., "Outcomes of adult living donor liver transplantation: comparison of the adult-to-adult living donor liver transplantation cohort study and the national experience," *Liver Transplantation*, vol. 17, no. 7, pp. 789–797, 2011.

[24] The Japanese Liver Transplantation Society, "Liver transplantation in Japan. Registry by the Japanese liver transplantation society," *Japanese Journal of Transplantation*, vol. 46, no. 6, pp. 524–536, 2011.

[25] M. G. Ghany, D. B. Strader, D. L. Thomas, and L. B. Seeff, "Diagnosis, management, and treatment of hepatitis C: an update," *Hepatology*, vol. 49, no. 4, pp. 1335–1374, 2009.

[26] P. A. Vagefi, N. L. Ascher, C. E. Freise et al., "Use of living donor liver transplantation varies with the availability of deceased donor liver transplantation," *Liver Transplantation*, vol. 18, no. 2, pp. 160–165, 2012.

[27] E. J. Gane, N. V. Naoumov, K. P. Qian et al., "A longitudinal analysis of hepatitis C virus replication following liver transplantation," *Gastroenterology*, vol. 110, no. 1, pp. 167–177, 1996.

[28] R. Sreekumar, A. Gonzalez-Koch, Y. Maor-Kendler et al., "Early identification of recipients with progressive histologic recurrence of hepatitis C after liver transplantation," *Hepatology*, vol. 32, no. 5, pp. 1125–1130, 2000.

[29] I. A. Hanouneh, A. E. Feldstein, A. J. McCullough et al., "The significance of metabolic syndrome in the setting of recurrent hepatitis C after liver transplantation," *Liver Transplantation*, vol. 14, no. 9, pp. 1287–1293, 2008.

[30] G. V. Papatheodoridis, S. G. Barton, D. Andrew et al., "Longitudinal variation in hepatitis C virus (HCV) viraemia and early course of HCV infection after liver transplantation for HCV cirrhosis: the role of different immunosuppressive regimens," *Gut*, vol. 45, no. 3, pp. 427–434, 1999.

[31] N. A. Shackel, J. Jamias, W. Rahman et al., "Early high peak hepatitis C viral load levels independently predict hepatitis C-related liver failure post-liver transplantation," *Liver Transplantation*, vol. 15, no. 7, pp. 709–718, 2009.

[32] C. Feray, L. Caccamo, G. J. Alexander et al., "European collaborative study on factors influencing outcome after liver transplantation for hepatitis C. European concerted action on viral hepatitis (EUROHEP) group," *Gastroenterology*, vol. 117, no. 3, pp. 619–625, 1999.

[33] H. E. Vargas, T. Laskus, L. F. Wang et al., "The influence of hepatitis C virus genotypes on the outcome of liver transplantation," *Liver Transplantation and Surgery*, vol. 4, no. 1, pp. 22–27, 1998.

[34] M. Berenguer, J. Crippin, R. Gish et al., "A model to predict severe HCV-related disease following liver transplantation," *Hepatology*, vol. 38, no. 1, pp. 34–41, 2003.

[35] N. Selzner, E. L. Renner, M. Selzner et al., "Antiviral treatment of recurrent Hepatitis C after liver transplantation: predictors of response and long-term outcome," *Transplantation*, vol. 88, no. 10, pp. 1214–1221, 2009.

[36] C. Féray, M. Gigou, D. Samuel et al., "Influence of the genotypes of hepatitis C virus on the severity of recurrent liver disease after liver transplantation," *Gastroenterology*, vol. 108, no. 4, pp. 1088–1096, 1995.

[37] D. G. Maluf, E. B. Edwards, R. T. Stravitz, and H. M. Kauffman, "Impact of the donor risk index on the outcome of hepatitis C virus-positive Liver transplant recipients," *Liver Transplantation*, vol. 15, no. 6, pp. 592–599, 2009.

[38] K. Rifai, M. Sebagh, V. Karam et al., "Donor age influences 10-year liver graft histology independently of hepatitis C virus infection," *Journal of Hepatology*, vol. 41, no. 3, pp. 446–453, 2004.

[39] J. F. Gallegos-Orozco, A. Yosephy, B. Noble et al., "Natural history of post-liver transplantation hepatitis C: a review of factors that may influence its course," *Liver Transplantation*, vol. 15, no. 12, pp. 1872–1881, 2009.

[40] A. P. Khapra, K. Agarwal, M. I. Fiel et al., "Impact of donor age on survival and fibrosis progression in patients with hepatitis C undergoing liver transplantation using HCV+ allografts," *Liver Transplantation*, vol. 12, no. 10, pp. 1496–1503, 2006.

[41] S. C. Rayhill, Y. M. Wu, D. A. Katz et al., "Older donor livers show early severe histological activity, fibrosis, and graft failure after liver transplantation for hepatitis C," *Transplantation*, vol. 84, no. 3, pp. 331–339, 2007.

[42] V. I. Machicao, H. Bonatti, M. Krishna et al., "Donor age affects fibrosis progression and graft survival after liver transplantation for hepatitis C," *Transplantation*, vol. 77, no. 1, pp. 84–92, 2004.

[43] A. W. Avolio, U. Cillo, M. Salizzoni et al., "Balancing donor and recipient risk factors in liver transplantation: the value of D-MELD with particular reference to HCV recipients," *American Journal of Transplantation*, vol. 11, no. 12, pp. 2724–2736, 2011.

[44] M. Selzner, A. Kashfi, N. Selzner et al., "Recipient age affects long-term outcome and hepatitis C recurrence in old donor livers following transplantation," *Liver Transplantation*, vol. 15, no. 10, pp. 1288–1295, 2009.

[45] P. S. Pang, A. Kamal, and J. S. Glenn, "The effect of donor race on the survival of black Americans undergoing liver transplantation for chronic hepatitis C," *Liver Transplantation*, vol. 15, no. 9, pp. 1126–1132, 2009.

[46] V. Saxena, J. C. Lai, J. G. O. 'Leary et al., "Donor-recipient race mismatch in African-American ant patients with chronic hepatitis C," *Liver Transplantation*, vol. 18, no. 5, pp. 524–531, 2012.

[47] T. Walter, J. Dumortier, O. Guillaud, V. Hervieu, J. Y. Scoazec, and O. Boillot, "Factors influencing the progression of fibrosis in patients with recurrent hepatitis C after liver transplantation under antiviral therapy: a retrospective analysis of 939 liver biopsies in a single center," *Liver Transplantation*, vol. 13, no. 2, pp. 294–301, 2007.

[48] J. C. Lai, E. C. Verna, R. S. Brown et al., "Hepatitis C virus-infected women have a higher risk of advanced fibrosis and graft loss after liver transplantation than men," *Hepatology*, vol. 54, no. 2, pp. 418–424, 2011.

[49] M. R. Charlton, A. Thompson, B. J. Veldt et al., "Interleukin-28B polymorphisms are associated with histological recurrence and

treatment response following liver transplantation in patients with hepatitis C virus infection," *Hepatology*, vol. 53, no. 1, pp. 317–324, 2011.

[50] P. G. Northup, C. K. Argo, D. T. Nguyen et al., "Liver allografts from hepatitis C positive donors can offer good outcomes in hepatitis C positive recipients: a us national transplant registry analysis," *Transplant International*, vol. 23, no. 10, pp. 1038–1044, 2010.

[51] J. I. Arenas, H. E. Vargas, and J. Rakela, "The use of hepatitis C-infected grafts in liver transplantation," *Liver Transplantation*, vol. 9, no. 11, pp. S48–S51, 2003.

[52] R. Ballarin, A. Cucchetti, M. Spaggiari et al., "Long-term follow-up and outcome of liver transplantation from anti-hepatitis C virus-positive donors: a European multicentric case-control study," *Transplantation*, vol. 91, no. 11, pp. 1265–1272, 2011.

[53] A. T. Burr, Y. Li, J. F. Tseng et al., "Survival after liver transplantation using hepatitis C virus-positive donor allografts: case-controlled analysis of the UNOS database," *World Journal of Surgery*, vol. 35, no. 7, pp. 1590–1595, 2011.

[54] K. D. S. Watt, E. R. Lyden, J. M. Gulizia, and T. M. McCashland, "Recurrent hepatitis C posttransplant: early preservation injury may predict poor outcome," *Liver Transplantation*, vol. 12, no. 1, pp. 134–139, 2006.

[55] P. W. Baron, D. Sindram, D. Higdon et al., "Prolonged rewarming time during allograft implantation predisposes to recurrent hepatitis C infection after liver transplantation," *Liver Transplantation*, vol. 6, no. 4, pp. 407–412, 2000.

[56] D. Brandman, A. Pingitore, J. C. Lai et al., "Hepatic steatosis at 1 year is an additional predictor of subsequent fibrosis severity in liver transplant recipients with recurrent hepatitis C virus," *Liver Transplantation*, vol. 17, no. 12, pp. 1380–1386, 2011.

[57] V. Subramanian, A. B. Seetharam, N. Vachharajani et al., "Donor graft steatosis influences immunity to hepatitis C virus and allograft outcome after liver transplantation," *Transplantation*, vol. 92, no. 11, pp. 1259–1268, 2011.

[58] J. R. Lake, "The role of immunosuppression in recurrence of hepatitis C," *Liver Transplantation*, vol. 9, no. 11, pp. S63–S66, 2003.

[59] P. A. Sheiner, M. E. Schwartz, E. Mor et al., "Severe or multiple rejection episodes are associated with early recurrence of hepatitis C after orthotopic liver transplantation," *Hepatology*, vol. 21, no. 1, pp. 30–34, 1995.

[60] M. Berenguer, V. Aguilera, M. Prieto et al., "Significant improvement in the outcome of HCV-infected transplant recipients by avoiding rapid steroid tapering and potent induction immunosuppression," *Journal of Hepatology*, vol. 44, no. 4, pp. 717–722, 2006.

[61] S. Brillanti, M. Vivarelli, N. de Ruvo et al., "Slowly tapering off steroids protects the graft against hepatitis C recurrence after liver transplantation," *Liver Transplantation*, vol. 8, no. 10, pp. 884–888, 2002.

[62] M. Vivarelli, P. Burra, G. L. Barba et al., "Influence of steroids on HCV recurrence after liver transplantation: a prospective study," *Journal of Hepatology*, vol. 47, no. 6, pp. 793–798, 2007.

[63] G. B. Klintmalm, G. L. Davis, L. Teperman et al., "A randomized, multicenter study comparing steroid-free immunosuppression and standard immunosuppression for liver transplant recipients with chronic hepatitis C," *Liver Transplantation*, vol. 17, no. 12, pp. 1394–1403, 2011.

[64] G. Sgourakis, A. Radtke, I. Fouzas et al., "Corticosteroid-free immunosuppression in liver transplantation: a meta-analysis

and meta-regression of outcomes," *Transplant International*, vol. 22, no. 9, pp. 892–905, 2009.

[65] C. Margarit, I. Bilbao, L. Castells et al., "A prospective randomized trial comparing tacrolimus and steroids with tacrolimus monotherapy in liver transplantation: the impact on recurrence of hepatitis C," *Transplant International*, vol. 18, no. 12, pp. 1336–1345, 2005.

[66] T. Kato, J. J. Gaynor, H. Yoshida et al., "Randomized trial of steroid-free induction versus corticosteroid maintenance among orthotopic liver transplant recipients with hepatitis C virus: impact on hepatic fibrosis progression at one year," *Transplantation*, vol. 84, no. 7, pp. 829–835, 2007.

[67] L. Lladó, J. Fabregat, J. Castellote et al., "Impact of immuno-suppression without steroids on rejection and hepatitis C virus evolution after liver transplantation: results of a prospective randomized study," *Liver Transplantation*, vol. 14, no. 12, pp. 1752–1760, 2008.

[68] P. Manousou, D. Samonakis, E. Cholongitas et al., "Outcome of recurrent hepatitis C virus after liver transplantation in a randomized trial of tacrolimus monotherapy versus triple therapy," *Liver Transplantation*, vol. 15, no. 12, pp. 1783–1791, 2009.

[69] "Cyclosporine a-based immunosuppression reduces relapse rate after antiviral therapy in transplanted patients with hepatitis C virus infection: a large multicenter cohort study," *Transplantation*, vol. 92, no. 3, pp. 334–340, 2011.

[70] P. Martin, R. W. Busuttil, R. M. Goldstein et al., "Impact of tacrolimus versus cyclosporine in hepatitis C virus-infected liver transplant recipients on recurrent hepatitis: a prospective, randomized trial," *Liver Transplantation*, vol. 10, no. 10, pp. 1258–1262, 2004.

[71] J. G. O'Grady, P. Hardy, A. K. Burroughs et al., "Randomized controlled trial of tacrolimus versus microemulsified cyclosporin (TMC) in liver transplantation: poststudy surveillance to 3 years," *American Journal of Transplantation*, vol. 7, no. 1, pp. 137–141, 2007.

[72] G. Levy, G. L. Grazi, F. Sanjuan et al., "12-month follow-up analysis of a multicenter, randomized, prospective trial in de novo liver transplantation recipients (LIS2T) comparing cyclosporine microemulsion (C2 monitoring) and tacrolimus," *Liver Transplantation*, vol. 12, no. 10, pp. 1464–1472, 2006.

[73] M. Berenguer, V. Aguilera, F. San Juan et al., "Effect of calcineurin inhibitors in the outcome of liver transplantation in hepatitis C virus-positive recipients," *Transplantation*, vol. 90, no. 11, pp. 1204–1209, 2010.

[74] M. Berenguer, A. Royuela, and J. Zamora, "Immunosuppression with calcineurin inhibitors with respect to the outcome of HCV recurrence after liver transplantation: results of a meta-analysis," *Liver Transplantation*, vol. 13, no. 1, pp. 21–29, 2007.

[75] W. D. Irish, S. Arcona, D. Bowers, and J. F. Trotter, "Cyclosporine versus tacrolimus treated liver transplant recipients with chronic hepatitis C: outcomes analysis of the UNOS/OPTN database," *American Journal of Transplantation*, vol. 11, no. 8, pp. 1676–1685, 2011.

[76] M. Berenguer, "Risk of extended criteria donors in hepatitis C virus-positive recipients," *Liver Transplantation*, vol. 14, supplement 2, pp. S45–S50, 2008.

[77] A. Nocito, A. M. El-Badry, and P. A. Clavien, "When is steatosis too much for transplantation?" *Journal of Hepatology*, vol. 45, no. 4, pp. 494–499, 2006.

[78] S. M. Strasberg, T. K. Howard, E. P. Molmenti, and M. Hertl, "Selecting the donor liver: risk factors for poor function after

orthotopic liver transplantation," *Hepatology*, vol. 20, no. 4, part 1, pp. 829–838, 1994.

[79] R. J. Ploeg, A. M. D'Alessandro, S. J. Knechtle et al., "Risk factors for primary dysfunction after liver transplantation—a multivariate analysis," *Transplantation*, vol. 55, no. 4, pp. 807–813, 1993.

[80] S. Feng, N. P. Goodrich, J. L. Bragg-Gresham et al., "Characteristics associated with liver graft failure: the concept of a donor risk index," *American Journal of Transplantation*, vol. 6, no. 4, pp. 783–790, 2006.

[81] J. Briceño, R. Ciria, M. Pleguezuelo et al., "Contribution of marginal donors to liver transplantation for hepatitis C virus infection," *Transplantation Proceedings*, vol. 39, no. 7, pp. 2297–2299, 2007.

[82] A. M. Cameron, R. M. Ghobrial, H. Yersiz et al., "Optimal utilization of donor grafts with extended criteria: a single-center experience in over 1000 liver transplants," *Annals of Surgery*, vol. 243, no. 6, pp. 748–753, 2006.

[83] R. Hernandez-Alejandro, K. P. Croome, D. Quan et al., "Increased risk of severe recurrence of hepatitis C virus in liver transplant recipients of donation after cardiac death allografts," *Transplantation*, vol. 92, no. 6, pp. 686–689, 2011.

[84] M. L. Shiffman, R. T. Stravitz, M. J. Contos et al., "Histologic recurrence of chronic hepatitis C virus in patients after living donor and deceased donor liver transplantation," *Liver Transplantation*, vol. 10, no. 10, pp. 1248–1255, 2004.

[85] A. Humar, K. Horn, A. Kalis, B. Glessing, W. D. Payne, and J. Lake, "Living donor and split-liver transplants in hepatitis C recipients: does liver regeneration increase the risk for recurrence?" *American Journal of Transplantation*, vol. 5, no. 2, pp. 399–405, 2005.

[86] D. G. Maluf, R. T. Stravitz, A. H. Cotterell et al., "Adult living donor versus deceased donor liver transplantation: a 6-year single center experience," *American Journal of Transplantation*, vol. 5, no. 1, pp. 149–156, 2005.

[87] M. W. Russo, J. Galanko, K. Beavers, M. W. Fried, and R. Shrestha, "Patient and graft surivival in hepatitis C recipients after adult living donor liver transplantation in the United States," *Liver Transplantation*, vol. 10, no. 3, pp. 340–346, 2004.

[88] A. Bozorgzadeh, A. Jain, C. Ryan et al., "Impact of hepatitis C viral infection in primary cadaveric liver allograft versus primary living-donor allograft in 100 consecutive liver transplant recipients receiving tacrolimus," *Transplantation*, vol. 77, no. 712, pp. 1066–1070, 2004.

[89] H. van Vlierberghe, R. Troisi, I. Colle, S. Ricciardi, M. Pract, and B. de Hemptinne, "Hepatitis C infection-related liver disease: patterns of recurrence and outcome in cadaveric and living-donor liver transplantation in adults," *Transplantation*, vol. 77, no. 2, pp. 210–214, 2004.

[90] T. D. Schiano, J. A. Gutierrez, J. L. Walewski et al., "Accelerated hepatitis C virus kinetics but similar survival rates in recipients of liver grafts from living versus deceased donors," *Hepatology*, vol. 42, no. 6, pp. 1420–1428, 2005.

[91] L. Guo, M. Orrego, H. Rodriguez-Luna et al., "Living donor liver transplantation for hepatitis C-related cirrhosis: no difference in histological recurrence when compared to deceased donor liver transplantation recipients," *Liver Transplantation*, vol. 12, no. 4, pp. 560–565, 2006.

[92] N. A. Terrault, M. L. Shiffman, A. S. F. Lok et al., "Outcomes in hepatitis C virus-infected recipients of living donor vs. deceased donor liver transplantation," *Liver Transplantation*, vol. 13, no. 1, pp. 122–129, 2007.

[93] M. Schmeding, U. P. Neumann, G. Puhl, M. Bahra, R. Neuhaus, and P. Neuhaus, "Hepatitis C recurrence and fibrosis progression are not increased after living donor liver transplantation: a single-center study of 289 patients," *Liver Transplantation*, vol. 13, no. 5, pp. 687–692, 2007.

[94] N. Selzner, N. Girgrah, L. Lilly et al., "The difference in the fibrosis progression of recurrent hepatitis C after live donor liver transplantation versus deceased donor liver transplantation is attributable to the difference in donor age," *Liver Transplantation*, vol. 14, no. 12, pp. 1778–1786, 2008.

[95] A. Jain, A. Singhal, R. Kashyap et al., "Comparative analysis of hepatitis C recurrence and fibrosis progression between deceased-donor and living-donor liver transplantation: 8-year longitudinal follow-up," *Transplantation*, vol. 92, no. 4, pp. 453–460, 2011.

[96] M. Charlton, E. Seaberg, R. Wiesner et al., "Predictors of patient and graft survival following liver transplantation for hepatitis C," *Hepatology*, vol. 28, no. 3, pp. 823–830, 1998.

[97] G. W. McCaughan and A. Zekry, "Mechanisms of HCV reinfection and allograft damage after liver transplantation," *Journal of Hepatology*, vol. 40, no. 3, pp. 368–374, 2004.

[98] R. J. Firpi, M. F. Abdelmalek, C. Soldevila-Pico et al., "One-year protocol liver biopsy can stratify fibrosis progression in liver transplant recipients with recurrent hepatitis C infection," *Liver Transplantation*, vol. 10, no. 10, pp. 1240–1247, 2004.

[99] M. Moeller, A. Zalawadia, A. Alrayes, G. Divine, K. Brown, and D. Moonka, "The impact of donor race on recurrent hepatitis C after liver transplantation," *Transplantation Proceedings*, vol. 42, no. 10, pp. 4175–4177, 2010.

[100] Y. Sugawara, S. Tamura, and N. Kokudo, "Liver transplantation in HCV/HIV positive patients," *World Journal of Gastrointestinal Surgery*, vol. 3, no. 2, pp. 21–28, 2011.

[101] J. C. Duclos-Vallee, C. Feray, M. Sebagh et al., "Survival and recurrence of hepatitis C after liver transplantation in patients coinfected with human immunodeficiency virus and hepatitis C virus," *Hepatology*, vol. 47, no. 2, pp. 407–417, 2008.

[102] J. C. Duclos-Vallee, B. Falissard, and D. Samuel, "Liver transplant outcomes in HIV-infected patients: a systematic review and meta-analysis with a synthetic cohort," *AIDS*, vol. 25, no. 13, pp. 1675–1676, 2011.

[103] A. Moreno, C. Cervera, J. Fortun et al., "Epidemiology and outcome of infections in human immunodeficiency virus/hepatitis C virus-coinfected liver transplant recipients: a FIPSE/GESIDA prospective cohort study," *Liver Transplantation*, vol. 18, no. 1, pp. 70–81, 2012.

[104] M. E. de Vera, I. Dvorchik, K. Tom et al., "Survival of liver transplant patients coinfected with HIV and HCV is adversely impacted by recurrent hepatitis C," *American Journal of Transplantation*, vol. 6, no. 12, pp. 2983–2993, 2006.

[105] J. Fung, B. Eghtesad, K. Patel-Tom, M. DeVera, H. Chapman, and M. Ragni, "Liver transplantation in patients with HIV infection," *Liver Transplantation*, vol. 10, no. 10, supplement 2, pp. S39–S53, 2004.

[106] K. Wojcik, M. Vogel, E. Voigt et al., "Antiviral therapy for hepatitis C virus recurrence after liver transplantation in HIV-infected patients: outcome in the Bonn cohort," *AIDS*, vol. 21, no. 10, pp. 1363–1365, 2007.

[107] N. M. Kemmer and K. E. Sherman, "Liver transplantation trends in the HIV population," *Digestive Diseases and Sciences*, vol. 56, no. 11, pp. 3393–3398, 2011.

[108] T. Fukuhara, A. Taketomi, T. Motomura et al., "Variants in IL28B in liver recipients and donors correlate with response to

peg-interferon and ribavirin therapy for recurrent hepatitis C," *Gastroenterology*, vol. 139, no. 5, article e3, pp. 1577–1585, 2010.

[109] D. Eurich, S. Boas-Knoop, M. Ruehl et al., "Relationship between the interleukin-28b gene polymorphism and the histological severity of hepatitis C virus-induced graft inflammation and the response to antiviral therapy after liver transplantation," *Liver Transplantation*, vol. 17, no. 3, pp. 289–298, 2011.

[110] C. M. Lange, D. Moradpour, A. Doehring et al., "Impact of donor and recipient IL28B rs12979860 genotypes on hepatitis C virus liver graft reinfection," *Journal of Hepatology*, vol. 55, no. 2, pp. 322–327, 2011.

[111] M. Coto-Llerena, G. Crespo, P. Gonzalez et al., "Determination of IL28B polymorphisms in liver biopsies obtained after liver transplantation," *Journal of Hepatology*, vol. 56, no. 2, pp. 355–358, 2012.

[112] H. R. Rosen, S. Chou, C. L. Corless et al., "Cytomegalovirus viremia: risk factor for allograft cirrhosis after liver transplantation for hepatitis C," *Transplantation*, vol. 64, no. 5, pp. 721–726, 1997.

[113] A. Humara, D. Kumar, J. Raboud et al., "Interactions between cytomegalovirus, human herpesvirus-6, and the recurrence of hepatitis C after liver transplantation," *American Journal of Transplantation*, vol. 2, no. 5, pp. 461–466, 2002.

[114] R. Teixeira, S. Pastacaldi, S. Davies et al., "The influence of cytomegalovirus viraemia on the outcome of recurrent hepatitis C after liver transplantation," *Transplantation*, vol. 70, no. 10, pp. 1454–1458, 2000.

[115] G. Nebbia, F. M. Mattes, E. Cholongitas et al., "Exploring the bidirectional interactions between human cytomegalovirus and hepatitis C virus replication after liver transplantation," *Liver Transplantation*, vol. 13, no. 1, pp. 130–135, 2007.

[116] A. Humar, K. Washburn, R. Freeman et al., "An assessment of interactions between hepatitis C virus and herpesvirus reactivation in liver transplant recipients using molecular surveillance," *Liver Transplantation*, vol. 13, no. 10, pp. 1422–1427, 2007.

[117] S. Baid, A. B. Cosimi, M. Lin Farrell et al., "Posttransplant diabetes mellitus in liver transplant recipients: risk factors, temporal, relationship with hepatitis C virus allograft hepatitis, and impact on mortality," *Transplantation*, vol. 72, no. 6, pp. 1066–1072, 2001.

[118] M. R. Foxton, A. Quaglia, R. Muiesan et al., "The impact of diabetes mellitus on fibrosis progression in patients transplanted for hepatitis C," *American Journal of Transplantation*, vol. 6, no. 8, pp. 1922–1929, 2006.

[119] A. A. AlDosary, A. S. Ramji, T. G. Elliott et al., "Post-liver transplantation diabetes mellitus: an association with hepatitis C," *Liver Transplantation*, vol. 8, no. 4, pp. 356–361, 2002.

[120] E. J. Gane, "Diabetes mellitus following liver transplantation in patients with hepatitis C virus: risks and consequences," *American Journal of Transplantation*, vol. 12, no. 3, pp. 531–538, 2012.

[121] B. J. Veldt, J. J. Poterucha, K. D. S. Watt et al., "Insulin resistance, serum adipokines and risk of fibrosis progression in patients transplanted for hepatitis C," *American Journal of Transplantation*, vol. 9, no. 6, pp. 1406–1413, 2009.

[122] D. N. Samonakis, C. K. Triantos, U. Thalheimer et al., "Immunosuppresion and donor age with respect to severity of HCV recurrence after liver transplantation," *Liver Transplantation*, vol. 11, no. 4, pp. 386–395, 2005.

[123] M. Charlton and E. Seaberg, "Impact of immunosuppression and acute rejection on recurrence of hepatitis C: results of the national institute of diabetes and digestive and kidney diseases liver transplantation database," *Liver Transplantation and Surgery*, vol. 5, no. 4, supplement 1, pp. S107–S114, 1999.

[124] U. P. Neumann, T. Berg, M. Bahra et al., "Long-term outcome of liver transplants for chronic hepatitis C: a 10-year follow-up," *Transplantation*, vol. 77, no. 2, pp. 226–231, 2004.

[125] J. D. Eason, S. Nair, A. J. Cohen, J. L. Blazek, and G. E. Loss, "Steroid-free liver transplantation using rabbit antithymocyte globulin and early tacrolimus monotherapy," *Transplantation*, vol. 75, no. 8, pp. 1396–1399, 2003.

[126] F. Filipponi, F. Callea, M. Salizzoni et al., "Double-blind comparison of hepatitis C histological recurrence rate in HCV+ liver transplant recipients given basiliximab+steroids or basiliximab+placebo, in addition to cyclosporine and azathioprine," *Transplantation*, vol. 78, no. 10, pp. 1488–1495, 2004.

[127] D. L. Segev, S. M. Sozio, E. J. Shin et al., "Steroid avoidance in liver transplantation: meta-analysis and meta-regression of randomized trials," *Liver Transplantation*, vol. 14, no. 4, pp. 512–525, 2008.

[128] Y. Calmus, J. R. Scheele, I. Gonzalez-Pinto et al., "Immunoprophylaxis with basiliximab, a chimeric anti-interleukin-2 receptor monoclonal antibody, in combination with azathioprine-containing triple therapy in liver transplant recipients," *Liver Transplantation*, vol. 8, no. 2, pp. 123–131, 2002.

[129] G. B. G. Klintmalm, W. K. Washburn, S. M. Rudich et al., "Corticosteroid-free immunosuppression with daclizumab in HCV+ liver transplant recipients: 1-year interim results of the HCV-3 study," *Liver Transplantation*, vol. 13, no. 11, pp. 1521–1531, 2007.

[130] P. Neuhaus, P. A. Clavien, D. Kittur et al., "Improved treatment response with basiliximab immunoprophylaxis after liver transplantation: results from a double-blind randomized placebo-controlled trial," *Liver Transplantation*, vol. 8, no. 2, pp. 132–142, 2002.

[131] D. R. Nelson, C. Soldevila-Pico, A. Reed et al., "Anti-interleukin-2 receptor therapy in combination with mycophenolate mofetil is associated with more severe hepatitis C recurrence after liver transplantation," *Liver Transplantation*, vol. 7, no. 12, pp. 1064–1070, 2001.

[132] A. Jain, R. Kashyap, A. J. Demetris, B. Eghstesad, R. Pokharna, and J. J. Fung, "A prospective randomized trial of mycophenolate mofetil in liver transplant recipients with hepatitis C," *Liver Transplantation*, vol. 8, no. 1, pp. 40–46, 2002.

[133] R. H. Wiesner, J. S. Shorr, B. J. Steffen, A. H. Chu, R. D. Gordon, and J. R. Lake, "Mycophenolate mofetil combination therapy improves long-term outcomes after liver transplantation in patients with and without hepatitis C," *Liver Transplantation*, vol. 11, no. 7, pp. 750–759, 2005.

[134] F. Sánchez-Bueno, M. L. Ortiz, J. Bermejo et al., "Prognostic factors for hepatitis C recurrence in patients undergoing orthotopic liver transplantation," *Transplant Immunology*, vol. 17, no. 1, pp. 47–50, 2006.

[135] T. M. Manzia, R. Angelico, L. Toti et al., "Long-term, maintenance MMF monotherapy improves the fibrosis progression in liver transplant recipients with recurrent hepatitis C," *Transplant International*, vol. 24, no. 5, pp. 461–468, 2011.

[136] A. Kornberg, B. Küpper, J. Wilberg et al., "Conversion to mycophenolate mofetil for modulating recurrent hepatitis C in liver transplant recipients," *Transplant Infectious Disease*, vol. 9, no. 4, pp. 295–301, 2007.

[137] A. Kornberg, B. Küpper, A. Tannapfel, M. Hommann, and J. Scheele, "Impact of mycophenolate mofetil versus azathioprine

on early recurrence of hepatitis C after liver transplantation," *International Immunopharmacology*, vol. 5, no. 1, pp. 107–115, 2005.

[138] M. Bahra, U. I. F. P. Neumann, D. Jacob et al., "MMF and calcineurin taper in recurrent hepatitis C after liver transplantation: impact on histological course," *American Journal of Transplantation*, vol. 5, no. 2, pp. 406–411, 2005.

[139] A. Zekry, M. Gleeson, S. Guney, and G. W. McCaughan, "A prospective cross-over study comparing the effect of mycophenolate versus azathioprine on allograft function and viral load in liver transplant recipients with recurrent chronic HCV infection," *Liver Transplantation*, vol. 10, no. 1, pp. 52–57, 2004.

[140] G. Germani, M. Pleguezuelo, F. Villamil et al., "Azathioprine in liver transplantation: a reevaluation of its use and a comparison with mycophenolate mofetil," *American Journal of Transplantation*, vol. 9, no. 8, pp. 1725–1731, 2009.

[141] T. Kawahara, S. Asthana, and N. M. Kneteman, "m-TOR inhibitors: what role in liver transplantation?" *Journal of Hepatology*, vol. 55, no. 6, pp. 1441–1451, 2011.

[142] S. Asthana, C. Toso, G. Meeberg et al., "The impact of sirolimus on hepatitis C recurrence after liver transplantation," *Canadian Journal of Gastroenterology*, vol. 25, no. 1, pp. 28–34, 2011.

[143] S. J. F. Harper, W. Gelson, I. G. Harper, G. J. M. Alexander, and P. Gibbs, "Switching to sirolimus-based immune suppression after liver transplantation is safe and effective: a single-center experience," *Transplantation*, vol. 91, no. 1, pp. 128–132, 2011.

[144] P. J. Gaglio, S. Malireddy, B. S. Levitt et al., "Increased risk of cholestatic hepatitis C in recipients of grafts from living versus cadaveric liver donors," *Liver Transplantation*, vol. 9, no. 10, pp. 1028–1035, 2003.

[145] M. Garcia-Retortillo, X. Forns, J. M. Llovet et al., "Hepatitis C recurrence is more severe after living donor compared to cadaveric liver transplantation," *Hepatology*, vol. 40, no. 3, pp. 699–707, 2004.

[146] P. J. Thuluvath and H. Y. Yoo, "Graft and patient survival after adult live donor liver transplantation compared to a matched cohort who received a deceased donor transplantation," *Liver Transplantation*, vol. 10, no. 10, pp. 1263–1268, 2004.

[147] N. Fausto and J. S. Campbell, "The role of hepatocytes and oval cells in liver regeneration and repopulation," *Mechanisms of Development*, vol. 120, no. 1, pp. 117–130, 2003.

[148] M. A. Zimmerman and J. F. Trotter, "Living donor liver transplantation in patients with hepatitis C," *Liver Transplantation*, vol. 9, no. 11, pp. S52–S57, 2003.

[149] K. M. Olthoff, "Hepatic regeneration in living donor liver transplantation," *Liver Transplantation*, vol. 9, no. 10, supplement 2, pp. S35–S41, 2003.

[150] G. T. Everson and J. Trotter, "Role of adult living donor liver transplantation in patients with hepatitis C," *Liver Transplantation*, vol. 9, no. 10, supplement 2, pp. S64–S68, 2003.

[151] R. Manez, R. Mateo, J. Tabasco, S. Kusne, T. E. Starzl, and R. J. Duquesnoy, "The influence of HLA donor-recipient compatibility on the recurrence of HBV and HCV hepatitis after liver transplantation," *Transplantation*, vol. 59, no. 4, pp. 640–642, 1995.

[152] B. Roche and D. Samuel, "Hepatitis C virus treatment pre- and post-liver transplantation," *Liver International*, vol. 32, supplement 1, pp. 120–128, 2012.

[153] J. A. Carrión, E. Martínez-Bauer, G. Crespo et al., "Antiviral therapy increases the risk of bacterial infections in HCV-infected cirrhotic patients awaiting liver transplantation: a

retrospective study," *Journal of Hepatology*, vol. 50, no. 4, pp. 719–728, 2009.

[154] X. Forns, M. García-Retortillo, T. Serrano et al., "Antiviral therapy of patients with decompensated cirrhosis to prevent recurrence of hepatitis C after liver transplantation," *Journal of Hepatology*, vol. 39, no. 3, pp. 389–396, 2003.

[155] J. S. Crippin, T. McCashland, N. Terrault, P. Sheiner, and M. R. Charlton, "A pilot study of the tolerability and efficacy of antiviral therapy in hepatitis C virus-infected patients awaiting liver transplantation," *Liver Transplantation*, vol. 8, no. 4, pp. 350–355, 2002.

[156] G. T. Everson, J. Trotter, L. Forman et al., "Treatment of advanced hepatitis C with a low accelerating dosage regimen of antiviral therapy," *Hepatology*, vol. 42, no. 2, pp. 255–262, 2005.

[157] R. M. Thomas, J. J. Brems, G. Guzman-Hartman, S. Yong, P. Cavaliere, and D. H. van Thiel, "Infection with chronic hepatitis C virus and liver transplantation: a role for interferon therapy before transplantation," *Liver Transplantation*, vol. 9, no. 9, pp. 905–915, 2003.

[158] G. T. Everson, N. A. Terrault, A. S. Lok et al., "A randomized controlled trial of pretransplant antiviral therapy to prevent recurrence of hepatitis C after liver transplantation," *Hepatology*.

[159] A. K. Shergill, M. Khalili, S. Straley et al., "Applicability, tolerability and efficacy of preemptive antiviral therapy in hepatitis C-infected patients undergoing liver transplantation," *American Journal of Transplantation*, vol. 5, no. 1, pp. 118–124, 2005.

[160] V. Mazzaferro, A. Tagger, M. Schiavo et al., "Prevention of recurrent hepatitis C after liver transplantation with early interferon and ribavirin treatment," *Transplantation Proceedings*, vol. 33, no. 1-2, pp. 1355–1357, 2001.

[161] S. Tamura, Y. Sugawara, N. Yamashiki, J. Kaneko, N. Kokudo, and M. Makuuchi, "Pre-emptive antiviral therapy in living donor liver transplantation for hepatitis C: observation based on a single-center experience," *Transplant International*, vol. 23, no. 6, pp. 580–588, 2010.

[162] A. Kuo, V. Tan, B. Lan et al., "Long-term histological effects of preemptive antiviral therapy in liver transplant recipients with hepatitis C virus infection," *Liver Transplantation*, vol. 14, no. 10, pp. 1491–1497, 2008.

[163] N. Chalasani, C. Manzarbeitia, P. Ferenci et al., "Peginterferon alfa-2a for hepatitis C after liver transplantation: two randomized, controlled trials," *Hepatology*, vol. 41, no. 2, pp. 289–298, 2005.

[164] N. Singh, T. Gayowski, C. F. Wannstedt et al., "Interferon-α for prophylaxis of recurrent viral hepatitis C in liver transplant recipients: a prospective, randomized, controlled trial," *Transplantation*, vol. 65, no. 1, pp. 82–86, 1998.

[165] N. Bzowej, D. R. Nelson, N. A. Terrault et al., "PHOENIX: a randomized controlled trial of peginterferon alfa-2a plus ribavirin as a prophylactic treatment after liver transplantation for hepatitis C virus," *Liver Transplantation*, vol. 17, no. 5, pp. 528–538, 2011.

[166] B. Roche, M. Sebagh, M. L. Canfora et al., "Hepatitis C virus therapy in liver transplant recipients: response predictors, effect on fibrosis progression, and importance of the initial stage of fibrosis," *Liver Transplantation*, vol. 14, no. 12, pp. 1766–1777, 2008.

[167] M. Berenguer, V. Aguilera, M. Prieto et al., "Worse recent efficacy of antiviral therapy in liver transplant recipients with

recurrent hepatitis C: impact of donor age and baseline cirrhosis," *Liver Transplantation*, vol. 15, no. 7, pp. 738–746, 2009.

[168] H. Rodriguez-Luna, A. Khatib, P. Sharma et al., "Treatment of recurrent hepatitis C infection after liver transplantation with combination of pegylated interferon α2b and ribavirin: an open-label series," *Transplantation*, vol. 77, no. 2, pp. 190–194, 2004.

[169] G. W. Neff, M. Montalbano, C. B. O'Brien et al., "Treatment of established recurrent hepatitis C in liver-transplant recipients with pegylated interferon-alfa-2b and ribavirin therapy," *Transplantation*, vol. 78, no. 9, pp. 1303–1307, 2004.

[170] A. S. Ross, A. K. Bhan, M. Pascual, M. Thiim, A. B. Cosimi, and R. T. Chung, "Pegylated interferon α-2b plus ribavirin in the treatment of post-liver transplant recurrent hepatitis C," *Clinical Transplantation*, vol. 18, no. 2, pp. 166–173, 2004.

[171] M. Babatin, L. Schindel, and K. W. Burak, "Pegylated-interferon alpha 2b and ribavirin for recurrent hepatities C after liver liver transplantation: from a Canadian experience to recommendations for therapy," *Canadian Journal of Gastroenterology*, vol. 19, no. 6, pp. 359–365, 2005.

[172] L. Castells, V. Vargas, H. Allende et al., "Combined treatment with pegylated interferon (α-2b) and ribavirin in the acute phase of hepatitis C virus recurrence after liver transplantation," *Journal of Hepatology*, vol. 43, no. 1, pp. 53–59, 2005.

[173] P. Toniutto, C. Fabris, E. Fumo et al., "Pegylated versus standard interferon-α in antiviral regimens for post-transplant recurrent hepatitis C: comparison of tolerability and efficacy," *Journal of Gastroenterology and Hepatology*, vol. 20, no. 4, pp. 577–582, 2005.

[174] M. Berenguer, A. Palau, A. Fernandez et al., "Efficacy, predictors of response, and potential risks associated with antiviral therapy in liver transplant recipients with recurrent hepatitis C," *Liver Transplantation*, vol. 12, no. 7, pp. 1067–1076, 2006.

[175] M. Biselli, P. Andreone, A. Gramenzi et al., "Pegylated interferon plus ribavirin for recurrent Hepatitis C infection after liver transplantation in naïve and non-responder patients on a stable immunosuppressive regimen," *Digestive and Liver Disease*, vol. 38, no. 1, pp. 27–32, 2006.

[176] I. Fernández, J. C. Meneu, F. Colina et al., "Clinical and histological efficacy of pegylated interferon and ribavirin therapy of recurrent hepatitis C after liver transplantation," *Liver Transplantation*, vol. 12, no. 12, pp. 1805–1812, 2006.

[177] S. Mukherjee and E. Lyden, "Impact of pegylated interferon α-2B and ribavirin on hepatic fibrosis in liver transplant patients with recurrent hepatitis C: an open-label series," *Liver International*, vol. 26, no. 5, pp. 529–535, 2006.

[178] U. Neumann, G. Puhl, M. Bahra et al., "Treatment of patients with recurrent hepatitis C after liver transplantation with peginterferon alfa-2B plus ribavirin," *Transplantation*, vol. 82, no. 1, pp. 43–47, 2006.

[179] E. Oton, R. Barcena, J. M. Moreno-Planas et al., "Hepatitis C recurrence after liver transplantation: viral and histologic response to full-dose peg-interferon and ribavirin," *American Journal of Transplantation*, vol. 6, no. 10, pp. 2348–2355, 2006.

[180] M. Angelico, A. Petrolati, R. Lionetti et al., "A randomized study on Peg-interferon alfa-2a with or without ribavirin in liver transplant recipients with recurrent hepatitis C," *Journal of Hepatology*, vol. 46, no. 6, pp. 1009–1017, 2007.

[181] J. A. Carrión, M. Navasa, M. García-Retortillo et al., "Efficacy of antiviral therapy on hepatitis C recurrence after liver transplantation: a randomized controlled study," *Gastroenterology*, vol. 132, no. 5, pp. 1746–1756, 2007.

[182] F. P. Picciotto, G. Tritto, A. G. Lanza et al., "Sustained virological response to antiviral therapy reduces mortality in HCV reinfection after liver transplantation," *Journal of Hepatology*, vol. 46, no. 3, pp. 459–465, 2007.

[183] P. Sharma, J. A. Marrero, R. J. Fontana et al., "Sustained virologic response to therapy of recurrent hepatitis C after liver transplantation is related to early virologic response and dose adherence," *Liver Transplantation*, vol. 13, no. 8, pp. 1100–1108, 2007.

[184] T. Zimmermann, W. O. Böcher, S. Biesterfeld et al., "Efficacy of an escalating dose regimen of pegylated interferon α-2a plus ribavirin in the early phase of HCV reinfection after liver transplantation," *Transplant International*, vol. 20, no. 7, pp. 583–590, 2007.

[185] I. A. Hanouneh, C. Miller, F. N. Aucejo, R. Lopez, M. K. Quinn, and N. N. Zein, "Recurrent hepatitis C after liver transplantation: on-treatment prediction of response to peginterferon/ribavirin therapy," *Liver Transplantation*, vol. 14, no. 1, pp. 53–58, 2008.

[186] F. Lodato, S. Berardi, A. Gramenzi et al., "Clinical trial: peginterferon alfa-2b and ribavirin for the treatment of genotype-1 hepatitis C recurrence after liver transplantation," *Alimentary Pharmacology and Therapeutics*, vol. 28, no. 4, pp. 450–457, 2008.

[187] S. Dinges, I. Morard, M. Heim et al., "Pegylated interferon-alpha2a/ribavirin treatment of recurrent hepatitis C after liver transplantation," *Transplant Infectious Disease*, vol. 11, no. 1, pp. 33–39, 2009.

[188] A. Jain, R. Sharma, C. Ryan et al., "Response to antiviral therapy in liver transplant recipients with recurrent hepatitis C viral infection: a single center experience," *Clinical Transplantation*, vol. 24, no. 1, pp. 104–111, 2010.

[189] S. C. Schmidt, M. Bahra, S. Bayraktar et al., "Antiviral treatment of patients with recurrent hepatitis c after liver transplantation with pegylated interferon," *Digestive Diseases and Sciences*, vol. 55, no. 7, pp. 2063–2069, 2010.

[190] W. Al-Hamoudi, H. Mohamed, F. Abaalkhail et al., "Treatment of genotype 4 hepatitis C recurring after liver transplantation using a combination of pegylated interferon alfa-2a and ribavirin," *Digestive Diseases and Sciences*, vol. 56, no. 6, pp. 1848–1852, 2011.

[191] K. S. Gurusamy, E. Tsochatzis, B. R. Davidson, and A. K. Burroughs, "Antiviral prophylactic intervention for chronic hepatitis C virus in patients undergoing liver transplantation," *Cochrane Database of Systematic Reviews*, no. 12, Article ID CD006573, 2010.

[192] B. J. Veldt, J. J. Poterucha, K. D. S. Watt et al., "Impact of pegylated interferon and ribavirin treatment on graft survival in liver transplant patients with recurrent hepatitis C infection," *American Journal of Transplantation*, vol. 8, no. 11, pp. 2426–2433, 2008.

[193] M. Berenguer, A. Palau, V. Aguilera, J. M. Rayón, F. S. Juan, and M. Prieto, "Clinical benefits of antiviral therapy in patients with recurrent hepatitis C following liver transplantation," *American Journal of Transplantation*, vol. 8, no. 3, pp. 679–687, 2008.

[194] R. J. Firpi, V. Clark, C. Soldevila-Pico et al., "The natural history of hepatitis C cirrhosis after liver transplantation," *Liver Transplantation*, vol. 15, no. 9, pp. 1063–1071, 2009.

[195] T. McCashland, K. Watt, E. Lyden et al., "Retransplantation for hepatitis C: results of a U.S. multicenter retransplant study," *Liver Transplantation*, vol. 13, no. 9, pp. 1246–1253, 2007.

[196] J. Martí, R. Charco, J. Ferrer et al., "Optimization of liver grafts in liver retransplantation: a European single-center experience," *Surgery*, vol. 144, no. 5, pp. 762–769, 2008.

[197] Y. Sugawara, M. Makuuchi, Y. Matsui et al., "Preemptive therapy for hepatitis C virus after living-donor liver transplantation," *Transplantation*, vol. 78, no. 9, pp. 1308–1311, 2004.

[198] Y. Kishi, Y. Sugawara, N. Akamatsu et al., "Splenectomy and preemptive interferon therapy for hepatitis C patients after living-donor liver transplantation," *Clinical Transplantation*, vol. 19, no. 6, pp. 769–772, 2005.

[199] S. Tamura, Y. Sugawara, N. Yamashiki, J. Kaneko, N. Kokudo, and M. Makuuchi, "Preemptive antiviral treatment for hepatitis C virus after living donor liver transplantation," *Transplantation Proceedings*, vol. 44, no. 3, pp. 971–973, 2012.

[200] Y. Ueda, Y. Takada, H. Haga et al., "Limited benefit of biochemical response to combination therapy for patients with recurrent hepatitis C after living-donor liver transplantation," *Transplantation*, vol. 85, no. 6, pp. 855–862, 2008.

[201] Y. Ueda, Y. Takada, H. Marusawa, H. Egawa, S. Ucmoto, and T. Chiba, "Individualized extension of pegylated interferon plus ribavirin therapy for recurrent hepatitis C genotype 1b after living-donor liver transplantation," *Transplantation*, vol. 90, no. 6, pp. 661–665, 2010.

[202] Y. Ueda, H. Marusawa, T. Kaido et al., "Effect of maintenance therapy with low-dose peginterferon for recurrent hepatitis C after living donor liver transplantation," *Journal of Viral Hepatitis*, vol. 19, no. 1, pp. 32–38, 2012.

[203] T. Ikegami, A. Taketomi, Y. Soejima et al., "The benefits of interferon treatment in patients without sustained viral response after living donor liver transplantation for hepatitis C," *Transplantation Proceedings*, vol. 41, no. 10, pp. 4246–4252, 2009.

[204] S. Eguchi, M. Takatsuki, A. Soyama et al., "Intentional conversion from tacrolimus to cyclosporine for HCV-positive patients on preemptive interferon therapy after living donor liver transplantation," *Annals of Transplantation*, vol. 12, no. 4, pp. 11–15, 2007.

[205] T. Kawaoka, N. Hiraga, S. Takahashi et al., "Prolongation of interferon therapy for recurrent hepatitis C after living donor liver transplantation: analysis of predictive factors of sustained virological response, including amino acid sequence of the core and NS5A regions of hepatitis C virus," *Scandinavian Journal of Gastroenterology*, vol. 45, no. 12, pp. 1488–1496, 2010.

[206] Y. Masuda, Y. Nakazawa, K. Matsuda et al., "Clinicopathological features of hepatitis C virus disease after living donor liver transplantation: relationship with in situ hybridisation data," *Pathology*, vol. 43, no. 2, pp. 156–160, 2011.

[207] S. Marubashi, K. Dono, H. Nagano et al., "Steroid-free living donor liver transplantation in adults: impact on hepatitis C recurrence," *Clinical Transplantation*, vol. 23, no. 6, pp. 904–913, 2009.

[208] L. B. Jeng, C. C. Lee, H. C. Chiang et al., "Indication for splenectomy in the Era of living-donor liver transplantation," *Transplantation Proceedings*, vol. 40, no. 8, pp. 2531–2533, 2008.

[209] T. Yoshizumi, A. Taketomi, Y. Soejima et al., "The beneficial role of simultaneous splenectomy in living donor liver transplantation in patients with small-for-size graft," *Transplant International*, vol. 21, no. 9, pp. 833–842, 2008.

30

Prognostic Factors for Long-Term Survival in Patients with Ampullary Carcinoma: The Results of a 15-Year Observation Period after Pancreaticoduodenectomy

Fritz Klein,[1] **Dietmar Jacob,**[2] **Marcus Bahra,**[1] **Uwe Pelzer,**[3] **Gero Puhl,**[1]
Alexander Krannich,[4] **Andreas Andreou,**[1] **Safak Gül,**[1] **and Olaf Guckelberger**[1]

[1] *Department of General, Visceral, and Transplantation Surgery, Charité Campus Virchow Universitätsmedizin Berlin, 13353 Berlin, Germany*
[2] *Department of General and Visceral Surgery, Bielefeld Evangelical Hospital, 33617 Bielefeld, Germany*
[3] *Department of Hematology/Oncology, Comprehensive Cancer Center, Charité Universitätsmedizin Berlin, 13353 Berlin, Germany*
[4] *Department of Biostatistics, Coordination Center for Clinical Trials, Charité Universitätsmedizin Berlin, 13353 Berlin, Germany*

Correspondence should be addressed to Fritz Klein; fritz.klein@charite.de

Academic Editor: Attila Olah

Introduction. Although ampullary carcinoma has the best prognosis among all periampullary carcinomas, its long-term survival remains low. Prognostic factors are only available for a period of 10 years after pancreaticoduodenectomy. The aim of this retrospective study was to identify factors that influence the long-term patient survival over a 15-year observation period. *Methods.* From 1992 to 2007, 143 patients with ampullary carcinoma underwent pancreatic resection. 86 patients underwent pylorus-preserving pancreaticoduodenectomy (60%) and 57 patients underwent standard Kausch-Whipple pancreaticoduodenectomy (40%). *Results.* The overall 1-, 5-, 10-, and 15-year survival rates were 79%, 40%, 24%, and 10%, respectively. Within a mean observation period of 30 (0–205) months, 100 (69%) patients died. Survival analysis showed that positive lymph node involvement ($P = 0.001$), lymphatic vessel invasion ($P = 0.0001$), intraoperative administration of packed red blood cells ($P = 0.03$), an elevated CA 19-9 ($P = 0.03$), jaundice ($P = 0.04$), and an impaired patient condition ($P = 0.01$) are strong negative predictors for a reduced patient survival. *Conclusions.* Patients with ampullary carcinoma have distinctly better long-term survival than patients with pancreatic adenocarcinoma. Long-term survival depends strongly on lymphatic nodal and vessel involvement. Moreover, a preoperative elevated CA 19-9 proved to be a significant prognostic factor. Adjuvant therapy may be essential in patients with this risk constellation.

1. Introduction

Ampullary carcinomas arise from the ampulla or papilla of Vater (the duodenal papilla) and account for 0.2% of tumors of the gastrointestinal tract. However, with a proportion of 7% to 9%, they represent the second largest proportion (after pancreatic carcinoma) of periampullary carcinomas, which include ampullary carcinomas and carcinomas of the pancreas, the distal bile duct, and the periampullary duodenum [1–3]. In contrast with other carcinomas of the periampullary region, ampullary carcinomas have a higher resection rate, a lower recurrence rate, and a better overall prognosis [3–6].

To date, the etiology of ampullary carcinoma has not been clearly identified. An adenoma-to-carcinoma sequence similar to that of colon carcinoma has been described for ampullary carcinoma [7].

In traditional terms, ampullary cancer is already distinguished from carcinomas of the pancreas, bile duct, and duodenum. For one thing, due to their anatomical location, ampullary tumors become clinically apparent early because of bile or pancreatic duct occlusion [8]. Thus, ampullary carcinomas are often diagnosed at an early tumor stage and, therefore, have a higher probability of successful surgical resection [4]. Secondly, the 5-year survival rate is reported with up to 39%, which is between that of duodenal carcinoma (59%) and carcinomas of the pancreas or bile duct (15% and 27%, resp.) [3, 9, 10]. A reason for the better overall prognosis may be the difference in the histological origin of ampullary carcinomas. As early as 1963, Whipple reported that ampullary cancers are more likely to be of the adenomatous type with less general lymphatic and blood vessel invasion [11]. Current histopathological studies have also suggested further subdivision of ampullary carcinomas based on their exact histopathological findings [12, 13]. For example, intestinal ampullary adenocarcinomas arise from the surrounding intestinal epithelial layer, whereas pancreatobiliary ampullary cancers originate in the endothelium of the distal bile duct or pancreatic duct [14, 15].

Computed tomography (CT) and magnetic resonance imaging cholangiopancreatography (MRCP) constitute the current clinical diagnostic methods of choice. Other methods, such as endosonography and endoscopic retrograde cholangiopancreatography (ERCP), allow for sample collection and thus permit further histological differentiation. A radical pancreaticoduodenectomy, performed either as a pylorus-preserving pancreatic head resection (PPPD) or a classic Whipple procedure (KW), is considered to be the gold standard therapy for ampullary carcinoma. Currently, endoscopic papillectomy is increasingly performed as an initial intervention in suspected benign papillary tumors [16, 17]. The decision to perform a subsequent pancreaticoduodenectomy may be based on the histopathological finding of the resected specimen. The resectability of ampullary carcinoma with a curative intention is 76.5% to 89.4% [2, 18]. Due to the rarity of this tumor, studies describing the long-term progress are scarce and are available only for up to 10 years after resection. Overall long-term survival still remains low. A major component in this issue is tumor recurrence. The aim of this retrospective study was to identify factors that influence the long-term survival in a large patient population over 15 years.

2. Patients and Methods

2.1. Preoperative Data. Between 1992 and 2007, 143 patients underwent resection of histologically verified ampullary cancer at our institution. Of these patients, 87 (61%) were men and 56 (39%) were women, with a median age of 64 (33–83) years. The median body mass index (BMI) in the patient group was 24.8 (13.5–38.8) kg/m^2. Forty-three (30%) patients presented with a Karnofsky index below 80%. Nicotine consumption was noted in 44 (31%) patients and regular alcohol consumption in 32 (22%) patients. Preoperative symptoms were apparent in 130 (91%) patients. Seventy-five (52%) patients presented with jaundice, and 88 (62%) patients had nonspecific epigastric pain. Twenty-nine (20%) patients described a weight loss of more than 10 kg in the three months preceding the presentation. Permanent nausea affected 29 (20%) patients, and a reduced performance status was experienced by 27 (19%) patients (Table 1). Twenty-one (15%) patients already presented with diabetes mellitus, of whom 15 (10%) were insulin-dependent and 6 (4%) were on

TABLE 1: Characteristics of the patients.

Number of patients	$n = 143$
Gender	
♂	87 (61%)
♀	56 (39%)
Median age: years (range)	64 (33–83)
Median body mass index (range)	24.8 (13.5–38.8)
Preoperative symptoms	
Jaundice	75 (52%)
Nonspecific epigastric pain	88 (62%)
10% reduction of body weight	29 (20%)
Nausea	29 (20%)
Reduced performance status	27 (19%)
Incidental finding	12 (8%)

oral antidiabetics. Thirteen (9%) patients had a history of pancreatitis. In the context of diagnosis, 121 (85%) patients had an abdominal CT, and a tumor was diagnosed in 56 cases (46% of all CT examinations). An endosonography was performed in 34 (24%) patients, with tumor findings in 22 (65% of all endosonographies) patients. Preoperative endoscopic retrograde cholangiography (ERC) was performed in 131 patients (92%), with evidence of tumor in 105 patients (73%). A papillotomy was undertaken in 57 patients (40%), and preoperative stent placement in the common bile duct was performed in 39 patients (27%). Preoperative laboratory chemical examinations gave a median CA 19-9 value of 23 U/L (1–9171), a bilirubin level of 1.7 mg/dL (0.2–44.4), and a γGT of 172 U/L (6–1865).

2.2. Surgical Procedure. In 86 (60%) patients a pylorus-preserving pancreaticoduodenectomy (PPPD) was performed and in 57 (40%) patients a Kausch-Whipple pancreaticoduodenectomy (KW) was performed. Pancreato-enteral anastomosis was performed as pancreatico jejunostomy in 123 patients (86%) or pancreaticogastrostomy in 20 patients (14%) using a mattress suture technique in 98 patients (69%) and Cattell duct-to-mucosa technique in 45 patients (31%). Due to tumor infiltration, partial portal vein resection has been performed in two (1%) patients. Reconstruction of the superior mesenteric artery was indicated in one patient (1%). The median operation time was 325 (182–785) minutes, with an average blood loss of 500 mL (100–3000). A total of 43 (30%) patients were intraoperatively substituted with packed red blood cells (PRBC). Pancreatic reconstruction was performed in 132 (92%) patients as pancreaticojejunostomy (PJ) and in 11 patients as pancreaticogastrostomy (PG) (8%). The operation was extended in nine (6%) patients, with four patients receiving a partial liver resection, two a splenectomy and partial colon resection, and one a nephrectomy. Intraoperative complications occurred in 4 (3%) patients; three patients had bleeding that was difficult to control and one patient experienced both myocardial infarction and cardiac arrhythmia. All of the operations were performed in line with tumor-surgical criteria by experienced visceral surgeons who were taking a curative approach. Both PPPD and KW were performed in accordance with international standards as en bloc dissection with lymphadenectomy along the hepatoduodenal ligament, celiac trunk, and superior mesenteric artery. The resection areas were classified intraoperatively as curative (R0) when no microscopic evidence of tumor cells was present histopathologically. The tumor stage was graded using the UICC classification of 2009 for ampullary cancers [19].

2.3. Standard Postoperative Care. Every patient received a nasogastric tube for gastric decompression. Amylase and/or lipase levels were monitored daily in the serum and in the intraoperatively placed abdominal drains (Degania Silicone Europe GmbH, Regensburg, Germany) on the first and fourth postoperative days. Radiological contrast imaging was performed on the fifth postoperative day over the nasogastric tube.

The diagnosis of a postoperative pancreatic fistula formation (POPF) was based on the definition of the International Study Group on Pancreatic Fistula (ISGPF) [20]. The levels of amylase in the intraoperatively placed drains were not available for all subjects in our database. The lipase levels in the drains had always been measured. We therefore slightly modified the ISGPF definitions and used amylase or lipase levels in the drains to define the existence of a POPF. Postpancreatectomy hemorrhage (PPH) and delayed gastric emptying (DGE) were also defined based on the International Study Group of Pancreatic Surgery (ISGPS) definitions. [21, 22]. However, the definitions of ISGPS for POPF, PPH, and DGE were not published until 2004 and 2007, respectively. Thus, incidences of POPF and PPH had to be retrospectively evaluated.

2.4. Statistics. The data were collected in a database (Microsoft Access 2.0, Microsoft Corporation, Seattle, USA) and evaluated retrospectively. Unless otherwise specified, the data are expressed as median and range. Survival analysis was determined by means of the Kaplan-Meier method (log-rank test) and specific risk factors by the Mann-Whitney U test using SPSS for Windows 14.0 (SPSS Inc. Chicago, IL, USA). A P value below 0.05 was considered to be significant.

3. Results

3.1. Postoperative Progress and Surgical Complications. The median length of hospital stay was 16 (9–100) days. The median stay in intensive care was 3 (1–74) days. Twelve (8%) patients developed POPF requiring operative revision in five cases. Insufficiency of the bile duct anastomosis occurred in two (1%) patients. In total, revision surgery was undertaken in 10 (7%) patients (Table 2). These revisions comprised four residual pancreatectomies and one new installation of the pancreatoenteral anastomosis (a pancreaticogastrostomy was followed by a pancreaticojejunostomy) and three revisions for wound dehiscence and two instances of PPH. Postoperative delayed gastric emptying occurred in 8 patients (6%). The perioperative lethality was 3.5%. The cause of death

TABLE 2: Operative and postoperative course.

Median operation time (minutes/range)	325 (182–785)
Median intraoperative blood loss (mL/range)	500 (100–3000)
Intraoperative complications	4 (3%)
Postoperative complications	34 (24%)
Wound infection	14 (10%)
Postpancreatectomy hemorrhage (PPH)	6 (4%)
Postoperative pancreatic fistula (POPF)	12 (8%)
Bile leak	2 (1%)
Delayed gastric emptying (DGE)	8 (6%)
Reoperation	10 (7%)
In-hospital mortality	5 (3.5%)

was sepsis in two patients, and one patient had surgically untreatable bleeding, cardiac decompensation from known cardiac insufficiency, or acute myocardial infarction. Within the observation period, 18 (13%) patients underwent in-patient readmission. Of these, 10 (7%) patients were operated on again for reasons unrelated to the underlying condition. Emerging diabetes mellitus was diagnosed in 9 (6%) patients, and 64 (45%) patients needed postoperative enzyme substitution at mealtimes. The total mortality was 69% in a median postoperative observation period of 30 months (0–205).

3.2. TNM. The histological examination of the pathological specimen and categorization by means of TNM classification resulted in a pTis stage in 2 (1%) patients and a pT1 stage in 14 (10%) patients. An almost identical number of patients had pT2 (53 patients; 37%) and pT3 stages (54 patients; 38%). In 20 (14%) patients a pT4 stage was diagnosed. Positive lymph node involvement (pN1) was evident in 69 (48%) cases. More than half of the patients were in a G2 stage (75 patients; 52%) of differentiation (pG), followed by stage G3 in 36% (52 patients). Fifteen (10%) patients presented with a G1 stage and 1 (1%) patient with a G4 stage. The tumor size was smaller than 2 cm in diameter in 53 patients (37%) and bigger than 2 cm in 90 patients (63%).

Microscopically detected tumor infiltration, detectable by microscopy (R1) of the resection margins or at the retropancreatic ablation level, was evidenced in 12 (8%) patients. Lymphatic invasion was present in 70 (49%) patients and vascular invasion in 17 (12%) patients in the final histology.

3.3. UICC Stages. As a result of classifying the 143 patients as per the UICC stages, 16 (11%) patients were stage 1a and 33 (23%) patients were stage 1b. Stage 2b, with 51 patients (35%), was the most frequent. In comparison, 20 patients (14%) were stage 2a and 16 (11%) and 7 (6%) patients were stages 3 and 4, respectively.

3.4. Survival and Prognostic Factors. After 1-, 5-, 10-, and 15-year periods, the overall survival of the examined patient population was 79%, 40%, 25%, and 10%, respectively, with a median survival term of 37 months (Figure 1). Survival analysis (log-rank) resulted in a significantly reduced survival for patients who had a reduced general condition ($P = 0.008$),

TABLE 3: Survival and prognostic factors with respect to survival-multivariate analysis.

	P value	Odds ratio (95% confidence interval)
No lymphatic invasion	$P = 0.000$	0.248 (0.145–0.425)
No intraoperative administration of PRBC	$P = 0.008$	0.510 (0.311–0.836)
Preoperatively elevated CA 19-9	$P = 0.023$	1.762 (1.081–2.870)

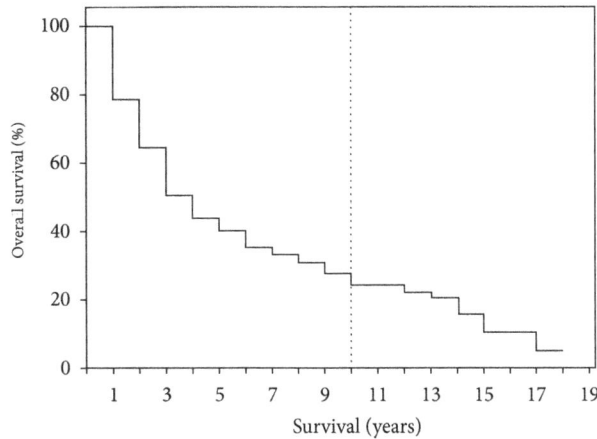

FIGURE 1: The overall survival for patients after the resection of ampullary carcinoma with curative intention.

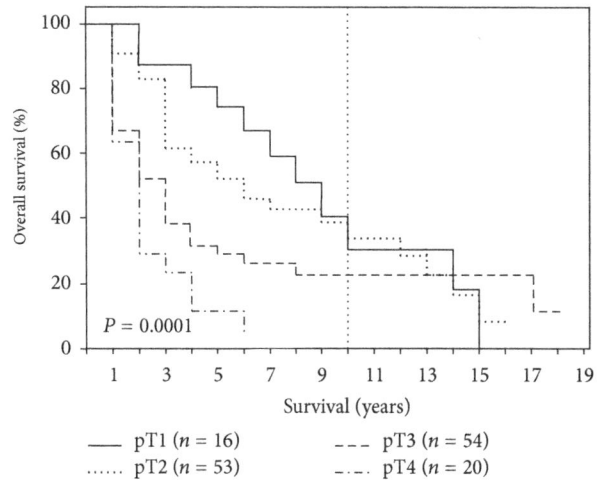

FIGURE 2: Survival depending on tumor stage (pT1, pT2, pT3, and pT4).

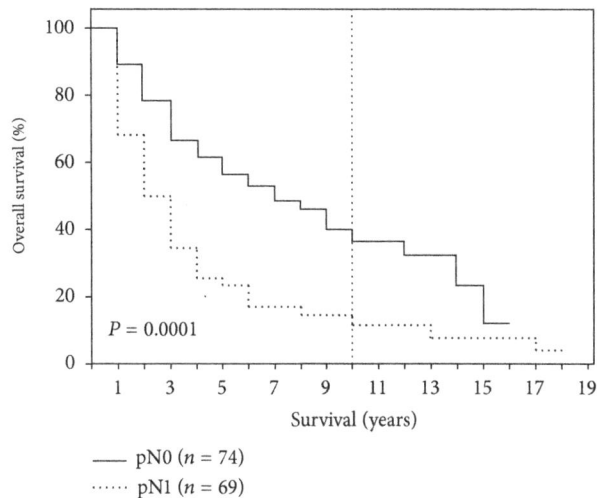

FIGURE 3: Survival according to lymph node status (pN0 versus pN1).

required intraoperative administration of PRBC ($P = 0.003$), had POPF ($P = 0.013$), had an advanced tumor stage ($P = 0.0001$) (Figure 2), had a pT4 tumor invasion depth ($P = 0.0001$), had a positive lymph node stage (0.0001) (Figure 3), had a pG4 tumor grade ($P = 0.0001$), had a microscopically or macroscopically positive resection margin ($P = 0.02$) (Figure 4), had vascular ($P = 0.008$) or lymphatic invasion ($P = 0.0001$) (Figure 5), and had a preoperatively elevated CA 19-9 ($P = 0.008$). There were no significant differences in regard of overall survival in patients who received a PPPD and patients who underwent classic Whipple procedure ($P - 0.222$). A tumor size smaller than 2 cm did not have a significant effect on overall survival ($P = 0.458$). Examining the risk factors with respect to survival, multivariate analysis revealed that the following are risk factors for poor prognosis: lymphatic invasion ($P = 0.000$), intraoperative administration of PRBC ($P = 0.008$), and a preoperatively elevated CA 19-9 ($P = 0.023$) (Table 3).

4. Discussion

In 1912, Hirschel conducted the first documented single-stage resection of an ampullary carcinoma in Heidelberg, Germany [23]. Since then, morbidity and mortality have been reduced continuously through modifications of the operative procedure and through general progress in diagnosis and peri- and postoperative management. However, long-term survival following curative resection of ampullary carcinoma remains low. The reported 5-year survival rates vary from 30 to 70% [4, 24–28]. In our study, the 5-year survival equaled 40% which is equivalent to the results of a retrospective study of a large American patient population by O'Connel et al. who reported a 5-year survival of 36.8% for a total of 3292 patients, however only 1301 of whom (40%) underwent primary surgical therapy [29]. The majority of current studies looking into the long-term follow-up of ampullary cancer are conducted multicentrically and examine the long-term results for up to a maximum of ten years following resection. The information on factors that influence the long-term prognosis following the resection of ampullary carcinomas is therefore limited. It should be noted that ampullary cancer does not occur frequently overall but constitutes a relevant proportion (20–40%) of all resected tumors of the periampullary region [2–4]. One reason for this situation is the high rate of resectability at the time of diagnosis, specified in the literature as up to

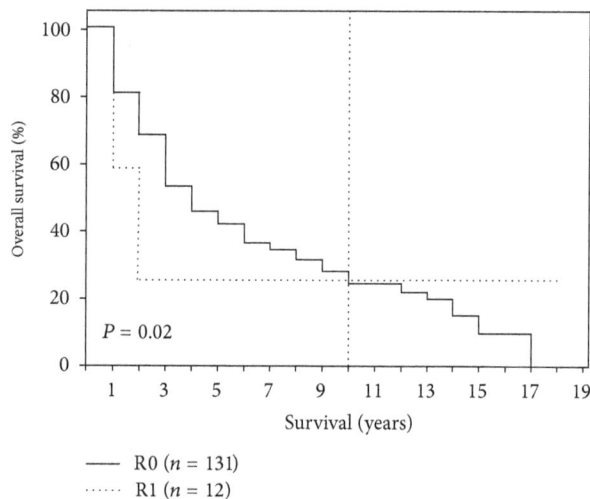

FIGURE 4: Survival depending on surgical radicality (R0 versus R1).

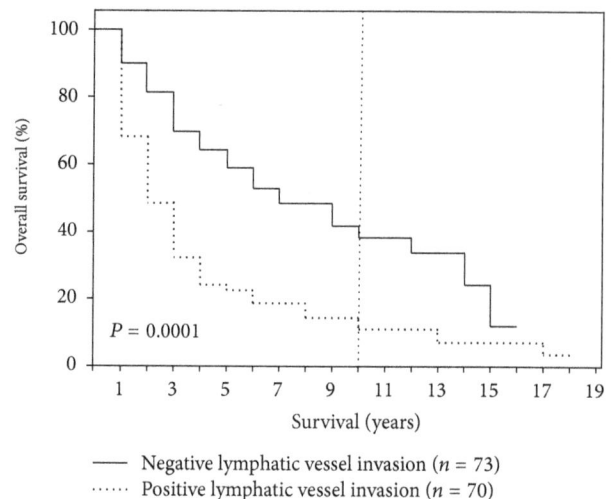

FIGURE 5: Survival depending on lymphatic vessel invasion (L0 versus L1).

80% which is significantly higher than for pancreatic head carcinoma (20%) [3, 30]. The anatomical location and the exophytic growth pattern of ampullary carcinomas, leading to early occlusion of the bile duct and therefore often-early clinical diagnosis, explain the high resectability rate and the positive results relative to the surgical radicality of the procedure [4–6]. This is underlined by the results of our study in which a total of 131 patients (92%) received R0 resection of the primary tumor with a 10-year survival of 25% and 15-year survival of 10%, respectively. In the survival analysis (log-rank), our study identified the following prognostic factors that were accompanied by a significantly reduced long-term survival: reduced general condition at the time of surgery, intraoperative administration of PRBC, POPF, tumor stage, substantial invasion depth of the tumor, lymph node stage, histological grading, resection border, vascular and lymphatic vessel invasion, and CA 19-9 levels higher than 37 U/L. There were no significant differences in regard of overall survival between patients who underwent PPPD in comparison to the classic Whipple procedure. A postpyloric resection approach therefore appears to be safe in patients with ampullary cancer.

In the multivariate analysis lymphatic vessel invasion, intraoperative administration of PRBCs, and an elevated CA 19-9 level were identified as independent risk factors for a reduced long-term survival. There is consensus in the literature for most carcinomas of the gastrointestinal tract (esophagus, stomach, and colorectum) regarding the influence of lymph node status on long-term prognosis. Aside from the results of our study, this hypothesis is substantiated by the results of Hurtuk et al., who noted the significant influence of positive lymph node involvement on long-term survival especially for ampullary and pancreatic carcinoma [31]. The 5-year survival reported in the literature is 0 to 30% when there is positive lymph node involvement and 39 to 78% in patients who lack lymph node involvement [32]. There is controversy over the extent of the lymphadenectomy. At our clinic, partial pancreaticoduodenectomy is performed

with a comprehensive lymphadenectomy, along the hepatoduodenal ligament, celiac trunk, and superior mesenteric artery. However, in a study in which the results from standard lymphadenectomy and extended lymphadenectomy were compared, there were no significant differences with respect to long-term survival (56 versus 60%) [33].

Beyond radical surgical approaches, also endoscopic treatment options for ampullary tumors exist such as endoscopic resection [34], photodynamic therapy [35], and electrofulguration [36]. Endoscopic resection can provide a safe and effective treatment option for benign ampullary tumors. If an ampullary tumor appears to be benign and the biopsy samples are negative for malignancy, endoscopic papillectomy should be considered as an initial intervention. The decision on whether to perform a subsequent pancreaticoduodenectomy should then be based on the histopathological findings. However, false negative rates of 40 to 85% have been reported for endoscopic biopsies and small ampullary cancers may be missed [37]. According to the results of our study, a tumor size smaller than 2 cm even in early tumor stages does not correlate with an improved survival. A delayed treatment may therefore be fatal. An accurate differentiation between benign and malignant lesions can only be achieved by radical pancreaticoduodenectomy. Prospective randomized trials will have to evaluate a possible benefit of endoscopic resection for small ampullary malignancies, for example, in patients with an increased operative risk score.

Howe et al. also identified lymph node metastases and a positive tumor cutting margin as risk factors for reduced long-term survival [4]. However, at the same time, these authors subdivided ampullary carcinomas into two subgroups by way of detailed histopathology and found that median survival of those tumors with a histologically verified pancreatobiliary origin was significantly lower in comparison to tumors with a histologically verified intestinal origin (22 months versus 60 months) [4]. Outerbridge reported back in 1913 that ampullary cancer could exhibit different histological origins [38]. Apart from origins in the duodenal mucosa, the epithelia of the common pancreatobiliary ductal system, pancreatic duct, or bile duct are possible points of origin. In clinical practice, due to the heterogeneity of the tumor and frequent, simultaneously present preneoplastic lesions, the exact histological origin can often be not clearly differentiated. In our study, we did not further classify ampullary carcinomas based on detailed histological findings. Kimura et al. (1994), who examined 53 patients with ampullary carcinoma, were one of the first to describe histological criteria that allow for more accurate allocation to either pancreatobiliary or intestinal origin [39]. These authors also reported that ampullary cancers of pancreatobiliary origin are more frequently accompanied by lymph node involvement and had a worse prognosis than carcinomas of an intestinal origin [39]. Zhou et al. reported in 2004 the use of cytokeratin and apomycin markers to assign ampullary cancers histologically and unambiguously to one of the two subgroups [13]. However, these methods are still not a popular standard today, even though Westgaard et al. showed that the histological subtype is an essentially more relevant prognostic factor than the otherwise typical affiliation to one of the anatomical subtypes of periampullary carcinomas [40].

Tumor recurrence after resection with curative intention remains a key problem in the long-term prognosis following radical resection. The tumor recurrence rate, as reported in the literature, varies from 28 to 44%. Examples of key manifestation regions are the liver and aortocaval lymph node metastases, as well as locoregional tumor recurrence [18, 26, 41]. Postoperative adjuvant chemotherapy [42] and radiochemotherapy [43, 44] have been shown to improve survival outcomes in patients with periampullary carcinomas. In current studies, however, patients considered for postoperative adjuvant therapy often had adverse prognostic factors, such as positive lymph node involvement, higher tumor stage, or poor tumor differentiation, compared with patients who were treated with surgery alone [45]. According to the results of our study, adjuvant therapy should be recommended for patients with positive tumor cutting margins or other risk constellations, such as lymph node involvement, tumor invasion into the surrounding tissue, or poorly differentiated tumor grade. However, there is an urgent need for further studies on the influence of adjuvant therapy on the long-term prognosis after the resection of ampullary cancer.

There are several limitations to the present study. Although the clinical data were prospectively collected, the study design and analysis are retrospective and are therefore subject to an inherent selection bias. Moreover, due to the rarity of this tumor entity, in an attempt to achieve a statistically relevant patient cohort, the patients included in this study were treated over a time period of 15 years. During this time surgical techniques, peri- and postoperative management, and the role of adjuvant therapy were not consistent with recent recommendations. However, to the best of our knowledge, this study is the first to investigate the factors that influence the long-term survival in a large patient population over a period of 15 years after the surgical treatment of ampullary carcinomas. This study may therefore help to guide future practice patterns and treatment recommendations.

5. Conclusion

The prognosis of ampullary carcinoma is clearly better than that of other carcinomas of the periampullary region. Nevertheless, the results of our study show that factors such as an increased tumor stage, considerable invasion depth of the tumor, positive lymph node involvement, blood vessel and lymphatic invasion of the tumor, and a CA 19-9 level higher than 37 U/L are accompanied by a reduced long-term prognosis. Subsequent adjuvant therapy remains essential especially in patients with this constellation of risk factors. However, additional studies are necessary to specify the role of adjuvant therapy in improving long-term results after the resection of ampullary carcinomas.

Authors' Contribution

Fritz Klein collected the data and wrote the paper. Dietmar Jacob designed and performed the research. Marcus Bahra collected the data. Gero Puhl collected the data. Andreas Andreou collected the data. Safak Gül collected the data. Olaf Guckelberger designed and performed the research. All of the authors contributed to the design and interpretation of the study and to further drafts.

References

[1] K. Yamaguchi and M. Enjoji, "Carcinoma of the ampulla of Vater. A clinicopathologic study and pathologic staging of 109 cases of carcinoma and 5 cases of adenoma," *Cancer*, vol. 59, no. 3, pp. 506–515, 1987.

[2] A. Nakase, Y. Matsumoto, K. Uchida, and I. Honjo, "Surgical treatment of cancer of the pancreas and the periampullary region: cumulative results in 57 institutions in Japan," *Annals of Surgery*, vol. 185, no. 1, pp. 52–57, 1977.

[3] C. J. Yeo, T. A. Sohn, J. L. Cameron, R. H. Hruban, K. D. Lillemoe, and H. A. Pitt, "Periampullary adenocarcinoma: analysis of 5-year survivors," *Annals of Surgery*, vol. 227, no. 6, pp. 821–831, 1998.

[4] J. R. Howe, D. S. Klimstra, R. D. Moccia, K. C. Conlon, and M. F. Brennan, "Factors predictive of survival in ampullary carcinoma," *Annals of Surgery*, vol. 228, no. 1, pp. 87–94, 1998.

[5] C. G. Willett, A. L. Warshaw, K. Convery, and C. C. Compton, "Patterns of failure after pancreaticoduodenectomy for ampullary carcinoma," *Surgery Gynecology and Obstetrics*, vol. 176, no. 1, pp. 33–38, 1993.

[6] P. Bucher, G. Chassot, Y. Durmishi, F. Ris, and P. Morel, "Long-term results of surgical treatment of Vater's ampulla neoplasms," *Hepato-Gastroenterology*, vol. 54, no. 76, pp. 1239–1242, 2007.

[7] K. Sahora, I. Kührer, D. Trenkwitz et al., "Pankreaskarzinom und periampulläres Karzinom," *Journal für Gastroenterologische und Hepatologische Erkrankungen*, vol. 7, no. 2, pp. 36–44, 2009.

[8] B. W. Miedema, M. G. Sarr, J. A. van Heerden et al., "Complications following pancreaticoduodenectomy: current management," *Archives of Surgery*, vol. 127, no. 8, pp. 945–950, 1992.

[9] K. W. Warren, D. S. Choe, J. Plaza, and M. Relihan, "Results of radical resection for periampullary cancer," *Annals of Surgery*, vol. 181, no. 5, pp. 534–540, 1975.

[10] F. Michelassi, F. Erroi, P. J. Dawson et al., "Experience with 647 consecutive tumors of the duodenum, ampulla, head of the pancreas, and distal common bile duct," *Annals of Surgery*, vol. 210, no. 4, pp. 544–556, 1989.

[11] A. O. Whipple, "A reminiscence: pancreaticduodenectomy," *Review of Surgery*, vol. 20, pp. 221–225, 1963.

[12] W. Kimura and K. Ohtsubo, "Incidence, sites of origin, and immunohistochemical and histochemical characteristics of atypical epithelium and minute carcinoma of the papilla of Vater," *Cancer*, vol. 61, no. 7, pp. 1394–1402, 1988.

[13] H. Zhou, N. Schaefer, M. Wolff, and H. P. Fischer, "Carcinoma of the ampulla of vater: comparative histologic/immunohistochemical classification and follow-up," *The American Journal of Surgical Pathology*, vol. 28, no. 7, pp. 875–882, 2004.

[14] K. Baczako, M. Büchler, H. G. Beger, C. J. Kirkpatrick, and O. Haferkamp, "Morphogenesis and possible precursor lesions of invasive carcinoma of the papilla of Vater: epithelial dysplasia and adenoma," *Human Pathology*, vol. 16, no. 3, pp. 305–310, 1985.

[15] I. C. Talbot, J. P. Neoptolemos, D. E. Shaw, and D. Carr-Locke, "The histopathology and staging of carcinoma of the ampulla of vater," *Histopathology*, vol. 12, no. 2, pp. 155–165, 1988.

[16] G. C. Harewood, N. L. Pochron, and C. J. Gostout, "Prospective, randomized, controlled trial of prophylactic pancreatic stent placement for endoscopic snare excision of the duodenal ampulla," *Gastrointestinal Endoscopy*, vol. 62, no. 3, pp. 367–370, 2005.

[17] S. Seewald, S. Omar, and N. Soehendra, "Endoscopic resection of tumors of the ampulla of Vater: how far up and how deep down can we go?" *Gastrointestinal Endoscopy*, vol. 63, no. 6, pp. 789–791, 2006.

[18] T. Todoroki, N. Koike, Y. Morishita et al., "Patterns and predictors of failure after curative resections of carcinoma of the ampulla of vater," *Annals of Surgical Oncology*, vol. 10, no. 10, pp. 1176–1183, 2003.

[19] L. H. Sobin, M. K. Gospodarowicz, C. Wittekind, and International Union against Cancer, *TNM Classification of Malignant Tumours*, Wiley, Blackwell, 7th edition, 2009.

[20] C. Bassi, G. Butturini, E. Molinari et al., "Pancreatic fistula rate after pancreatic resection: the importance of definitions," *Digestive Surgery*, vol. 21, no. 1, pp. 54–59, 2004.

[21] M. N. Wente, J. A. Veit, C. Bassi et al., "Postpancreatectomy hemorrhage (PPH)—an international study group of pancreatic surgery (ISGPS) definition," *Surgery*, vol. 142, no. 1, pp. 20–25, 2007.

[22] M. N. Wente, C. Bassi, C. Dervenis et al., "Delayed gastric emptying (DGE) after pancreatic surgery: a suggested definition by the international study group of pancreatic surgery (ISGPS)," *Surgery*, vol. 142, no. 5, pp. 761–768, 2007.

[23] D. W. Crist and J. L. Cameron, "The current status of the Whipple operation for periampullary carcinoma," *Advances in Surgery*, vol. 25, pp. 21–49, 1992.

[24] M. A. Talamini, R. C. Moesinger, H. A. Pitt et al., "Adenocarcinoma of the ampulla of Vater: a 28-year experience," *Annals of Surgery*, vol. 225, no. 5, pp. 590–600, 1997.

[25] J. P. Duffy, O. J. Hines, J. H. Liu et al., "Improved survival for adenocarcinoma of the ampulla of Vater: fifty-five consecutive resections," *Archives of Surgery*, vol. 138, no. 9, pp. 941–950, 2003.

[26] V. Bettschart, M. Q. Rahman, F. J. F. Engelken, K. K. Madhavan, R. W. Parks, and O. J. Garden, "Presentation, treatment and outcome in patients with ampullary tumours," *The British Journal of Surgery*, vol. 91, no. 12, pp. 1600–1607, 2004.

[27] A. Di Giorgio, S. Alfieri, F. Rotondi et al., "Pancreatoduodenectomy for tumors of Vater's ampulla: report on 94 consecutive patients," *World Journal of Surgery*, vol. 29, no. 4, pp. 513–518, 2005.

[28] K. M. Brown, A. J. Tompkins, S. Yong, G. V. Aranha, and M. Shoup, "Pancreaticoduodenectomy is curative in the majority of patients with node-negative ampullary cancer," *Archives of Surgery*, vol. 140, no. 6, pp. 529–533, 2005.

[29] J. B. O'Connell, M. A. Maggard, J. Manunga Jr. et al., "Survival after resection of ampullary carcinoma: a national population-based study," *Annals of Surgical Oncology*, vol. 15, no. 7, pp. 1820–1827, 2008.

[30] R. D. Kim, P. S. Kundhal, I. D. McGilvray et al., "Predictors of failure after pancreaticoduodenectomy for ampullary carcinoma," *Journal of the American College of Surgeons*, vol. 202, no. 1, pp. 112–119, 2006.

[31] M. G. Hurtuk, C. Hughes, M. Shoup, and G. V. Aranha, "Does lymph node ratio impact survival in resected periampullary malignancies?" *The American Journal of Surgery*, vol. 197, no. 3, pp. 348–352, 2009.

[32] H. P. Hsu, Y. S. Shan, Y. H. Hsieh, T. M. Yang, and P. W. Lin, "Predictors of recurrence after pancreaticoduodenectomy in ampullary cancer: comparison between non-, early and late recurrence," *Journal of the Formosan Medical Association*, vol. 106, no. 6, pp. 432–443, 2007.

[33] C. J. Yeo, J. L. Cameron, K. D. Lillemoe et al., "Pancreaticoduodenectomy with or without distal gastrectomy and extended retroperitoneal lymphadenectomy for periampullary adenocarcinoma—part 2: randomized controlled trial evaluating survival, morbidity, and mortality," *Annals of Surgery*, vol. 236, no. 3, pp. 355–368, 2002.

[34] K. F. Binmoeller, S. Boaventura, K. Ramsperger, and N. Soehendra, "Endoscopic snare excision of benign adenomas of the papilla of Vater," *Gastrointestinal Endoscopy*, vol. 39, no. 2, pp. 127–131, 1993.

[35] R. Lambert, T. Ponchon, A. Chavaillon, and F. Berger, "Laser treatment of tumors of the papilla of Vater," *Endoscopy*, vol. 20, no. 1, pp. 227–231, 1988.

[36] E. Shemesh, S. Nass, and A. Czerniak, "Endoscopic sphincterotomy and endoscopic fulguration in the management of adenoma of the papilla of Vater," *Surgery Gynecology and Obstetrics*, vol. 169, no. 5, pp. 445–448, 1989.

[37] M. K. Jung, C. M. Cho, S. Y. Park et al., "Endoscopic resection of ampullary neoplasms: a single-center experience," *Surgical Endoscopy*, vol. 23, no. 11, pp. 2568–2574, 2009.

[38] G. Outerbridge, "Carcinoma of the papilla of Vater," *Surgery*, vol. 57, pp. 402–426, 1913.

[39] W. Kimura, N. Futakawa, S. Yamagata et al., "Different clinicopathologic findings in two histologic types of carcinoma of papilla of Vater," *Japanese Journal of Cancer Research*, vol. 85, no. 2, pp. 161–166, 1994.

[40] A. Westgaard, S. Tafjord, I. N. Farstad et al., "Pancreatobiliary versus intestinal histologic type of differentiation is an independent prognostic factor in resected periampullary adenocarcinoma," *BMC Cancer*, vol. 8, article 170, 2008.

[41] M. Kayahara, T. Nagakawa, T. Ohta, H. Kitagawa, and I. Miyazaki, "Surgical strategy for carcinoma of the papilla of

Vater on the basis of lymphatic spread and mode of recurrence," *Surgery*, vol. 121, no. 6, pp. 611–617, 1997.

[42] H. Oettle, S. Post, P. Neuhaus et al., "Adjuvant chemotherapy with gemcitabine vs observation in patients undergoing curative-intent resection of pancreatic cancer: a randomized controlled trial," *The Journal of the American Medical Association*, vol. 297, no. 3, pp. 267–277, 2007.

[43] S. S. Sikora, P. Balachandran, K. Dimri et al., "Adjuvant chemoradiotherapy in ampullary cancers," *European Journal of Surgical Oncology*, vol. 31, no. 2, pp. 158–163, 2005.

[44] J. H. Klinkenbijl, J. Jeekel, T. Sahmoud et al., "Adjuvant radiotherapy and 5-fluorouracil after curative resection of cancer of the pancreas and periampullary region: phase III trial of the EORTC gastrointestinal tract cancer cooperative group," *Annals of Surgery*, vol. 230, no. 6, pp. 776–784, 1999.

[45] S. Bhatia, R. C. Miller, M. G. Haddock, J. H. Donohue, and S. Krishnan, "Adjuvant therapy for ampullary carcinomas: the Mayo clinic experience," *International Journal of Radiation Oncology Biology Physics*, vol. 66, no. 2, pp. 514–519, 2006.

31

Pancreatic Cancer: 80 Years of Surgery—Percentage and Repetitions

Birgir Gudjonsson

The Medical Clinic, Álfheimum 74, 104 Reykjavik, Iceland

Correspondence should be addressed to Birgir Gudjonsson; bghav@simnet.is

Academic Editor: Pablo Ramírez

Objective. The incidence of pancreatic cancer is estimated to be 48,960 in 2015 in the US and projected to become the second and third leading causes of cancer-related deaths by 2030. The mean costs in 2015 may be assumed to be $79,800 per patient and for each resection $164,100. Attempt is made to evaluate the results over the last 80 years, the number of survivors, and the overall survival percentage. *Methods.* Altogether 1230 papers have been found which deal with resections and reveal survival information. Only 621 of these report 5-year survivors. Reservation about surgery was first expressed in 1964 and five-year survival of nonresected survivors is well documented. *Results.* The survival percentage depends not only on the number of survivors but also on the subset from which it is calculated. Since the 1980s the papers have mainly reported the number of resections and survival as actuarial percentages, with or without the actual number of survivors being reported. The actuarial percentage is on average 2.75 higher. Detailed information on the original group (TN), number of resections, and actual number of survivors is reported in only 10.6% of the papers. Repetition occurs when the patients from a certain year are reported several times from the same institution or include survivors from many institutions or countries. Each 5-year survivor may be reported several times. *Conclusion.* Assuming a 10% resection rate and correcting for repetitions and the life table percentage the overall actual survival rate is hardly more than 0.3%.

1. Introduction

Resections for pancreatic adenocarcinoma which Whipple et al. [1] initiated after earlier attempts by Codivilla [2] and Kausch [3] have now been carried out for 80 years. Opinions still differ as to the results. Some authors claim a survival percentage of up to 22% and are widely quoted and extol the benefits and success of resections [4] while others doubt that anyone survives pancreatic cancer [5].

2. Incidence, Economics

The incidence of pancreatic cancer has been estimated at 48,960 in 2015 in the US and is the fourth leading cause of death from cancer for both sexes [6]. It is projected to increase to 62,000 in the year 2020 and to 88,000 for both sexes in 2030 and to surpass breast, prostate, and colorectal cancers to become the second and third leading causes of cancer-related deaths by 2030 [7].

The cost of treatment of pancreatic cancer is of concern in many countries. O'Neill and colleagues studied the total direct medical cost of patients 66 years and older who were diagnosed from 2000 to 2007 in the US. The mean total direct cost was $65,500, for resectable locoregional disease cost was $134,700, and for unresectable locoregional or distant disease cost was $65,300 and $49,000, respectively [8]. Lea and Stahlgren had earlier pointed out the difference in the cost of resections versus bypass [9].

Assuming 2.5% inflation over 8 years, the mean cost in 2015 would be $79,800, for resections $164,100, for unresectable (or bypasses) disease $79,500, and for distant disease $59,700. With the estimated number of patients in 2015 the overall cost would be close to $4 billion.

3. Methods and Evaluation of Results

There is a growing concern that reports of success in medical research are inflated [10].

Here an attempt is made to evaluate the results over the last 80 years, the number of survivors, and the overall survival percentage.

This author has continued to scrutinize the literature on surgery from the onset, initially using the *Index Medicus* and then Ovid/PubMed until the end of 2014, with cross-references. Approximately 1230 papers have been found in 15 languages in approximately 200 journals from 44 countries which deal with resections and reveal at least some survival information. A total of 40.5% of the papers originated in the US, 19.3% from Japan, 7.3% from Germany, 5.3% from Italy, and 4% from France and the UK. These have been inserted into a database.

Papers on the surgical aspects of pancreatic cancer differ as to the approach and the composition of the patient group and the method of reporting. A few emphasize only the technical aspects and the mortality with limited or no survival information and indiscriminately cover patients with various malignant and benign pathologies which may require pancreatoduodenal resection, but without clearly separating each pathology group or presenting separate survival information. Only papers with separate pathologic information on patients were selected for analysis for this paper. Analysis of the database reveals that, of these 1230 papers, 609 do not report any 5-year survivors, some seem to be mainly technical, and some report only up to a 3-year survival rate. A total of 621 papers report 5-year survivors and will be examined further in detail in this paper. Special attention has been paid to the origin of each paper, the time period each study covered, patient composition, the subset of patients used for calculations, and the statistical method used.

4. Reservation, Nonresected Survivors

The first reservation about the effect of surgery on this disease was expressed by Glenn and Thorbjarnarson [11] in 1964, again by Gallitano et al. [12] in 1968 whose only 5-year survivor was "nonresected," and then strongly by Crile Jr. in 1970 [13], whose only survivor was also nonresected. He challenged the value of resection for pancreatic cancer, followed by Shapiro in 1975 [14]. Crile Jr.'s criticism was directed at the then high mortality rate and the survival calculations which were carried out and might count only those who survived the operation and in ignorance of the nonresected survivors.

The presence of nonresected survivors has been disputed [15], but it is a major issue in the debate on survival. It was first pointed out by Cattell and Young in 1957 [16] and, as above, later by Gallitano and Crile Jr. The data were summarized by the present author in a paper in 1995 [17] and a letter in 1996 [18]. In a review by the present author published in 1978 only 65 five-year survivors could be found in the literature, of whom 8 were nonresected [19]. In a review published in 1987, 165 survivors could be found, but 12 of these were nonresected [20]. In this review 41 reports have been found from 31 institutions in 12 countries, many from eminent institutions and renowned authors, thereof 17 from the US, two from Yale [19, 20], two from the University Texas MD Anderson [12, 21], and two from Harvard MGH [22, 23], as well as from the University of Chicago [24], the Dana Farber Cancer Clinic [25], and Thomas Jefferson [26], to mention a few.

Nonresected survival is a fact and should be kept in mind in assessing overall therapeutic results. Initially reports detailed the course of all patients diagnosed at a particular institution but in recent decades reports have concentrated only on resected patients, completely ignoring any nonresected survivors. Nonresected survivors would therefore not be found.

5. Survival Calculations

The survival percentage depends not only on the number of survivors but on the subset from which the number is calculated.

A few earlier studies started by examining the respective tumor registries and disclosed that only about 35–68% of patients in tumor registries had histologic confirmation. Survival calculations have been based on the original number of patients with histologic diagnoses at a particular institution, previously called the total number (TN), the approximately 80% of cases that were surgically explored, the cases that were resected, or location, size, or R status of the tumor, or even only those patients who survived the operation.

Overall survival success must be based on the original group diagnosed with pancreatic cancer (the TN or total number) and the number of survivors and not only on a small subgroup of the cases. Different methods of calculation have been used to enumerate the results, that is, actual versus the actuarial, projected, or estimated percentage.

Initially most papers revealed the TN, the number of resections, and simply the number of survivors, whereas later authors also presented actual percentage figures. In the late 1980s the papers started reporting only the number of resections and survival as actuarial percentages, usually calculated with the Kaplan-Meier method with or without the actual number of survivors being reported [27].

Sir Hill pointed out in his book in 1937 that when a "large number of patients is lost sight of" the outcome might be erroneously high. This warning is reemphasized in later editions [28]. In a frequently quoted paper 11 survivors out of 201 are claimed as proof of 22% survival [4].

As indicated in Table 1 the original number TN of patients studied in a report is only revealed in 90 or 14.5% of the papers and in these the actual number of survivors is stated in only 49. In the remaining 41 with a documented TN and actuarial calculation the actual number of survivors is stated in 17, in addition to life table curves. Detailed information on the original TN group studied, number of resections, and actual number of survivors is therefore reported in only 66 or 10.6% of all papers on pancreatic cancer. In the remaining 89.4% some form of estimate or calculation is required to assess survival percentage. In 531 papers there is no information on the original number of patients from which the number of resections was drawn, although in 102 of these the number of survivors is stated or confirmed by inquiry.

In 424 of these 531 reports with survival calculations by actuarial methods 378 are by the Kaplan-Meier method and 48 by other or unclear methods, though KM is also very likely. The number of survivors is stated in 147 of the reports or 34.6%, but not in the remaining 277 or 65.3%.

TABLE 1: Survival information.

Categories of reports	Number of reports	Reports with/without survivors	Reports with/without stated TN	Reports with actual survival calculations	Reports with actuarial calculations and stated number of survivors	Reports with actuarial calculation and survivors confirmed by inquiry	Reports with actuarial calculations and estimated number of survivors
TN number of reports	1230						
Reports with survivors		621					
Reports with stated TN of patients			90				
Actual survival calculations				49			
Actuarial calculations with stated number of survivors					17		
Actuarial calculation with survivors confirmed by inquiry						7	
Reports with estimated number of survivors							17
Reports with estimated TN of patients			531				
Actual survival calculations				102			
Reports with actuarial calculation and stated number of survivors					146		
Survivors confirmed by inquiry						57	
Estimated number of survivors							226
Reports without survivors		609					

Author	Years	60	70	80	90	00	10		Srv
U Kiel/ Hamburg									
Henne-Bruns D [39]	1988–96				------				2 ?
Henne-Bruns D [40]	1988–98				-------				6 ?
Hannover M S									
Klempnauer J [41]	1971–93			---------------					12 s
Klempnauer J [42]	1971–93			---------------					10 s
Klempnauer J [43]	1971–93			---------------					12 s
Humboldt U									
Wenger FA [44]	1981–96				-----------				7 ??
Von Wolff H [45]	1979–85			-----					3 s
Joh Gutenberg U									
Böttger TC [46]	1978–87			------					2 ??
Böttger TC [47]	??–92	???		--------------					1 ?
K Mannheim U Heidelberg									
Trede M [48]	1972–83		--------						5 s
Richter A [49]	1972–98			------------------					31 s
Richter A [50]	1972–00			--------------------					16 ?
Hartel M [51]	1980–01				---------------				19 ??
Trede M [52]	1985–89				-----				11 i
U Erlangen									
Gall FP [53]	1969–84		------------						1 s
Gall FP [54]	1969–87		------------						7 ?
Tannapfel A [55]	1972–87		-----------						10 i
U Heidelberg									
Kleef J [56]	2001–05					---			1 ?
Welsch T [57]	2001–08					-----			30 ??
Hartwig W [58]	2001–09					------			35 ??
Hartwig W [59]	2001–09					-------			16 ??
Strobel O [60]	2001–09					------			1 ??
Pausch T [61]	2001–10					-------			45 ?
U Mainz									
Rückert K [62]	1964–76		--------						4 s
Kümmerle F [63]	1964–82		-----------						10 s
Kümmerle K [64]	1964–84		------------						9 s

Graphs are approximate
s: stated number of survivors
i: number of survivors obtained by inquiry
?: number of patients estimated from actuarial calculations.

FIGURE 1: Repetitions Germany sample. See [40–65].

A total of 240 inquiries were sent to authors where the actual number of patients was not reported and only 58 replies were obtained. The actual number of survivors with actuarial calculation is therefore known in 205 of the 424 reports or 48.3%. The actuarial and actual percentage figures can therefore be compared, as demonstrated previously [29, 30], and reveal that the actuarial percentage is on average 2.75 higher than the actual percentage. This figure has therefore been used to estimate the number of survivors and the survival percentage in the relevant studies where only the actuarial percentage has been published.

The resection rate has been debatable and varies and can only be assessed accurately if the original group is large and well defined. Tertiary referral centers cannot know the size of the original group from which their resection group is drawn. Of the studies published in the last 5 years, 156 of 161 or 97% report only the number of resections and the percentages. In an earlier study by this author the resection rate was 10.8%. In earlier US studies [31, 32] the rate was, respectively, 8.4%

and 12%. In 2 European nationals [33, 34] the rate was from 8% to 12% over the last 5 years. In a recent report from the surgical service at a European university hospital [35] the resection rate was 11.6%. It is therefore practical to assume that the resection rate is 10% in the studies where the original TN of the group is not reported in order to estimate the TN accordingly and divide the percentage by 2.5–3 where the actuarial KM only has been published.

After totaling the numbers in the 621 studies with survivors with the above correction, but without further adjustment, the TN comes to 1,731,834, the number of resected patients comes to 162,207, and the number of survivors comes to 11,300, for an apparent survival percentage of 0.77%.

After totaling the number of patients in all the 1230 reports, the original TN comes to 3,188,543, the number of resected patients to 284,298, and the number of survivors to 11,330. The overall survival percentage would then be only 0.45%.

Author	Years	60	70	80	90	00	10	Srv
Catholic Univ								
Civello IM [65]	1981–96			----------				1 s
Alfieri S [66]	1985–95			--------				2 s
Magistrelli P [67]	1987–94			-----				4 i
Magistrelli P [68]	1988–03			----------				8 ?
Magistrelli P [69]	1988–97			------				4 s
Magistrelli P [70]	1988–98			--------				5 s
Morganti AG [71]	1990–96			------				3 s
Mattiucci GC [72]	2001–07					-----		3 ??
St Raffaele								
Reni M [73]	1985–98			---------				5 i
Di Carlo V [74]	1990–95			-----				2 i
Di Carlo V [75]	1990–97			------				4 ?
U Milano								
Taschieri AM [76]	1980–93			----------				4 ?
Taschieri AM [77]	19??–96		??--					10 ?
U Verona								
Serio G [78]	1970–93		------------------					3 ?
Crippa S [79]	1990–08				-------------			52 s
Malleo G [80]	1990–08				-------------			48 ??
Iacono C [81]	1992–96				-----			2 s
Barugola G [82]	1997–06				-------			10 i
Barugola G [83]	2001–08					-----		17 i
U Pisa								
Mosca F [84]	1980–93			----------				5 ?
Mosca F [85]	1980–94			----------				5 s
U Padua								
Pedrazzoli S [86]	1968–92	------------------						3 s
Sperti C [87]	1970–87	--------------						7 s
Sperti C [88]	1970–92	-------------------						7 s
Sperti C [89]	1970–92	-------------------						9 s
Sperti C [90]	1970–93	--------------------						3 s

Graphs are approximate

s: stated number of survivors

i: number of survivors obtained by inquiry

?: number of patients estimated from actuarial calculations.

FIGURE 2: Repetitions Italy sample. See [66–91].

6. Repetitions

Repetition of reporting the same survivors in different papers was first pointed out in 1978 [17]. It occurs in various ways, such as when papers include survivors from many different institutions or known databases in a specific country or even when a study includes patients from many countries. Thus 92 of the 620 studies with 5-year survivors are from many institutions in a specific country or 14.8% and 10 of these from many countries or 1.6%.

Repetition occurs, though mainly when the patient population and survivors from a certain year are reported several times from the same institution. As can be seen in Figures 1–5, repetition has occurred up to 6–8 times in Germany, Italy, and Japan and up to 20 times in the US.

Examination of reports from a single institution covering the entire study period and stating the number of survivors and then adding up the number of patients from all the studies, including those with an estimated number of survivors, reveals that the total number reported is over 10 times larger than the number reported in the studies with a documented number of survivors.

Each paper may at times reveal some new information but only infrequently is it disclosed that the patients have been reported before.

There is no scientific method to assess the number of repetitions accurately but each reported 5-year survivor and thereby respective resection and the TN seems to be reported 3–5 times. Dividing the number of reported survivors and respective resections and TN by 4, the overall number of 5-year survivors is hardly more than 2,800, the number of resections 40,500, and the original TN number of patients 433,000.

Repetitions occur also in the "no-survivor" group of reports, but not as frequently. It may be assumed that all published reports with or without survivors are drawn from a TN of approx. 1,000,000 patients and with fewer than 3,000 survivors, of whom a significant number were nonresected, meaning that the overall survival rate was no more than approximately 0.3%.

Author	Years	70	80	90	00	10		Srv	
Hiroshima U									
Murakami Y [91]	1990–06			-----------				3	s
Murakami Y [92]	1992–08			-----------				3	s
Murakami Y [93]	1994–09			-----------				8	??
Murakami Y [94]	1996–10			-----------				6	s
Murakami Y [95]	2002–09			------				7	s
Kanazawa U									
Kayahara M [96]	1970–95	--------------------------						2	s
Nagakawa T [97]	1973–90	-----------						7	s
Kayahara M [98]	1973–91	-------------						9	s
Nagakawa T [99]	1973–95	---------------						8	s
Nagakawa T [100]	1973–97	-----------------						10	s
Nagakawa T [101]	1974–99	-------------------------						15	s
Nagakawa T [102]	1980–95	-----------						3	s
Kumamoto U									
Hiraoka T [103]	1969–88	----------------						4	i
Hiraoka T [104]	1984–97		---------					4	i
Takamori H [105]	1984–99		----------					3	?
Takamori H [106]	1984–99		----------					6	s
Takamori H [107]	1984–99		----------					3	?
Kyoto U									
Nakase A [108] 57 inst	1949–74	---------						8	s
Manabe T [109]	1966–87	---------------						5	s
Manabe T [110]	1966–87	---------------						5	?
Manabe T [111]	1969–87	-----------						5	?
Kokubo M [112]	1980–97		-------------					5	i
Imamura M [113]	1981–97		-------------					6	s
Hosotani R [114]	1982–95		--------					5	s
Doi R [115]	1980–99		--------------					2	s
Doi R [116] 19 inst	19??–02		????-------					1	s
Nagasaki U									
Tsuchiya R [117] 19 inst	19??–79	??-------						4	s
Tsuchiya R [118] 441 inst	1966–80	------------						35	s
Tsuchiya R [119] 441 inst	1966–83	----------------						9	i
Tsuchiya R [120] 441 inst	1975–84	--------						11	i
Nanashima A [121]	1994–08			----------				4	?
Nagoya U									
Nimura Y [122]	2000–03				---			9	s
Nakao A [123]	1981–00		--------------					17	?
Nakao A [124]	1981–03		----------------					11	i
Nakao A [125]	1981–05		-----------------					12	i
Yamada S [126]	2001–10				-------			16	??
Osaka Ctr Adult Dis, Med f Ca, CSM									
Ishikawa O [127]	1960–94	---------------------						14	s
Matsui Y [128]	1963–75	------						1	s
Miyata M [129]	1974–89	-----------						4	?
Satake K [130] 59 inst	1980–90		--------					23	??
Ishikawa O [131]	1981–93		----------					9	?
Ishikawa O [132]	1981–95		----------					20	?
Ishikawa O [133]	1984–89		----					4	i
Ishikawa O [134]	1985–89		---					7	i
Ohigashi H [135]	1995–02			------				5	s
Ohigashi H [136]	2002–07				----			5	??
Takahashi H [137]	2002–09				-----			21	??
Takahashi H [138]	2002–11				--------			36	??
Sendai U									
Motoi F [139]	1989–08			-------------				13	?
Sato T [140]	1960–76	----------						1	s
Sato T [141]	1960–76	----------						2	s
Matsuno S [142]	1960–85	----------------						2	s
Shibata C [143]	1983–98		----------					5	i

FIGURE 3: Continued.

Author	Years	70	80	90	00	10	Srv
Tochigi U							
Sata N [144]	2001–05				------		78 ?
Yoshizawa K [145]	1976–95	---------------					4 s
Hishinuma S [146]	1985–04		-------------------------				1 s
Hishinuma S [147]	1987–03		----------------------				31 s
Ogata Y [148]	1988–00		-----------------				2 s
Tokyo Nat Ca Ctr							
Ozaki H [149]	1983–89	------					4 s
Shimada K [150]	1990–03			-----------			40 s
Shimada K [151]	1990–04			-----------			7 s
Yachida S [152]	1990–99			---------			16 ?
Shimada K [153]	1990–04			-----------			22 ?
Shimada K [154]	1999–03			----			12 ?
Oguro S [155]	2001–09			-----------			44 ??

Graphs are approximate
s: stated number of survivors
i: number of survivors obtained by inquiry
?: number of patients estimated from actuarial calculations.

FIGURE 3: Repetitions Japan sample. See [92–156].

Author	Years	40	50	60	70	80	90	00	10	Srv
Miller EM [156]	1936–45	------								1 s
Mongé JJ [157]	1941–62	---------------								8 s
ReMine WH [158]	1942–68	--------------------								2 s
Pliam MB [159]	1942–73	----------------------								2 s
Edis AJ [160]	1951–75		------------------							3 s
Van Heerden JA [161]	1951–78		--------------------							1 i
Van Heerden JA [162]	1951–85		--------------------------							3 s
Dalton RR [163]	1963–87			-----------------						1 i
Van Heerden JA [164]	1972–82				-------					1 s
Foo ML [165]	1974–86				--------					2 s
Schnelldorfer T [166]	1981–01					---------------				62 s
Fatima J [167]	1981–07					------------------				43 ?
Khan S [168]	1981–07					------------------				41 ?
Khan S [169]	1981–07					------------------				39 ?
Nitecki SS [170]	1981–91					---------				10 i
Spencer MP [171]	1982–87					-----				2 s
Billings BJ [172]	1985–02					-----------				2 s
Hsu CC and JH [173]	1985–05					---------------				58 ?
Christein JD [174]	1987–03					----------				4 s
Farnell MB [175]	1997–03						-----			6 ?
Al-Haddad [176]	1998–05						-----			1 i
Barton JG [177]	2000–07							-----		18 ?
Croome KP [178]	2008–13								-----	1 s

Graphs are approximate
s: stated number of survivors
i: number of survivors obtained by inquiry
?: number of patients estimated from actuarial calculations.

FIGURE 4: Repetitions Mayo Clinic. See [157–179].

7. Mortality, Positive Margins, and Nodes

Mortality during the first 20 years, 1945–1965, was on average 25.2% with a single report of 62.5%. During the next 20 years or up to 1984 mortality was on average 19.9% with the highest rate at 52%. In 1985–1994 it lowered to 9.8%. In subsequent 5-year periods mortality was reduced to 6.8% and then 4.6% and during the last 5 years 4% with a high of 33%. Aside from the 33%, the average is now 3.7%. The overall mortality rate has therefore greatly reduced.

The majority of surgeons in recent decades have reported the number of positive margins and nodes and numbers over

Author	Years	70	80	90	00	10	Srv	
Crist DW [179]	1969–86	----------------------					6	s
Crist DW [180]	1969–86	----------------------					6	i
Cameron JL [181]	1969–90	------------------------------					5	?
Cameron JL [182]	1969–03	--					30	?
Yeo CJ [4]	1970–92	---------------------------------					22	s
Yeo CJ [183]	1970–94	-----------------------------------					11	s
DiGiuseppe JA [184]	1970–94	-----------------------------------					11	s
Riall TS [185]	1970–99	--					93	s
Makary MA [186]	1970–05	--					103	?
Winter JM [187]	1970–06	---					85	?
Reddy S [188]	1970–07	--					85	?
Nordback IH [189]	1972–89	--------------------------					1	s
Allison DC [190]	1975–88	----------------------					3	s
Allison DC [191]	1975–92	--------------------------					17	s
He J [192]	1975–09	--					110	s
McGuire GE [193]	1979–90	---------------					1	?
Lin JW [194]	1981–02	-----------------------------					40	?
Sohn TA [195]	1984–99	-------------------------					33	s
Hsu CC and MCl [173]	1985–05	-------------------------------					58	?
Lillemoe KD [196]	1986–94	-------------					1	s
Yeo CJ [197]	1990–96	---------					20	?
Sohn TA [198]	1991–97	----------					20	?
Hristov B [199]	1993–05	-----------------					14	?
Gleisner AL [200]	1995–05	--------------					44	?
Asiyanbola B [201]	1995–05	--------------					11	?
Tsai S [202]	1995–05	--------------					48	?
Yeo CJ [203]	1996–01	--------					14	?
Yeo CJ [204]	1996–01	--------					14	?
Riall TS [205]	1996–01	--------					17	?
Emick DM [206]	1996–03	----------					93	i
Nathan H and SEER [207]	1998–04	------					171	?

Graphs are approximate
s: stated number of survivors
i: number of survivors obtained by inquiry
?: number of patients estimated from actuarial calculations.

FIGURE 5: Repetitions Johns Hopkins University. See [38, 180–207].

60–70% frequently quoted [36–38]. It is of great interest that even in the most experienced hands only 16% of cases were both margins and nodes negative [38].

Tumor cells can be found in the bone marrow in up to 50% of cases [39].

8. Discussion and Conclusion

Pancreatic cancer is thus both a costly and devastating disease and has usually spread beyond its boundaries at time of diagnosis and treatment and is thus a systemic disease. The literature on pancreatic surgery, while purporting to report the facts, is nevertheless inaccurate.

The use of actuarial calculation methods exaggerates the percentage and thereby the number of presumed survivors in a particular study.

Reporting the same patients repeatedly without any qualification gives a false impression of success.

Life table curves should be accompanied by the actual number of survivors. The course of nonresected patients should be studied.

Surgical skills are imperative for the care and palliation of pancreatic cancer patients including possible resections, but they have had only a minimal impact on the survival rate.

It is of importance for the medical profession that published results are indisputable.

Disclosure

The paper is based on 45 years of continuous study of the cancer of pancreas with previous communications and papers.

Competing Interests

The author declares that they have no competing interests.

Acknowledgments

The author thanks Terry G. Lacy Ph.D. for reviewing the manuscript.

References

[1] A. O. Whipple, W. B. Parsons, and C. R. Mullins, "Treatment of carcinoma of the ampulla of Vater," *Annals of Surgery*, vol. 102, no. 4, pp. 763–776, 1935.

[2] J. M. Howard and W. Hess, *History of the Pancreas: Mysteries of a Hidden Organ*, Kluwer Academic/Plenum Publishers, New York, NY, USA, 2002.

[3] W. Kausch, "Das Carcinom der Papilla duodeni und seine radikale Entfernung," *Beitrage zur Klinischen Chirurgie*, vol. 78, pp. 439–486, 1912.

[4] C. J. Yeo, J. L. Cameron, K. D. Lillemoe et al., "Pancreaticoduodenectomy for cancer of the head of the pancreas: 201 patients," *Annals of Surgery*, vol. 221, no. 6, pp. 721–733, 1995.

[5] M. Carpelan-Holmström, S. Nordling, E. Pukkala et al., "Does anyone survive pancreatic ductal adenocarcinoma? A nationwide study re-evaluating the data of the Finnish Cancer Registry," *Gut*, vol. 54, no. 3, pp. 385–387, 2005.

[6] R. L. Siegel, K. D. Miller, and A. Jemal, "Cancer statistics, 2015," *CA Cancer Journal for Clinicians*, vol. 65, no. 1, pp. 5–29, 2015.

[7] L. Rahib, B. D. Smith, R. Aizenberg, A. B. Rosenzweig, J. M. Fleshman, and L. M. Matrisian, "Projecting cancer incidence and deaths to 2030: the unexpected burden of thyroid, liver, and pancreas cancers in the United States," *Cancer Research*, vol. 74, no. 11, pp. 2913–2921, 2014.

[8] C. B. O'Neill, C. L. Atoria, E. M. O'Reilly, J. Lafemina, M. C. Henman, and E. B. Elkin, "Costs and trends in pancreatic cancer treatment," *Cancer*, vol. 118, no. 20, pp. 5132–5139, 2012.

[9] M. S. Lea and L. H. Stahlgren, "Is resection appropriate for adenocarcinoma of the pancreas?. A cost-benefit analysis," *The American Journal of Surgery*, vol. 154, no. 6, pp. 651–654, 1987.

[10] J. P. A. Ioannidis, "Why most published research findings are false," *PLoS Medicine*, vol. 2, no. 8, article e124, 2005.

[11] F. Glenn and B. Thorbjarnarson, "Carcinoma of the pancreas," *Annals of Surgery*, vol. 159, pp. 945–958, 1964.

[12] A. Gallitano, H. Fransen, and R. G. Martin, "Carcinoma of the pancreas. Results of treatment," *Cancer*, vol. 22, no. 5, pp. 939–944, 1968.

[13] G. Crile Jr., "The advantages of bypass operations over radical pancreatoduodenectomy in the treatment of pancreatic carcinoma," *Surgery Gynecology and Obstetrics*, vol. 130, no. 6, pp. 1049–1053, 1970.

[14] T. M. Shapiro, "Adenocarcinoma of the pancreas: a statistical analysis of biliary bypass vs whipple resection in good risk patients," *Annals of Surgery*, vol. 182, no. 6, pp. 715–721, 1975.

[15] T. A. Gordon and J. L. Cameron, "Management of patients with carcinoma of the pancreas," *Journal of the American College of Surgeons*, vol. 181, no. 6, pp. 558–560, 1995.

[16] R. B. Cattell and W. C. Young, "Long survival in a case of carcinoma of the pancreas," *The Lahey Clinic Bulletin*, vol. 10, no. 5, pp. 131–134, 1957.

[17] B. Gudjonsson, "Carcinoma of the pancreas: critical analysis of costs, results of resections, and the need for standardized reporting," *Journal of the American College of Surgeons*, vol. 181, no. 6, pp. 483–503, 1995.

[18] B. Gudjonsson, "Letter to the editor," *Journal of the American College of Surgeons*, vol. 183, pp. 290–291, 1996.

[19] B. Gudjonsson, E. M. Livstone, and H. M. Spiro, "Cancer of the pancreas. Diagnostic accuracy and survival statistics," *Cancer*, vol. 42, no. 5, pp. 2494–2506, 1978.

[20] B. Gudjonsson, "Cancer of the pancreas. 50 years of surgery," *Cancer*, vol. 60, no. 9, pp. 2284–2303, 1987.

[21] M. H. G. Katz, P. W. T. Pisters, D. B. Evans et al., "Borderline resectable pancreatic cancer: the importance of this emerging stage of disease," *Journal of the American College of Surgeons*, vol. 206, no. 5, pp. 833–846, 2008.

[22] J. Tepper, G. Nardi, and H. Suit, "Carcinoma of the pancreas: review of MGH experience from 1963 to 1973. Analysis of surgical failure and implications for radiation therapy," *Cancer*, vol. 37, no. 3, pp. 1519–1524, 1976.

[23] I. T. Konstantinidis, A. L. Warshaw, J. N. Allen et al., "Pancreatic ductal adenocarcinoma: is there a survival difference for R1 resections versus locally advanced unresectable tumors? What is a "true" R0 resection?" *Annals of Surgery*, vol. 257, no. 4, pp. 731–736, 2013.

[24] F. Michelassi, F. Erroi, P. J. Dawson et al., "Experience with 647 consecutive tumors of the duodenum, ampulla, head of the pancreas, and distal common bile duct," *Annals of Surgery*, vol. 210, no. 4, pp. 544–556, 1989.

[25] M. K. Krzyzanowska, J. C. Weeks, and C. C. Earle, "Treatment of locally advanced pancreatic cancer in the real world: population-based practices and effectiveness," *Journal of Clinical Oncology*, vol. 21, no. 18, pp. 3409–3414, 2003.

[26] M. Mohiuddin, F. Rosato, D. Barbot, A. Schuricht, W. Biermann, and R. Cantor, "Long-term results of combined modality treatment with I-125 implantation for carcinoma of the pancreas," *International Journal of Radiation Oncology, Biology, Physics*, vol. 23, no. 2, pp. 305–311, 1992.

[27] E. L. Kaplan and P. Meier, "Nonparametric estimation from incomplete observations," *Journal of the American Statistical Association*, vol. 53, pp. 457–481, 1958.

[28] A. B. Hill, *Principles of Medical Statistics*, The Lancet Limited, London, UK, 1971.

[29] B. Gudjonsson, "Survival statistics gone awry: pancreatic cancer, a case in point," *Journal of Clinical Gastroenterology*, vol. 35, no. 2, pp. 180–184, 2002.

[30] B. Gudjonsson, "Pancreatic cancer: survival, errors and evidence," *European Journal of Gastroenterology and Hepatology*, vol. 21, no. 12, pp. 1379–1382, 2009.

[31] T. P. Wade, K. S. Virgo, and F. E. Johnson, "Distal pancreatectomy for cancer: results in U.S. Department of Veterans Affairs Hospitals, 1987–1991," *Pancreas*, vol. 11, no. 4, pp. 341–344, 1995.

[32] S. B. Edge, R. E. Schmieg Jr., L. K. Rosenlof, and M. C. Wilhelm, "Pancreas cancer resection outcome in American university centers in 1989-1990," *Cancer*, vol. 71, no. 11, pp. 3502–3508, 1993.

[33] S. W. Nienhuijs, S. A. van den Akker, E. de Vries, I. H. de Hingh, O. Visser, and V. E. Lemmens, "Nationwide improvement of only short-term survival after resection for pancreatic cancer in the netherlands," *Pancreas*, vol. 41, no. 7, pp. 1063–1066, 2012.

[34] J. K. Bjerregaard, M. B. Mortensen, K. R. Schönnemann, and P. Pfeiffer, "Characteristics, therapy and outcome in an unselected and prospectively registered cohort of pancreatic cancer patients," *European Journal of Cancer*, vol. 49, no. 1, pp. 98–105, 2013.

[35] J. Kat'uchová, J. Bober, and J. Radoňak, "Postoperative complications and survival rates for pancreatic cancer patients," *Wiener Klinische Wochenschrift*, vol. 123, no. 3-4, pp. 94–99, 2011.

[36] C. G. Willett, K. Lewandrowski, A. L. Warshaw, J. Efird, and C. C. Compton, "Resection margins in carcinoma of the head of the pancreas: Implications for radiation therapy," *Annals of Surgery*, vol. 217, no. 2, pp. 144–148, 1993.

[37] V. J. Picozzi, R. A. Kozarek, and L. W. Traverso, "Interferon-based adjuvant chemoradiation therapy after pancreaticoduodenectomy for pancreatic adenocarcinoma," *American Journal of Surgery*, vol. 185, no. 5, pp. 476–480, 2003.

[38] J. L. Cameron, D. W. Crist, J. V. Sitzmann et al., "Factors influencing survival after pancreaticoduodenectomy for pancreatic cancer," *The American Journal of Surgery*, vol. 161, no. 1, pp. 120–125, 1991.

[39] K. Z'graggen, B. A. Centeno, C. Fernandez-Del Castillo, R. E. Jimenez, J. Werner, and A. L. Warshaw, "Biological implications of tumor cells in blood and bone marrow of pancreatic cancer patients," *Surgery*, vol. 129, no. 5, pp. 537–546, 2001.

[40] D. Henne-Bruns, I. Vogel, J. Lüttges, G. Klöppel, and B. Kremer, "Ductal adenocarcinoma of the pancreas head: survival after regional versus extended lymphadenectomy," *Hepato-Gastroenterology*, vol. 45, no. 21, pp. 855–866, 1998.

[41] D. Henne-Bruns, I. Vogel, J. Lüttges, G. Klöppel, and B. Kremer, "Surgery for ductal adenocarcinoma of the pancreatic head: staging, complications, and survival after regional versus extended lymphadenectomy," *World Journal of Surgery*, vol. 24, no. 5, pp. 595–602, 2000.

[42] J. Klempnauer, G. J. Ridder, H. Bektas, and R. Pichlmayr, "Surgery for exocrine pancreatic cancer. Who are the 5- and 10-year survivors?" *Oncology*, vol. 52, no. 5, pp. 353–359, 1995.

[43] J. Klempnauer, G. J. Ridder, and R. Pichlmayr, "Prognostic factors after resection of ampullary carcinoma: multivariate survival analysis in comparison with ductal cancer of the pancreatic head," *British Journal of Surgery*, vol. 82, no. 12, pp. 1686–1691, 1995.

[44] J. Klempnauer, G. J. Ridder, H. Bektas, and R. Pichlmayr, "Extended resections of ductal pancreatic cancer-impact on operative risk and prognosis," *Oncology*, vol. 53, no. 1, pp. 47–53, 1996.

[45] F. A. Wenger, F. Peter, J. Zieren, A. Steiert, C. A. Jacobi, and J. M. Müller, "Prognosis factors in carcinoma of the head of the pancreas," *Digestive Surgery*, vol. 17, no. 1, pp. 29–35, 2000.

[46] H. Wolff and H. Lippert, "Das pankreaskarzinom aus der sicht des chirurgen," *Zbl Chirurgie*, vol. 112, pp. 1–11, 1987.

[47] T. Bottger, J. Zech, W. Weber, K. Sorger, and T. Junginger, "Relevant factors in the prognosis of ductal pancreatic carcinoma," *Acta Chirurgica Scandinavica*, vol. 156, no. 11-12, pp. 781–788, 1990.

[48] T. C. Böttger, S. Störkel, S. Wellek, M. Stöckle, and T. Junginger, "Factors influencing survival after resection of pancreatic cancer. A DNA analysis and a histomorphologic study," *Cancer*, vol. 73, no. 1, pp. 63–73, 1994.

[49] M. Trede, G. G. Schwall, and H.-D. Saeger, "Survival after pancreatoduodenectomy: 118 consecutive resections without an operative mortality," *Annals of Surgery*, vol. 211, no. 4, pp. 447–458, 1990.

[50] A. Richter, M. Niedergethmann, D. Lorenz, J. W. Sturm, M. Trede, and S. Post, "Resection for cancers of the pancreatic head in patients aged 70 years or over," *European Journal of Surgery*, vol. 168, no. 6, pp. 339–344, 2002.

[51] A. Richter, M. Niedergethmann, J. W. Sturm, D. Lorenz, S. Post, and M. Trede, "Long-term results of partial pancreaticoduodenectomy for ductal adenocarcinoma of the pancreatic head: 25-year experience," *World Journal of Surgery*, vol. 27, no. 3, pp. 324–329, 2003.

[52] M. Hartel, M. Niedergethmann, M. Farag-Soliman et al., "Benefit of venous resection for ductal adenocarcinoma of the pancreatic head," *European Journal of Surgery*, vol. 168, no. 12, pp. 707–712, 2002.

[53] M. Trede, "The surgical treatment of pancreatic carcinoma," *Surgery*, vol. 97, no. 1, pp. 28–35, 1985.

[54] F. P. Gall, H. Kessler, and P. Hermanek, "Surgical treatment of ductal pancreatic carcinoma," *European Journal of Surgical Oncology*, vol. 17, no. 2, pp. 173–181, 1991.

[55] F. P. Gall and H. Kessler, "Das Frühcarcinom des exokrinen Pankreas: Diagnose und Prognose," *Der Chirurg*, vol. 58, pp. 78–83, 1987.

[56] A. Tannapfel, C. Wittekind, and G. Hünefeld, "Ductal adenocarcinoma of the pancreas—histopathological features and prognosis," *International Journal of Pancreatology*, vol. 12, no. 2, pp. 145–152, 1992.

[57] J. Kleeff, M. K. Diener, K. Z'graggen et al., "Distal pancreatectomy: risk factors for surgical failure in 302 consecutive cases," *Annals of Surgery*, vol. 245, no. 4, pp. 573–582, 2007.

[58] T. Welsch, L. Degrate, S. Zschäbitz, S. Hofer, J. Werner, and J. Schmidt, "The need for extended intensive care after pancreaticoduodenectomy for pancreatic ductal adenocarcinoma," *Langenbeck's Archives of Surgery*, vol. 396, no. 3, pp. 353–362, 2011.

[59] W. Hartwig, T. Hackert, U. Hinz et al., "Multivisceral resection for pancreatic malignancies. Risk-analysis and long-term outcome," *Annals of Surgery*, vol. 250, no. 1, pp. 81–87, 2009.

[60] W. Hartwig, T. Hackert, U. Hinz et al., "Pancreatic cancer surgery in the new millennium: better prediction of outcome," *Annals of Surgery*, vol. 254, no. 2, pp. 311–319, 2011.

[61] O. Strobel, V. Berens, U. Hinz et al., "Resection after neoadjuvant therapy for locally advanced, 'unresectable' pancreatic cancer," *Surgery*, vol. 152, no. 3, pp. S33–S42, 2012.

[62] T. Pausch, W. Hartwig, U. Hinz et al., "Cachexia but not obesity worsens the postoperative outcome after pancreatoduodenectomy in pancreatic cancer," *Surgery*, vol. 152, no. 3, pp. S81–S88, 2012.

[63] K. Rückert and F. Kümmerle, "Totale duodenopankreatektomie als regeloperation beim pankreazcarcinoma," *Der Chirurg*, vol. 49, pp. 162–166, 1978.

[64] F. Kümmerle and K. Rückert, "Surgical treatment of pancreatic cancer," *World Journal of Surgery*, vol. 8, no. 6, pp. 889–894, 1984.

[65] F. Kümmerle and K. Rückert, "Role of surgical treatment in pancreatic carcinoma," *Digestive Diseases*, vol. 4, no. 1, pp. 33–42, 1986.

[66] I. M. Civello, D. Frontera, G. Viola, G. Cina, G. Sganga, and F. Crucitti, "Extensive resection in pancreatic cancer: review of the literature and personal experience," *Hepato-Gastroenterology*, vol. 45, no. 23, pp. 1877–1893, 1998.

[67] S. Alfieri, A. G. Morganti, A. Di Giorgio et al., "Improved survival and local control after intraoperative radiation therapy and postoperative radiation therapy: a multivariate analysis of 46 patients undergoing surgery for the pancreatic head," *Archives of Surgery*, vol. 136, no. 3, pp. 343–347, 2001.

[68] P. Magistrelli, A. Antinori, A. Crucitti et al., "Il trattamento chirurgico resettivo del carcinoma pancreatico," *Tumori*, vol. 85, pp. S22–S26, 1999.

[69] P. Magistrelli, A. Antinori, A. Crucitti et al., "Prognostic factors after surgical resection for pancreatic carcinoma," *Journal of Surgical Oncology*, vol. 74, no. 1, pp. 36–40, 2000.

[70] P. Magistrelli, R. Coppola, G. Tonini et al., "Apoptotic index or a combination of Bax/Bcl-2 expression correlate with survival after resection of pancreatic adenocarcinoma," *Journal of Cellular Biochemistry*, vol. 97, no. 1, pp. 98–108, 2006.

[71] P. Magistrelli, R. Masetti, R. Coppola et al., "Pancreatic resection for periampullary cancer in elderly patients," *Hepato-Gastroenterology*, vol. 45, no. 19, pp. 242–247, 1998.

[72] A. G. Morganti, V. Valentini, G. Macchia et al., "Adjuvant radiotherapy in resectable pancreatic carcinoma," *European Journal of Surgical Oncology*, vol. 28, no. 5, pp. 523–530, 2002.

[73] G. C. Mattiucci, E. Ippolito, G. R. D'Agostino et al., "Long-term analysis of gemcitabine-based chemoradiation after surgical resection for pancreatic adenocarcinoma," *Annals of Surgical Oncology*, vol. 20, no. 2, pp. 423–429, 2013.

[74] M. Reni, M. G. Panucci, A. J. M. Ferreri et al., "Effect on local control and survival of electron beam intraoperative irradiation for resectable pancreatic adenocarcinoma," *International Journal of Radiation Oncology Biology Physics*, vol. 50, no. 3, pp. 651–658, 2001.

[75] V. Dicarlo, G. Balzano, A. Zerbi, and E. Villa, "Pancreatic cancer resection in elderly patients," *British Journal of Surgery*, vol. 85, no. 5, pp. 607–610, 1998.

[76] V. Di Carlo, A. Zerbi, G. Balzano, and V. Corso, "Pylorus-preserving pancreaticoduodenectomy versus conventional Whipple operation," *World Journal of Surgery*, vol. 23, no. 9, pp. 920–925, 1999.

[77] A. M. Taschieri, M. Elli, M. Cristaldi, G. Montecamozzo, T. Porretta, and P. G. Danelli, "Pancreasectomia totale vs pancreasectomia parziale nel trattamento chirurgico del carcinoma della testa del pancreas," *Chirurgia Italiana*, vol. 46, pp. 44–50, 1994.

[78] A. M. Taschieri, M. Elli, M. Rovati et al., "Surgical treatment of pancreatic tumors invading the spleno-mesenteric-portal vessels. An Italian multicenter survey," *Hepato-Gastroenterology*, vol. 46, no. 25, pp. 492–497, 1999.

[79] G. Serio, C. Icono, G. Prati, E. Facci, G. Falezza, and A. Gorla, "La chirurgia resettiva per neoplasie pancreatiche negli ultimi venti anni," *Chirurgia Italiana*, vol. 46, pp. 1–10, 1994.

[80] S. Crippa, S. Partelli, G. Zamboni et al., "Poorly differentiated resectable pancreatic cancer: is upfront resection worthwhile?" *Surgery*, vol. 152, no. 3, pp. S112–S119, 2012.

[81] G. Malleo, G. Marchegiani, R. Salvia, G. Butturini, P. Pederzoli, and C. Bassi, "Pancreaticoduodenectomy for pancreatic cancer: the verona experience," *Surgery Today*, vol. 41, no. 4, pp. 463–470, 2011.

[82] C. Iacono, S. Accordini, L. Bortolasi et al., "Results of pancreaticoduodenectomy for pancreatic cancer: extended versus standard procedure," *World Journal of Surgery*, vol. 26, no. 11, pp. 1309–1314, 2002.

[83] G. Barugola, S. Partelli, S. Marcucci et al., "Resectable pancreatic cancer: who really benefits from resection?" *Annals of Surgical Oncology*, vol. 16, no. 12, pp. 3316–3322, 2009.

[84] G. Barugola, S. Partelli, S. Crippa et al., "Outcomes after resection of locally advanced or borderline resectable pancreatic cancer after neoadjuvant therapy," *American Journal of Surgery*, vol. 203, no. 2, pp. 132–139, 2012.

[85] F. Mosca, P. C. Giulianotti, T. Balestracci et al., "La duodenocefalopancreasectomia con conservazione del piloro (PPPD) nel carcinoma pancreatico e periampollare," *Chirurgia Italiana*, vol. 46, pp. 59–67, 1994.

[86] F. Mosca, P. C. Giulianotti, T. Balestracci et al., "Long-term survival in pancreatic cancer: pylorus-preserving versus Whipple pancreatoduodenectomy," *Surgery*, vol. 122, no. 3, pp. 553–566, 1997.

[87] S. Pedrazzoli, C. Sperti, and C. Pasquali, "Previsione della resecabilita e del rischio chirurgico del carcinoma pancreatic; fattori che condizionano la sopravvivenza dopo intervento resettivo," *Chirurgia Italiana*, vol. 46, pp. 30–38, 1994.

[88] C. Sperti, B. Bonadimani, C. Pasquali et al., "Ductal adenocarcinoma of the pancreas. Clinicopathological features and survival," *Tumori*, vol. 79, no. 5, pp. 325–330, 1993.

[89] C. Sperti, C. Pasquali, A. Piccoli, and S. Pedrazzoli, "Survival after resection for ductal adenocarcinoma of the pancreas," *British Journal of Surgery*, vol. 83, no. 5, pp. 625–631, 1996.

[90] C. Sperti, C. Pasquali, A. Piccoli, and S. Pedrazzoli, "Recurrence after resection for ductal adenocarcinoma of the pancreas," *World Journal of Surgery*, vol. 21, no. 2, pp. 195–200, 1997.

[91] C. Sperti, C. Pasquali, and S. Pedrazzoli, "Ductal adenocarcinoma of the body and tail of the pancreas," *Journal of the American College of Surgeons*, vol. 185, no. 3, pp. 255–259, 1997.

[92] Y. Murakami, K. Uemura, T. Sudo et al., "Postoperative adjuvant chemotherapy improves survival after surgical resection for pancreatic carcinoma," *Journal of Gastrointestinal Surgery*, vol. 12, no. 3, pp. 534–541, 2008.

[93] Y. Murakami, K. Uemura, T. Sudo et al., "Number of metastatic lymph nodes, but not lymph node ratio, is an independent prognostic factor after resection of pancreatic carcinoma," *Journal of the American College of Surgeons*, vol. 211, no. 2, pp. 196–204, 2010.

[94] Y. Murakami, K. Uemura, T. Sudo, Y. Hashimoto, Y. Yuasa, and T. Sueda, "Prognostic impact of para-aortic lymph node metastasis in pancreatic ductal adenocarcinoma," *World Journal of Surgery*, vol. 34, no. 8, pp. 1900–1907, 2010.

[95] Y. Murakami, K. Uemura, T. Sudo et al., "Long-term results of adjuvant gemcitabine plus S-1 chemotherapy after surgical resection for pancreatic carcinoma," *Journal of Surgical Oncology*, vol. 106, no. 2, pp. 174–180, 2012.

[96] Y. Murakami, K. Uemura, T. Sudo et al., "Benefit of portal or superior mesenteric vein resection with adjuvant chemotherapy for patients with pancreatic head carcinoma," *Journal of Surgical Oncology*, vol. 107, no. 4, pp. 414–421, 2013.

[97] M. Kayahara, T. Nagakawa, K. Ueno et al., "Distal pancreatectomy. Does it have a role for pancreatic body and tail cancer," *Hepato-Gastroenterology*, vol. 45, no. 21, pp. 827–832, 1998.

[98] T. Nagakawa, I. Konishi, K. Ueno et al., "Surgical treatment of pancreatic cancer-the japanese experience," *International Journal of Pancreatology*, vol. 9, no. 1, pp. 135–143, 1991.

[99] M. Kayahara, T. Nagakawa, K. Ueno, T. Ohta, Y. Tsukioka, and I. Miyazaki, "Surgical strategy for carcinoma of the pancreas head area based on clinicopathologic analysis of nodal involvement and plexus invasion," *Surgery*, vol. 117, no. 6, pp. 616–623, 1995.

[100] T. Nagakawa, M. Nagamori, F. Futakami et al., "Results of extensive surgery for pancreatic carcinoma," *Cancer*, vol. 77, no. 4, pp. 640–645, 1996.

[101] T. Nagakawa, I. Konishi, K. Ueno, T. Ohta, M. Kayahara, and I. Miyazaki, "Extended radical pancreatectomy for carcinoma of the head of the pancreas," *Hepato-Gastroenterology*, vol. 45, no. 21, pp. 849–854, 1998.

[102] T. Nagakawa, H. Sanada, M. Inagaki et al., "Long-term survivors after resection of carcinoma of the head of the pancreas: significance of histologically curative resection," *Journal of Hepato-Biliary-Pancreatic Surgery*, vol. 11, no. 6, pp. 402–408, 2004.

[103] T. Nagakawa, K. Ueno, T. Ohta et al., "Evaluation of long-term survivors after pancreatoduodenectomy for pancreatoduodenal

carcinoma," *Hepato-Gastroenterology*, vol. 42, no. 2, pp. 117–122, 1995.

[104] T. Hiraoka, R. Uchino, K. Kanemitsu et al., "Combination of intraoperative radiation with resection of cancer of the pancreas," *International Journal of Pancreatology*, vol. 7, no. 1–3, pp. 201–207, 1990.

[105] T. Hiraoka and K. Kanemitsu, "Value of extended resection and intraoperative radiotherapy for resectable pancreatic cancer," *World Journal of Surgery*, vol. 23, no. 9, pp. 930–936, 1999.

[106] H. Takamori, T. Hiraoka, K. Kanemitsu, and T. Tsuji, "Pancreatic liver metastases after curative resection combined with intraoperative radiation for pancreatic cancer," *Hepato-Gastroenterology*, vol. 51, no. 59, pp. 1500–1503, 2004.

[107] H. Takamori, T. Hiraoka, K. Kanemitsu, T. Tsuji, C. Hamada, and H. Baba, "Identification of prognostic factors associated with early mortality after surgical resection for pancreatic cancer—under-analysis of cumulative survival curve," *World Journal of Surgery*, vol. 30, no. 2, pp. 213–218, 2006.

[108] H. Takamori, T. Hiraoka, K. Kanemitsu et al., "Long term outcomes of extended radical resection combined with intraoperative radiation therapy for pancreatic cancer," *Journal of Hepato-Biliary-Pancreatic Surgery*, vol. 15, no. 6, pp. 603–607, 2008.

[109] A. Nakase, Y. Matsumoto, K. Uchida, and I. Honjo, "Surgical treatment of cancer of the pancreas and the periampullary region: cumulative results in 57 institutions in Japan," *Annals of Surgery*, vol. 185, no. 1, pp. 52–57, 1977.

[110] T. Manabe, G. Ohshio, N. Baba et al., "Radical pancreatectomy for ductal cell carcinoma of the head of the pancreas," *Cancer*, vol. 64, no. 5, pp. 1132–1137, 1989.

[111] T. Manabe and T. Tobe, "Progress in the diagnosis and treatment of pancreatic cancer—The Kyoto University experience," *Hepato-Gastroenterology*, vol. 36, no. 6, pp. 431–436, 1989.

[112] T. Manabe, G. Ohshio, N. Baba, and T. Tobe, "Factors influencing prognosis and indications for curative pancreatectomy for ductal adenocarcinoma of the head of the pancreas," *International Journal of Pancreatology*, vol. 7, no. 1–3, pp. 187–193, 1990.

[113] M. Kokubo, Y. Nishimura, Y. Shibamoto et al., "Analysis of the clinical benefit of intraoperative radiotherapy in patients undergoing macroscopically curative resection for pancreatic cancer," *International Journal of Radiation Oncology Biology Physics*, vol. 48, no. 4, pp. 1081–1087, 2000.

[114] M. Imamura, R. Hosotani, and M. Kogire, "Rationale of the so-called extended resection for pancreatic invasive ductal carcinoma," *Digestion*, vol. 60, no. 1, pp. 126–129, 1999.

[115] R. Hosotani, M. Kogire, S. Arii, Y. Nishimura, M. Hiraoka, and M. Imamura, "Results of pancreatectomy with radiation therapy for pancreatic cancer," *Hepato-Gastroenterology*, vol. 44, no. 18, pp. 1528–1535, 1997.

[116] R. Doi, H. Ikeda, H. Kobayashi, M. Kogire, and M. Imamura, "Carcinoma in the remnant pancreas after distal pancreatectomy for carcinoma," *European Journal of Surgery, Supplement*, vol. 168, no. 588, pp. 62–65, 2003.

[117] R. Doi, M. Imamura, R. Hosotani et al., "Surgery versus radiochemotherapy for resectable locally invasive pancreatic cancer: final results of a randomized multi-institutional trial," *Surgery Today*, vol. 38, no. 11, pp. 1021–1028, 2008.

[118] R. Tsuchiya, T. Oribe, and T. Noda, "Size of the tumor and other factors influencing prognosis of carcinoma of the head of the pancreas," *American Journal of Gastroenterology*, vol. 80, no. 6, pp. 459–462, 1985.

[119] R. Tsuchiya, T. Noda, N. Harada et al., "Collective review of small carcinomas of the pancreas," *Annals of Surgery*, vol. 203, no. 1, pp. 77–81, 1986.

[120] R. Tsuchiya, N. Harada, T. Tsunoda, T. Miyamoto, and K. Ura, "Long-term survivors after operation on carcinoma of the pancreas," *International Journal of Pancreatology*, vol. 3, no. 6, pp. 491–496, 1988.

[121] R. Tsuchiya, T. Tsunoda, and T. Yamaguchi, "Operation of choice for resectable carcinoma of the head of the pancreas," *International Journal of Pancreatology*, vol. 6, no. 4, pp. 295–306, 1990.

[122] A. Nanashima, S. Tobinaga, T. Abo et al., "Evaluation of surgical resection for pancreatic carcinoma at a Japanese single cancer institute," *Hepato-Gastroenterology*, vol. 59, no. 115, pp. 911–915, 2012.

[123] Y. Nimura, M. Nagino, S. Takao et al., "Standard versus extended lymphadenectomy in radical pancreatoduodenectomy for ductal adenocarcinoma of the head of the pancreas," *Journal of Hepato-Biliary-Pancreatic Sciences*, vol. 19, no. 3, pp. 230–241, 2012.

[124] A. Nakao, "Debate: extended resection for pancreatic cancer; the affirmative case," *Journal of Hepato-Biliary-Pancreatic Surgery*, vol. 10, no. 1, pp. 57–60, 2003.

[125] A. Nakao, S. Takeda, M. Sakai et al., "Extended radical resection versus standard resection for pancreatic cancer: the rationale for extended radical resection," *Pancreas*, vol. 28, no. 3, pp. 289–292, 2004.

[126] A. Nakao, S. Takeda, S. Inoue et al., "Indications and techniques of extended resection for pancreatic cancer," *World Journal of Surgery*, vol. 30, no. 6, pp. 976–982, 2006.

[127] S. Yamada, T. Fujii, A. Nakao et al., "Aggressive surgery for borderline resectable pancreatic cancer: evaluation of national comprehensive cancer network guidelines," *Pancreas*, vol. 42, no. 6, pp. 1004–1010, 2013.

[128] O. Ishikawa, H. Ohigashi, S. Imaoka et al., "Minute carcinoma of the pancreas measuring 1 cm or less in diameter—collective review of Japanese case reports," *Hepato-Gastroenterology*, vol. 46, no. 25, pp. 8–15, 1999.

[129] Y. Matsui, Y. Aoki, O. Ishikawa et al., "Ductal carcinoma of the pancreas. Rationales for total pancreatectomy," *Archives of Surgery*, vol. 114, no. 6, pp. 722–726, 1979.

[130] M. Miyata, K. Nakao, T. Takao et al., "An appraisal of pancreatectomy for advanced cancer of the pancreas based on survival rate and postoperative physical performance," *Journal of Surgical Oncology*, vol. 45, no. 1, pp. 33–39, 1990.

[131] K. Satake, H. Nishiwaki, H. Yokomatsu et al., "Surgical curability and prognosis for standard versus extended resection for T1 carcinoma of the pancreas," *Surgery Gynecology and Obstetrics*, vol. 175, no. 3, pp. 259–265, 1992.

[132] O. Ishikawa, "Surgical technique, curability and postoperative quality of life in an extended pancreatectomy for adenocarcinoma of the pancreas," *Hepato-Gastroenterology*, vol. 43, no. 8, pp. 320–325, 1996.

[133] O. Ishikawa, H. Ohigashi, Y. Sasaki et al., "Adjuvant therapies in extended pancreatectomy for ductal adenocarcinoma of the pancreas," *Hepato-Gastroenterology*, vol. 45, no. 21, pp. 644–650, 1998.

[134] O. Ishikawa, H. Ohigashi, S. Imaoka et al., "Preoperative indications for extended pancreatectomy for locally advanced pancreas cancer involving the portal vein," *Annals of Surgery*, vol. 215, no. 3, pp. 231–236, 1992.

[135] O. Ishikawa, H. Ohigashi, S. Imaoka et al., "Is the long-term survival rate improved by preoperative irradiation prior to Whipple's procedure for adenocarcinoma of the pancreatic head?" *Archives of Surgery*, vol. 129, no. 10, pp. 1075–1080, 1994.

[136] H. Ohigashi, O. Ishikawa, H. Eguchi et al., "Feasibility and efficacy of combination therapy with preoperative full-dose gemcitabine, concurrent three-dimensional conformal radiation, surgery, and postoperative liver perfusion chemotherapy for T3-pancreatic cancer," *Annals of Surgery*, vol. 250, no. 1, pp. 88–95, 2009.

[137] H. Ohigashi, O. Ishikawa, H. Eguchi et al., "Feasibility and efficacy of combination therapy with preoperative and postoperative chemoradiation, extended pancreatectomy, and postoperative liver perfusion chemotherapy for locally advanced cancers of the pancreatic head," *Annals of Surgical Oncology*, vol. 12, no. 8, pp. 629–636, 2005.

[138] H. Takahashi, H. Ohigashi, O. Ishikawa et al., "Perineural invasion and lymph node involvement as indicators of surgical outcome and pattern of recurrence in the setting of preoperative gemcitabine-based chemoradiation therapy for resectable pancreatic cancer," *Annals of Surgery*, vol. 255, pp. 95–102, 2012.

[139] H. Takahashi, H. Ohigashi, K. Gotoh et al., "Preoperative gemcitabine-based chemoradiation therapy for resectable and borderline resectable pancreatic cancer," *Annals of Surgery*, vol. 258, no. 6, pp. 1040–1050, 2013.

[140] F. Motoi, T. Rikiyama, Y. Katayose, S.-I. Egawa, and M. Unno, "Retrospective evaluation of the influence of postoperative tumor marker status on survival and patterns of recurrence after surgery for pancreatic cancer based on RECIST guidelines," *Annals of Surgical Oncology*, vol. 18, no. 2, pp. 371–379, 2011.

[141] T. Sato, Y. Saitoh, N. Noto, and S. Matsuno, "Follow up studies of radical resection for pancreaticoduodenal cancer," *Annals of Surgery*, vol. 186, no. 5, pp. 581–588, 1977.

[142] T. Sato, Y. Saitoh, N. Noto, and S. Matsuno, "Factors influencing the late results of operation for carcinoma of the pancreas," *The American Journal of Surgery*, vol. 136, no. 5, pp. 582–586, 1978.

[143] S. Matsuno and T. Sato, "Surgical treatment for carcinoma of the pancreas. Experience in 272 patients," *The American Journal of Surgery*, vol. 152, no. 5, pp. 499–503, 1986.

[144] C. Shibata, M. Kobari, T. Tsuchiya et al., "Pancreatectomy combined with superior mesenteric-portal vein resection for adenocarcinoma in pancreas," *World Journal of Surgery*, vol. 25, no. 8, pp. 1002–1005, 2001.

[145] N. Sata, K. Kurashina, H. Nagai et al., "The effect of adjuvant and neoadjuvant chemo(radio)therapy on survival in 1,679 resected pancreatic carcinoma cases in Japan: report of the national survey in the 34th annual meeting of Japanese Society of Pancreatic Surgery," *Journal of Hepato-Biliary-Pancreatic Surgery*, vol. 16, no. 4, pp. 485–492, 2009.

[146] K. Yoshizawa, H. Nagai, K. Kurihara, N. Sata, T. Kawai, and K. Saito, "Long-term survival after surgical resection for pancreatic cancer," *Hepato-Gastroenterology*, vol. 48, no. 40, pp. 1153–1156, 2001.

[147] S. Hishinuma, Y. Ogata, M. Tomikawa, I. Ozawa, K. Hirabayashi, and S. Igarashi, "Patterns of recurrence after curative resection of pancreatic cancer, based on autopsy findings," *Journal of Gastrointestinal Surgery*, vol. 10, no. 4, pp. 511–518, 2006.

[148] S. Hishinuma, Y. Ogata, M. Tomikawa, and I. Ozawa, "Stomach-preserving distal pancreatectomy with combined resection of the celiac artery: radical procedure for locally advanced cancer of the pancreatic body," *Journal of Gastrointestinal Surgery*, vol. 11, no. 6, pp. 743–749, 2007.

[149] Y. Ogata and S. Hishinuma, "The impact of pylorus-preserving pancreatoduodenectomy on surgical treatment for cancer of the pancreatic head," *Journal of Hepato-Biliary-Pancreatic Surgery*, vol. 9, no. 2, pp. 223–232, 2002.

[150] H. Ozaki, T. Kinoshita, T. Kosuge et al., "An aggressive therapeutic approach to carcinoma of the body and tail of the pancreas," *Cancer*, vol. 77, no. 11, pp. 2240–2245, 1996.

[151] K. Shimada, Y. Sakamoto, S. Nara, M. Esaki, T. Kosuge, and N. Hiraoka, "Analysis of 5-year survivors after a macroscopic curative pancreatectomy for invasive ductal adenocarcinoma," *World Journal of Surgery*, vol. 34, no. 8, pp. 1908–1915, 2010.

[152] K. Shimada, Y. Sakamoto, T. Sano, T. Kosuge, and N. Hiraoka, "Reappraisal of the clinical significance of tumor size in patients with pancreatic ductal carcinoma," *Pancreas*, vol. 33, no. 3, pp. 233–239, 2006.

[153] S. Yachida, N. Fukushima, M. Sakamoto, Y. Matsuno, T. Kosuge, and S. Hirohashi, "Implications of peritoneal washing cytology in patients with potentially resectable pancreatic cancer," *British Journal of Surgery*, vol. 89, no. 5, pp. 573–578, 2002.

[154] K. Shimada, Y. Sakamoto, T. Sano, and T. Kosuge, "Prognostic factors after distal pancreatectomy with extended lymphadenectomy for invasive pancreatic adenocarcinoma of the body and tail," *Surgery*, vol. 139, no. 3, pp. 288–295, 2006.

[155] K. Shimada, Y. Sakamoto, T. Sano, and T. Kosuge, "The role of paraaortic lymph node involvement on early recurrence and survival after macroscopic curative resection with extended lymphadenectomy for pancreatic carcinoma," *Journal of the American College of Surgeons*, vol. 203, no. 3, pp. 345–352, 2006.

[156] S. Oguro, K. Shimada, Y. Kishi, S. Nara, M. Esaki, and T. Kosuge, "Perioperative and long-term outcomes after pancreaticoduodenectomy in elderly patients 80 years of age and older," *Langenbeck's Archives of Surgery*, vol. 398, no. 4, pp. 531–538, 2013.

[157] E. M. Miller and O. T. Clagett, "Survival five years after radical pancreatoduodenectomy for carcinoma of the head of the pancreas," *Annals of Surgery*, vol. 134, no. 6, pp. 1013–1017, 1951.

[158] J. J. Monge, E. S. Judd, and R. P. Gage, "Radical pancreatoduodenectomy: a 22-year experience with the complications, mortality rate and survival rate," *Annals of Surgery*, vol. 160, pp. 711–722, 1964.

[159] W. H. ReMine, J. T. Priestley, E. S. Judd, and J. N. King, "Total pancreatectomy," *Annals of Surgery*, vol. 172, no. 4, pp. 595–604, 1970.

[160] M. B. Pliam and W. H. ReMine, "Further evaluation of total pancreatectomy," *Archives of Surgery*, vol. 110, no. 5, pp. 506–512, 1975.

[161] A. J. Edis, P. D. Kiernan, and W. F. Taylor, "Attempted curative resection of ductal carcinoma of the pancreas. Review of Mayo Clinic experience, 1951–1975," *Mayo Clinic Proceedings*, vol. 55, no. 9, pp. 531–536, 1980.

[162] J. A. van Heerden, W. H. ReMine, L. H. Weiland, D. C. McIlrath, and D. M. Ilstrup, "Total pancreatectomy for ductal adenocarcinoma of the pancreas. Mayo clinic experience," *The American Journal of Surgery*, vol. 142, no. 3, pp. 308–311, 1981.

[163] J. A. Van Heerden, D. C. McIlrath, D. M. Ilstrup, and L. H. Weiland, "Total pancreatectomy for ductal adenocarcinoma of the pancreas: an update," *World Journal of Surgery*, vol. 12, no. 5, pp. 658–661, 1988.

[164] R. R. Dalton, M. G. Sarr, J. A. Van Heerden, and T. V. Colby, "Carcinoma of the body and tail of the pancreas: is curative resection justified?" *Surgery*, vol. 111, no. 5, pp. 489–494, 1992.

[165] J. A. Van Heerden, "Pancreatic resection for carcinoma of the pancreas: whipple versus total pancreatectomy-an institutional perspective," *World Journal of Surgery*, vol. 8, no. 6, pp. 880–888, 1984.

[166] M. L. Foo, L. L. Gunderson, D. M. Nagorney et al., "Patterns of failure in grossly resected pancreatic ductal adenocarcinoma treated with adjuvant irradiation ± 5 fluorouracil," *International Journal of Radiation Oncology, Biology, Physics*, vol. 26, no. 3, pp. 483–489, 1993.

[167] T. Schnelldorfer, A. L. Ware, M. G. Sarr et al., "Long-term survival after pancreatoduodenectomy for pancreatic adenocarcinoma: is cure possible?" *Annals of Surgery*, vol. 247, no. 3, pp. 456–462, 2008.

[168] J. Fatima, T. Schnelldorfer, J. Barton et al., "Pancreatoduodenectomy for ductal adenocarcinoma: implications of positive margin on survival," *Archives of Surgery*, vol. 145, no. 2, pp. 167–172, 2010.

[169] S. Khan, G. Sclabas, K. Reid-Lombardo et al., "Does body mass index/morbid obesity influence outcome in patients who undergo pancreatoduodenectomy for pancreatic adenocarcinoma?" *Journal of Gastrointestinal Surgery*, vol. 14, no. 11, pp. 1820–1825, 2010.

[170] S. Khan, G. Sclabas, K. R. Lombardo et al., "Pancreatoduodenectomy for ductal adenocarcinoma in the very elderly; is it safe and justified?" *Journal of Gastrointestinal Surgery*, vol. 14, no. 11, pp. 1826–1831, 2010.

[171] S. S. Nitecki, M. G. Sarr, T. V. Colby, and J. A. Van Heerden, "Long-term survival after resection for ductal adenocarcinoma of the pancreas: is it really improving?" *Annals of Surgery*, vol. 221, no. 1, pp. 59–66, 1995.

[172] M. P. Spencer, M. G. Sarr, and D. M. Nagorney, "Radical pancreatectomy for pancreatic cancer in the elderly: is it safe and justified?" *Annals of Surgery*, vol. 212, no. 2, pp. 140–143, 1990.

[173] B. J. Billings, J. D. Christein, W. S. Harmsen et al., "Quality-of-life after total pancreatectomy: is it really that bad on long-term follow-up?" *Journal of Gastrointestinal Surgery*, vol. 9, no. 8, pp. 1059–1067, 2005.

[174] C. C. Hsu, J. M. Herman, M. M. Corsini et al., "Adjuvant chemoradiation for pancreatic adenocarcinoma: The Johns Hopkins Hospital-Mayo Clinic collaborative study," *Annals of Surgical Oncology*, vol. 17, no. 4, pp. 981–990, 2010.

[175] J. D. Christein, M. L. Kendrick, C. W. Iqbal, D. M. Nagorney, and M. B. Farnell, "Distal pancreatectomy for resectable adenocarcinoma of the body and tail of the pancreas," *Journal of Gastrointestinal Surgery*, vol. 9, no. 7, pp. 922–927, 2005.

[176] M. B. Farnell, R. K. Pearson, M. G. Sarr et al., "A prospective randomized trial comparing standard pancreatoduodenectomy with pancreatoduodenectomy with extended lymphadenectomy in resectable pancreatic head adenocarcinoma," *Surgery*, vol. 138, no. 4, pp. 618–630, 2005.

[177] M. Al-Haddad, J. K. Martin, J. Nguyen et al., "Vascular resection and reconstruction for pancreatic malignancy: a single center survival study," *Journal of Gastrointestinal Surgery*, vol. 11, no. 9, pp. 1168–1174, 2007.

[178] J. G. Barton, T. Schnelldorfer, C. M. Lohse et al., "Patterns of pancreatic resection differ between patients with familial and sporadic pancreatic cancer," *Journal of Gastrointestinal Surgery*, vol. 15, no. 5, pp. 836–842, 2011.

[179] K. P. Croome, M. B. Farnell, F. G. Que et al., "Total laparoscopic pancreaticoduodenectomy for pancreatic ductal adenocarcinoma. Oncologic advances over open approaches," *Annals of Surgery*, vol. 260, no. 4, pp. 633–640, 2014.

[180] D. W. Crist, J. V. Sitzmann, and J. L. Cameron, "Improved hospital morbidity, mortality, and survival after the Whipple procedure," *Annals of Surgery*, vol. 206, no. 3, pp. 358–365, 1987.

[181] D. W. Crist and J. L. Cameron, "Current status of pancreaticoduodenectomy for periampullary carcinoma," *Hepato-Gastroenterology*, vol. 36, no. 6, pp. 478–485, 1989.

[182] J. L. Cameron, T. S. Riall, J. Coleman, and K. A. Belcher, "One thousand consecutive pancreaticoduodenectomies," *Annals of Surgery*, vol. 244, no. 1, pp. 10–15, 2006.

[183] C. J. Yeo, T. A. Sohn, J. L. Cameron, R. H. Hruban, K. D. Lillemoe, and H. A. Pitt, "Periampullary adenocarcinoma: analysis of 5-year survivors," *Annals of Surgery*, vol. 227, no. 6, pp. 821–831, 1998.

[184] J. A. DiGiuseppe, C. J. Yeo, and R. H. Hruban, "Molecular biology and the diagnosis and treatment of adenocarcinoma of the pancreas," *Advances in Anatomic Pathology*, vol. 3, no. 3, pp. 139–155, 1996.

[185] T. S. Riall, J. L. Cameron, K. D. Lillemoe et al., "Resected periampullary adenocarcinoma: 5-year survivors and their 6- to 10-year follow-up," *Surgery*, vol. 140, no. 5, pp. 764–772, 2006.

[186] M. A. Makary, J. M. Winter, J. L. Cameron et al., "Pancreaticoduodenectomy in the very elderly," *Journal of Gastrointestinal Surgery*, vol. 10, no. 3, pp. 347–356, 2006.

[187] J. M. Winter, J. L. Cameron, K. A. Campbell et al., "1423 pancreaticoduodenectomies for pancreatic cancer: a single-institution experience," *Journal of Gastrointestinal Surgery*, vol. 10, no. 9, pp. 1199–1211, 2006.

[188] S. Reddy, C. L. Wolfgang, J. L. Cameron et al., "Total pancreatectomy for pancreatic adenocarcinoma: evaluation of morbidity and long-term Survival," *Annals of Surgery*, vol. 250, no. 2, pp. 282–287, 2009.

[189] I. H. Nordback, R. H. Hruban, J. K. Boitnott, H. A. Pitt, and J. L. Cameron, "Carcinoma of the body and tail of the pancreas," *The American Journal of Surgery*, vol. 164, no. 1, pp. 26–31, 1992.

[190] D. C. Allison, K. K. Bose, R. H. Hruban et al., "Pancreatic cancer cell DNA content correlates with long-term survival after pancreatoduodenectomy," *Annals of Surgery*, vol. 214, no. 6, pp. 648–656, 1991.

[191] D. C. Allison, S. Piantadosi, R. H. Hruban et al., "DNA content and other factors associated with ten-year survival after resection of pancreatic carcinoma," *Journal of Surgical Oncology*, vol. 67, no. 3, pp. 151–159, 1998.

[192] J. He, B. H. Edil, J. L. Cameron et al., "Young patients undergoing resection of pancreatic cancer fare better than their older counterparts," *Journal of Gastrointestinal Surgery*, vol. 17, no. 2, pp. 339–344, 2013.

[193] G. E. McGuire, H. A. Pitt, K. D. Lillemoe, J. E. Niederhuber, C. J. Yeo, and J. L. Cameron, "Reoperative surgery for periampullary adenocarcinoma," *Archives of Surgery*, vol. 126, no. 10, pp. 1205–1212, 1991.

[194] J. W. Lin, J. L. Cameron, C. J. Yeo, T. S. Riall, and K. D. Lillemoe, "Risk factors and outcomes in postpancreaticoduodenectomy pancreaticocutaneous fistula," *Journal of Gastrointestinal Surgery*, vol. 8, no. 8, pp. 951–959, 2004.

[195] T. A. Sohn, C. J. Yeo, J. L. Cameron et al., "Resected adenocarcinoma of the pancreas—616 patients: results, outcomes, and prognostic indicators," *Journal of Gastrointestinal Surgery*, vol. 4, no. 6, pp. 567–579, 2000.

[196] K. D. Lillemoe, J. L. Cameron, C. J. Yeo et al., "Pancreaticoduo-denectomy: does it have a role in the palliation of pancreatic cancer?" *Annals of Surgery*, vol. 223, no. 6, pp. 718–728, 1996.

[197] C. J. Yeo, J. L. Cameron, T. A. Sohn et al., "Six hundred fifty consecutive pancreaticoduodenectomies in the 1990s: pathology, complications, and outcomes," *Annals of Surgery*, vol. 226, no. 3, pp. 248–260, 1997.

[198] T. A. Sohn, K. D. Lillemoe, J. L. Cameron, J. J. Huang, H. A. Pitt, and C. J. Yeo, "Surgical palliation of unresectable periampullary adenocarcinoma in the 1990s," *Journal of the American College of Surgeons*, vol. 188, no. 6, pp. 658–669, 1999.

[199] B. Hristov, S. Reddy, S. H. Lin et al., "Outcomes of adjuvant chemoradiation after pancreaticoduodenectomy with mesenterico-portal vein resection for adenocarcinoma of the pancreas," *International Journal of Radiation Oncology Biology Physics*, vol. 76, no. 1, pp. 176–180, 2010.

[200] A. L. Gleisner, L. Assumpcao, J. L. Cameron et al., "Is resection of periampullary or pancreatic adenocarcinoma with synchronous hepatic metastasis justified?" *Cancer*, vol. 110, no. 11, pp. 2484–2492, 2007.

[201] B. Asiyanbola, A. Gleisner, J. M. Herman et al., "Determining pattern of recurrence following pancreaticoduodenectomy and adjuvant 5-flurouracil-based chemoradiation therapy: effect of number of metastatic lymph nodes and lymph node ratio," *Journal of Gastrointestinal Surgery*, vol. 13, no. 4, pp. 752–759, 2009.

[202] S. Tsai, M. A. Choti, L. Assumpcao et al., "Impact of obesity on perioperative outcomes and survival following pancreatico-duodenectomy for pancreatic cancer: a large single-institution study," *Journal of Gastrointestinal Surgery*, vol. 14, no. 7, pp. 1143–1150, 2010.

[203] C. J. Yeo, J. L. Cameron, K. D. Lillemoe et al., "Pancreaticoduodenectomy with or without distal gastrectomy and extended retroperitoneal lymphadenectomy for periampullary adenocarcinoma, part 2: randomized controlled trial evaluating survival, morbidity, and mortality," *Annals of Surgery*, vol. 236, no. 3, pp. 355–368, 2002.

[204] C. J. Yeo, "The whipple operation: is a radical resection of benefit?" *Advances in Surgery*, vol. 37, pp. 1–27, 2003.

[205] T. S. Riall, J. L. Cameron, K. D. Lillemoe et al., "Pancreaticoduodenectomy with or without distal gastrectomy and extended retroperitoneal lymphadenectomy for periampullary adenocarcinoma-part 3: update on 5-year survival," *Journal of Gastrointestinal Surgery*, vol. 9, no. 9, pp. 1191–1206, 2005.

[206] D. M. Emick, T. S. Riall, J. L. Cameron et al., "Hospital readmission after pancreaticoduodenectomy," *Journal of Gastrointestinal Surgery*, vol. 10, no. 9, pp. 1243–1253, 2006.

[207] H. Nathan, C. L. Wolfgang, B. H. Edil et al., "Peri-operative mortality and long-term survival after total pancreatectomy for pancreatic adenocarcinoma: a population-based perspective," *Journal of Surgical Oncology*, vol. 99, no. 2, pp. 87–92, 2009.

Permissions

The contributors of this book come from diverse backgrounds, making this book a truly international effort. This book will bring forth new frontiers with its revolutionizing research information and detailed analysis of the nascent developments around the world.

We would like to thank all the contributing authors for lending their expertise to make the book truly unique. They have played a crucial role in the development of this book. Without their invaluable contributions this book wouldn't have been possible. They have made vital efforts to compile up to date information on the varied aspects of this subject to make this book a valuable addition to the collection of many professionals and students.

This book was conceptualized with the vision of imparting up-to-date information and advanced data in this field. To ensure the same, a matchless editorial board was set up. Every individual on the board went through rigorous rounds of assessment to prove their worth. After which they invested a large part of their time researching and compiling the most relevant data for our readers.

The editorial board has been involved in producing this book since its inception. They have spent rigorous hours researching and exploring the diverse topics which have resulted in the successful publishing of this book. They have passed on their knowledge of decades through this book. To expedite this challenging task, the publisher supported the team at every step. A small team of assistant editors was also appointed to further simplify the editing procedure and attain best results for the readers.

Apart from the editorial board, the designing team has also invested a significant amount of their time in understanding the subject and creating the most relevant covers. They scrutinized every image to scout for the most suitable representation of the subject and create an appropriate cover for the book.

The publishing team has been an ardent support to the editorial, designing and production team. Their endless efforts to recruit the best for this project, has resulted in the accomplishment of this book. They are a veteran in the field of academics and their pool of knowledge is as vast as their experience in printing. Their expertise and guidance has proved useful at every step. Their uncompromising quality standards have made this book an exceptional effort. Their encouragement from time to time has been an inspiration for everyone.

The publisher and the editorial board hope that this book will prove to be a valuable piece of knowledge for researchers, students, practitioners and scholars across the globe.

Contributors

Mohamad T. Badawy, Hosam El-Din Soliman, Magdy El-Gendy and Tarek Ibrahim
Liver Transplant Department, National Liver Institute, Menoufiya University, Shebeen El-Koum, Egypt

Brian R. Davidson
University Department of Surgery and Liver Transplant Unit, Royal Free Hospital Trust and Royal Free and University College School of Medicine, Hampstead Campus, Pond Street, London NW3 2QG, UK

Mohamed Ghazaly
Liver Transplant Department, National Liver Institute, Menoufiya University, Shebeen El-Koum, Egypt
University Department of Surgery and Liver Transplant Unit, Royal Free Hospital Trust and Royal Free and University College School of Medicine, Hampstead Campus, Pond Street, London NW3 2QG, UK

S. A. Jackson, B. M. T. Fox, J. D. Mitchell, S. Aroori, M. J. Bowles, E. M. Armstrong and J. F. Shirley
Plymouth Hospitals NHS Trust, Derriford Hospital, Derriford Road, Plymouth, Devon PL6 8DH, UK
Plymouth University, Peninsula College of Medicine and Dentistry, John Bull Building, Plymouth, Devon PL6 8BU, UK

M. G. Wiggans D. A. Stell
Plymouth Hospitals NHS Trust, Derriford Hospital, Derriford Road, Plymouth, Devon PL6 8DH, UK

Ibrahim Abdelkader Salama, Hany Abdelmeged Shoreem, Sherif Mohamed Saleh, Osama Hegazy and Tarek Ibrahim
Department of Hepatobiliary Surgery, National Liver Institute, Menophyia University, Shiben Elkom, Egypt

Mohamed Housseni
Department of Radiology, National Liver Institute, Menophyia University, Shiben Elkom, Egypt

Mohamed Abbasy and Gamal Badra
Department of Hepatology, National Liver Institute, Menophyia University, Shiben Elkom, Egypt

Kristoffer Watten Brudvik
Centre for Molecular Medicine Norway, University of Oslo, 0318 Oslo, Norway
Biotechnology Centre, University of Oslo, 0317 Oslo, Norway
Department of Hepato-Pancreato-Biliary Surgery, Oslo University Hospital, 0424 Oslo, Norway

Simer Jit Bains
Centre for Molecular Medicine Norway, University of Oslo, 0318 Oslo, Norway
Biotechnology Centre, University of Oslo, 0317 Oslo, Norway

Lars Thomas Seeberg, Knut Jørgen Labori, Anne Waage and Bjørn Atle Bjørnbeth
Department of Hepato-Pancreato-Biliary Surgery, Oslo University Hospital, 0424 Oslo, Norway

Kjetil Taskén
Centre for Molecular Medicine Norway, University of Oslo, 0318 Oslo, Norway
Biotechnology Centre, University of Oslo, 0317 Oslo, Norway
Department of Infectious Diseases, Oslo University Hospital, 0424 Oslo, Norway

Einar Martin Aandahl
Centre for Molecular Medicine Norway, University of Oslo, 0318 Oslo, Norway
Biotechnology Centre, University of Oslo, 0317 Oslo, Norway

Department of Transplantation Surgery, Oslo University Hospital, 0424 Oslo, Norway

Arash Nickkholgh, Zhanqing Li, Xue Yi, Elvira Mohr, Rui Liang, Saulius Mikalauskas, Markus W. Büchler and Peter Schemmer
Department of General and Transplant Surgery, Ruprecht-Karls University, 69120 Heidelberg, Germany

Marie-Luise Gross
Institute of Pathology, Ruprecht-Karls University, 69120 Heidelberg, Germany

Markus Zorn
Central Laboratory, Ruprecht-Karls University, 69120 Heidelberg, Germany

Steffen Benzing
Fresenius Kabi Deutschland GmbH, 61440 Oberursel, Germany

Heinz Schneider
Health Econ AG, 4051 Basel, Switzerland

Laith H. Jamil, Kanwar R. S. Gill, Daniela Scimeca, Massimo Raimondo, Timothy A. Woodward and Michael B. Wallace
Division of Gastroenterology and Hepatology, Mayo Clinic, Jacksonville, FL 32224, USA

Ana M. Chindris and Shon E. Meek
Division of Endocrinology, Mayo Clinic, Jacksonville, FL 32224, USA

John A. Stauffer and Horacio J. Asbun
Department of Surgery, Mayo Clinic, Jacksonville, FL 32224, USA

Michael G. Heckman
Biostatistics Unit, Mayo Clinic, Jacksonville, FL 32224, USA

Justin H. Nguyen
Department of Transplantation, Mayo Clinic, Jacksonville, FL 32224, USA

M. J. Bowles and S. Aroori
Hepatobiliary Surgery, Plymouth Hospitals NHS Trust, Derriford Hospital, Derriford Road, Plymouth, Devon PL6 8DH, UK

G. Shahtahmassebi
School of Science and Technology, Nottingham Trent University, Nottingham NG1 4BU, UK

M. G. Wiggans and D. A. Stell
Hepatobiliary Surgery, Plymouth Hospitals NHS Trust, Derriford Hospital, Derriford Road, Plymouth, Devon PL6 8DH, UK
Peninsula College of Medicine and Dentistry, University of Exeter and Plymouth University, John Bull Building, Plymouth, Devon PL6 8BU, UK

Per Lindnér, Magnus Rizell and Lo Hafström
Transplant Institute, Institute of Clinical Sciences, Sahlgrenska Academy at University of Gothenburg, Sahlgrenska University Hospital, SE-413 45 Gothenburg, Sweden

Jennifer K. Plichta, Gerard J. Abood and Gerard V. Aranha
Department of Surgery, Loyola University Health Systems, 2160 S. First Avenue, Maywood, IL 60153, USA

Anjali S. Godambe and Sherri Yong
Department of Pathology, Loyola University Health Systems, 2160 S. First Avenue, Maywood, IL 60153, USA

Zachary Fridirici
Stritch School of Medicine, Loyola University Medical Center, 2160 S. First Avenue, Maywood, IL 60153, USA

James M. Sinacore
Department of Preventive Medicine, Loyola University Medical Center, 2160 S. First Avenue, Maywood, IL 60153, USA

Christoph Czerny
Center for Cell Death, Injury and Regeneration, Departments of Pharmaceutical and Biomedical Sciences, Medical University of South Carolina, Charleston, SC 29425, USA
Departement of Trauma Surgery, J.W. Goethe University Frankfurt am Main, 60590 Frankfurt am Main, Germany

Tom P. Theruvath, Eduardo N. Maldonado and Zhi Zhong
Center for Cell Death, Injury and Regeneration, Departments of Pharmaceutical and Biomedical Sciences, Medical University of South Carolina, Charleston, SC 29425, USA

Mark Lehnert and Ingo Marzi
Departement of Trauma Surgery, J.W. Goethe University Frankfurt am Main, 60590 Frankfurt am Main, Germany

John J. Lemasters
Center for Cell Death, Injury and Regeneration, Departments of Pharmaceutical and Biomedical Sciences, Medical University of South Carolina, Charleston, SC 29425, USA
Biochemistry and Molecular Biology, Medical University of South Carolina, MSC 140, Charleston, SC 29425, USA

Lei Yuan, Youlei Zhang, Yi Wang, Wenming Cong and Mengchao Wu
Second Department of Hepatic Surgery, Eastern Hepatobiliary Surgery Hospital, Second Military Medical University, 225 Changhai Road, Shanghai 200438, China

Denis Ehrl, Katharina Rothaug, Bernhard Hofer and Horst-Günter Rau
Department of Visceral, Thoracic und Vascular Surgery, Clinic of Dachau, 85221 Dachau, Germany

Peter Herzog
Department of Radiology, Clinic of Dachau, Krankenhausstrare 15, 85221 Dachau, Germany

Christine S. M. Lau
Department of Surgery, Saint Barnabas Medical Center, Livingston, NJ 07039, USA
Saint George's University School of Medicine, True Blue, Grenada

Krishnaraj Mahendraraj
Department of Surgery, Saint Barnabas Medical Center, Livingston, NJ 07039, USA

Ronald S. Chamberlain
Department of Surgery, Saint Barnabas Medical Center, Livingston, NJ 07039, USA
Saint George's University School of Medicine, True Blue, Grenada
Department of Surgery, New Jersey Medical School, Rutgers University, Newark, NJ 07103, USA

Anne-Frédérique Manichon, Marion Durieux-Millon and Agnés Rode
Department of Radiology, Croix Rousse Hospital, Grande rue de la Croix-Rousse, 69004 Lyon Cedex 04, France

Brigitte Bancel
Department of Pathology, Croix Rousse Hospital, 103 Grande rue de la Croix-Rousse, 69004 Lyon Cedex 04, France

Christian Ducerf and Jean-YvesMabrut
Department of Digestive Surgery, Croix Rousse Hospital, 103 Grande rue de la Croix-Rousse, 69004 Lyon Cedex 04, France

Marie-Annick Lepogam
Site Laccasagne, 162 Avenue Laccassagne, 69424 Lyon, France

Maxwell A. Thompson and Lindsey Glueckert
University of Alabama at Birmingham, Birmingham, AL 35294, USA

David T. Redden
Biostatistics Division, School of Public Health, University of Alabama at Birmingham, Birmingham, AL 35294, USA

A. Blair Smith, Jack H. Crawford and Keith A. Jones
Department of Anesthesia, University of Alabama at Birmingham, Birmingham, AL 35294, USA

Devin E. Eckhoff, Stephen H. Gray, Jared A. White and Derek A. DuBay
Liver Transplant and Hepatobiliary Surgery, University of Alabama at Birmingham, 701 ZRB, 1530 3rd Avenue South, Birmingham, AL 35294-0007, USA

Joseph Bloomer
Transplant Hepatology, University of Alabama at Birmingham, Birmingham, AL 35294, USA

D.Hipps, F. Ausania, D. M. Manas, J. D. G. Rose and J. J. French
Hepato-Pancreato-Biliary and Transplant Surgery Unit, Freeman Hospital, Newcastle Upon Tyne NE7 7DN, UK

S. Rehman, S. K. P. John and J. J. French
Department of Hepatobiliary and Transplantation Surgery, The Freeman Hospital, Newcastle upon Tyne NE7 7DN, UK

D. M. Manas and S. A. White
Department of Hepatobiliary and Transplantation Surgery, The Freeman Hospital, Newcastle upon Tyne NE7 7DN, UK
The Liver Research Group, The University of Newcastle, Leech Building, Framlington Place, Newcastle upon Tyne NE1 7RP, UK

Jordan J. Nostedt, Daniel T. Skubleny, A. M. James Shapiro and David L. Bigam
Department of Surgery, Division of General Surgery, University of Alberta Hospital, 2D4.41W.M.C, 8440-112 St., Edmonton, AB, Canada T6G 2B7

Sandra Campbell
JohnW. Scott Health Sciences Library, University of Alberta, 2K3.28W.M.C, 8440-112 St., Edmonton, AB, Canada T6G 2B7

Darren H. Freed
Department of Physiology, University of Alberta, 7-55 Medical Sciences Building, Edmonton, AB, Canada T6G 2H7
Department of Biomedical Engineering, University of Alberta, 1098 Research Transition Facility, 8308-114 St., Edmonton, AB, Canada T6G 2V2
Department of Surgery, Division of Cardiac Surgery, University of Alberta and 4A7.056 Mazankowski Alberta Heart Institute, 11220-83 Ave, Edmonton, AB, Canada T6G 2B7

Martin de Santibañes and Eduardo de Santibañes
Department of Hepato-Biliary-Pancreatic Surgery and Liver Transplant Unit, Hospital Italiano de Buenos Aires, Perón 4190, 1181 Buenos Aires, Argentina

Agustin Dietrich
Department of General Surgery, Hospital Italiano de Buenos Aires, Per'on 4190, 1181 Buenos Aires, Argentina

T.Malinka, F. Klein, J. Pratschke and M. Bahra
Department of Surgery, Charité Campus Mitte and Charité Campus Virchow Klinikum, Charité-Universitätsmedizin Berlin, Berlin, Germany

T. Denecke
Department of Radiology, Charité Campus Virchow Klinikum, Charité-Universitätsmedizin Berlin, Berlin, Germany

U. Pelzer
Department of Hematology/Oncology/Tumor Immunology, Campus Virchow Klinikum, Charité-Universitätsmedizin Berlin, Berlin, Germany

Saleem Ahmed
Department of General Surgery, Tan Tock Seng Hospital, Singapore 308433
Ministry of Health Holdings, 1 Maritime Square, Singapore 099253

Nurun Nisa de Souza
Duke-NUS Graduate Medical School, 8 College Road, Singapore 169857
Singapore Clinical Research Institute, 31 BiopolisWay, Singapore 138669

Wang Qiao
Ministry of Health Holdings, 1 Maritime Square, Singapore 099253

Meidai Kasai
Department of Gastroenterological Surgery, Sendai Kousei Hospital, 8-15 Hirosemachi, Aoba-ku, Sendai-shi, Miyagi 9800873, Japan

Low Jee Keem and Vishal G. Shelat
Department of General Surgery, Tan Tock Seng Hospital, Singapore 308433

Vijayaragavan Muralidharan, Linh Nguyen, Jonathan Banting and Christopher Christophi
Department of Surgery, The University of Melbourne and Austin Hospital, Lance Townsend Building Level 8, Studley Road, Heidelberg, Melbourne, VIC 3084, Australia

Yuichiro Uchida, Hiroaki Furuyama, Daiki Yasukawa, Yasuhisa Ando, Toshiyuki Hata, Takafumi Machimoto and Tsunehiro Yoshimura
Department of Gastrointestinal and General Surgery, Tenri Yorozu Hospital, 200 Mishima-cho, Tenri, Nara 632-8552, Japan

Hiroto Nishino
Division of Hepato-Biliary-Pancreatic and Transplant Surgery, Graduate School of Medicine, Kyoto University, 54 Shogoin-kawahara-cho, Kyoto 606-8507, Japan

SimonMoosburner, Joseph M. G. V. Gassner, Maximilian Nösser, Julian Pohl, DavidWyrwal, Felix Claussen, Johann Pratschke and Igor M. Sauer
Department of Surgery, Campus Charité Mitte | Campus Virchow-Klinikum, Experimental Surgery and Regenerative Medicine, Charité –Universitätsmedizin Berlin 13353, Germany

Paul V. Ritschl and Nathanael Raschzok
Department of Surgery, Campus Charité Mitte | Campus Virchow-Klinikum, Experimental Surgery and Regenerative Medicine, Charité–Universitätsmedizin Berlin 13353, Germany
BIH Charité Clinician Scientist Program, Berlin Institute of Health (BIH), Berlin 10178, Germany

Duska Dragun
Berlin Institute of Health and Department of Nephrology and Critical Care Medicine, Charité Universitätsmedizin, Berlin 13353, Germany

Jordan Levy
Division of General Surgery, Jewish GeneralHospital, McGill University, Montreal, QC, CanadaH3T 1E2

Geva Maimon
Lady Davis Institute for Medical Research, Montreal, QC, Canada H3T 1E2

Mehdi Tahiri, Tsafrir Vanounou and Simon Bergman
Division of General Surgery, Jewish GeneralHospital, McGill University, Montreal, QC, CanadaH3T 1E2
Lady Davis Institute for Medical Research, Montreal, QC, Canada H3T 1E2

Gendong Tian, Yuan Guo, Mujian Teng and Jie Li
Hepatobiliary and Liver Transplantation Department, The Affiliated Qianfoshan Hospital, Shandong University, No. 16766 Jingshi Road, Jinan, Shandong 250014, China

Qiong Chen
General Surgery Department, The First People's Hospital of Jinan City, No. 132 Minghu Road, Jinan, Shandong 250014, China

K. S. Norman
Department of Surgery, University of Hawaii John A. Burns School of Medicine, Honolulu, HI 96813, USA

S. R. Domingo
Department of Surgery, University of Hawaii John A. Burns School of Medicine, Honolulu, HI 96813, USA
Queens Medical Center, Honolulu, HI 96813, USA

L. L. Wong
Department of Surgery, University of Hawaii John A. Burns School of Medicine, Honolulu, HI 96813, USA
University of Hawaii Cancer Center, Honolulu, HI 96813, USA

Fritz Klein, Igor Maximilian Sauer, Johann Pratschke and Marcus Bahra
Department of Surgery, Charité-Universitätsmedizin Berlin, Augustenburger Platz 1, 13353 Berlin, Germany

Nobuhisa Akamatsu
Department of Hepato-Biliary-Pancreatic Surgery, Saitama Medical Center, Saitama Medical University, 1981 Tsujido-cho, Kamoda, Kawagoe, Saitama 350-8550, Japan
Artif zcial Organ and Transplantation Division, Department of Surgery, Graduate School of Medicine, University of Tokyo, 7-3-1 Hongo, Bunkyo-ku, Tokyo 113-8655, Japan

Yasuhiko Sugawara
Artif zcial Organ and Transplantation Division, Department of Surgery, Graduate School of Medicine, University of Tokyo, 7-3-1 Hongo, Bunkyo-ku, Tokyo 113-8655, Japan

Fritz Klein, Marcus Bahra, Gero Puhl, Andreas Andreou, Safak Gül and Olaf Guckelberger
Department of General, Visceral, and Transplantation Surgery, Charité Campus Virchow Universitätsmedizin Berlin, 13353 Berlin, Germany

Dietmar Jacob
Department of General and Visceral Surgery, Bielefeld Evangelical Hospital, 33617 Bielefeld, Germany

Uwe Pelzer
Department of Hematology/Oncology, Comprehensive Cancer Center, Charité Universitätsmedizin Berlin, 13353 Berlin, Germany

Alexander Krannich
Department of Biostatistics, Coordination Center for Clinical Trials, Charité Universitätsmedizin Berlin, 13353 Berlin, Germany

Birgir Gudjonsson
The Medical Clinic, Álfheimum 74, 104 Reykjavik, Iceland

Index